Handbook of
Experimental Pharmacology

Continuation of Handbuch der experimentellen Pharmakologie

Vol. 61

Chemotherapy of Viral Infections

Contributors

M. J. Bartkoski, Jr. · S. Bridges · P. E. Came · H. J. Eggers
P. H. Fischer · H. Friedman · M. Green · C. Gurgo · J. Hay
B. D. Korant · J. J. McSharry · L. R. Overby · F. Pancic
N.-H. Park · D. Pavan-Langston · C. J. Pfau · L. M. Pfeffer
W. H. Prusoff · J. L. Schulman · P. B. Sehgal · S. Specter
B. A. Steinberg · I. Tamm · D. R. Tershak · F. H. Yin

Editors

P. E. Came and L. A. Caliguiri

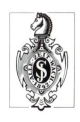

Springer-Verlag Berlin Heidelberg New York 1982

Dr. Paul E. Came

Sterling-Winthrop Research Institute, Rensselaer, NY 12144/USA

Dr. Lawrence A. Caliguiri

Department of Microbiology, University of Pittsburgh,
School of Medicine, Pittsburgh, PA 15261/USA

With 133 Figures

ISBN 3-540-11347-9 Springer-Verlag Berlin Heidelberg New York
ISBN 0-387-11347-9 Springer-Verlag New York Heidelberg Berlin

Library of Congress Cataloging in Publication Data. Main entry under title: Chemotherapy of viral infections.
(Handbook of experimental pharmacology; vol. 61) Bibliography: p. Includes index. 1. Virus diseases – Chemotherapy.
2. Antiviral agents – Testing. I. Bartkoski, M.J. (Michael J.) II. Came, Paul E. III. Caliguiri, Lawrence. IV. Series.
[DNLM: 1. Viruses – Pathogenicity. 2. Antiviral agents – Pharmacodynamics. 3. Virus diseases – Drug therapy.
4. Antiviral agents – Therapeutic use. W1 HA51L v. 61/QV 268.5 C517] QP905.H3 vol. 61 [RC114.5] 615'.1s. 81-23320.
ISBN 0-387-11347-9. [616.9'25061]. AACR2

Printed in Germany.

The use of registered names, trademarks, etc. in this publication does not imply, even in the absence of a specific
statement, that such names are exempt from the relevant protective laws and regulations and therefore free for
general use.

Typesetting, printing, and bookbinding: Brühlsche Universitätsdruckerei, Giessen.
2122/3130-543210

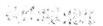

Dedicated to

Bette, Paula, and Heather
and Maggy, Laura, and Anne

Preface

Exciting events in the basic disciplines of virology, immunology, and pharmacology continue to advance the understanding of the pathogenesis and control of virus diseases. At the same time, the rational development of antiviral agents is attracting, to an increasing extent, the interest of workers in other disciplines. Improvements in technology facilitate the definition of potential target sites for antiviral intervention and unmask new viral and host genes. The outcome is a further steady development of new antiviral agents which approach the "magic bullets" first proposed by PAUL EHRLICH. Remarkable advances in protein synthetic methods that yield polypeptides which inhibit active sites of viral proteins have aided substantially in the basic and clinical study of these antiviral agents. In addition, the extremely rapid progression in recombinant DNA techniques, leading to the synthesis of large quantities of gene products, is also increasing our opportunities at a dashing pace. New information and developing technology facilitate research on the mechanism of action, toxicity, pharmacokinetics, and pharmacodynamics of new agents. The list of clinically effective antiviral agents is expanding and the number of potentially useful compounds is growing rapidly.

This book is a combined theoretical text and practical manual which, it is hoped, will be of use to all who have an interest in virus diseases, particularly scientists, physicians and graduate students. There are two major divisions of the volume: the first part deals with antiviral agents which are clinically effective and the second discusses compounds which are not, at present, widely used as chemotherapeutic agents, but are either currently under study as possible drugs or are used to elucidate the mechanism of virus replication. These major sections are preceded by a comprehensive chapter on current models of pathogenesis of virus disease produced by all the major groups of viruses. This updated coverage highlights the diversity of the important pathogens and offers insight into possible means of their control.

We have asked that the contributors of chapters consider the efforts and attempts of the chemists to cite important aspects of structure–activity relationships. The pharmacologic interactions including half-life, tissue distribution, and excretion rate are discussed where appropriate. The available results of clinical trials for various compounds are also discussed.

It is our goal to discuss the recent advances in historical perspective and to add a better understanding of antiviral compounds or drugs, per se. As the reader will learn, some of the chemicals which have never become drugs are the very compounds that supplied the impetus and optimism to continue the search. It is our hope that this volume will provide an awareness of previous contributions, investigations of newer agents suitable for chemotherapy of virus infections, and the excitement of the current work with the anticipation of the viral therapeutics of the future – the seat and cause of the pharmacology of antiviral agents.

We thank our colleagues who have made contributions to this work and made this volume possible, and acknowledge the valuable assistance of Ms. KATHLEEN CAVANAGH and Ms. MARY FRAZIER who provided editorial assistance in addition to excellent secretarial skills.

PAUL E. CAME
LAWRENCE A. CALIGUIRI

List of Authors

Dr. M. J. BARTKOSKI, Jr., Department of Microbiology, Uniformed Services University of the Health Sciences, 4301 Jones Bridge Road, Bethesda, MD 20014/USA

Dr. S. BRIDGES, Centro di Endocrinologia e Oncologia Sperimentale del C.N.R., Istituto di Patologia Generale, Via Sergio Pansini, 5, I-80131 Naples

Dr. P. E. CAME, Sterling-Winthrop Research Institute, Rensselaer, NY 12144/ USA

Professor Dr. H. J. EGGERS, Institut für Virologie der Universität Köln, Fürst-Pückler-Straße 56, D-5000 Köln 41

Dr. P. H. FISCHER, Department of Human Oncology, Wisconsin Clinical Cancer Center, University of Wisconsin, Madison, WI 53792/USA

Dr. H. FRIEDMAN, Department of Medical Microbiology, College of Medicine, University of South Florida, 12901 North 30th Street, Tampa, FL 33612/USA

Dr. M. GREEN, Institute for Molecular Virology, St. Louis University School of Medicine, 3681 Park Avenue, St. Louis, MO 63310/USA

Dr. C. GURGO, Centro di Endocrinologia e Oncologia Sperimentale des C.N.R., Via Sergio Pansini, 5, I-80131 Naples

Professor Dr. J. HAY, Department of Microbiology, Uniformed Services University of the Health Sciences, 4301 Jones Bridge Road, Bethesda, MD 20014/USA

Dr. B. D. KORANT, Central Research and Development Department, Experimental Station, E.I. du Pont de Nemours & Co. Inc., Wilmington, DE 19898/USA

Professor Dr. J. J. MCSHARRY, Department of Microbiology and Immunology, The Neil Hellman Medical Research Building, Albany Medical College of Union University, New Scotland Avenue, Albany, NY 12208/USA

Dr. L. R. OVERBY, Experimental Biology, Abbott Diagnostics Division, Abbott Laboratories, North Chicago, IL 60064/USA

Dr. F. PANCIC, Department of Microbiology, Sterling-Winthrop Research Institute, Columbia Turnpike, Rensselaer, NY 12144/USA

Dr. N.-H. PARK, Eye Research Institute of Retina Foundation, Department of Ophthalmology, Harvard Dental School, 20 Staniford Street, Boston, MA 02114/USA

Professor Dr. D. PAVAN-LANGSTON, Eye Research Institute of Retina Foundation and Department of Ophthalmology, Harvard Dental School, 20 Staniford Street, Boston, MA 02114/USA

Dr. C. J. PFAU, Biology Department, Rensselaer Polytechnic Institute, Troy, NY 12181/USA

Dr. L. M. PFEFFER, The Rockefeller University, 1230 York Avenue, New York, NY 10021/USA

Dr. W. H. PRUSOFF, Department of Pharmacology, Yale University, Sterling Hall, School of Medicine, 333 Cedar Street, New Haven, CT 06510/USA

Prof. Dr. J. L. SCHULMAN, Department of Microbiology, Mt. Sinai School of Medicine, City University of New York, New York, NY 10029/USA

Dr. P. B. SEHGAL, The Rockefeller University, 1230 York Avenue, New York, NY 10021/USA

Dr. S. SPECTER, Department of Medical Microbiology, College of Medicine, University of South Florida, 12901 North 30th Street, Tampa, FL 33612/USA

Dr. B. A. STEINBERG, Department of Microbiology, Sterling-Winthrop Research Institute, Division of Sterlin Drug Inc., Rensselaer, NY 12144/USA

Dr. I. TAMM, The Rockefeller University, 1239 York Avenue, New York, NY 10021/USA

Professor Dr. D. R. TERSHAK, Microbiology and Molecular Physics, S101 Frear Building, Department of Microbiology and Cell Biology, Biochemistry and Biophysics, The Pennsylvania State University, University Park, PA 16802/USA

Dr. F. H. YIN, Central Research and Development Department, Experimental Station, E.I. DuPont de Nemours & Co., Wilmington, DE 19898/USA

Contents

Part A

CHAPTER 2

Pyrimidine Nucleosides with Selective Antiviral Activity.
P. H. FISCHER and W. H. PRUSOFF. With 1 Figure

CHAPTER 3

Purines. N.-H. PARK and D. PAVAN-LANGSTON. With 9 Figures

CHAPTER 4

Amantadine and Its Derivatives. J. L. SCHULMAN. With 1 Figure

CHAPTER 5

The Thiosemicarbazones. C. J. PFAU. With 24 Figures

CHAPTER 6

Interferon and Its Inducers. P. B. SEHGAL, L. M. PFEFFER, and I. TAMM.
With 5 Figures

CHAPTER 7

Immunotherapy and Immunoregulation. H. FRIEDMAN and S. SPECTER

Part B

CHAPTER 8

Guanidine. D. R. TERSHAK, F. H. YIN, and B. D. KORANT. With 9 Figures

CHAPTER 10

Arildone: A β-Diketone. J. J. McSharry and F. Pancic. With 12 Figures

CHAPTER 11

Phosphonoacetic Acid. L. R. OVERBY. With 9 Figures

CHAPTER 12

Natural Products. P. E. Came and B. A. Steinberg. With 17 Figures

CHAPTER 13

Rifamycins. C. Gurgo, S. Bridges, and M. Green. With 2 Figures

List of Abbreviations

ABPP	2-amino-5-bromo-6-phenyl-4-pyrimidinol	BVdUrd	E-5-(2-bromovinyl)-2'-deoxyuridine
ADCC	antibody-dependent cellular cytotoxicity	CA	chorioallantoic
5'-AdThd	5'-aminodeoxythymidine	cAMP	cyclic adenosine mono-phosphate
AHF	Argentinian hemorrhagic fever	CFA	complete Freund's adjuvant
AIdUDP	5-iodo-5'-amino-2',5'-dideoxyuridine diphosphate	CF$_3$dUMP	5-trifluoromethyl-2'-deoxy-uridine monophosphate
AIdUrd	5-iodo-5'-amino-2,5'-dideoxyuridine	CF$_3$dUrd	5-trifluoromethyl-2'-deoxy-uridine
AIdUTP	5-iodo-5'-amino-2,5'-dideoxy-uridine triphosphate	CF$_3$dUTP	5-trifluoromethyl-2'-deoxy-uridine triphosphate
AIPP	2-amino-5-iodo-6-phenyl-4-pyrimidinol	CID	cytomegalovirus inclusion disease
AMP	adenosine monophosphate	CJD	Creutzfeldt-Jakob disease
AMV	avian myeloblastosis virus	CMP	cytomegalovirus
Ara-A	arabinofuranosyladenine	CPE	cytopathic effect
Ara-ADP	arabinofuranosyladenine diphosphate	cpm	counts per minute
Ara-AMP	arabinofuranosyladenine monophosphate	dATP	deoxyadenine triphosphate
Ara-ATP	arabinofuranosyladenine triphosphate	dCTP	deoxycytidine triphosphate
Ara-C	arabinofuranosylcytosine	dCyd	deoxycytidine
Ara-Hx	arabinofuranosylhypoxan-thine	DEV	duck embryo vaccine
		dGTP	deoxyguanosine triphosphate
Ara-HxMP	arabinofuranosylhypoxan-thine monophosphate	DHAdt	5,6-dihydro-5-azathymidine
		DI	defective interfering (particles)
Ara-T	arabinofuranosylthymine	DMSO	dimethylsulfoxide
Ara-TMP	arabinofuranosylthymine monophosphate	DNA	deoxyribonucleic acid
		DNAP	Dane particle associated RNA polymerase
Ara-TTP	arabinofuranosylthymine triphosphate	DNase	deoxyribonuclease
ATP	adenosine triphosphate	dNMP-PA	deoxynucleotide mono-phosphate phosphonoacetate
		dpm	disintegrations per minute
BCG	bacille Calmette–Guérin	DRB	5,6-dichloro-1-β-D-ribofuranosylbenzimidazole
BEV	baboon endogenous virus		
BHF	Bolivian hemorrhagic fever	dThd	deoxythymidine
BHK	baby hamster kidney (cells)	dTMP	deoxythymidine mono-phosphate
BL	Burkitt's lymphoma		
BRU-PEL	*Brucella abortus* preparation	dTTP	deoxythymidine triphosphate
BSA	bovine serum albumin	EA	early antigen
BTV	Bluetongue virus	EBNA	Epstein–Barr nuclear antigen
		EBV	Epstein–Barr virus

EDTA	ethylenediaminetetracetic acid	LCM	lymphocytic chorio-meningitis
EEE	Eastern equine encephalo-myelitis	LHA	lower hemagglutinin
EIBT	N_1-ethylisatin-β-thiosemicarbazone	LPS	lipopolysaccharide
EMC	encephalomyocarditis	MA	membrane antigen
EtdUrd	5-ethyl-2'-deoxyuridine	MCMV	murine cytomegalovirus
		MDMP	2-(4-methyl-2,6-dinitro-vanilino)-N-methylpropion-amide
2'F-Ara-IC	1-(2-deoxy-2-fluoro-β-D-arabinofuranosyl)-5-iodo-cytosine		
		MDP	muramyl dipeptide
FCS	fetal calf serum	MEM	minimum essential medium
F_3dThd	trifluorothymidine	MER	methanol-extracted residue
FMDV	foot-and-mouth disease virus	MHV	mouse hepatitis virus
FPA	p-fluorophenylalanine	MIBT	N-methylisatin-β-thiosemi-carbazone
FSV	feline sarcoma virus		
FUDR	fluorodeoxyuridine	MIC	minimum inhibitory concentration
GMK	green monkey kidney (cells)	MLV	murine leukemia virus
		MMdUrd	5-methoxymethyl-2'-deoxyuridine
HA	hemagglutinin		
HBB	2-(α-hydroxybenzyl)-benzimidazole	MMTV	murine mammary tumor virus
		m.o.i.	multiplicity of infection
HB_cAg	hepatitis B core antigen	MRB	5-methyl-2-D-ribobenzimid-azole
HB_eAg	hepatitis B enzyme antigen		
HBIG	hepatitis B immune globulin	mRNA	messenger ribunucleic acid
HB_sAg	hepatitis B surface antigen		
HDCS	human diploid cell strain	NA	neuraminidase
HDL	high density lipoprotein	NCV	noncapsid viral (protein)
HFI	human fibroblast interferon	NDV	Newcastle diseases virus
HLA	human leukocyte antigen	NK	natural killer (cells)
HLI	human leukocyte interferon	NP	nucleoprotein
hnRNA	heterogeneous nuclear riboncleic acid	NPC	nasopharyngeal carcinoma
HPLC	high pressure liquid chromatography	opv	oral poliovirus vaccine
HPV	human papillomavirus	PAS	periodic acid–Schiff
HSV	herpes simples virus	PEG	polyethylene glycol
HVA	hepatitis virus A	pfu	plaque forming unit
HVB	hepatitis virus B	PML	progressive multifocal leukoencephalopathy
IBT	isatin-β-thiosemicarbazone	PPi	inorganic pyrophosphate (phosphodiesterase)
IBV	infectious bronchitis virus		
IdCyd	5-iodo-2'-deoxycytidine	PrdUrd	5-propyl-2'-deoxyuridine
IdUMP	5-iodo-2'-deoxyuridine monophosphate	PVM	pneumonia virus of mice
IdUrd	5-iodo-2'-deoxyuridine	RF	replicative form
IgG	immunoglobulin α	RI	replicative intermediate
IgG	immunoglobulin γ	RLV	Rauscher leukemia virus
IgM	immunoglobulin μ	RNA	ribonucleic acid
IMP	inosine monophosphate	RNP	ribonuclear protein (complex)
ipv	inactivated poliovirus vaccine	RSV	respiratory synctial virus
ISG	immune serum globulin		
		SDS	sodium dodecylsulfate
K	killer (cells)	SFV	Semliki Forest virus
KTS	kethoxal-bis-thiosemi-carbazone	SGOT	serum glutamate-oxalo-acetate transaminase

SMON	subacute myelo-optico-neuropathy	TPCK	L-1-tosylamide-2-phenylethyl-chloromethyl ketone
SRBC	sheep red blood cells	tRNA	transfer ribonucleic acid
SSPE	subacute sclerosing para-encephalitis	TSC	thiosemicarbazone
SSV	simian sarcoma virus	UHA	upper hemagglutinin
SV	simian virus	UMP	uridine monophosphate
SVP	subviral particles		
		VA	virus-associated
TCID$_{50}$	tissue culture median infective dose	VCA	viral capsid antigen
		VIG	vaccinia immune globulin
TCT	γ-thiochromanone-1-thio-semicarbazone	VPg	genome-linked viral protein
		VSV	vesicular stomatitis virus
TdT	deoxynucleotidyl transferase	VZIG	varicella zoster immune globulin
TGE	transmissible gastroenteric (virus of swine)		
		VZV	varicella zoster virus
TK	thymidine kinase		
TLCK	N-α-p-tosyl-L-lysinechloro-methyl ketone	WEE	Western equine encephalo-myelitis
TMV	tobacco mosaic virus	WT	wild-type (virus)

CHAPTER 1

Pathogenesis of Viral Infections

J. HAY and M. J. BARTKOSKI, JR.

A. Introduction

This introductory chapter is an attempt to combine our knowledge of the general features of viral replication studied at the molecular level (usually in cell culture) with some information on the course and outcome of infection (insofar as it can be studied) in the whole animal. A comprehensive review of molecular virologic studies would be so diverse that it would be beyond the scope of this chapter and would probably be superfluous for the majority of readers. However, some remarks on the underlying principles of the immune response to viral infection and on viral pathogenesis seem to be appropriate, along with some specific comments on integration of viral DNA into cell genomes and on defective interfering particles. Paradoxically, the host's immune response to virus infection can play several roles: it can provide both short- and long-term assistance in combating the infection, but also may be at least partially responsible for development of disease symptoms.

Three types of antibody are involved in the antiviral humoral immune response. The first of these which an infecting virus may encounter is IgA, secreted locally onto mucous surfaces of the gut and respiratory tract in response to the presence of virus at that site. Viremia, which may or may not (depending on the virus) follow from initial virus infection, leads to major production of IgG and IgM, the former persisting for long periods and the latter quickly disappearing. These immunoglobulins will prevent (by neutralization) the spread of cell-released virus throughout the body via body fluids. Cell-to-cell transmission of virus, on the other hand, is probably prevented by cell-mediated responses which have been programmed to recognize viral antigens and lyse cells carrying them. This may involve T-lymphocytes and/or macrophages in a number of complex interactions whose relative importance for a given disease is not well worked out.

Contributions to the pathogenesis of a disease can be made in several ways: nephritis can result from the deposition in the kidney of antibody–antigen (virus) complexes with complement to give a cell-mediated inflammatory response, or virus which grows in lymphocytes (such as cytomegalovirus) may set up a markedly lymphoproliferative condition. These are just two examples of what is likely to be, once our knowledge of these cell-mediated responses in general is more developed, a major feature of viral pathogenesis. A further factor in the spread of virus infection is interferon, which is induced in variable amounts by different viruses and to which individual viruses are differentially susceptible.

Virus can enter the organism by a number of routes. Infection through contact with respiratory tissues is frequent and normally gives rise to fairly localized virus multiplication and consequent local symptoms: the rhinoviruses are a good example of this category. Other viruses, which have structures that can survive the gut environment, infect and multiply in the gastrointestinal tract, and may spread to other body sites to multiply further and cause disease signs there. Genital contact and insect bites are two other important sources of virus infection.

When virus spreads in the body, it usually does so via the blood, reaching special target organs (e.g., hepatitis) or spreading less specifically (e.g., disseminated zoster). In some cases viremia may be maintained over long periods by chronic infections of the reticuloendothelial system. The skin (and mucous membranes) is a target organ for several different viruses, and multiplication of virus at sites on the body surface (via viremia) combines with the immune response to give characteristic rashes. Central nervous system infections can be set up by direct virus growth along nerves (e.g., rabies) or by virus growth in tissues adjacent to the central nervous system (e.g., in the choroid plexus).

The period between initial contact with the virus and the onset of obvious signs of disease is the incubation period, and this can be a variable length of time, depending on the virus. For most infections it is in the range of 2–3 days to 2–3 weeks, and is a direct consequence of the route of pathogenesis in the host. The incubation period is also a useful parameter to bear in mind for each virus infection, since it usually determines the treatment that is likely to be useful.

Most of what has been outlined so far has dealt with acute virus infections, characterized by virus multiplication, developing and disappearing over a relatively short period. However, several viruses can establish a persistent infection, in which virus may be shed over long periods at low levels, or latent infections, in which the virus escapes detection. In these cases the virus may be reactivated to cause an acute infection at a later date. Slow virus infections produce chronic fatal progressive illnesses over long periods, normally through degeneration of nerve tissue.

I. Defective Interfering Particles

Defective interfering (DI) particles can be produced by a large number of virus groups (and conceivably by all viruses) and are formed in cell culture after multiple passage, usually at high multiplicity of infection (m.o.i.) or in the infected host animal as a consequence of natural infection. These particles are defective in that they contain viral genome material with deletions, both large and small. Indeed, the genome need not code for any recognizably normal virus polypeptide, but must be able to be replicated (enzyme recognition site) and to be packaged in the virus particle (packaging sequences). DI particles cannot replicate in the absence of helper (usually standard) virus but will interfere with the normal replication of standard virus.

It was postulated by Huang and Baltimore (1970) that production of DI virus was a natural means of modulating virus infections. This has been amply demonstrated both in the animal and in cell culture; it is quite feasible to prevent the onset of disease (e.g., with influenza) with DI preparations in infected animals. The mechanism of interference is not entirely understood; however, it probably involves direct interference at the level of virus replication as well as the immune response and interferon production. In addition to preventing acute infection, DI virus may be a major factor in the establishment of persistent infections in cases in which standard virus infection is usually acute. While the mechanism of this change is again obscure, it is significant that the cell has a role in the formation of DI virus.

II. Integration of Viral Genomes

Another mechanism of achieving a persistent infection in animal cells is demonstrated by several groups of viruses which are capable of integrating their genome into the genome of the host cell. The retroviruses are RNA viruses which can integrate their genetic information into germ line cells of susceptible species through a DNA intermediate. In this way, the "provirus" is passed on from generation to generation; although gene expression is usually quite severely repressed, and induction of the provirus usually quite difficult.

All the DNA viruses which replicate in the nuclei of cells, of course, share this ability to become integrated into cell DNA and this has been shown to take place during normal lytic infection. The extent of this integration detected appears to be increasing as technology develops; however, a role for integration of viral DNA in lytic infections has not been defined.

On the other hand, as a feature of cell transformation by DNA viruses, integration seems to have an important part to play: either it ensures that modification or expression of cellular genes is heritably based, or that viral genes are stably present, in the correct copy number and appropriately controlled. Generally, transformed cells which are able to cause tumors in susceptible animals carry integrated viral sequences with them into the tumor cells. One hypothesis to explain "abortively transformed" cells is that true integration was never established to give stable association of viral and cell DNA, but this has not been rigorously shown.

Another function of integrated genomes may well be in the establishment of a latent (or persistent) infection: in this case the whole genome is integrated, as opposed to cell transformation, in which only part of the viral DNA complement is required. Inherent in the latency model is a means by which the integrated genome can be activated and allowed to be replicated in the cell. Much work, it is clear, still remains to be done to explain the phenomenon. What follows this general introduction is a description of the many virus types important in human disease.

B. Adenoviruses

Adenoviruses have, in all likelihood, been the cause of outbreaks of acute respiratory disease in military recruit populations for many years, but only recently have they been diagnosed as such (DINGLE and LANGMUIR 1968). Most children have, by the end of their first year, been infected with an adenovirus, and in about one-half of these, obvious disease is seen, normally a rather nonspecific respiratory illness (FOX et al. 1969).

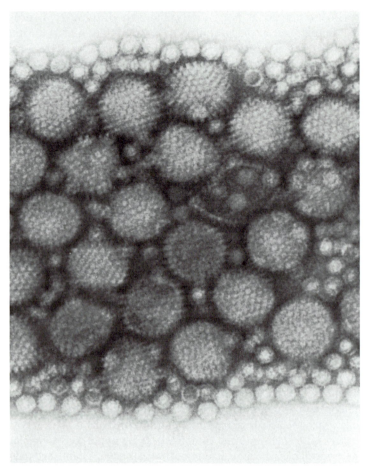

Fig. 1. Adenovirus type 18 (80 nm diameter) preparation banded on a CsCl density gradient. The preparation is contaminated with adeno-associated virus, a parvovirus (20 nm diameter). (Courtesy of C. Garon and J. Rose)

I. Structure and Replication

Adenoviruses have a unique structure, an icosahedron of 252 capsomeres, 240 hexons with 12 penton proteins (which consist of a base and a fiber) surrounding a nucleoprotein core structure and having no envelope (Fig. 1). The 240 hexon proteins have 3 identical polypeptides (molecular weight about 10^5 daltons) and carry the type-specific as well as type-common antigens (Maizel et al. 1968; Wilcox and Ginsberg 1963). The fiber contains three polypeptides (molecular weight about 60,000 daltons), and is phosphorylated and glycosylated (Ishibashi and Maizel 1974; Russel et al. 1972), while the penton base protein has four or five polypeptides of molecular weight 70,000–80,000 daltons associated noncovalently with the fiber (Maizel et al. 1968). Three basic core proteins (V, VII, X) are complexed with DNA in the center of the particle (Laver 1970) and several other minor polypeptides can also be found associated with the virus structure (GINSBERG and YOUNG 1977). An endonuclease, specific for DNA, is also present in the virion.

The viral DNA is a linear double strand of molecular weight $20-25 \times 10^6$ daltons and the strands can be separated. The human adenoviruses contain 31 serotypes which have 5 DNA homology subgroups (A–E), (GREEN et al. 1979 a). Subgroup C (type 1, 2, 5, 6) is the most common cause of childhood infection. Recently, it has been suggested that intermediate strains of adenovirus exist, which carry a single type of neutralizing antigen, but hemagglutinins of two different strains (HIERHOLZER et al. 1980). The DNA has an inverted terminal repetition which allows formation of single-stranded circles (GARON et al. 1972; ARRAND and ROBERTS 1979).

In subgroup C adenovirus, the 5′ terminus of the DNA is covalently bound to a protein of molecular weight 55,000 daltons (REKOSH et al. 1977; a fourth core protein). It increases infectivity of viral DNA in vitro (SHARP et al. 1976) but is not related (structurally) to any of the viral proteins recognized so far (HARTER et al. 1979).

The fiber of the virus particle attaches to the surface of a susceptible cell, but the identity of the specific recognition site is not clear (LEVINE and GINSBERG 1967). The particle passes through the plasma membrane of the host cell and then starts to disintegrate; the pentons are removed first and the capsid follows to leave the core structure. The uncoating process may be host specified (SUSSENBACH 1967). Migration to the nucleus follows, where replication is initiated by transcription from the viral DNA; whether this is carried out on naked DNA or on a still partially coated molecule is not known. The naked viral DNA is infectious at about 10^9 pfu μmol^{-1} (GRAHAM and VAN DER EB 1973).

The host cell's RNA polymerase II (presumably unmodified) produces initially five distinct "early" transcriptional units, which can be synthesized in the presence of cycloheximide (NEVINS et al. 1979; Fig. 2). Each of these is produced with different kinetics with the unit for the 72,000 dalton DNA-binding protein appearing last, conceivably a reflection of that protein's controlling role in gene expression. All of the mRNAs corresponding to these early DNA regions appear to be the product of posttranscriptional splicing (BERK and SHARP 1978) and several sizes of mRNA are generated from each region. The early 1B region, for example, encodes three mRNAs and three proteins, protein IX, a 15,000, and a 52,000 dalton polypeptide (HALBERT et al. 1979). The final number of early adenovirus polypeptides is still in doubt; there may be as many as seven polypeptides encoded by the transforming region (the left-hand end, 0–11 map units on the genome, see Fig. 2) alone (HALBERT et al. 1979). At about 6 h postinfection, DNA synthesis starts and is followed by the production of late mRNA species, all formed from a very large transcription unit reaching from 16 to 99 units on the genome, under the influence of a single promoter region (ZIF and EVANS 1978; Fig. 2). While late transcription occurs, only some of the early transcription units decline in production, e.g., unit 4 (NEVINS and WINKLER 1980). These late mRNAs all have the same 5′ end (which is "capped") and appear to be polyadenylated before splicing (NEVINS and DARNELL 1978). The viral transcipts appear as mRNAs in the cytoplasm and at late times consist chiefly of structural polypeptides: the first of them to appear is the hexon protein, and all are made in great excess (GREEN 1970). As late transcription

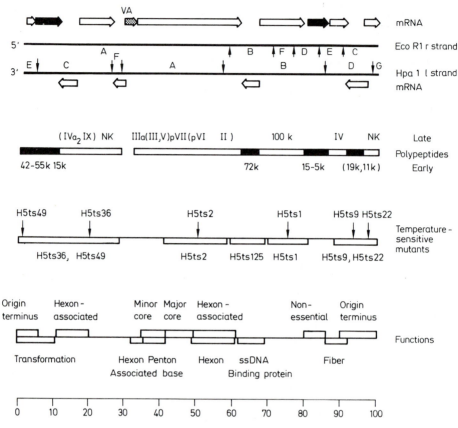

Fig. 2. The adenovirus genome is shown by horizontal lines, 0–100 units, in each part of the figure. In the map of mRNA sequences, the two lines represent the r and l strands of Ad2 DNA; the vertical lines indicate sites of cleavage by Eco R1 and Hpa 1. The arrows above and below the genome depict the regions to which mRNA is complementary; genes for the nonmessenger RNA, VA RNA, are indicated by the *stippled area*. In this, and the map of polypeptides shown below, *solid areas* indicate early viral gene products, whereas *open areas* show late products. In the polypeptide map, parentheses indicate uncertainty in order. (Flint 1977)

starts, a large increase in the amount of viral RNA produced takes place with viral DNA (or its replication) playing a major role. However, it does not seem that a DNA replicative intermediate is the target for late transcription (Brison et al. 1979).

Viral DNA synthesis cannot start without early protein synthesis, but it is not yet clear how many early products are required: genetic studies suggest three, one of which is the 72,000 dalton DNA-binding protein (Van der Vliet and Levine 1973). It has been possible to isolate nucleoprotein complexes from adenovirus-infected cells which will elongate and terminate viral DNA synthesis, but not initiate it (Wilhelm et al. 1976). Viral DNA in such complexes has been shown to be associated with several proteins which may assist in DNA synthesis in vivo. Among them are the viral 72,000 dalton DNA-binding protein, the cellular DNA polymerase α and γ (but not β), a DNA ligase, and the cell's RNA polymerase II (ARENS et al. 1977). Presumably this list is incomplete since the system does not initiate, and genetic studies suggest more than one viral product is involved: as a corollary, not all of the above activities may be necessary in vivo. Initiation of DNA synthesis needs the 72,000 dalton DNA-binding protein, possibly also the 55,000 dalton terminal protein (REKOSH et al. 1977), and takes place at the terminus of one strand of the molecule. The subsequent elongation displaces a parental strand which is independently used as a template in the subsequent continuous synthesis of the second new strand (WINNAKER 1978). The inverted terminal repeat has been sequenced (STERNBERGH et al. 1977) and has clusters of GC and AT-rich regions analogous to those seen in other DNA initiation sites, but the mechanism of initiation (e.g., involvement of RNA primer, etc.) and of successful completion of adenovirus DNA molecules remains obscure.

The various components of the virus structure gather in the nucleus where a likely sequence of events is capsid proteins → capsid structures, light intermediate (7–11 S DNA) → heavy intermediate (34 S DNA) → young virions (36 S DNA) → mature virions (34 S DNA); (D'HALLUIN et al. 1978). During these steps, two proteins are associated with and then leave the structure (50,000 and 39,000 dalton, possibly scaffolding proteins), while precursors to the core proteins V and VII are cleaved (EVERITT et al. 1977). Empty capsids have recently been shown to associate with one molecule of viral DNA in vitro (TIBBETTS and GIAM 1979). The inclusion bodies seen in adenovirus-infected cells appear to be aggregates of excess structural proteins and viral DNA, and mature adenovirions are only seen in the cytoplasm when the nuclear membrane has been breached to allow release of virus. Release from the cell presumably depends on rupture of the cytoplasmic membrane. Adenoviruses catalyze a rather slow decrease in cell functions after infection and the penton fiber protein has been characterized as responsible for these processes.

The human adenoviruses, while not as yet implicated in human oncogenesis, have the property of causing tumor formation and cell transformation in rodents and rodent cells. On the basis of oncogenicity, the following subgroups of the adenovirus serotypes can be recognized: A – highly oncogenic (high frequency of tumor formation in newborn rodents); B – weakly oncogenic (low frequency of tumor formation), and C, D, E which do not cause tumors directly, but can transform cells in tissue culture (GREEN et al. 1979a). The transforming region of the DNA is at the extreme left-hand end and probably ranges from about 8% to 4.5% of the adenovirus genome (DIJKEMA et al. 1979). Although there is much similarity among members of one group (MARKEY et al. 1979), different subgroups have different transforming sequences which may explain the old observation that different T antigens are made by the different groups (HEUBNER 1967). A number of candidate transformation proteins have been described with molecular weights in the range 10–65,000 daltons (LEWIS et al. 1976; GREEN et al. 1979) and seem to be similar in size among the virus group examined.

The mechanism (or mechanisms) for tumor formation is thus not well understood, but viral sequences do seem to persist in transformed cells. Transformed cells also frequently contain copies of viral DNA sequences other than those at the extreme left-hand end (GALLIMORE et al. 1974).

In view of the easily demonstrable oncogenic potential of human adenoviruses, interest has been aroused in their possible involvement in human oncogenic disease. It was recently reported that "normal" human placenta and liver and various primate tissues had adenovirus DNA sequences, including the left-hand end of the adenovirus genome (Jones et al. 1979). On the other hand, Green et al. (1979c) examined a large number of normal and tumoral human tissues for adenovirus DNA sequences with no apparent success. In the same study, multiple copies of the adenovirus genome were shown to be present in tonsil tissue from which it is possible to cultivate adenovirus. Restriction enzyme analysis of the DNA from tonsils showed unusual patterns which suggested that some of the viral DNA might be integrated into the cell genome. Also, since adenovirus frequently becomes latent in tonsil tissue, this finding may have a bearing on the mechanism of latency establishment by adenovirus.

In the course of adenovirus infection, incomplete or defective particles may accompany normal infectious virions; these usually retain some viral functions (e. g., cell-killing ability) but may not be infectious (Mak 1971). Some particles have a DNA genome derived from host cell DNA (Tjia et al. 1977) and others, viral DNA with deletions (Mak et al. 1979). The former type of particle probably resulted from aberrations in the final assembly process in the infected cell. Generation of at least one class of incomplete DNA molecule has been proposed to take place via DNA replication read-through past looped-out regions related to possible splicing mechanisms (Mak et al. 1979). The role of adenovirus defective particles in normal infection has not been elucidated.

Adenovirus mutants have been isolated from a number of laboratories (for review see Ginsberg and Young 1977) and both complementation and recombination have been demonstrated to occur. Recombination maps for adenovirus type 5 (Ad5; Williams et al. 1974; Ginsberg and Young 1977) and adenovirus type 2 (Ad2; Bégin and Weber 1975) have been constructed and give remarkably good correlation (two factor crosses) with each other (2,5) and with the physical maps of the genome which have been constructed. There are 13 complementation groups of Ad2 and Ad12 (Bégin and Weber 1975; Shiroki and Shimojo 1974) and mutants within one complementation group seem to cluster on the recombination map. Adenovirus–SV40 hybrids can be isolated from monkey cells (normally nonpermissive for adenovirus) upon coinfection with the two viruses. Sequences of the SV40 early region can replace part of the AD2 genome and presumably supply a helper function.

Ad2-infected cells produce, in large amounts late in infection, virus-associated (VA) RNA with a major (1) and a minor (2) component (Harris and Roeder 1978) which has the same 156 nucleotides as (1) plus an extra 38–40 at the 3' end. These RNAs have no certain function but a recent hypothesis suggests (Murray and Holliday 1979) that their role may involve binding across a splice point of heterogeneous nuclear RNA to allow formation of the true message.

II. Adenovirus Infections

The endemic adenoviruses (group C, types, 1, 2, 5, 6) tend to infect children to give respiratory infections; infection with types 3 and 7, on the other hand, frequently leads to pharyngoconjunctival fever, which occurs in epidemics. Acute respiratory disease (ARD) in recruits is usually caused by Ad4 (or Ad7) in epidemics (DUDDING et al. 1973) and epidemic keratoconjunctivitis is frequently caused by Ad8 (GRAYSTON et al. 1964).

Transmission occurs via several routes to give characteristic disease: for example, eye infections can be acquired in swimming pools. The most frequent route of spread, however, is a fecal–oral one, to give respiratory illness. In general, illness is acute and self-limiting in terms of symptoms, but the virus may continue to be shed for long periods after symptoms have disappeared. Viremia may develop in some cases and result in the formation of a rash which can be confused with rubella (GUTEKÜNST and HEGGIE 1961). Tonsils are a source of virus in about one-half of the child population, and adenovirus is presumed to inhabit this tissue in a latent form, although no one knows exactly what the state of the virus is under these circumstances (EVANS 1958). Type-specific antibody is produced upon infection, and is protective. Young children (with residual maternal antibody) seem less prone to adenovirus infections, a probable reflection of the protective power of circulating antibody.

The incubation period appears to be about 1 week, and in the rare fatal case of adenovirus infection, virus is present in essentially all body organs. An interesting correlation appeared during the New York Virus Watch program: mumps infection appeared to stimulate the production of adenovirus, conceivably by triggering the release of the latent state (FOX et al. 1969).

Vaccination against adenovirus infection has been shown to be successful, but has been limited to the military population. Inactivated monkey-cell-grown virus preparations were used initially but suffered from variable potency and contamination problems (PIERCE et al. 1968). Now a live vaccine is used, presented in a capsule whose contents are released only in the gastrointestinal tract, to give reliable immunity without respiratory tract infection. Since there is still concern about a possible role of adenovirus in tumorigenesis and since the virus is spread quite effectively through populations (STANLEY and JACKSON 1969), there are no plans at present to use the vaccine on children or the general population.

C. Arenaviruses

The arenaviruses are a recently characterized group of viruses which derive their name (Latin *harenosus, sandy*) from the electron-dense granules (host ribosomes) found in variable numbers in the virus particles (CARTER et al. 1973; FARBER and RAWLS 1975). The viruses in this group include lymphocytic choriomeningitis (LCM) virus, Lassa fever virus, and the Tacaribe group of viruses (Machupo, Junin, Tacaribe, Tamiami, Parana, Latino, Pichinde, and Atmapari). Of these viruses only Lassa fever, Machupo, Junin, and LCM are known to cause human disease; LCM virus causing a sporadic, and relatively mild meningoencephalitis, while the other three may cause a serious, highly fatal hemorrhagic fever.

The virions of the arenaviruses are pleomorphic in shape, approximately 80–130 μm in diameter (MURPHY and WHITFIELD 1975) and its outer shell is a unit membrane derived from the host cell through budding (Fig. 3). The genome con-

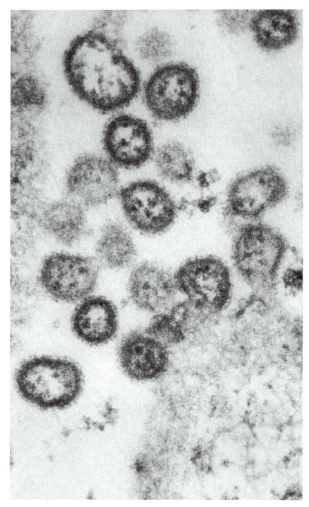

Fig. 3. Arenaviruses. Photograph shows Lassa fever virus in first cell passage after isolation from a patient in Sierra Leone. The envelope, surface projection layers, and internal ribosomes are well resolved. (Courtesy of F. A. Murphy) × 121,000

sists of two major size classes of RNA, L (molecular weight 3.2×10^6 daltons) and S(molecular weight 1.6×10^6 daltons; Faber and Rawls 1975), as well as variable amounts of host cell RNA species (Vezza et al. 1978). As a consequence of their segmented genome these viruses show a high frequency of genetic recombination (Vezza and Bishop 1977). There appear to be four main structural proteins, two of which are glycoproteins, probably representing components of the viral envelope (Ramos et al. 1972) and the virion is also reported to contain a RNA polymerase (Carter et al. 1974). The replication cycle of the arenaviruses is not well defined, but high multiplicity passage of undiluted stocks of virus may lead to the production of DI particles (Huang and Baltimore 1977). Studies with macrophages from mice infected with LCM virus demonstrated that these cells were resistant to infection with a homologous, but not a heterologous virus (MIMS and SUBRAHMANYAN 1966). A quantitative assay for these DI particles based on interference with infectious center formation by wild-type virus has been worked out (WELSH and PFAU 1972). The DI particles cannot be separated from the wild-type virus (WELSH et al. 1972) but the variability in host response to arenavirus infection may indicate an important role for these particles in normal infection (WOODWARD and SMITH 1975).

Rodents appear to be the natural host of the arenaviruses. The virus population in nature is maintained by chronic infection of the host, usually by perinatal inoculation; the result is chronic lifetime infection, with many animals showing a total lack of immunologic response. In contrast, inoculation of adult animals results in an acute (often fatal) disease with a normal immunologic response. Infection of humans (as is the case with many diseases) is accidental and the disease is acquired after coming into contact with excreta from an infected animal. Infection of humans with LCM, as with all arenaviruses, is classified as a zoonosis. The spread of LCM in most human cases is not well documented, but is throught to be through infected aersols and contact with infected rodent urine (FARMER and JANEWAY 1942; HIMAN et al. 1975). Person-to-person spread has not been shown except for Lassa fever (MONATH 1975). LCM infection begins with fever, chills, and myalgia which may occur after an incubation period of 5–10 days, with symptoms of meningitis usually starting 15–23 days after exposure (MANDELL et al. 1979). There is no specific treatment available but human deaths are rare.

LCM infection in mice is a classic example of a virus-induced immunopathologic disease, and for this reason its pathogenesis deserves special mention. The virus is transmitted congenitally to every mouse in an infected colony. The mice are born "normal" and remain "normal" for most of their lives. Throughout this time they have persistent viremia and viruria and nearly all cells in the animal are infected. Circulating free antibody is not detectable as the virus circulates in the bloodstream in the form of a virus–IgG complex which is infectious. Late in life these mice may show "late" disease. This late disease is due to the deposition of the antigen–antibody (virus–IgG) complexes in the glomeruli, resulting in glomerulonephritis. In the adult mice, a different response is seen. Intracerebral inoculation results in the stimulation of the immune response, causing a fatal choriomeningitis with no evidence of neuronal damage. Immune suppression of the adult mice protects against death due to the virus, even though viral growth is similar in both suppressed and nonsuppressed animals. Further work has suggested that cell-mediated rather than humoral immunity is responsible for the lesions. A similar relationship between virus and natural host may be true for many of the arenaviruses.

Lassa fever and the remaining arenaviruses which infect humans, in contrast to LCM infection, may produce a fatal hemorrhagic fever. Lassa fever is primarily a disease of West Africa (FRAME et al. 1970; BUCKLEY and CASALS 1970), but has spread to other areas of the world, resulting in sporadic outbreaks (LEIFER et al. 1970). Lassa fever virus, unlike other arenaviruses, may on occasion be spread in groups such as health care workers owing to their intimate contact with infected patients. The spread in these nosocomial outbreaks may be through parenteral inoculation of infected fluids, close contact, or airborne spread (MONATH 1975). The symptoms of Lassa fever range from a mild or subclinical disease to a fulminant, often fatal condition. Following an incubation period of 1–2 weeks symptoms including fever, chills, malaise, myalgia, and diarrhea begin (MONATH and CASALS 1975). By the end of the first week the symptoms worsen and mouth lesions, exudative pharyngitis, and pulmonary symptoms appear. Edema, along with a petechial rash of neck and face, may occur. In the second week of symptoms a shock syndrome may appear, characterized by loss of intracellular mass through capillary leakage, vasoconstriction, hypotension, kidney failure, and pulmonary edema; myocarditis may also be present. There are hemorrhages, but of insufficient amount to produce the shock. At this point, either the patient dies or convalescence begins. Mortality in hospitalized cases averages about 36%. The diagnosis may be made serologically or by virus isolation, but this should be attempted only in a maximum containment laboratory.

Machupo and Junin viruses, the cause of Bolivian hemorrhagic fever (BHF) and Argentinian hemorrhagic fever (AHF), respectively, have similar clinical symptoms as well as being antigenically related (JOHNSON 1977). The diseases are often multisystem, involving the renal, hematopoietic, and clotting systems. Fever is high and sustained for 5–8 days. Patients often appear to be intoxicated and very sick, with fever, malaise, and myalgia (MANDELL et al. 1979; JOHNSON 1977). As the illness progresses, significant hemorrhagic as well as neurologic manifestations may be seen. Mortality averages 10%–20%.

Infection by arenaviruses may be prevented by blocking transmission, from rodents or infected persons. Rodent control has been shown to work for both BHF and lymphocytic choriomeningitis (HINMAN et al. 1975; MACKENZIE 1965). Treatment is supportive and may be lifesaving. Vaccines are available for Junin and Machupo virus and may be of some benefit. No vaccine is available for LCM or Lassa fever (JOHNSON 1975).

D. Coronaviruses

The coronaviruses belong to the family Coronaviridae. The human strains of this family are morphologically similar to the infectious bronchitis virus (IBV) of chickens, mouse hepatitis virus (MHV), and transmissible gastroenteritis virus (TGE) of swine (TYRRELL et al. 1968a). The term corona refers to the crown-like appearance of the particle surface projections (TYRRELL et al. 1968b). The first human strain was isolated in 1965 from a patient suffering from a cold (TYRRELL and BYNOE 1965) but the virus proved resistant to growth in common tissue culture and grew only after several passages in organ culture (TYRRELL and BYNOE 1965). The newer isolates of the virus have proved equally difficult to grow, and only two human strains, 229E and OC43 have been adapted to tissue culture (MCINTOSH 1979).

The coronaviruses are enveloped RNA viruses, approximately 80–120 mm in diameter, with helical nucleocapsids (Fig. 4). The genome has been shown to be composed of a single-stranded, nonsegmented, RNA of positive polarity (messenger sense) and having a molecular weight of $5–6 \times 10^6$ daltons (LAI and STOHLMAN 1978). A molecular weight in excess of 8×10^6 daltons has also been reported (LOMNICZI and KENNEDY 1977; TANNOCK 1973; MACNAUGHTON and

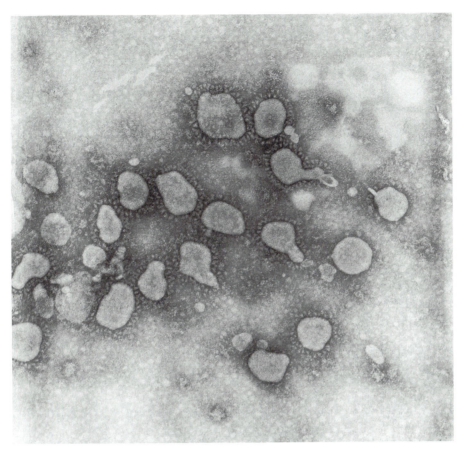

Fig. 4. Coronaviruses. Negatively stained preparation showing corona effect produced by surface projections. (KAPIKIAN, 1969) × 144,000

MADGE 1977). The genomic RNA is both polyadenylated and infectious (SCHOCHETMAN et al. 1977; WEGE et al. 1978).

The structural polypeptides of the coronaviruses are made up of two envelope glycoproteins E1 and E2 and a third nucleocapsied protein N of molecular weight 23, 180, and 50,000 daltons respectively (STURMAN et al. 1980). El lies within the lipoprotein envelope (STURMAN 1977), E2 may be found in two forms (180 and 90,000 daltons) and the 180,000 dalton from can be cleaved into the 90,000 dalton form by trypsin (STURMAN and HOLMES 1977).

During replication, as many as six different RNA species may be synthesized, five of which are subgenomic while the other is the whole genome. All six RNA species are synthesized in roughly constant proportions and are polyadenylated (STERN and KENNEDY 1980). Human coronavirus 229E replication was shown to be sensitive to actinomycin D (KENNEDY and JOHNSON-LUSSENBURG 1978) while other coronaviruses were not (MALLUCI 1965). DI particles have not been demonstrated, but one suspects that this is because the proper experiments have not been done. The virus matures by budding from internal cellular membranes and not from the plasma membrane (McIntosh 1974). It must be pointed out that all the work so far collected on the molecular biology and physical characterization of the coronaviruses has been performed on coronaviruses other than human strains.

Coronaviruses appear to be a major cause of common respiratory infection in all age groups (Monto 1976), responsible for up to 15% of all colds (McIntosh 1979). The coronaviruses are probably transmitted by the respiratory route (Stair et al. 1972) as no other route of transmission has been shown, but animal coronaviruses are infectious by the fecal–oral route (Stair et al. 1972). In the United States, periodicity, with epidemics occuring at 2–3-year intervals, has been demonstrated (Monto 1974).

The incubation period for coronaviruses is relatively short, ranging from 2 to 4 days (Bradburne et al. 1967; Tyrrell et al. 1968a) and the duration of the illness is from 6 to 7 days. Infections mainly involve the surface of the respiratory tract, meaning that IgA probably plays a direct role in protection (Monto 1976) and coronavirus are characterized by a high rate of reinfection (Monto and Lim 1974). Coronaviruses have been reported isolated from the stools of patients with diarrhea, raising the possibility of the involvement of these viruses in human gastroenteritis, as is the case with some animal coronaviruses (Stair et al. 1972). However, a definitive role for these agents in gastroenteritis has not been discovered.

E. Viral Hepatitis

Acute inflammation of the liver can be caused by a number of human viruses, such as some of the herpesviruses, coxsackievirus, mumps virus, and yellow fever virus, but *viral hepatitis* is usually considered to describe infections with hepatitis A virus (HAV), hepatitis B virus (HBV), or neither – the so-called non-A and non-B hepatitis.

Viral hepatitis is a major health problem worldwide, particularly in countries with poor public health and sanitation. In the United States, 60,000 cases annually are reported and this is generally accepted as a small fraction of the true occurrence (Center for Disease Control 1977). It appears to have been a recognized health problem for 2,500 years (Zuckerman 1976) but its infectious nature was not taken seriously until the 1940s when injection equipment was implicated in the spread of hepatitis. In the mid 1960s, two events took place which have laid the foundation for our current knowledge of viral hepatitis. It had been recognized that two forms of the disease existed, one with a short and the other with a long incubation period. Blumberg (1977) discovered "Australia antigen" in the serum of multiply transfused patients and subsequent work demonstrated that this was a serologic marker for the long-incubation hepatitis or hepatitis B; blood which was positive for Australia antigen (now known to be the surface antigen HBsAg) could transmit hepatitis B infection. The second discovery was that, as had been suspected, two distinct forms of the disease could be recognized (Krugman et al. 1967) on the basis of the general clinical and immunologic picture: hepatitis A or "infectious" hepatitis and hepatitis B or "serum" hepatitis.

I. Hepatitis A

The infectious agent of hepatitis A appears to be a picornavirus (BRADLEY et al. 1978), and it is excreted in large quantities into the environment from stools of infected individuals. Not all of these infected individuals will show signs of disease, however, and it may be that the majority of those shedding virus have mild or asymptomatic infection. Spread of the virus by the fecal–oral route had been demonstrated in 1945 when feces was fed to volunteers who subsequently (average of 4 weeks) developed the disease. Natural transmission appears to be via contaminated water and food (there have been several outbreaks of shellfish-related disease, but no evidence for a nonhuman host) and by close personal contact.

The primary site of infection is probably not the liver, since virus is shed well before any clinical or molecular evidence of liver damage is apparent, but the sequence of events leading to hepatocyte damage is not clear. The virus (which is stable in the intestinal environment) enters the body via the gastrointestinal tract and presumably reaches the liver through the blood. However, liver damage may result not from direct infection of liver cells but from an immune reaction to the presence of virus or viral antigens (MURPHY et al. 1978). Infections with hepatitis A tend to be mild but a small number of people (about 50/year in the United States) die of fulminant hepatitis (FRANCIS and MAYNARD 1979).

The HAV is an unenveloped cubic particle of about 27 nm diameter with three major structural polypeptides (CONLEPIS et al. 1978). Since the genome has been shown to be single-straded RNA (apparently somewhat smaller than poliovirus RNA; SIEGL and FROSNER 1978) and the particle polypeptides similar in size to those seen in the enteroviruses, HAV has been judged to be a picornavirus. It is, like the enteroviruses, resistant to heat, acid, and organic solvents. Infected individuals have antibody to hepatitis A (there is only one serotype) and sensitive serologic tests for this now exist; as a corollary, human immune serum can be used prophylactically. No vaccine is available at present, since the virus has yet to be grown successfully in cell or tissue culture.

II. Hepatitis B

The onset of hepatitis B is usually associated with a long period (weeks to months) of fatigue and malaise, and the overall course of the disease is normally more severe than for hepatitis A, leading to significant mortality in older age groups (Fig. 5). HBV also causes both chronic acute and chronic persistent hepatitis. The standard route of infection is from infected serum via vaccination, transfusion, injection, drug abuse, etc., but it is becoming increasingly clear that various forms of intimate contact help to spread infection too. Infectious virus has been found in blood, semen, and saliva (ALTER et al. 1977) and, once released into the environment, it is apparently quite stable. Contact with objects contaminated by these body fluids may be sufficient, even days after the event, to cause infection.

Three factors appear to be important in the pathogenesis of HBV infection. First, the immunocompetence of the host (PRINCE et al. 1978) inversely determines the chronic status of the disease. Second, the route of infection plays an important role in establishing the infection, e.g., subcutaneous injection is particularly effi-

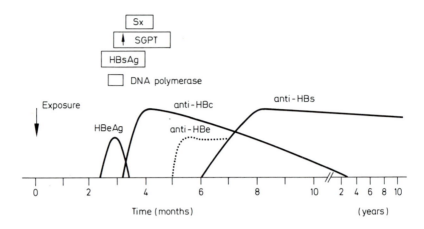

Acute viral hepatitis B

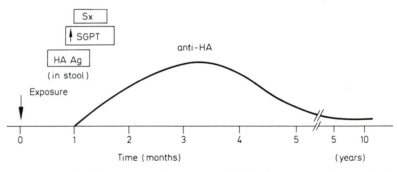

Acute viral hepatitis A

Fig. 5. Representative time course of appearance of clinical symptoms (if present), liver enzyme elevation, viral antigens, and antibodies in acute hepatitis B and A. Persons are infectious for hepatitis B during the period when HB$_s$Ag, DNA polymerase and HB$_e$Ag are present in serum. For hepatitis A, the period of infectivity corresponds to the presence of hepatitis antigen (HA Ag) in feces. (Reed and Boyer 1979)

cient (Barker et al. 1975). Third, the source of virus is crucial: many individuals whose blood contains viral antigens are not infectious and the best test of infectivity seems to be the level of HBeAg (Seeff et al. 1978).

A month or more after infection is normally required before signs of virus replication are detectable: the first of these is the presence of HBsAg in the blood, a result of replication of the virus at some unknown site or sites (Krugman and Giles 1973). Normally, an additional month elapses before signs of liver damage are obvious, but there is no clear correlation between the level of infectious virus in the blood and the severity of hepatic damage. It has recently been postulated that the pathogenicity of the virus stems from the host's immune response to infected hepatocytes (CHISARI et al. 1978). This model proposes that both humoral and suppressor T-cell-mediated mechanisms interact with the infected cell; preponderance of the latter mechanism allows infected cells to survive owing to the lessening of the immune response, while the opposite reaction results in massive destruction of hepatocytes. In this latter case, severe acute illness develops: in the former, a chronic carrier state is the result.

The virus particle (dane particle) is 42 nm in diameter, infecting humans and a few other primates and is a most unusual type of virus – a woodchuck analog has recently been isolated, (SUMMERS et al. 1978) but cannot be grown at present in cell culture. The viral DNA is a partially single-stranded circle (HRUSKA et al. 1977) of molecular weight about 1.6×10^6 daltons and can be converted to an intact double strand (3,200 base pairs) by the DNA polymerase activity present in the virion. These circles are formed by the annealing of single-stranded cohesive ends (about 300 bases long; SATTLER and ROBINSON 1979). Recently, particles of varying antigenic subtypes have been shown to possess distinctive restriction enzyme cleavage sites (SIDDIQUI et al. 1979). One of the antigenic structures associated with the virion is the HBsAg with both group-specific and type-specific determinants, and it may also form 22 nm spherical or tubular particles with no nucleic acid, which occur in sera. Two other antigens are the internal virion antigen HBeAg and the core antigen HBcAg, located internally to the coat of the virion (ALMEIDA et al. 1971). All these antigens occur in infected patients' sera and the HBeAg occurs as a small molecule distinct from the 27 nm HBcAg or the HBsAg forms. The HBeAg is most frequently (when seen in conjunction with HBsAg) a signal in serum of present disease and high infectivity (ELEFTHERIOU et al. 1975). The antigen is present both in Dane particles and cores, but needs to be activated (proteolysis or detergent treatment) before activity can be seen. Two core polypeptides (19,000 and 45,000 daltons) are associated with the antigenicity (TAKAHASHI et al. 1979). A recent study, in which a primary liver carcinoma cell line (from a patient with hepatitis B infection) producing small amounts of HBsAg was examined, indicates that the whole HBV genome is present in an integrated form in these cells and that all sequences are transcribed (MARION et al. 1980), although only the HBsAg appeared to be produced in a detectable form. The suspicion that a link exists between HBV and liver carcinoma (SZMUNESS 1978) may be strengthened by this observation. Dane particles have a complex antigenic structure with group-specific (a) and type-specific determinants (d,y,w,r), so that the complete description of particle might be HBsAg/adr, for example. The particle is a double-shelled structure and the outer coat (where resides the HBsAg) has two polypeptides (P1 and P2); both are probably the same polypeptide, P2 being a glycoprotein. Other polypeptides up to about 100,000 daltons have also been described in surface antigen preparations (SHI and GERIN 1977). Several successful attempts have been made recently to clone sequences from HBV DNA into bacterial vectors. It has been possible to obtain expression of the HBcAg in *Escherichia coli* such that the product is immunologically active in rabbits, establishing the feasibility, at least, of vaccine production from viral antigen synthesis in prokaryotic cells (PASEK et al. 1979). The cloned product has molecular weight 21,000 daltons, close to that found in vivo. Preliminary data suggest that the HBsAg may also be effectively produced in a somewhat modified system (PASEK et al. 1979).

F. Herpesviruses

There are five human herpesviruses, herpes simplex types 1 and 2, cytomega-lovirus, varicella zoster virus, and Epstein–Barr virus. All cause widespread infec-tions, with occasionally quite serious consequences and all have the property of re-maining latent in the infected host, sometimes for the lifetime of that host. A variety of stimuli can resurrect the virus from its latent state (in which it is normally undetectable) to give recurrent infections which may be quite frequent (in the case of herpes simplex, for example) and either localized or more generalized. There is also evidence that members of this group are involved in oncogenesis.

I. Herpes Simplex Viruses 1 and 2

Herpes simplex viruses (HSV) exist as two genotypes distinguisable by routes of transmission and sites of infection. HSV-2 is spread by genital contact and tends to infect sites below the waist, usually the genitalia, while HSV-1 is spread by other means (e.g., oral contact) and is normally found above the waist. The correlations with site of occurence are not absolute, however. Infection with both genotypes is widespread, HSV-1 being acquired in childhood, HSV-2 somewhat later; HSV-1 infections are also more prevalent than HSV-2 although the latter infection often represents serious problems (social and otherwise) for the people involved. Both infections are characterized by latent states and more or less frequent recurrences.

Based on electron microscopic data, the herpes virion has four major structural components: core, capsid, tegument, and envelope (O'Callaghan and Randall 1976). The core has a cylindrical protein structure around which the DNA is wound as a toroid (Furlong et al. 1972) and the whole is encased in the capsid, a 162 capsomer icosahedron (Wildy 1967, Fig. 6). Between capsid and envelope is the amorphous tegument layer (Roizman et al. 1975) and the envelope, in the electron microscope, is indistinguishable from the cell's nuclear membrane. There may be as many as 30 polypeptides in the particle, and Roizman et al. (1975) have summarized the probable location of many of them in the four components recog-nized. The major virus glycoproteins are found on the envelope, are derived from four unique polypeptides (Spear 1976), and appear to be necessary for successful infection and for the cell fusion reaction typical of some HSV strains. Sulfation may accompany glycosylation and several virion proteins appear to be phosphory-lated (Gibson and Roizman 1974). Two polyamines, spermine and spermidine, are associated with the nucleocapsid and the envelope, respectively (Gibson and Roiz-man 1971).

Both HSV-1 and HSV-2 DNA have a molecular weight of about 100×10^6 dal-tons and have a linear double-stranded configuration with 67% and 69% guanosine plus cytosine content, respectively (Kieff et al. 1971). The linear duplex is susceptible to alkali fragmentation, probably owing both to nicks and to ribonu-cleotides present in the DNA; whether alkali treatment yields random single strands or defined pieces of viral DNA is still a matter for controversy (Frenkel and Roizman 1972; Wilkie 1973). The genome has a terminal redundancy which allows formation of double-stranded circles after, for example, λ exonuclease di-gestion (Grafstrom et al. 1974). The most interesting feature of HSV DNA, how-

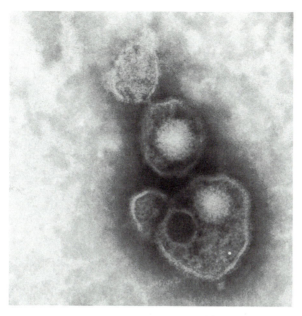

Fig. 6. Herpes simplex virus (capsid diameter 100 nm). Shown is a full enveloped particle (center) (Courtesy of D. H. WATSON)

ever, is the existence of two sets of internally inverted repeat sequences, duplicating sequences in the termini of the duplex (Fig. 7), postulated by SHELDRICK and BER-THELOT 1974). A consequence of this structure is that intramolecular rearrangement may occur to generate four forms of the HSV genome (Fig. 7). That these four forms exist in infected cells and in virons (in more or less equal proportion) was demonstrated by restriction enzyme cleavage and by partial denaturation mapping (HAYWARD et al. 1975; DELIUS and CLEMENTS 1976). Whether all four forms are functional is not yet clear and it is suspected that not all are (ROIZMAN 1979). There are several other insertions, deletions, redundancies, etc., whose importance is ill defined. Other herpesviruses have different structures. Cytomegalovirus (CMV) looks like HSV-1 and HSV-2, except that it is larger, while Epstein–Barr virus (EBV) is radically different (Fig. 7). Varicella zoster virus (VZV) DNA appears to be the smallest of this group and to have one internal inverted region (STRAUS et al. 1981).

The herpesvirus particle enters the cell either by pinocytosis or by membrane fusion and moves to the cell nucleus to become an active transcription substrate, presumably as some uncoated entity: some association of input DNA with the cellular nuclear proteins has been suggested (WAGNER and SUMMERS 1978). Infection leads to disruption of all polysomes, cell RNA synthesis inhibition, and degradation of cell mRNA (WAGNER and ROIZMAN 1969b; NISHOKA and SILVERSTEIN 1977). Viral message on cytoplasmic polysomes (about 10–33 S) seeems to be derived from larger precursor RNAs (WAGNER and ROIZMAN 1969a) and to account for esentially all genome sequences late in infection. Early RNA is largely representative of about 40% of coding sequences, with, probably, less abundant RNA spe-

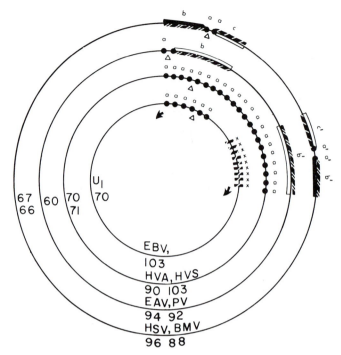

Fig. 7. Comparison of the structures of several known herpesvirus DNAs shown in a circular arrangement. The triangles denote the positions of the termini of the linear molecules. The *full circles*, shown out of proportion to their true size, represent the a sequences. The *full*, *open*, and *striated segments* of the circular representations are meant to indicate the terminal sequences that are inverted internally. The numbers below each circle give the molecular weights of the DNAs in millions. The numbers on the left indicate the approximate molecular weights of the unique sequences of L components (U$_L$). EBV Epstein–Barr virus; HVA *Herpesvirus ateles;* HVS *Herpesvirus saimiri;* EAV equine abortion virus; PV pseudorabies virus; HSV herpes simplex virus; BMV bovine mamillitis virus. (Roizman 1979)

cies accounting for up to another 40% (Swanstrom and Wagner 1974; Kozak and Roizman 1974). Evidence for restricted cytoplasmic sequences being dependent on processing from more extensive transcription in the nucleus has been presented, but is not generally agreed upon (Clements and Hay 1977). A subset of early RNA is immediate early RNA, which is produced in the absence of viral protein synthesis and has been mapped physically to restricted regions of the genome (Clements et al. 1977). Thus, at least three levels of control seem to operate: first, "on–off" control; second, abundance control; and third, control by specific nuclear retention of certain sequences. mRNA is capped (Bartkoski and Roizman 1976), can be polyadenylated, and is produced by the cell's RNA polymerase II (Alwine et al. 1974). Recently, some limited splicing has been demonstrated (R. J. Watson, personal communication 1980).

There may be well over 100 polypeptides in infected cells (H. S. Marsden and L. Haar, personal communication 1980) of which perhaps 30 are structural. Honess and Roizman (1974) have divided the synthesis of viral polypeptides into three main groups, α, β, γ, regulated by an interlocking cascade scheme: α polypeptides

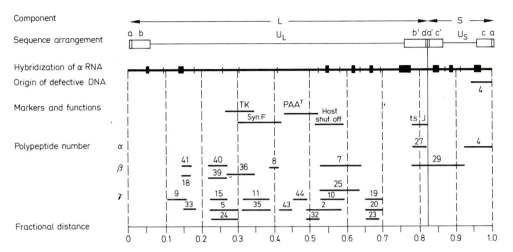

Fig. 8. Location of templates specifying HSV markers, functions, and polypeptides determined from an analysis of HSV-1 × HSV-2 recombinants. U_L and U_S are the long and short unique regions of the DNA; TK is thymidine kinase; PAA^r is the resistance locus for phosphonoacetate; Syn is a locus for syncytium formation; F and J are temperature-sensitive mutants of HSV-1. (MORSE et al. 1978)

are made first (from immediate early or α mRNA) and regulate the switch to later modes of synthesis (PRESTON 1979); γ polypeptides represent structural polypeptides and their synthesis is not (qualitatively) dependent on viral DNA synthesis, although a class of proteins which seems to be progeny DNA-dependent has been described (POWELL et al. 1975); β polypeptides include enzymes, DNA-binding proteins, etc.

Several enzyme activities have been shown to be induced by herpes simplex virus infection, and some of them have been shown to be virus coded. Pyrimidine deoxynucleoside kinase (DUBBS and KIT 1964), DNA polymerase, and alkaline deoxyribonuclease (KEIR and GOLD 1963) have all been mapped physically on the genome, and other induced activities include ribonucleotide reductase, deoxythymidylate kinase (part of the pyrimidine deoxynucleoside kinase activity), RNase H, nucleoside phosphotransferase, uridine, and choline kinases, protein kinase, and deoxynucleoside triphosphatase. No evidence for altered or new RNA polymerase II activity has been forthcoming, although it has been looked for.

Much effort has recently gone into physical and functional mapping of viral polypeptides, and Fig. 8 shows the data of MORSE et al. (1978) more or less identical with that of MARSDEN et al. (1978) and PRESTON et al. (1978). Viral DNA synthesis, judged by the number of viral mutants deficient in that function, is likely to be dependent on several viral activities, one of which is a DNA polymerase activity (PURIFOY and POWELL 1977), although cell functions are also implicated (YANAGI et al. 1978). It takes place in the nucleus, by a mechanism which is currently uncertain, although ROIZMAN (1979) has proposed a plausible model. Viral structural polypeptides can migrate from the cytoplasm to form capsids in the nucleus; these can become associated with viral DNA and enter the cytoplasm, acquiring a nuclear membrane-derived envelope on the way. The virus leaves the cell either by budding or via channels in the membranes of infected cells.

Like most other animal viruses, herpesvirus accumulates DI particles when virus stocks are passaged in tissue culture or in the animal. Tandem repeats of DNA from herpes simplex, either from short, S regions (Frenkel et al. 1976) or from the middle of long, L regions (Cuifo and Hayward 1980) form molecules of about whole genome size and their bouyant densities may be higher or the same as wild-type virus. Defective molecules derived from L also have a short (200 base pairs) region derived from the right-hand end of S. The existence of initiation sites for DNA synthesis in both L and S is suggested by these data.

II. Herpes Simplex Virus Infections

Infection with HSV often leads to a productive lytic cycle, but can also result in transformation of cells in culture in a persistent infection in vitro or in latency in vivo. Latent infections with HSV occur as a result of a primary infection and virus can be reactivated from its latent state to give recurrent lytic phases of viral multiplication. Later HSV-1 infections in humans were traced to the trigeminal ganglion by the nerve section experiments of Carter and Kilbourne, 1952. Using the mouse model, Stevens and Cook (1971) found that infection of the footpad resulted in acute sensory ganglion infection; in surviving animals, latent infections had been established, but no direct demonstration of virus or viral products was apparent. However, explantation and in vitro cultivation leads to production of infectious virus and, in addition to mouse ganglia, herpes simplex virus has been thus recovered from rabbit trigeminal ganglia (Stevens 1972) and human trigeminal ganglia (HSV-1; Baringer and Swoveland 1973) and sacral ganglia (HSV-2; Baringer 1975). Recent evidence suggests that a particular HSV-1 strain infects each individual and that, after replication, this virus may become latent at more than one ganglionic site (Lonsdale et al. 1979). It is not known how virus is transported neurally, but an intra-axonal mechanism has been proposed (Lavail and Lavail 1972). Which cell type harbors the latent virus has not been agreed upon; on the one hand the neuron itself has been suggested (Cook et al. 1974), and on the other the satellite cells (A McLennan and G. Darby, personal communication 1980). Similarly, whether the latency represents a tiny amount of viral replication (essentially undetectable) in a few cells or a total lack of viral multiplication (e.g., viral DNA integrated into the cell genome and quite nonfunctional) is not yet clear. In the mouse, antiviral IgG seems to be of importance in preventing reactivation, but cellular immunity may also play a role (Nahmias and Roizman 1973). Some human ganglia also harbor defective viral genomes and these may play a role in other disease processes, currently not understood (Brown et al. 1979).

Several herpes viruses can cause tumors after direct inoculation in a host; herpes simplex virus does not appear to do this with any great frequency, although HSV-2 may have a function in the formation of cervical carcinoma. Seroepidemiologic surveys (Adam et al. 1974) were supported by the findings that cervical carcinoma tissue harbors HSV-2 sequences (Frenkel et al. 1972) and although a series of negative findings were subsequently reported (Pagano 1975), very recent data lends support to the original experiments (R. EGLIN and G. B. CLEMENTS, personal communication 1981).

Both "biochemical" and "morphological" transformation have been described with herpes simplex virus, the prerequisite, in both cases, being virus which is unable to replicate properly, (e.g., UV-inactivated, temperature-sensitive *(ts)* mutant, DNA fragment). Biochemical transformation involves the sequestration of viral thymidine kinase (TK) gene sequences in an expressible form in cells and was originally described for LTK⁻ cells by MUNYON et al. (1971). Other regions (not just the TK gene) of the viral DNA are co-transferred and this system should be generally useful in the (selectable) transfer of genes to a mammalian cell. The TK genes have been mapped to a region of the HSV-1 and HSV-2 genome around 0,300 fractional length; biochemically transformed cells are not oncogenic.

Morphological transformation was first carried out by DUFF and RAPP (1971) in hamster cells, and both HSV-1 and HSV-2-transformed cells were oncogenic in newborn hamsters. An analogous rat system was described by MACNAB (1974) using *ts* mutants. Fragments of viral DNA can be used to transform cells morphologically and, using this assay, the transforming regions of HSV-1 and HSV-2 have been located. A number of polypeptides seen in normal infections with HSV have been detected in transformed cells, and some specific tumor-related antigens are also cataloged (AURELIAN et al. 1975) but no HSV "T antigen" is obvious at present.

The characteristic pattern of herpes simplex virus infection is, as we have already mentioned, a primary infection followed by recurrences at the body surface served by a specific nerve. Primary episodes can be varied, and induce infection of the oral (HSV-1 mainly) and genital (HSV-2 mainly) regions, herpetic keratitis, skin herpes, respiratory herpes, and herpes encephalitis. Neonatal herpes infections occur usually via passage through an infected birth canal. All of these are likely to result in recurrent infections of the same general area as the primary infection by transmission of the virus from latently infected ganglia to the surface of the body served by the corresponding nerve endings. Respiratory herpes does not usually recur and encephalitis is most often a fatal primary infection. There is no known animal vector and transmission takes place through direct contact, e.g., oral contact for oral herpes and genital contact for genital herpes. Primary infections are usually inapparent, but in special cases, like severe undernourishment, the disease may be severe. In these cases, virus replicates at the site of infection to give viremia which allows further multiplication in certain organs, resulting in a second wave of viremia and yet further organ involvement (BECKER et al. 1968; in the neonate this often affects the brain. Commonly, viremia is unusual and the replication at the initial site (or in local lymph tissue) would seem to be the major source of virus necessary to establish the infection. Both humoral antibody responses and involvement of cell-mediated mechanisms are common responses to primary infections (NAHMIAS and ROIZMAN 1973; NAHMIAS et al. 1976).

Recurrent infections tend to be less severe than primary ones but there have been reports of encephalitis presenting as a recurrent infection (CRAIG and NAHMIAS 1973). Recurrences tend to occur in the presence of humoral antibodies and of functioning cell-mediated responses, while both nonspecific and specific mechanisms are capable of halting cell-to-cell spread of virus (LODMELL et al. 1973).

III. Cytomegalovirus

Cytomegalovirus (CMV) infections are ubiquitous and are acquired during the childhood years generally, although acquisition is often asymptomatic. Congenital infections are serious in many cases and are considered to the major problems associated with this virus infection. Primary infection can be followed by bouts of virus shedding (recurrence) although circulating antibody levels are high.

The virus is a typical herpesvirus when viewed in the electron microscope, but the particle contains a DNA molecule (double-stranded, linear) which is much larger (150×10^6 daltons) than all the other human herpesviruses. Defective virus contains much smaller DNA, some of which has a molecular weight of about 100×10^6 daltons (DeMarchi et al. 1978; Stinski et al. 1979). The genome-sized molecule is internally arranged in a fashion analogous to that of HSV, with long and short unique regions bounded by inverted repeat sequences. The particle has about 35 recognizable polypeptides, some modified (Stinski 1977), not all of which may necessarily be virus specified.

One of the difficulties in analysis of events after infection of cells with CMV is that all DNA, RNA, and protein synthesis can be stimulated (Furukawa et al. 1975), although cell DNA synthesis stimulation is not seen in cells actively replicating CMV (DeMarchi and Kaplan 1977). An early and a late phase of protein synthesis are discernable, and the late proteins seem to correlate with structural polypeptides (Stinski 1978). Early proteins (at least ten) are made in the absence of viral DNA synthesis (and in nonpermissive cells) but late proteins need progeny viral DNA. CMV induces cellular RNA polymerases I, II, and III (Tanaka et al. 1978) and its own DNA polymerase activity (Huang 1976), although no thymidine kinase seems to be virus specified. Several *ts* mutants of CMV have been isolated and their properties suggest that at least four complementation groups are involved in viral DNA synthesis, which, in turn, is not needed for cell DNA synthesis stimulation (Yamanishi and Rapp 1979).

Inactivated CMV can induce oncogenic transformation of hamster embryo fibroblasts (Albrecht and Rapp 1973) and in human fibroblasts a persistent infection can be set up in vitro (Geder et al. 1976; Mocarski and Stinski 1979), but what factor or factors control restriction is uncertain. Interestingly, a fraction of the persistently infected cells mentioned previously become transformed after passage and can cause tumors in mice.

Extensive secretion of CMV in body fluids over long periods in the absence of symptoms and in the presence of circulating antibody is common, and the virus is spread through populations with ease. This is particularly true in groups which live in close proximity to one another, e.g., in nursing homes or boarding schools. Congenital infection (to give cytomegalovirus inclusion disease, CID) is more common following primary natural infection (Stern and Tucker 1973). The reason for this, presumably, is that viremia is more likely in a primary infection and thus spread to other organs (including the placenta) is favored. However, it is clear that such events do not always have a serious outcome, although CID has a 1% live birth frequency with 10% serious sequelae (Starr et al. 1970). Primary infection in the young adult can lead to an infectious mononucleosis type of illness whose pathogenesis may be an immunologic interaction. Similar to that suggested for Epstein–

Barr virus (SHELDON et al. 1973) and hepatitis due to CMV is also found. CMV can be contracted via blood transfusion or organ transplant, but the source of infection in these cases is still vague. The immune response to CMV is long-lasting in most cases, but the roles of humoral versus cell-mediated antibody have not been fully assessed.

IV. Varicella Zoster Virus

Varicella zoster virus (VZV) is the agent of two common diseases, one generally of childhood, chickenpox, and the other generally of older people, zoster. The second is a classical herpes recurrent infection resulting from an initial primary infection (the chickenpox). The virus is particularly infectious in populations (in school classrooms, for example) and children may acquire chickenpox from recurrent zoster lesions. Paradoxically, VZV has been extraordinarily difficult to grow in cell culture systems, which explains why the molecular biology of the virus is still in such a primitive state.

The virus particle is typical of herpes viruses and is easily distinguished from smallpox virus in the electron microscope (rash from both infections can be confused). The viral DNA (about 47% guanine plus cytosine, linear double-stranded) is the smallest of the human herpesviruses, around 80×10^6 daltons, and has been shown to be infectious, as have the other human herpesviruses (DUMAS et al. 1980; STRAUS et al. 1981). The DNA exists in two forms differentiated by the orientation of a unique set of sequences (5.8×10^6 daltons), bounded by invertible repeat regions (each 3.5×10^6 daltons; STRAUS et al. 1981). DNA from both chickenpox and from zoster isolates appear to have some sequence differences, but are equally infectious in vitro. Analysis of viral DNA from separate virus isolates (from both zoster and chickenpox) show clear variations in restriction enzyme digest patterns and imply that "molecular epidemiology" may be feasible (S. E. STRAUS and J. HAY, unpublished work 1981). The events which characterize the infectious cycle have not been defined for VZV, although a DNA polymerase activity as well as a thymidine kinase activity and a deoxyribonuclease activity (CHENG et al. 1979) have been reported. The virus specificity of these enzymes is presumably the reason for the ability of antiviral agents such as acycloguanosine to modify VZV infections. Under special circumstances, both varicella and zoster may be life-threatening. Leukemia and other malignancies may lead to disseminated varicella in children, and Hodgkin's disease reactivates zoster at rates higher than in normal patients.

In the normal host with operative immune mechanisms, one attack of varicella is not likely to be followed by a second and the incubation period of the disease is about 2 weeks. The virus probably enters the body via the oropharynx, upper respiratory tract or, rarely, the skin. Multiplication in situ leads to a spread of infection followed by several cycles of further multiplication. The ensuing viremia allows dissemination and skin lesions start to appear. These are contained by humoral as well as cell-mediated responses.

An aftermath of varicella is the persistence of VZV in the body. It has been proposed that the virus sequesters itself in sensory ganglia, and there is evidence to support that contention (ESIRI and TOMLINSON 1972). Overt infection is triggered by some unusual circumstance and virus appears at the nerve endings in characteristic vesicles. One attack of zoster is normal and more than two very rare (JUEL-JENSEN and MacCALLUM 1972). It is tempting to equate the latency and reactivation of herpes simplex with that of zoster, but at present, this is not wholly justified. Quite often the virus replication seems to be more widespread than simply in those cells close to sensory nerve endings and dissemination of the virus (with serious consequences) is a recognized difficulty with reactivity in patients with Hodgkin's disease.

V. Epstein–Barr Virus

Epstein–Barr virus (EBV) is the fifth member of the herpesvirus group. Infection with the virus is worldwide in distribution, usually causing a subclinical infection in early childhood. When infection occurs in late adolescence or early adulthood the result is normally heterophile-positive infectious mononucleosis (HENLE et al. 1968; NIEDERMAN et al. 1968). The virus was first identified in cultured lymphoblasts from Burkitt's lymphoma (EPSTEIN et al. 1964), and has since been implicated as the causal agent of both this lymphoma and nasopharyngeal carcinoma.

EBV has the characteristic morphology of the herpesvirus group (Fig. 6). The virions are approximately 100–150 nm in diameter and consist of an icosahedral mucleocapsid surrounded by a lipid envelope. The DNA of EBV is linear, approximately 1×10^8 daltons in molecular weight (1.7×10^5 base pairs; PRITCHETT et al. 1975; HAYWARD and KIEFF 1977). The bouyant density of the DNA is 1.718 g/cm^2, indicating a guanosine plus cytosine content of 57%–58% (PRITCHETT et al. 1975). At both ends of the DNA are a series (1–12) of tandem repeats of a 500 base pair sequence and both ends of the DNA contain sequences which are direct repetitions of each other (GIVEN and KIEFF 1978, 1979). In addition, internally there are 1–12 reiterations of a 3,200 base pair sequence of relatively high guanine plus cytosine content (RYMO and FORSBLUM 1978; GIVEN and KIEFF 1979; HAYWARD et al. 1980). These repeats are arranged in an adjacent tandem array with all copies in the same orientation (HAYWARD et al. 1980). Thus, the arrangement of terminal and internal repeats indicates that EBV DNA, like other mammalian herpesviruses, is divisible into a large (L) segment and a smaller (S) segment (HAYWARD et al. 1980), although the arrangement of these repetitive sequences within the EBV S segment is different from all other herpesvirus genomes so far described (HAYWARD et al. 1980). An interesting observation relating to the possible function of the internal repeats is that the DNA of EBV strains that transform cord blood lymphocytes have 8–12 copies of the repeat, while nontransforming strains have only 3–4 (HAYWARD et al. 1980).

The host range of EBV is very limited. In vitro cultivation has been shown only in B-lymphocytes, possibly because they alone have proper receptors for the virus (JONDAL and KLEIN 1973). That the restriction for growth of EBV is at an early event (adsorption, penetration, or uncoating) is shown in experiments in which microinjection of EBV DNA into normally nonpermissive cells allowed for transcription of some viral products (GRAESSMAN et al. 1980). As if this restricted host range were not enough of a problem for experimentalists, only a minority of the cells in these "producer" lines actually produces virus (ROIZMAN and KIEFF 1974). It is believed that the natural target cells in vivo for primary infection by EBV are epithelial cells of the ororhinopharynx (DE THÉ 1979; LEMON et al. 1977), and makes some sense of the association of EBV with nasopharyngeal carcinoma, an epithelial tumor.

Several antigens have been detected in EBV-infected cells and used as markers for infection of cell lines: EBNA, EBV-specific nuclear antigen; EA, early antigen (the production of these two antigens is not prevented by blocking DNA synthesis (HENLE et al. 1970; GERGELY et al. 1971); VCA, viral capsid antigen, and MA, membrane antigen.

Compared with the herpes simplex viruses, little is known of the regulation of events during infection. The virus-specific RNA is adenylated (HAYWARD and KIEFF 1976) and appears to be processed differently in permissive and nonpermissive (restringent) infections (HAYWARD and KIEFF 1976; ORELLANA and KIEFF 1977). In restringent infection about 16%–30% of the DNA is represented by RNA of which only 5%–7% is adenylated and found on polyribosomes, while in the permissive system 45% of the DNA is represented by RNA; all of these sequences associate with polyribosomes (HAYWARD and KIEFF 1976; ORELLANA and KIEFF 1977; THOMAS-POWELL et al. 1979). Whether this selective polyadenylation is related to the restriction is unknown. An analysis of the EBV-specific RNA in Burkitt's lymphoma tissue indicated adenylated RNA homologous to 3%–6% of the EBV DNA (DAMBAUGH et al. 1979). EBV has also been shown to code for its own DNA polymerase (ALLANDEEN and BERTINO 1978; DATTA et al. 1980), nuclease (CLOUGH 1979), and to be sensitive to phosphonoacetic acid, properties shared with other herpesviruses; no general agreement exists as to the induction of a virus-specific thymidine kinase.

The major route of transmission of infectious mononucleosis in young adults is through intimate oral contact (HOAGLAND 1955; SAWYER et al. 1971; EVANS and NIEDERMAN 1977) and the incubation period is 4–7 weeks (HOAGLAND 1964; EVANS 1960). Virus shedding occurs during acute illness and from weeks to months after onset (EVANS and NIEDERMAN 1977). After invasion of the nasopharynx, the virus enters the blood stream; here B-lymphocytes are infected and proliferate, leading to immune stimulation and proliferation of T-cells, the atypical cells characteristic of the disease (PURTILO 1976). The proliferation of B-cells is thought to be held in check by a T-cell-cytotoxic response and by antibody production (PEARSON and ORR 1976). Recovery from illness results in disappearance of these atypical lymphocytes and presence of both humoral and cell-mediated immune functions specific for EBV (SCHOOLEY and DOLIN 1979). The virus, however, is not eliminated from the host; thus EBV is similar to other members of the herpesvirus group in its ability to remain "latent." The immune responses are thought to play a role both in Burkitt's lymphoma and in fatal infectious mononucleosis (PURTILO et al. 1977).

The characteristic clinical picture consists of fever, pharyngitis, and cervical lymphadenopathy, accompanied by splenomegaly and/or hepatomegaly. Abnormalities in liver function are a regular occurrence (EVANS and NIEDERMAN 1977; SCHOOLEY and DOLIN 1979); serious complications (e.g., fatal infectious mononucleosis) are rare (BAR et al. 1974; PURTILO et al. 1977). The vast majority of the cases resolve spontaneously in 2–3 weeks and the prostration associated with the illness is usually gradual in its course. The disease results in the production of circulating antibodies against viral antigens as well as unrelated antigens; these latter antibod-

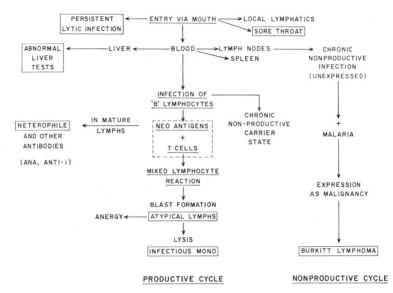

Fig. 9. Hypothetical pathogenesis of EBV infection. (Evans and Niederman 1977)

ies being the heterophile antibodies. Diagnosis is based on the typical clinical picture with fever, sore throat, and lymphadenopathy in addition to heterophile antibodies. In heterophile-negative cases, antibodies to EBV must be demonstrated. A flow diagram of our current understanding of EBV pathogeneiss is presented in Fig. 9.

EBV has been associated with two malignant human tumors, the African type Burkitt's lymphoma (BL) and nasopharyngeal carcinoma (NPC) of a particular type encountered in people of Southern Chinese extraction (Fenner and White 1976; Epstein and Achong 1977). The association between EBV and BL is based upon the regular presence of viral products in tumor cells and a specific EBV immune profile of the patients. The tumor tissue of Burkitt's lymphoma consists of B-lymphocytes of a single clone (Wright 1972; Fialkow et al. 1973), which are infected with EBV. Tumor tissue usually contains multiple copies of the EBV genome (Zur Hausen et al. 1970; Nonoyama and Pagano 1973) and the EBV DNA in this tumor tissue is found in the form of a closed circular episome (Kaschka-Dierich et al. 1976; Lindahl et al. 1976); whether any viral DNA is actually integrated into the host genome is not known (Dambaugh et al. 1979).

There are many different kinds of epidemiologic data linking EBV to African BL. The data suggest an etiologic role for the virus and imply that endemic malaria in these areas may be a cofactor. For example, patients with BL were shown to have higher levels of antibodies against a variety of EBV antigens (EA, VCA, MA) than unaffected patients in the same area (De Thé 1979). A simple relationship of EBV to BL is difficult to understand since EBV is widespread, while BL has a very limited geographic distribution (Burkitt and Wright 1966). Nevertheless, the data from the best prospective study to date (De Thé et al. 1978) suggest a strong association of BL and EBV, particularly in cases characterized by EBV DNA in tumor cells, and high VCA titers. The risk of developing BL was estimated to be 30 times greater in children with high VCA titers and these titers may reflect the severity of the original primary infection, owing either to dose or host response. It is known that with other oncogenic viruses oncogenic potential is enhanced when the virus is given to newborn infants (GROSS 1970), and such may be the case with EBV (DE THÉ 1977). The data supporting a relationship of EBV to NPC is similar to that for BL. Patients with NPC have high VCA titers (HENLE et al. 1970) and DNA has been demonstrated in biopsy material (ZUR HAUSEN et al. 1970). Of particular interest has been the observation that the tumor cells in NPC are epithelial (WOLF et al. 1973) as opposed to lymphoid as in BL. As with BL, NPC is remarkably restricted in distribution though EBV is widespread, suggesting that genetic and/or environmental factors are also involved in tumor induction.

G. Orthomyxoviruses

Three types of influenza virus have been described; A, B, and C. Every 2–3 years major outbreaks of influenza A occur with high attack rates (40%) in the 5–14 year age group, declining progressively with age; conversely, the mortality rate increases with age. Total excess deaths in the United States per 100,000 attributable to pneumonia following influenza infection in recent outbreaks has been less than 10, but this still represents a significant number of avoidable deaths. Influenza B, on the other hand, causes disease with a lower attack rate and less mortality than influenza A, major outbreaks generally appearing only every 4–7 years. Influenza C, with poorly defined epidemiology, is a relatively minor problem for children.

I. Influenza A and B Viruses

Influenza A virus isolated from successive outbreaks demonstrates two types of variation. "Antigenic shift" occurs when a strain of virus appears which is either not, or only remotely, related antigenically to the virus of the preceding outbreak. This occurred in 1947, with the emergence of the A_1/Fm/1/47 prototype (FRANCIS et al. 1947) and again in 1957 when A_2/Japan/305/57 appeared (MEYER et al. 1957). Between these bouts of distinct change in the virus isolates a more subtle "antigenic drift" is evident which results from small changes in virus polypeptides and is driven, presumably, by the rising levels of antibody present in the population as infections with a given subtype become more widespread. Antigenic shift releases a virus strain for which little or no immune protection exists in the population, and is a major factor in the relative severity of outbreaks every 10–15 years. An attractive theory for the development of new antigenically shifted virus is that recombination between certain animal and human influenza viruses can occur in which virulence for the human population is combined with an antigenic component of the animal virus in a new virus subtype (KILBOURNE 1968; LAVER and WEBSTER 1973). Influenza B was first associated (retrospectively) with an outbreak in 1936 (FRANCIS 1940) and, while it seems to drift antigenically, no large shifts have been evident.

The basic architecture of the particle is shown in Fig. 10 in which nucleoprotein is surrounded by a lipid membrane, coated on the inside by a matrix protein and

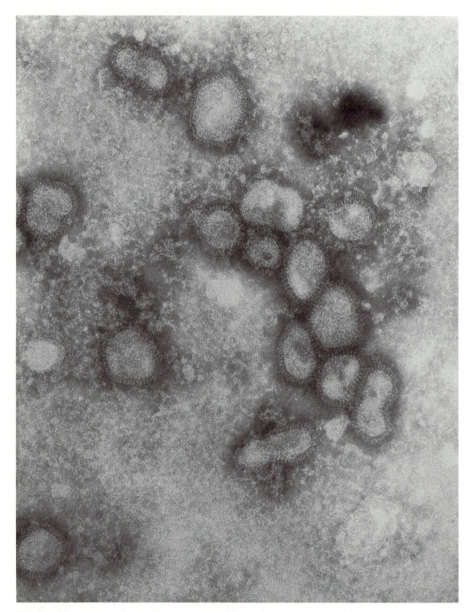

Fig. 10. Electron micrograph of influenza A virions. (Madeley 1972) × 200,000

externally by spikes of neuraminidase (NA) and hemagglutinin (HA), both glycoproteins. The whole virion is about 100 nm in diameter. The NA recognizes neuraminic acid on cell surface mucoproteins, converting mucous to a thin liquid and
exposing cell surface receptors, while HA allows recognition and attachment to the
mucoproteins. The genome RNA (negative polarity) is present in several segments:
for influenza A and B there are eight segments, varying in total molecular weight

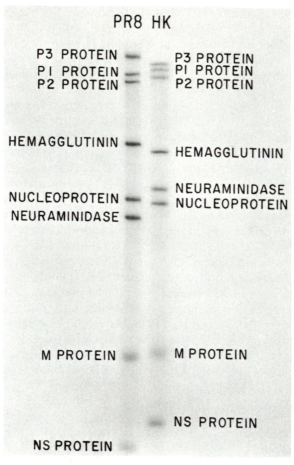

Fig. 11. Map of influenza virus genome. Polyacrylamide gel of the RNAs of A/PR/8/34 and A/HK/8/68 viruses (PR8 and HK viruses) showing identification of the eight genes with respect to their gene products. (PALESE et al. 1978)

from 5 to 7×10^6 daltons, while influenza C seems to have half that number (PALESE and SCHULMAN 1976; PONS 1976; MCGEOCH et al. 1976). This property of the RNA allows "recombinants" (products of the reassortment of the RNA segments) to be isolated and the generation of specific recombinants along with the use of *ts* mutants and in vitro polypeptide synthesis have allowed the assignment of each RNA segment to production of a specific virus polypeptide (PALESE et al. 1978; Fig. 11).

Virus is able to enter susceptible cells either by vacuolation of virus or by the uptake of nucleoproteins directly following fusion of particles with the cell plasma membrane. As with all negative-strand viruses, the first step in intracellular replication is the production of RNA complementary to virion RNA, to form functional mRNAs. Production of mRNA is under the control of the particle-associated RNA polymerase activity and seems to be associated with proteins P1 and P3

(Palese et al. 1974; Ritchey and Palese 1977). Each mRNA is employed as a template for new virion RNA synthesis and requires P2 and the nucleoprotein (NP). The precise mode of interaction of the RNA and polypeptide components in the infected cell is not clear, but evidence suggests that there is a coordinated packaging mechanism which results in the formation of particles with a single copy of each segment of RNA (Laver and Downie 1976). Virulence factor for influenza have not been assigned to specific polypeptides but a potential *ts* live vaccine candidate has defects in proteins P3 and in NP (Palese and Ritchey 1977) which appear to be directly connected to attenuation of the virus in humans.

The primary step in uncoating influenza virus appears to be the removal of the outer envelope which releases the nucleoprotein active in primary transcription. The eight segments of influenza virus genome RNA are transcribed into new virion RNA individually (Pons and Rochovansky 1979). Initial transcription of the influenza genome is catalyzed by the particle-associated RNA polymerase which in vitro produces polyadenylated incomplete transcripts which seem identical to in vivo message (McGeoch and Kitron 1975). Two classes of RNA complementary to genome RNA (cRNA) appear in vivo, mRNA (capped) which is the smaller, is located on polysomes and is made at different times from the other cRNA class, the putative precursor of new virion RNA (Skehel and Hay 1978). The control of virus protein production would seem to be at the level of control of transcription into mRNA species (Skehel and Hay 1978). An RNA polymerase activity can be isolated from infected cells, which contains NP and P polypeptides (Caliguiri and Compans 1974) and which probably is analogous to the virion activity.

The production of new virion RNA needs functional protein systhesis in the infected cell (Hay et al. 1977) and continuous nucleoplasmic RNA synthesis for transcription to occur (Spooner and Barry 1977). The influenza viruses are unique in their need for active DNA transcription without, apparently, the formation of viral DNA; this seems to relate to the role of host message in transferring a cap structure to influenza mRNA.

The eight RNA fragments of both influenza A and B have been assigned to the production of the individual proteins of influenza: the two surface glycoproteins HA and NA; the two internal NP and M (matrix) proteins; NS (nonstructure) proteins of unknown function; and three P proteins involved, probably, in the synthesis of virus-specific RNA (Racaniello and Palese 1979). HA can be divided into two parts, coded by the same gene: HA1 which binds to cell receptors and HA2 which is involved in insertion of HA into the membrane of the particle. Recently, it has been suggested that certain segments of RNA may code for two functional mRNA molecules (Lamb and Choppin 1979). Antigenic shift, as we have seen, usually means that a new type of HA has appeared (perhaps accompanied by a new type of NA). About 16 different types of HA can be distinguished antigenically in virus isolated from human and other animals (Laver and Webster 1979). Recently the HA gene has been cloned in the plasmid pBR 322, and the sequence data suggest that there are major changes in amino acid sequence among "shifted" strains (Jou et al. 1980), probably so major that the different subtypes would have to have existed already. Drift, on the other hand, looks like a series of single base changes in the RNA (Gerhart and Webster 1978) affecting, probably, HA1. It is still not clear, however, which feature or features of the biology of influenza viruses make them prone to such frequent antigenic variation, a situation not seen with other animal RNA viruses.

The precursor to the viral envelope is a patch of cell plasma membrane which has been modified externally by the addition of spikes of HA and NA, and internally with a coating of M protein. Meanwhile, the ribonucleoprotein (RNP) which has formed in the cytoplasm migrates to these altered membrane patches and the particle is formed by budding at that point. Final release may be aided by neuraminidase activity. Influenza A maturation is blocked in HeLa cells, probably owing to a defect in a late event involving the cell membrane in maturation of the virus (CALIGUIRI and HOLMES 1979).

II. Influenza C Virus

Influenza C differs from A and B in a number of respects. It has a different neuraminidase (KENDALL 1975) and a different carbohydrate composition in the structural glycoproteins as well as some host range pecularities; on the other hand it does have a segmented genome (between six and nine pieces is the current estimate, (PETRI et al. 1979; COMPANS et al. 1977). As we have seen, influenza A and B need host nuclear functions for replication and recent evidence (PETRI et al. 1979) suggests that the same is true for influenza C, perhaps emphasizing the close similarity between C and the other two types.

It is over 25 years since the classic description by VON MAGNUS (1954) of influenza particles with low infectivity and the capacity to interfere with normal infection and normal HA activity. Only recently have the physical and clinical properties of DI influenza particles come under serious scrutiny. DI particles have altered morphology and polypeptide composition compared with wild-type virus (LENARD and COMPANS 1975) and recent evidence suggests that general features of their genetic makeup are smaller quantities of the larger RNA segments and the presence of new small RNA segments. However, the entire complement of genome RNA is present, unlike most other DI systems. There is evidence that at least some (and perhaps all) of the new small RNAs are derived from part of other genome segments (NAYAK et al. 1978; NAKAJIMA et al. 1979).

III. Influenza Infections

Infection in humans probably occurs when air containing droplets of infected respiratory secretions is inhaled into the upper respiratory tract; the general spread can then be either upward, if mucociliary action prevails, or downward, if mucosal secretions swamp the action (MIMS 1976; SWEET and SMITH 1980). The virus seems to be localized to the respiratory tract during the infectious cycle, and secretions from these tissues may have as many as 10^6 infectious particles/ml. Peak virus production starts 1–2 days after infection and carries on for the next 2–3 days, although symptoms of the disease (fever, malaise, respiratory problems) may persist for longer (STUART-HARRIS 1965). The most feared complication is pneumonia, about one-fifth of which is directly viral while the majority of cases are related to bacterial infections. This increased susceptibility to bacterial infection is felt to be due to hindered disposal of inhaled bacteria caused by mechanical damage of the respiratory epithelium after virus infection (STUART-HARRIS 1979).

A program of annual vaccination of those considered to be at special risk from infections of the lower respiratory tract has been in force for several years. The killed vaccine preparations are available as whole virus or subunit (for children) and are usually polyvalent for the strains of influenza expected to be incubating in any one year (for 1979–1980 it was A/Brazil/78; A/Texas/77; B/Hong Kong/72). Most of the side effects of vaccination are akin to a mild dose of influenza, but rare complications such as immediate allergic responses or the Guillian–Barré syndrome may also occur. Vaccination seems to be of real benefit to the recipient, affording a high level of protection. In the U.S.S.R., a live vaccine has been in use for some time with results similar to those obtained with killed material. Potential advantages of live vaccine are better production of local immunity and use of smaller doses.

H. Human Papillomavirus

The human papillomavirus (HPV), commonly called the human wart virus, belongs to the papovavirus group. More common members of this group include SV40 of monkeys, polyomavirus of mice, and Shope papillomavirus of rabbits. Human papilloma virus is the only authentic human tumor virus, producing a transmissible benign neoplastic disease (warts).

The virus is an unenveloped, icosahedral particle, approximately 45–55 nm in diameter (Fig. 12). The DNA is in the form of a superhelical, closed, circular structure of approximately 5×10^6 daltons molecular weight. Essentially nothing is known of the replication strategy of the virus as it has never been reproducibly grown in tissue culture. Reports of growth of the virus in tissue culture (EISINGER et al. 1975) have appeared, but have not been corroborated. Until recently it was believed that only one type of human wart virus existed (GOLDSCHMIDT and KLIGMAN 1958). Recent experiments in which viral DNA was purified from virus particles extracted from wart tissue has indicated the existence of several genetically different strains. In these experiments, viral DNA was cleaved with restriction endonucleases. What emerged in the examination of 30 isolates were 3 strains (HPV-1–3) which were closely related, and HPV-4, different from the others in both base composition and antigenicity (GISSMAN and ZUR HAUSEN 1976; GISSMAN et al. 1977). These data indicated that HPV-4 predominated in warts with rather low particle production and HPV-1–3) in warts with high particle production. HPV-1 was found in more than 60% of the warts. A result of particular interest in these studies was that DNA from HPV-1 or HPV-4 failed to hybridize to DNA from different types of warts, indicating the existence of further types of papilloma viruses.

The pathogenesis of human warts is poorly understood. Human transmission experiments indicate an incubation period of 1–20 months. The location of the virus during the incubation is unknown. Warts are classified into major categories depending on their location or appearance: verruca vulgaris (common warts), verruca plana (flat warts), plantar warts, condyloma acuminatum (venereal warts), and filiform warts. Human warts seem to be the consequence of an infection of a single basal cell. Thus, each wart is probably a clonal descendent of a single in-

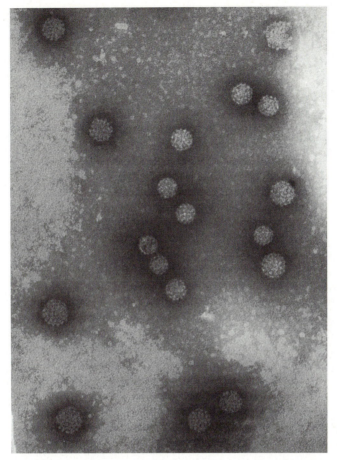

Fig. 12. Polyoma virus (45 nm diameter) and papilloma virus (human wart; 55 nm diameter) in a mixed preparation. (Courtesy of L. V. CRAWFORD)

fected cell (SAMBROOK 1977). The different clinical forms of warts are usually diagnosed by their gross appearance. Although warts may persist for years, most warts spontaneously resolve within 2 years; therapy is usually not instituted unless pain or discomfort results from the wart's presence. There are some data to suggest that certain types of warts (condylomata acuminatum and laryngeal warts) have an increased risk for malignant conversion (ZUR HAUSEN et al. 1978). The reason for this malignant transformation is unknown, but has been attributed to secondary factors (local irritation, etc.) rather than differences in the oncogenic properties of the viruses involved (ZUR HAUSEN et al. 1978).

J. Paramyxoviruses

Paramyxoviruses do not cause extensive cell destruction in vitro and persistent infections are readily established. Syncytium formation (cell fusion) is another characteristic feature of this group of viruses which, unlike the influenza viruses, do not

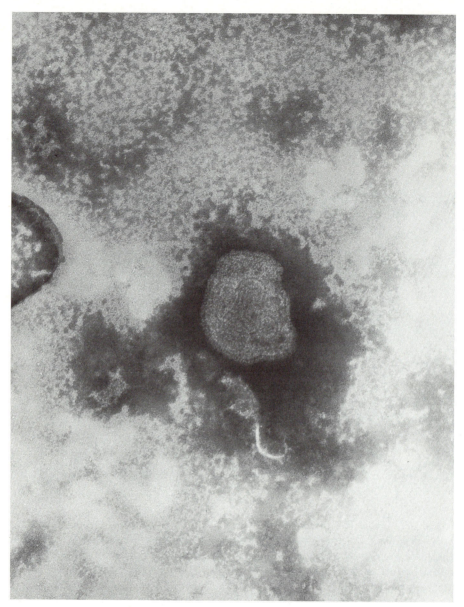

Fig. 13. Electron micrograph of parainfluenza 3 virus. (Madeley 1978) × 200,000

need an intact cell nucleus for complete growth. Measles, mumps, and respiratory syncytial virus (RSV) have one serotype, while parainfluenza virus has five. Measles has no neuraminidase, while RSV has no hemagglutin, no neuraminidase, no hemolysin, and does not hemadsorb. In addition, RSV particle morphology is different from the other members of the paramyxovirus group: it should probably be considered as a separate virus group. Measles, mumps, and the parainfluenza viruses are the viruses with which we are most concerned in this section: however, much of the molecular biology of paramyxovirus replication has been carried out with Newcastle disease virus (NDV), Sendai virus, and simian virus 5 (SV5).

Paramyxovirus particles vary somewhat in size and shape: the most common are 150–200 nm diameter, but much larger (5–600 nm) forms and filamentous particles can often be seen (Fig. 13). The internal nucleocapsid is helical ribonucleoprotein and is surrounded by a lipid and glycoprotein-containing envelope. The ribonucleoprotein contains the virion RNA, a single strand of negative polarity (antimessage) with only one segment present and this differentiates the paramyxoviruses from the (segmented) orthomyxoviruses like influenza. The sedimentation coefficient of the RNA is 50 S, corresponding to a molecular weight of $5–5.6 \times 10^6$ daltons (KOLAKOFSKY et al. 1975). Some RNA annealing to genome RNA has been detected in virions, but its significance is obscure (KOLAKOFSKY and BRUTSCHI 1975). The RNA is not infectious and the virion contains an RNA polymerase activity which is presumably needed for successful infection.

Structural polypeptides of the virus consist of five virus-specific proteins, a glycoprotein G (80,000 daltons, P2 (70,000 daltons), NP (60,000 daltons), F_1 (41,000 daltons), and M (31,000 daltons) (STALLCUP et al. 1979; GRAVES et al. 1978). Three other proteins are also found in the virus, L [a high molecular weight protein of undefined origin, (150,000–200,000 daltons, actin (43,000 daltons), and F_2 (15,000 daltons)], a probable relative of F_1 (STALLCUP et al. 1979; TYRRELL and NORRBY 1978; SCHEID and CHOPPIN 1977). The G and F_1 polypeptides are associated with the external structure of the envelope, while M was confirmed to be the matrix protein of measles. Viral RNA seems to exist in contact with L and NP, with varying amounts of P2 and M present, to form the nucleocapsid (STALLCUP et al. 1979). The F polypeptide (F_1 and F_2; SCHEID and CHOPPIN 1977) and the G polypeptide are both glycosylated and the former is probably hemolysin, while the latter is hemagglutinating (NORRBY and GOLLMAR 1975). By analogy with other paramyxoviruses, the L polypeptide is probably involved in RNA polymerase activity (BUETTI and CHOPPIN 1977) and the M protein may also play a role in the regulation of transcription (MARX et al. 1974). Finally, the M protein appears to differ between wild-type measles and SSPE virus in electrophoretic mobility (HALL et al. 1978).

Measles virus particles recognize and attach to surface receptors on susceptible cells by a means different from the other paramyxoviruses: measles does not recognize neuraminic acid, but possesses a neuraminidase activity (NORRBY 1962). As mentioned previously, the virus has a hemolysis function. Internalization of measles virus is presumably carried out by the same mechanism as for other members of the group; both viropexis and membrane fusion mechanisms have been proposed, with the weight of evidence favoring the latter scheme.

A transcription complex containing virion polypeptides can be isolated from paramyxovirus-infected cells and this complex will transcribe virion RNA into complementary RNA species to form mRNA (BUETTI and CHOPPIN 1977). Messages appear to be of 35 S and 18 S and, are of sufficient size to code for all of the viral polypeptides. Formation of new virion RNA needs prior protein synthesis in infected cells and it is uncertain whether the same enzymes form both message and new viral genomes. It does seem, however, that message production occurs from a single inititation site to give separate mRNA molecules for each polypeptide. Viral message is polyadenylated and capped, the enzymes for which, in addition to others which may be required (e.g., protein kinase) may be of viral origin (COLONNO and STONE 1976).

Paramyxovirus polypeptides appear to be made in relative amounts consistent with the quantities of specific mRNAs produced in infected cells; in this respect, the negative-strand viruses in general seem to follow the strategy of uninfected and DNA virus-infected animal cells (COLLINS and BRATT 1973). It seems likely that the control of mRNA abundance is achieved through the use of a single promoter, with the most abundant message being read proximal to the promoter and the least abundant most distal. This "polarity" of reading from a single promoter may be followed by specific cleavage events to form individual messages or other mechanisms may operate (e.g., further promoters are functional only when message has been read from an earlier one; GLAZIER et al. 1977). However this may be, the gene order obtained from UV mapping is (in Sendai) 3′-NP-F-M,P-HN-L-5′. HN would be equivalent to G in measles virus and F to F_1 and F_2. Newly formed virion RNA and nucleocapsid proteins self-assemble in the cytoplasm as individual units or aggregates and migrate to the inner surface of the plasma membrane at points at which the M protein (internally) and the glycoproteins (externally) have become incorporated. Arrival of nucleocapsid at the plasma membrane seems to trigger the formation of external spikes on that part of the membrane; the virion then buds out from the surface.

One recurring problem in the analysis of cells infected with measles virus is that the background of synthesis of host proteins remains high (measles is a poor inhibitor of cell synthesis) and the yield of virus from infected cells is not large. Four immunoprecipitable virus polypeptides (H, P, NP, and M) have recently been made in vitro (NIVELEAU and WILD 1979) and approaches like this may help to solve some of the problems encountered. Recombination with paramyxoviruses (as with all negative polarity RNA viruses) has not been detected, but complementation between mutants is a normal occurrence. There are five complementation groups for NDV and measles (TSIPIS and BRATT 1976; BRESHKIN et al. 1977) and seven for Sendai and RSV (PORTER et al. 1974; GIMENEZ and PRINGLE 1978).

I. Measles Infection

Reported measles cases in the United States before the introduction of vaccine (1963) amounted to 400,000/year. In all likelihood, however, the true incidence was much greater, probably involving, in one form or another, the entire child population. After a 10–12-day incubation period most of those infected develop fever and upper respiratory tract infection symptoms with conjunctivitis, followed by a rash; however, complications are quite common. These range from otitis media and pneumonia caused by subsequent bacterial infection to encephalitis and subacute sclerosing panencephalitis (SSPE). In encephalitis cases there are frequent neurologic sequelae and it may be that in some measles cases not diagnosed as encephalitis, mild neurologic sequelae may be present (FULGITINI et al. 1967). SSPE is a rare disease, invariably fatal, which can develop some time after a measles infection. It is characterized by a slow development of neuronal degeneration and very high levels of measles antibody in serum, and specifically, in the cerebrospinal fluid. The virus involved is probably a variant of wild-type measles virus.

Virus administered to the nose or the lower respiratory tract is efficiently infectious (KRESS et al. 1961) and aerosol transmission from infected people is probably the main source. The respiratory mucosa is normally the best source of disseminated virus, but measles will grow in most body tissues. Respiratory secretions are infectious until antibody can be produced and urine remains infectious for a few days longer. There is viremia during the prodromal period, but the study of sequence of spread and release of virus has been hampered by the difficulty of early diagnosis and of efficient virus growth in vitro. However, the Koplik's spots which appear in the oral mucosa toward the end of the prodromal period contain virus (SURINGA et al. 1970), as do the cells in the macule of the measles rash. Levels of virus in the body quickly fall after the rash is evident, but some virus must occasionally persist for a time in SSPE for example, in at least part of the population. It has recently been shown that infection of marmosets offers a laboratory model for distinguishing differences in virulence of natural and attenuated strains of measles virus (ALBRECHT et al. 1980). This should allow, for the first time, a characterization of factors (route of inoculation, virus strain, etc.) important in the pathogenesis of the disease. The vaccine in current use is a highly attenuated live vaccine which causes a mild or inapparent noncommunicable infection. Earlier attempts to control measles with killed vaccine led to hypersensitization of some recipients with subsequent problems, and early types of live vaccine also caused too high a level of reaction. The incidence of measles has not, however, fallen to levels which were predicted in the early days of vaccine use (SPENCER et al. 1967), probably for a number of reasons. The chief one seems to be the failure to reach a high enough percentage of susceptible people (especially in disadvantaged areas), but a second factor may be that the immunity conferred by the vaccine is less reliable than in natural infection and significant numbers are becoming susceptible again (CHERRY et al. 1972).

II. Persistent Measles Infection

In a recent study, it has been shown that both the vaccine strain (Edmonston) and an SSPE isolate of measles virus can persistently infect a variety of cell types in vitro (neural and nonneural) (LUCAS et al. 1978). When this occurs, virus production becomes thermolabile despite the fact that the virus itself is not temperature sensitive. Thus, a feature of the cell (or the virus–cell interaction) is different in persistent (in contrast to lytic) infection. In hamster cells persistently infected with measles virus, a similar phenomenon occurs which has been traced to temperature-sensitive production of structural polypeptides and temperature-sensitive failure of structural proteins to become associated with infected cell membranes (FISHER and RAPP 1979).

SSPE patients have high levels of circulating antibody (serum and cerebrospinal fluid) against all the major virion polypeptides of measles virus, except the membrane protein M (HALL et al. 1979) and cells cultured from the brain of an SSPE patient do not produce any M protein (HALL and CHOPPIN 1979). Such a failure in production would result in a failure to complete new infectious virus particles and could conceivably, lead to an abortive infection. The basis for the failure to produce M (transcription or posttranscription) is not clear. Persistent infections in HeLa cells seem to be associated with the production of viral mutants (WECHS-LER et al. 1979). These cells produced altered structural proteins (M and possibly H and NP) and virus obtained from them is temperature sensitive, continuing to express polypeptide defects in subsequent normal infections. Defective interfering particles from either wild-type measles virus or from an SSPE isolate show both homotypic and heterotypic interference, another indication of the relatedness of the two viruses (FERGUSON and MURPHY 1980).

III. Mumps Infection

Mumps is primarily a disease of young school-age children and is generally self-limiting. A wide range of responses to infection reflects the ability of the virus to cause generalized infections with a preference for glandular and nervous tissue. Virus is transmitted via aerosols from infected throat or salivary gland secretions and is somewhat less contagious than measles. After uptake into the respiratory tract, mumps virus multiplies locally and in lymph glands, causing viremia which disseminates the virus widely, e.g., to the testes (orchitis is a quite frequent complication of mumps infection). The virus is present in urine and has been isolated from other human body fluids. The common syndrome is swelling of the parotid gland or glands, but an assortment of other syndromes is found (PHILIP et al. 1959). Mumps is the most common cause of viral encephalitis in the United States and deafness is an important residual complication of the disease.

Among military populations, mumps has always been a major public health problem, and vaccination was first used with any real success by the Finnish armed forces, who treated servicemen with a killed vaccine to give a greater than 90% reduction in the incidence of the disease (PENTTINEN et al. 1968). The vaccine in current use in the United States was introduced in 1967 and has proved to be a useful, well-tolerated live vaccine. Vaccination usually produces a mild (or subclinical) infection which is noncommunicable and has few side effects. It is too early yet to know whether immunity conferred by the vaccine is permanant, but continued protection over 10 years has been reported. The vaccine is normally given as a trivalent preparation (measles, mumps, rubella), thus while mumps itself is not regarded as a first priority public health problem, its association with these two other vaccines has made the use of mumps vaccine widespread. It has yet to be established whether childhood mumps vaccination will prevent adult infections and their attendant, quite serious, complications.

IV. Parainfluenza Infection

All four types of parainfluenza virus (parainfluenza 1, 2, 3, and 4 viruses) cause lower respiratory tract infections in young children and upper tract infections in older children and adults. Parainfluenza 3 virus appears to be the most effective in spreading through populations (CHANOCK et al. 1963) and is second only to respiratory syncytial virus as a source of pneumonia and bronchiolitis. Parainfluenza 3 infection is endemic; infant infection can occur in the presence of maternal antibodies and reinfection of older children and adults has been described. The virus is spread via direct contact or by droplet dispersion and presumably replicates in the respiratory tissues. While viremia has been reported (GROSS et al. 1973), little clinical sign of disseminated disease is apparent. Clinical signs vary from mild afebrile upper respiratory tract infection to serious (life-threatening) lower respiratory tract disease.

Both parainfluenza 1 and 2 are associated with croup, a function presumably of the severe inflammatory response of the glottal tissues, and disease tends to be epidemic on a 2-year cycle, with parainfluenza 2 responsible for less serious problems than parainfluenza 1. Maternal antibody prevents parainfluenza 1 and 2 infection. Parainfluenza 4 virus is not often encountered and disease associated with it is usually trivial. All of these lesser parainfluenza viruses have antigenically related animal counterparts; for example, Sendai virus shares antigens with parainfluenza 1 virus and SV5 with parainfluenza 2 virus.

K. Picornaviruses

In humans and in other animals, the picornaviruses constitute one of the largest and most important sources of virus disease. The common cold and, of course, poliomyelitis are problems of which all are aware, even if, in the latter case, the false impression abounds that the disease has disappeared, thanks to effective vaccination programs. In the domestic animal world, there are few more feared infections than foot-and-mouth disease: it follows, therefore, that both medical and veterinary research has traditionally focused on the various members of this family, resulting in the current quite detailed state of knowledge of replication of picornaviruses (PEREZ-BERCOFF 1979).

Four genera; enterovirus, cardiovirus, rhinovirus, and aphthovirus (foot-and-mouth) make up the Picornaviridae family and share many common features. Picornaviruses are very stable to inactivation by several agents, for example, but acid lability (correlated with bouyant density) distinguishes the aphthoviruses (unstable below pH 7) from the rhinoviruses (unstable below pH 5) and the cardioviruses and enteroviruses (stable to pH 4 or less; NEWMAN et al. 1973).

I. Structure and Replication

The picornaviruses (Fig. 14) all have a capsid with cubic symmetry and no envelope surrounding single-stranded RNA of positive (message) polarity. In the capsid are four polypeptides, VP1–4; VP1, 2, and 3 have molecular weights of about 30,000 daltons, while VP4 is about one-third as large. The 60 subunit model for the virion is now generally accepted (BALTIMORE 1971) with each of the polypeptides present in equivalent molar amounts.

The capsid structure is put together in a series of steps (REUKERT 1976). These steps start with the assembly of a precursor chain (1), cleavage and rearrangement of an intermediate (2), assembly of the intermediate and insertion of the RNA (3), and finally (4) cleavage and rearrangement of the complete shell. The protein activity involved in steps 2 and 4 can be detected in cell-free extracts 2–3 h after infection (ESTEBAN and KERR 1974) but it is difficult to demonstrate the process of

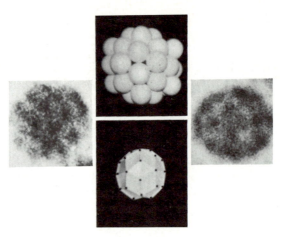

Fig. 14. Electron micrograph of a purified preparation of poliovirus negatively stained. (Courtesy of H. Mayor) × 300,000

virion assembly in vitro, although reconstitution of some infectivity from dissociated particles has been reported (Drzeniek and Billelo 1972). Minor species of polypeptide also occur in picornavirus capsids, including VP0 (the uncleaved VP2 plus VP4), the viral component of the RNA polymerase activity and the uncleaved VP1 and VP3 (Reukert et al. 1969; Ziola and Scraba 1974; Sangar et al. 1976).

The viral RNA of molecular weight about 2.8×10^6 daltons, is replicated via an intermediate involving a complementary RNA strand. The replicative intermediate (RI) is generally thought to be involved in the process of producing several new viral RNA strands and recent work suggests that the basic structure is a double-stranded one (Meyer et al. 1978). Replication of the viral RNA takes place via an RNA polymerase activity, at least a component of which is virus coded (Flanagan and Baltimore 1979). Also important in RNA replication is the VPg protein which is found covalently bound to the 5′ end of viral RNA during replication, to virion RNA but not to functional messages (Lee et al. 1977; Golini et al. 1978; Sangar 1979). It is not certain that this is a virus-coded protein, but it is attached to the virus RNA through a tyrosine-0^4-phosphodiester link to uridine monophosphate (UMP; Ambros and Baltimore 1979). VPg can be removed from the RNA by an enzyme (cellular) which leaves the RNA intact, and at least one function for VPg seems to be in initiation of RNA replication (Caliguiri 1974; Nomoto et al. 1977). Even with VPg removed, however, the 5′ end of picornavirus mRNA is quite different from most other eukaryotic mRNAs in that it has no "cap" structure (Shatkin 1976). On the other hand, the 3′ end of the RNA seems quite oridnary, with a poly(A) tract of between 40 and 100 bases, apparently genetically determined (Yogo and Wimmer 1973); infectivity of viral RNA is related to the presence of a suitable poly(A) sequence (Hruby and Roberts 1976). A second homopolymer tract, poly(C), is found internally in the cardioviruses and aphthoviruses, a point of differentiation between these and the other two picornavirus genera (Brown et al. 1974). This tract is located close to the 5′ end of the RNA and may be related to virulence of the virus in vivo (Harris and Brown 1977).

The genetic information for the RNA polymerase activity or activities seems to include the sequence for the protease activity (protein 22 in encephalomyocarditis virus) and possibly the VPg protein (PALMENBERG et al. 1979). The poliovirus noncapsid viral protein (NCVP4) is capable of elongation of a RNA chain but cannot initiate new synthesis in vitro without a primer (FLANAGAN and BALTIMORE 1979): it also has poly(U) polymerase activity. Partial purification of a soluble complex which will copy poliovirus RNA without a primer indicates (DASGUPTA et al. 1979) that both NCVP4 and NCVP2 are needed for this activity: this preparation seems to prefer poliovirus RNA to others tested.

Picornavirus mRNA is translated into a single large precursor polypeptide, the result of a single initiation site for protein synthesis: a second ribosome binding seems to occur in vitro in poliovirus RNA (JENSE et al. 1978). A series of specific cleavages occur (at the time of translation) to give several primary products (detectable in vivo) which can be further cleaved. At least some of these proteolytic steps are catalyzed by a virus-coded enzyme [to yield VP0, VP3, and VP4 in poliovirus (KORANT 1979), for example] but others may be cell-specific processes. A control scheme for the balancing of RNA and protein production in poliovirus-infected cells has been put forward by COOPER (1977).

Almost 20 years ago recombination among poliovirus mutants was described, yet the mechanism behind this unique (for nonsegmented RNA viruses) property of the picornaviruses remains obscure (COOPER 1977). A consistent genetic map based on recombination shows that structural polypeptides map at the 5' end of the genome, while the 3' end is taken up with RNA-polymerizing activities. Pactamycin mapping, which, owing to preferential inhibition of translation initiation, allows ordering (5'→3') of gene functions in a picornavirus RNA, agrees with the genetic map and gives rather more detail on the individual polypeptides (SUMMERS and MAIZEL 1971). Recently, the center of the poliovirus genome has been shown to code for a protease activity.

II. Picornavirus Infections

Many of the picornaviruses have a very restricted host range, like poliovirus, which can only infect humans and some laboratory primates. The primary reason for this seems to be the lack of a suitable receptor on the surface of cells. Permissive–nonpermissive cell hybrids have been constructed which show that chromosome 19 of human cells codes for at least part of the receptor molecule for poliovirus (MILLER et al. 1974). In susceptible cells, the cytopathic effect caused by enteroviruses is extensive, the cells quickly becoming detached from the growing surface. Virus spreads by dissemination into culture medium. While intact virus in incapable of attachment to nonsusceptible cells, the extracted viral RNA can infect a wide range of cell types. Ability (or lack of it) to recognize specific cell surfaces through a receptor would seem to be a major factor in determining the pathogenicity of the picornaviruses. Interference experiments suggest that different receptors exist for the various groups of picornaviruses and even for specific members inside these groups (CROWELL 1976). Attachment per se may only account for part of the ability of a picornavirus to infect a cell successfully; however, examples are known of cells which have receptors for virus but never show signs of infection. What follows

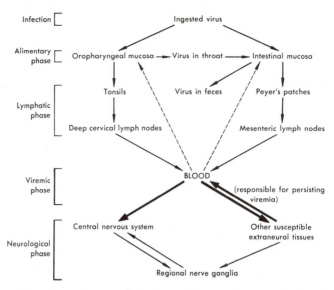

Fig. 15. A model for the pathogenesis of poliomyelitis based on a synthesis of data obtained in humans and chimpanzees. (Davis et al. 1973)

attachment on the cell surface presumably is another cell-specific parameter of which we know little, although it does seem to involve partial "uncoating" of the particle with, perhaps, some loss of polypeptide (Crowell and Philipson 1971).

Of the four capsid polypeptides, VP4 is probably exposed on the virion so as to interact with the cell surface receptor or receptors (Wetz and Habermehl 1979) although VP3 may also play an important role on the virion surface (Wetz and Habermehl 1979). The crucial factors in neurovirulence of poliovirus are still unknown, but a recent analysis of the Sabin vaccine strain of polio has shown several amino acid alterations in VP1, VP3, and VP4 (Kew et al. 1980). Whether these alterations relate directly to loss of virulence has yet to be established. The nature of the receptor on the cell surface is not known, but seems to be a complex of several types of macromolecule firmly inserted in the cell membrane: inactivation by chymotrypsin needs protein synthesis to restore activity and a soluble extract with some biologic activity against coxsackievirus B3 has recently been prepared (Crowell and Siak 1978).

Virus is spread from host to host usually via infected body fluids (e.g., fecal–oral for most enteroviruses, from nasal secretion for rhinoviruses), and subclinical virus shedders are common. In rhinovirus infection, virus probably has to reach the nasal (or conjunctival) mucosa for efficient infection (Hendley et al. 1973) when localized edema and hyperemia follow with the production of fluid. Virus production takes about 3 days to peak and shedding of virus for several days ensues (Douglas 1970). Initial replication of the enteroviruses is probably in the lymph tissue of the gut and the pharynx, from where virus enters the blood and is distributed to target organs or for further replication in the reticuloendothelial system. Neurovirulent poliovirus will multiply in and kill certain cell types in the brain and spinal cord (Melnick 1976; Fig. 15).

Over the past 25 years the incidence of poliomyelitis has decreased dramatically owing to the widespread use of vaccination: in the United States there were 18,000 cases of paralytic disease in 1954 and less than 20 in 1973–1978: The formalin-inactivated poliovirus vaccine (ipv) (Salk) alone was used until 1963 when the trivalent live attenuated oral poliovirus vaccine (opv) (Sabin) was introduced. Each primary vaccination (three doses) with opv will produce long-lasting immunity to all 3 poliovirus types in more than 95% of those vaccinated.

The opv is the preferred vaccine in the United States for a number of reasons; it is well tolerated, simple to administer, produces good intestinal immunity, causes fortuitous immunization of some contacts of vaccinees and has removed paralytic poliomyelitis as a disease in the United States. Some countries still use ipv, though, and there is little apparent difference between the effectiveness of opv and currently available ipv. Indeed, ipv is preferred over opv for patients with immunodeficiency difficulties. In very rare cases, some paralysis has followed the administration of opv in healthy individuals, but both opv and ipv remain among the best tolerated of all vaccines. The success of the vaccination programs has led to a feeling among the population that polio has disappeared and that vaccination is no longer necessary. Unhappily, this is not true: wild poliovirus strains (the cause of significant acquired immunity in the past) no longer circulate as they once did, and unvaccinated children run the risk of being involved in an outbreak of a kind reminiscent of the prevaccination period.

L. Reoviruses

The family Reoviridae is primarily defined by the presence of a segmented, double-stranded RNA genome, and is composed of six genera, Orthoreovirus, orbivirus, cypovirus, phytoreovirus, fijivirus, and rotavirus (JOKLIK et al. 1980). Within the six genera, possible human pathogens are found only in three genera, orthoreovirus, orbivirus, and rotavirus. This section will be primarily concerned with orthoreovirus and orbivirus; the rotaviruses will be covered separately. While all the groups are classified as Reoviridae, on the basis of the presence of a segmented double-stranded RNA genome, their relationship ends there. There appears to be no antigenic relationship between genera, the number of genome segments vary from 12 to 2, and virion structure is different (JOKLIK et al. 1980a). The name reovirus is a siglum for "respiratory enteric orphan"; when these viruses were first isolated they were not found in association with any disease (FENNER and WHITE 1976). Since that time new viruses have been discovered in a variety of animal species, but the name has stuck.

The reoviruses contain double-stranded RNA, which is enclosed in a characteristic double capsid shell structure of icosahedral symmetry (SHATKIN et al. 1977; Fig. 16). The orbiviruses appear to possess a single capsid (FENNER and WHITE 1976). The double-stranded RNA (ds RNA) of the reoviruses (types 1, 2, 3) consists of ten molecules in three categories of molecular weight: large RNA, L1–3, $2.3–2.7 \times 10^6$ daltons; medium RNA, M1–3, $1.3–1.6 \times 10^6$ daltons, and small RNA, S1, $0.6–0.9 \times 10^6$ daltons, the total molecular weight being about 15×10^6 daltons (SHATKIN et al. 1977). The nature of the arrangement of the ten segments within the genome is unknown. The plus strand (same polarity as mRNA) of each

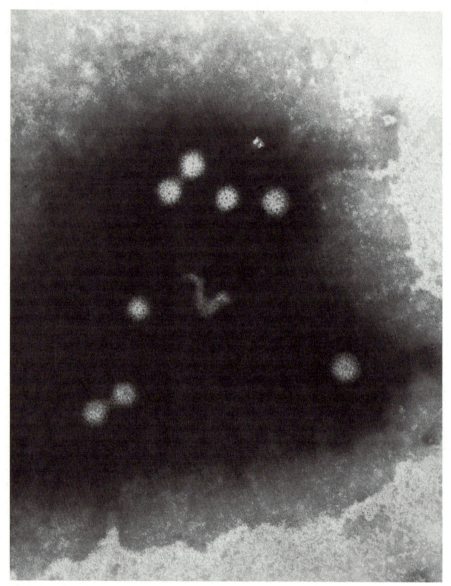

Fig. 16. Reovirus type 3. Particles demonstrate the characteristic double-shell structure of reovirions. (Madeley 1978) × 200,000

dsRNA segment has been shown to be "capped" at the 5′ end (Furuichi et al. 1975 a) and each segment serves as a monocistronic message for the production of a unique polypeptide (Both et al. 1975).

The polypeptides of reoviruses fall into three size classes λ, μ, and δ (Zweerink et al. 1971; Shatkin et al. 1976) which are composed of seven capsid proteins, $\lambda 1$–2, $\mu 1$–2, $\delta 1$–3. All are primary gene products except $\mu 2$ which is derived from $\mu 1$

(ZWEERINK et al. 1971). Three proteins $\sigma3$, $\mu2$, and $\sigma1$ constitute the outer shell of the virion and account for about 65% of the virion protein (JOKLIK 1974); $\lambda1$, $\lambda2$, $\delta2$, and μl make up the core proteins (JOKLIK 1974). A recent report (CARTER 1979) indicates that some structural proteins may contain a covalently linked oligoadenylate moiety, the function of which is unknown.

Reovirions also contain approximately 3,500 molecules of single-stranded oligonucleotide composed of two classes; one class, pyrimidine-rich heteropolymers 3–8 nucleotides long (BELLAMY and HOLE 1970; NICHOLS et al. 1972; STOLTZFUS and BANERJEE 1972), and a second class composed of polyadenylic acid 10–20 bases long (STOLTZFUS and BANERJEE 1972; NICHOLS et al. 1972; CARTER et al. 1974a). They do not appear to be necessary for infectivity (CARTER et al. 1974) and are thought to be products of abortive transcription (NICHOLS et al. 1972; STOLTZFUS and BANERJEE 1972).

Reoviruses enter the cell by phagocytosis, become enclosed in phagocytic vesicles which then fuse with liposomes (DALES et al. 1965). In the liposomes the virions are converted to subviral particles (SVP) by removal of the outer protein shell (SILVERSTEIN and DALES 1968), a process which activates a virion-associated polymerase (SILVERSTEIN et al. 1970). Transcription of the dsRNA is by a conservative mechanism (SKEHEL and JOKLIK 1969), viral plus strands being synthesized from only one strand. These plus strands serve as both mRNA and as templates for synthesis of minus strand RNA to form dsRNA (SKEHEL and JOKLIK 1969; ACS et al. 1971). Parental genomes remain in SVPs for the entire replication cycle (ZWEERINK et al. 1972). These SVPs contain the enzymes responsible for methylating (capping) reovirus mRNA (SHATKIN 1974), however, these mRNA molecules produced during infection do not contain poly(A) (STOLTZFUS et al. 1973). Two recent reports have demonstrated that progeny SVPs are not capable of "capping" mRNA, therefore, leaving early mRNA "capped" and later mRNA "uncapped" (SKUP and MILLWARD 1980; ZARBL et al. 1980). This may be the mechanism for reovirus inhibition of host protein synthesis (SKUP and MILLWARD 1980; ZARBL et al. 1980). The processes involved in the final maturation of reoviruses are poorly understood, but the virus particles are probably released when the infected cell lyses (JOKLIK 1974).

The human reoviruses have not been proven to have a causal relationship to any disease, but are, however, frequently isolated from people with respiratory infection, and gastroenteritis. They are also frequently recovered from healthy individuals. Infection of volunteers has shown the virus to occur both in the respiratory and gastrointestinal tract and a recent report has shown that reovirus is capable of inducing diabetes mellitus in mice, raising the possibility of a similar situation in humans owing to the ubiquity of reovirus infections (ONODERA et al. 1978). Orbiviruses are responsible for Colorado tick fever (caused by Colorado tick fever virus). The onset of the disease is sudden, characterized by fever, chills, and generalized aches, but serious complications are limited almost exclusively to children. The disease is transmitted by the bite of an infect tick (FENNER and WHITE 1976).

Despite the lack of major epidemiologic importance, reoviruses have been important in defining some molecular factors in viral virulence. A recent publication indicated that the S1 gene was responsible for the differing cell tropisms seen among the three types and also was the major determinant of neurovirulence

(WEINER et al. 1977, 1980). The type 1 S1 gene was shown to be responsible for ependymal damage with subsequent hydrocephalus and the type 3 S1 gene was responsible for neuronal necrosis and neurovirulence (WEINER et al. 1977, 1980). The authors postulated that these differences were due to the specific interaction of σ1, the outer capsid polypeptide (the S1 gene product) with receptors on either ependymal or neuronal cells (WEINER et al. 1977, 1980). The S1 gene has also been shown to be the predominant gene determining the specificity of cytotoxic T-cells (FINBERG et al. 1979) and the gene responsible for the type-specific hemagglutination observed with these viruses (WEINER et al. 1978).

M. RNA Tumor Viruses

During the past decade, research on RNA tumor viruses, their replication, transforming capabilities, and possible role or roles in human cancers has been of primary interest in molecular virology. The attractiveness of this group of viruses stems from their ability to cause (in many animal species) a variety of types of tumors (leukemia, sarcomas, etc.), from the finding that the genome of these viruses may be a part of the "normal" genome of many animals (PANEM et al. 1975), and from the feeling that by studying these viruses we may begin to understand the interactions which lead to cell transformation. However, despite a clear role in animal tumors, there is still no definitive proof that any of these viruses are related to any human cancers.

The RNA tumor viruses have been classified as a family called Retroviridae. This family contains viruses with similar structural and physical characteristics, but not necessarily oncogenic potential. The family is defined by four major characteristics: (a) the architecture of the virion; (b) a diploid single-stranded RNA genome of positive polarity; (c) the presence of reverse transcriptase in the virion; and (d) a requirement for a DNA intermediate in viral replication (BISHOP 1978). Within this group the viruses are classified into genera based on morphological characteristics. The first genus, oncornavirus C, contains the C particles (Fig. 17). This is the largest genus and contains many of the sarcoma and leukemia agents. These particles are released in an immature form and mature, following release, into C particles. The second genus oncornavirus B, contains the viruses which were formerly classified as having B-type morphology. This group contains the mouse mammary tumor viruses. The third genus, oncornavirus D, contains viruses with morphology intermediate between A and B and contains two subfamilies Lentiviridae and Spumaviridae. The two subfamilies contain the viruses of the Retroviridae family with unknown natural oncogenic potential. There also exists one other morphological group, the A particles, which appear to be nucleocapsids or immature forms of B and D particles. The RNA tumor viruses are often further subdivided on the basis of their ability to transform fibroblasts in vitro; those which can are designated sarcoma viruses and those which cannot are designated leukemia viruses (JOKLIK et al. 1980b). The sarcoma viruses contain the avian sarcoma viruses which can both transform and replicate without helper functions and mammalian sarcoma viruses which transform, but are defective for replication. The leukemia viruses contain genes essential for replication, but not for transformation.

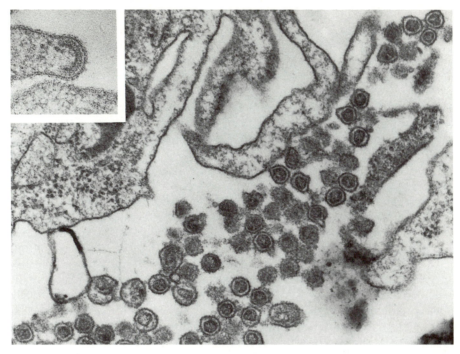

Fig. 17. RNA tumor virus. The large micrograph illustrates mature type C virions at the surface of a mouse cell grown in tissue culture. The small *inset* depicts a type C virion budding from the plasma membrane. In these budding virions, and in recently detached virions, the electron-dense nucleoid and intermediate layers can be distinguished, while in mature virions they have condensed into a single irregular layer under the limiting membrane. The mechanism of synthesis and release of retroviruses is generally not cytolytic, and many cell lines produce virus indefinitely. (Courtesy of J. Dahlberg) × 70,000

It is believed that they become transforming viruses by picking up transforming sequences from the host cell (Joklik et al. 1980).

The RNA tumor viruses are enveloped particles having a coiled nucleocapsid in an icosahedral shell. They are approximately 150 nm in diameter. The genome of the RNA tumor viruses is diploid (Coffin and Billeter 1976). It consists of a 60–70 S complex composed of two identical RNA subunits which are terminally redundant (Haseltine et al. 1977) approximately 35 S in size, and having a molecular weight of 3×10^6 daltons. Subunits are linked together via their 5' ends, through a palindromic sequence (Haseltine et al. 1977). The individual subunit RNA species are also adenylated (Lai and Duesberg 1972; Gillespie et al. 1972; Ross et al. 1972), capped (Furuichi et al. 1975b), and messenger RNA species produced during infection are spliced molecules (Mellon and Duesberg 1977). A tRNA molecule from the host cell is linked near the 5' end and serves as a primer for replication (Dahlberg et al. 1974). The genome of these viruses encodes four genes whose order is 5'-*gag-pol-env-src*-3'. The *gag* gene codes for a polyprotein which gives rise to several structural proteins of the viral coat, the *pol* gene codes for the DNA polymerase (reverse transcriptase), the *env* gene specifies the envelope glycoproteins, and the *src* (sarcoma) gene codes for the function responsible for the transformation of host cells (Duesberg et al. 1976).

The replication of RNA tumor viruses has been shown to proceed via an integrated DNA intermediate. The idea of a DNA intermediate in retrovirus replication was first suggested by Temin (1964) and several years later the enzymatic activity responsible for this reaction was discovered (Baltimore 1970; Temin and Mizutani 1970). The enzyme, since termed reverse transcriptase (RNA-dependent DNA polymerase), explained the conceptual problem of how a viral RNA molecule could transform, by allowing the RNA genome to be transcribed into a double-stranded DNA genome.

After entry into the cell, the polymerase becomes activated (Baltimore 1970; Temin and Mitzutani 1970) and transcribes the viral RNA into DNA, via single- and then double-stranded DNA intermediates (Bishop and Varmus 1975). The viral DNA circularizes, migrates to the nucleus, and integrates (Hatanaka et al. 1971; Gianni and Weinberg 1975; Takano and Hatanaka 1975). The integration appears to be obligatory for both transformation and progeny production (Guntaka et al. 1975; Roa and Bose 1974). It appears that while the viral genome may integrate into the host genome at several sites, only sites which contain specific neighboring cellular DNA sequences allow viral expression (O'Rear et al. 1980). It was also shown that cell death in the acute phase of infection is the result of integration of infectious DNA at multiple sites and that only cells with integration at a single site survive (Battula and Temin 1978). These retrovirus proviral sequences have also been shown to resemble transposable elements in bacteria (Shimotohno et al. 1980). The virus matures in the cytoplasm and receives its envelope by budding through the plasma membrane (Dalton 1962).

As mentioned earlier, those retroviruses which carry the *src* gene can transform fibroblasts and induce sarcomas in animals. However, the gene responsible for leukemia induction has not been found (Rosenberg and Baltimore 1976; Graf et al. 1976). A functional gene product of the *src* gene is essential for morphological transformation (Sefton et al. 1980). The gene product is a 60,000 dalton phosphoprotein, with protein kinase activity (Brugge and Erikson 1977; Levinson et al. 1978; Rübsamen et al. 1979) which is essential for transforming activity (Selfton et al. 1980). Finally, it appears that the *src* genes from a variety of avian sarcoma virus strains encode a polymorphic family of *src* proteins (Beemon et al. 1979). This and similar data have led to the hypothesis that the *src* genes were derived from the genomes of various species of origin of those viruses (Stehelin et al. 1976; Scolnick et al. 1973).

N. Rhabdoviruses

Rabies infection of humans, once established, is invariably fatal; although one case of recovery is quite well documented (Hattwick et al. 1972) it remains a celebrated exception to a general rule. It is a rare disease in the United States (only 1–2 cases/ year) but more prevalent in some other countries, and has declined in the United States, probably owing to the great decrease in rabies amongst the domestic (cat and dog) animal population. At the same time, rabies in the wild animal population has not diminished and is a constant source of potential disease.

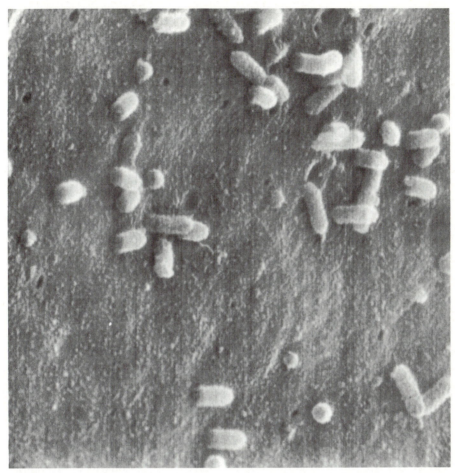

Fig. 18. High resolution scanning electron micrograph of vesicular stomatitis virus maturing at the surface of a BHK-21 cell. (Courtesy of M. DuBois-Dalcq) × 132,000

I. Structure and Replication

The structure of rabies virus is that of a typical rhabdovirus (Fig. 18). The bullet-shaped enveloped virion contains two membrane proteins (M_1 and M_2) which are not glycosylated, and a glycoprotein G. The nucleocapsid consists of a single strand of negative-polarity RNA which is not infectious on its own and is associated with a phosphoprotein (N). The RNA has a molecular weight of about 4.6×10^6 daltons and is associated in the virion with an RNA polymerase activity (Flamand et al. 1978); a fifth polypeptide (L) is also found in virions and in infected cells and is probably part of the RNA polymerase activity (Kawai 1977). The ability of rabies virions to transcribe RNA in vitro is very low compared with vesicular stomatitis virus (VSV), however.

The virion surface contains spikes, which seem largely to be composed of the G protein, the major factor in the neutralizing antigenic activity of the virus (Wik-

tor et al. 1973). Spikes also seem to be the source of the very weak hemagglutinating activity of rabies virus and the recognition point on the virus surface for susceptible cells. Having recognized and bound to the cell, the virion gains entry either
by fusion of its envelope with the cell membrane or by phagocytosis (Simpson et
al. 1969; Heine and Schnaitman 1969). Either way, the nucleocapsid appears in
the cytoplasm of the infected cell and is then functional as a transcriptional unit,
forming the mRNA species for virus protein production. Then messages (capped
and polyadenylated) individually corresponding to each of the five polypeptides
found in VSV-infected cells and are derived from the entire sequence of the virion
RNA with the exception of a small number of intervening sequences (Clewley and
Bishop 1979).

In VSV, the gene order on virion RNA is 3'-N-NS-M-G-L-5' as determined by
UV inactivation and in vitro transcription (Abraham and Banerjee 1976; Ball
and White 1976) with production of transcripts, dependent on the synthesis of the
previous ones in sequence. The mRNA for N polypeptide starts 51 nucleotides in
from the 3' end of virion RNA and is preceded by a leader RNA and a short A-rich
sequence which is not transcribed. Other data suggest that an A-rich sequence specifies the end of all transcripts in VSV, either by terminating transcriptase activity
or via processing (Keene et al. 1980). Of course, during replication of the virus
RNA to give new genomic material these A-rich sequences must be copied and thus
some suppression mechanism must exist to ensure faithful reproduction of the
virus genome. The simplest concept for formation of new genome RNA is via a
replicative intermediate containing intact genome-sized RNA of positive polarity.
It has not been possible, so far, to make the full-length plus strand in vitro, suggesting that the suppression mechanism outlined earlier only operates in infected cells.

Defective interfering (DI) particles of VSV contain various bits of RNA, and
have been suggested to originate via premature termination of minus strands with
copyback synthesis at their own 5' end to give panhandle structures with 3' polymerase initiation sites (Perrault and Leavitt 1977). Both glycoprotein and matrix protein are rapidly incorporated into infected cell cytoplasmic membranes
while the nucleocapsid is generated separately from its component RNA and polypeptides. How the two components of the virion recognize each other is not clear
but, depending on the cell type, budding and final assembly are able to take place
both at intracytoplasmic membranes and from the outher surface of the cell.

In general, rabies virus replication seems to follow the broad scheme set out
above for VSV, but it has yet to be shown that rabies virus has a virion transcriptase (Bishop and Flamand 1975) or that it can multiply in enucleate cells (Wiktor
and Koprowski 1974); this could indicate a fundamental difference between the
strategy of these two rhabdoviruses. No recombination can be detected between
rhabdovirus mutants, although resumptive "recombinants" can be isolated which
subsequently fail to breed true (because of polyploid particle formation?). However, complementation has been widely studied and is an effective way of defining
the functional areas of the viral genome. There are five (Cocal, New Jersey strains)
or six (Indiana strain) complementation groups for VSV, but no complementation
of rabies mutants has so far been described. Indiana group I mutants probably
have a transcriptase defect, group III a matrix protein defect, and group V a glycoprotein defect (Pringle 1977).

In 1970, HUANG and BALTIMORE suggested that defective particles may play a role in the pathogenesis of slow virus diseases. This idea was confirmed 3 years later when it was shown that defective VSV particles injected into mouse brain would, upon challenge with large doses of normal virus, cause a slow virus disease rather than the more common rapid, fatal infection (DOYLE and HOLLAND 1973). The same defective particles protected mice against low doses of VSV, however. Persistent infection may also be established in cell cultures by means of large amounts of defective particles; in this case, the course of the persistent infection and its establishment was accompanied by the accumulation of spontaneous *ts* mutants, which may behave as conditionally defective interfering particles. Low input multiplicities of *ts* mutant can also trigger persistent infections in cell cultures, presumably by a similar mechanism (YOUNGNER et al. 1976).

In a similar vein, a VSV *ts* mutant has been shown to cause delayed death and neurologic symptoms when injected into newborn hamsters. In this experiment, virus was localized in the brain, while infection with wild-type VSV usually causes a rapid disseminated disease. This effect appears, however, not to be related to a specific (genetic) feature of a mutant, but rather to the ability of the animal to survive infection long enough; the virus seems to be poorly cleared from the central nervous system (STANNERS and GOLDBERG 1975). Two mutants of VSV cause a disease in mice similar to the spongiform encephalopathies (RABINOWTZ et al. 1976). One of these, *ts*G31, when taken from the brain of an infected mouse, is no longer identical to the original mutant. It appears to have lost the ability to synthesize normal viral proteins, but makes unique high molecular weight species. Nor can this central nervous system isolate inhibit host protein synthesis effectively (HUGHES et al. 1979) although it still retains the *ts* character of its parent. It has also been shown, using the mutants of VSV, that not only did the disease process vary depending on the mutant, but the expression of neurovirulence was intimately tied to the host employed (DAL CANTO et al. 1979). Infection of newborn mice with certain rabies virus *ts* mutants much reduces their virulence and incubation period. Animals injected with one of the mutants, *ts*2, conferred resistance to challenge by wild-type rabies virus (CLARK and KOPROWSKI 1971).

It was proposed that DI particles were generated in infected cells as part of the host cells defense against virus. Support for this view comes from work with defective particles of VSV, whose generation is dependent on an actinomycin D-sensitive (directly or indirectly) host function: this host role in formation of DI particles of VSV does not apply to replication of already formed defective particles, however, and different cell types seem to be capable of the formation of quite different types of defective particle (KANG and ALLEN 1978).

II. Rabies Virus Infection

While a bite is the most frequently encountered means of human infection from an animal, a lick may be enough to infect a scratch and cause disease. Infection of humans is not productive for the virus, as humans do not usually transmit the virus to keep the infective cycle turning. Nevertheless, the virus persists in nature by being secreted from the salivary glands of animals whose nervous system it has infected to the extent that they are driven to dash about and bite other animals.

A bite from a rabid animal may not cause disease (low dose of virus, no skin breakage, etc.) and the incubation time in those individuals who have been successfully inoculated with the virus is extremely variable. Often, 6 months or more will pass before symptoms appear: there is a correlation, too, between the site of inoculation and the length of incubation. Generally, the further away from the head the bite is, the longer the incubation period.

Other means of infection with rabies have been described (e.g., airborne, Constantine 1962); ingestion of rabid animal flesh, Fischman and Ward 1968) but, for humans, the bite appears to be the usual route. There is probably some virus replication at the site of inoculation (Murphy et al. 1973b) from where the virus spreads to ganglia via the peripheral nerves. Thorough cleansing of the wound area is one of the best means of reducing the risk of infection and amputation of an infected limb is efficacious for some time after inoculation (in the mouse; Baer and Cleary 1972). The virus grows in infected ganglia and quickly spreads throughout the central nervous system. Viremia is not normally at a level high enough to suggest that it is an important factor in pathogenesis but almost all of the organs in the body eventually become infected, perhaps via the nerve supply. As soon as symptoms are seen in humans, antivirus antibody can be detected in the cerebrospinal fluid (Bell et al. 1966) and virus antigen is present in a number of different tissues. In biting animals, the salivary gland titer of the virus is usually very high (higher than in the central nervous system, for example). In the human infection, the course of obvious disease lasts 4–10 days, starting with fever and general malaise, and ending with various neurologic problems and death. Whether the effect on the host is a direct result of infection or an indirect consequence mediated through an immunologic response is in doubt (Tighor et al. 1974), nor is it clear why the infection has such a long incubation period.

Preexposure vaccination of high-risk groups (e.g., veterinarians) has been carried out for some time, using the inactivated duck embryo vaccine (DEV), with reasonable (80%–90%) success (seroconversion). The same vaccine is used for postexposure treatment, and is usually effective because of the long incubation time of the disease. However, a high frequency of local reaction to the vaccine plus a low frequency of more serious (neurologic) considerations has led to the development of a human diploid cell strain vaccine (HDCS). It is still not generally available (it may be obtained from the Center for Disease Control, Atlanta, Georgia), but is more effective (greater seroconversion and lower rate of adverse reactions) and is likely to supersede the DEV soon. Antirabies globulin is frequently used to treat bites (locally) soon after inoculation.

O. Rotaviruses

Rotaviruses have emerged only recently as a cause of acute gastroenteritis in children (Flewett et al. 1973) although the initial isolation of the virus type was from calves with diarrhea (Mebus et al. 1969). Infection of humans with rotaviruses is worldwide and a wide variety of animal species are susceptible to infection (McNulty 1978).

I. Structure and Replication

The virus particle is about 70 nm in diameter and, intact, appears to be a double-shelled sphere (Fig. 19). The morphology resemble that of reoviruses and seems to be the same for rotaviruses from different species (WOODE et al. 1976). Negatively stained preparations have a dense core structure (about 40 nm) and it has been pro-

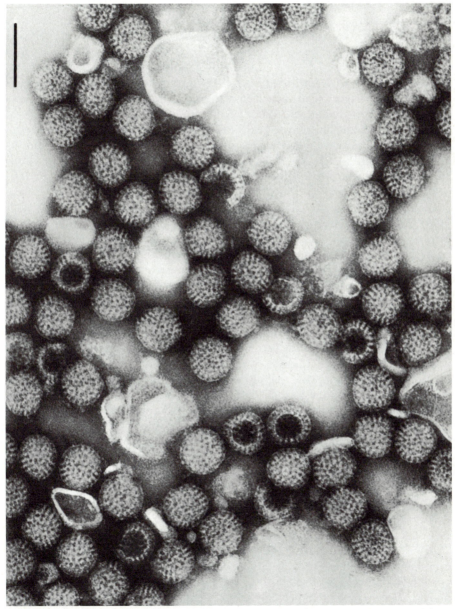

Fig. 19. Rotavirus particles observed by electron microscopy in a stool filtrate prepared from an infant with acute gastroenteritis. *Bar* = 100 nm. (KAPIKIAN et al. 1974)

posed (STANNARD and SCHOUB 1977; ESPARZA and GIL 1978) that the structure of both inner and outer shells is the same, with subunits arranged as an open mesh around 5- and 6-coordinated holes, although the number of holes has not been agreed upon. Removal of the outer core gives a 60 nm (roughly) orbivirus-like particle, which is usually seen (with intact particles) in preparations of virus from infected animals. Human rotaviruses appear to be assembled in the cytoplasm of infected cells, from tangles of fibrous virus precursor material (HOLMES et al. 1975) outside the cisternae. Some particles appear to bud through the endoplasmic reticulum and can obtain an envelope in the process; the virus particles are released from infected cells after the cells lyse.

The virus particle contains a group-specific antigen (KAPIKIAN et al. 1976) associated with the single-shelled structure (60 nm) and convalescent sera will agglutinate such particles. The outer shell of the virion is associated with species-specific antigenic activity and with a hemagglutinin (FAUVEL et al. 1978) and at least two serotypes of human rotavirus exist (THOULESS et al. 1978). No serologic relationships exist, however, between the rotaviruses and human reoviruses and orbiviruses (KAPIKIAN et al. 1976). The RNA in rotavirus particles occurs as a double-stranded structure, present as eleven fragments (molecular weight about 0.5–1.9×10^6 daltons; $11–12 \times 10^6$ daltons total) whose migration behavior in gel electrophoresis can be used to differentiate at least three human strains (KALICA et al. 1978). Single- and double-shelled virus particles (the former have very low infectivity) can be separated by density; the double-shelled particles have eight polypeptides, the single-shelled four, and there are probably three others in infected cells.

Comparison of various animal rotaviruses shows a remarkable similarity in the polypeptides they produce; also, there appear to be about as many polypeptides as there are RNA genome fragments. The major polypeptide of the outer shell is a glycoprotein (RODGER et al. 1977) and the calf virion is relatively acid stable and insensitive to $CHCl_3$ and ether as well as a variety of proteases. Heat or versene treatment of virions allows the expression of a particle RNA polymerase activity which copies the genome RNA into single-stranded material in vitro (COHEN 1977).

Rotaviruses do not grow well in tissue culture as a rule and do not seriously inhibit cell protein synthesis: this tends to make studies of the molecular biology difficult. This is in contrast to their in vivo ability to spread easily from animal to animal. However, it has been shown that the simian rotavirus SA11 grows well in homologous cell culture and seems to exhibit a wide and varied host range in vitro, although fetal calf serum contains an inhibitor of its growth (ESTES et al. 1979). Virus yield in a number of cell lines does not correlate with obvious cytopathic effect.

Replication of rotavirus in cell culture can give rise to the production of coreless particles, suggesting that lack of effective virus production in such a system may be a function of the failure of the cell to allow complete virus replication rather than a simple failure to adsorb the virus (MCNULTY et al. 1976). In addition, however, the suggestion has been made that a lactase activity is important for the uncoating and adsorbing of rotavirus to epithelial cells in vivo (HOLMES et al. 1976) and it has been shown that proteolytic enzymes may assist in the infection process via appropriate modification of the surface of rotavirus particles (THEIL et al. 1977). A plaque assay is available in simian cells (MATSUMO et al. 1977).

II. Rotavirus Infections

Rotavirus infection is ubiquitous, infecting young children (0.5–3 years) to give a diarrheal illness, chiefly during the winter, similar to the seasonal incidence of respiratory syncytial virus. Adults may acquire the disease from infected children and can seroconvert without obvious signs of illness. Rotavirus infection is usually confirmed by direct electron microscope identification of virus from stools or by immunologic testing of stool material, either directly or after culture in mammalian cells. Both radioimmunoassay and enzyme linked immunosorbant assay tests have been worked out (MIDDLETON et al. 1977; ELLENS and DeLEEUW 1977) and may be more suitable for widespread use than traditional methods. A few days after the onset of disease in humans, seroconversion takes place and this can be also used as a diagnostic tool (complement fixation, immunofluorescence; DAVIDSON et al. 1975); it is not clear though, what role circulating, as opposed to local, antibody plays in the prevention and control of disease.

Direct inoculation of the human virus into calf small intestine can cause (after passage in vivo) both diarrhea and virus shedding with seroconversion and it is possible that in nature rotaviruses of different animal strains may cross-infect (MEBUS et al. 1976). In this animal model, the pathogenesis of the virus was as follows: viral antigens appeared in epithelial cells of the lower small intestine very soon after the start of diarrhea; over the next several hours, degenerative changes in the villi took place with disappearance of the viral antigens; 2 days later, all was normal again (MEBUS et al. 1977). Virus appeared in the feces for the first 2 days only. Thus, this infection is a very rapid process, probably spreading in a cephalocaudal direction: circulating antibody may not be protective. While virus forms chiefly in the villous epithelial cells of the small intestine, it has also been isolated from other tissues (lung, stomach, etc.). Virus replication causes shedding of celles and their replacement by immature epithelial cells which may be resistant to infection (HOLMES et al. 1976). The pathogenicity of the virus may be related to the impaired capacity of these immature cells to process dietary sugars successfully, leading to changes in tonicity and increased loss of water in the feces, and may be exacerbated by bacterial production of fatty acids and a consequent inflammatory effect (McNULTY 1978). No human vaccine is available at present and it is not clear that the available attenuated calf vaccine works at all well (ACRES and RADSOTIS 1976).

P. Poxviruses

Since smallpox can kill about one-half of the people it infects given the appropriate circumstances, it is no surprise that it has long been considered one of the real scourges of the human race. All the more reason, therefore, to congratulate those involved in the complete eradication of the disease, which was recently achieved after much work. Eradication was always a possibility with the disease, since the virus appears to have no latent or persistent state and there appears to be no animal reservoir. Whether a poxvirus of another species can (sooner or later) fill the void occupied by smallpox is not known at present, but is a possibility we should not entirely discount. For these reasons we shall not discuss smallpox in detail since, with any luck, we may not have to deal with it again in human populations.

The Poxviridae have six main groupings based on a variety of criteria, (Fenner et al. 1974) and the orthopoxvirus (vaccinia–variola subgroup) can be further divided into four groupings on the basis of polypeptides in infected cells and of restriction enzyme cleavage of DNA (Harper et al. 1978; Esposito et al. 1978).

I. Structure and Replication

The particle is a complex (brick-shaped) entity with a biconcave core (lateral bodies in the concavities) and an envelope, (Fig. 20) containing DNA of molecular weight about $125–130 \times 10^6$ daltons (vaccinia) while other poxviruses possess genomes of much greater length (about 180×10^6 daltons; Gafford et al. 1978). The particle also contains lipid, carbohydrate, and protein. The DNA is a linear double strand, with 95% of its sequences unique and perhaps 4% as highly reiterated sequences

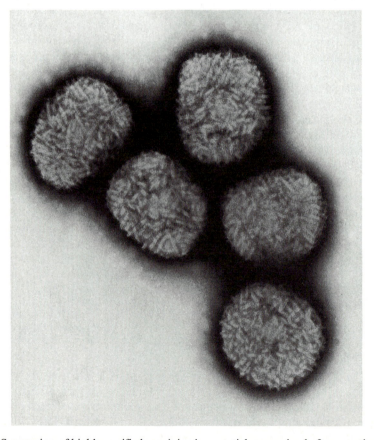

Fig. 20. Suspension of highly purified vaccinia virus particles examined after negative staining with phosphotungstate. The surface of each particle is convoluted into characteristic tubular ridges (Gold and Dales 1968) × 120,000

(GRADY and PAOLETTI 1977). The vaccinia genome also contains cross-links at or near the molecular termini which do not allow separation of two single strands of the viral DNA (BERNS and SILVERMAN 1970). The virion may contain as many as 100 polypeptides judged by two-dimensional polyacrylamide gel electrophoresis (ESSANI and DALES 1979) a number of which are modified by glycosylation or phosphorylation. Vertebrate poxviruses show a group-specific antigen but its identity is not clear, while an antigenic difference does seem to exist between virus particles found inside infected cells and those which are naturally exported from the cell (APPLEYARD et al. 1971). As a rule, vaccinia virus is not well released from infected cells and the majority of particles remain intracellular. Unlike other DNA animal viruses, the poxvirus particles contain a number of enzyme activities, mostly affecting nucleic acid metabolism. There are three deoxyribonucleosides, nucleoside triphosphatases, a reversible DNA ligating activity, a protein kinase, an RNA polymerase with poly(A) adding activity, and capping enzymes. The RNA polymerase was presumed to be necessary since poxvirus replicated, it was thought, wholly in the cytoplasm of infected cells: recent data have shown that the nucleus is required for complete vaccinia replication, however (PENNINGTON and FOLLETT 1974). The particle also has a hemagglutinin activity associated with one of the glycoproteins (PAYNE 1979).

The extracellular form of the virus appears to penetrate the infected cell largely by membrane fusion (PAYNE 1979) and is then uncoated in the cytoplasm in a two-stage process. The first part removes the lipid and one-half of the protein (JOKLIK 1964) and the second part needs a virus product or products, producing deoxyribonuclease-sensitive DNA. RNA synthesis is started using the particle RNA polymerase activity which transcribes a limited fraction of the genome and translation produces virus-specific early products including enzymes and presumably the uncoating activity for the second stage. About one-third to one-half of the genome is transcribed early (PAOLETTI and GRADY 1977); later, the entire genome is represented by transcripts, although the synthesis of some early products (i.e., enzymes) rapidly declines at late times. The mRNAs can be capped and polyadenylated (MOSS et al. 1976) and appear likely to be produced from high molecular weight precursors. At least part of this process can be duplicated in vitro and cleavage appears to be via an endogenous viral RNAse activity associated with cores. Recently a population of low molecular weight RNAs has been described after vaccinia infection which act as precursor to the cap and polyadenylation of mature mRNAs (PAOLETTI et al. 1980). Early protein synthesis declines quickly after DNA is synthesized, signalling the late phase of polypeptide production, chiefly virion components. It is not clear which RNA polymerase is responsible for the later transcription events. Viral DNA synthesis occurs within discrete foci in the cytoplasm and appears to involve the viral DNA polymerase activity, although recent data suggest that isolated nuclei in vitro may be capable of some viral DNA replication (LA COLLA and WEISSBACH 1976). Assembly of virus particles takes place in cytoplasmic factories where DNA is produced. Both cupule and spherical structures can be seen in the electron microscope (EASTERBROOK 1972) which develop into virus particles; these may further develop into an intracellular double-membrane-coated virion which can migrate to the cell surface. This particle fuses one membrane with the cytoplasmic membrane and is released minus one membrane: this form seems likely to be responsible for the dissemination of poxvirus infection (Payne and Kristensson 1979) both in vivo and in vitro.

Poxvirus infection generally leads to cell death rather rapidly and a cell-fusion factor appears to be associated with certain members of the group (Appleyard et al. 1962). In keeping with these biologic parameters, host cell molecular synthesis (DNA, RNA, and protein) also appear to be efficiently depressed after infection (Moss 1974). In other circumstances, however, poxviruses can stimulate cell proliferation and, in a kind of persistent infection, cause cell alterations reminiscent of transformation with other viruses (Koziorowska et al. 1971).

Recently, L. Payne (personal communication 1980) has suggested that the form of vaccinia virus responsible for both in vitro and in vivo spread of infection is the extracellular enveloped form of the virus; for example, treatment of mice with antienvelope serum would protect them from lethal vaccinia infection whereas inactivated intracellular virus antiserum would not. The major human problem arising from poxvirus infection is, as we have pointed out, smallpox. The various host responses to infection have been categorized (Christie 1969) and much of the epidemiologic and descriptive clinical picture has been obtained in India where the disease (until very recently) was part of everyday life and surrounded by various religious implications.

There are several different types of smallpox, some with characteristic lesions and some (e.g., hemorrhagic smallpox) with an almost certain prognosis of death. Incubation periods are of the order of 2 weeks and vaccination in most cases allows a 90% reduction in fatality rate. The standard vaccination for smallpox is, of course, vaccinia virus, which multiplies locally to express smallpox cross-reacting antigens but does not, normally, disseminate. A second attack of smallpox is rare and vaccination protects for about 5 years or so. Levels of circulating antibody are a major factor in the prevention of disease (vaccination quickly after exposure can protect) although local control via interferon and some T-cell-mediated response are also likely.

II. Poxvirus Infections

The studies of Fenner (1948) using mousepox virus in mice has provided us with a clear basis for understanding the pathogenesis of poxviruses. The general picture of pathogenesis has been described by Downie (1970). The virus enters via the respiratory route, undergoes primary replication in lymph nodes and spreads to a number of organs where a secondary replication takes place to give a viremia which leads to skin and mucous membrane infection (Fig. 21). Virus localized in the skin or the mucous membranes multiplies, in the first case to give macules, papules, a pustule owing to recruitment of polymorphonuclear cells, and finally a crusted lesion under which the epithelium can reform. In the second case, the lesion remains open and a great deal of infectious virus is released. Deep scars are often the result of a secondary bacterial infection. High levels of circulating infectivity usually mean severe consequences and in hemorrhagic disease, vast amounts of virus can be found in skin with evidence of virus replication in internal organs which are not normal sites for virus multiplication.

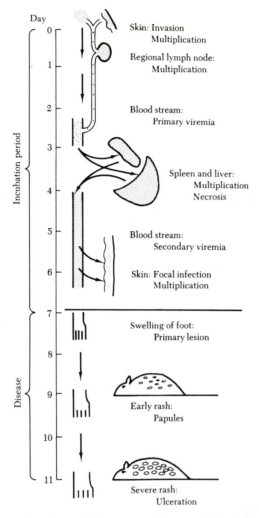

Day

0 — Skin: Invasion
        Multiplication

1 — Regional lymph node:
        Multiplication

2 — Blood stream:
        Primary viremia

3 —

4 — Spleen and liver:
        Multiplication
        Necrosis

5 — Blood stream:
        Secondary viremia

6 — Skin: Focal infection
        Multiplication

7 — Swelling of foot:
        Primary lesion

8 —

9 — Early rash:
        Papules

10 —

11 — Severe rash:
        Ulceration

Incubation period

Disease

Fig. 21. Scheme illustrating the possible sequence of events during the incubation period and development of signs of disease in mousepox. (FENNER 1948)

Q. Togaviruses and Bunyaviruses

The togaviruses and bunyaviruses were formerly classified along with many other viruses under the broad heading of arboviruses (arthropod-borne viruses). In recent years, it has become apparent that the arboviruses are composed of a very heterogeneous group of unrelated viruses. These viruses have now been classified into the following families: Togaviridae, Bunyaviridae, Reoviridae, and Rhabdoviridae (FENNER 1976). In this section we will be concerned only with the Togaviridae and Bunyaviridae, two families composed of RNA viruses which vary widely in physical characteristics.

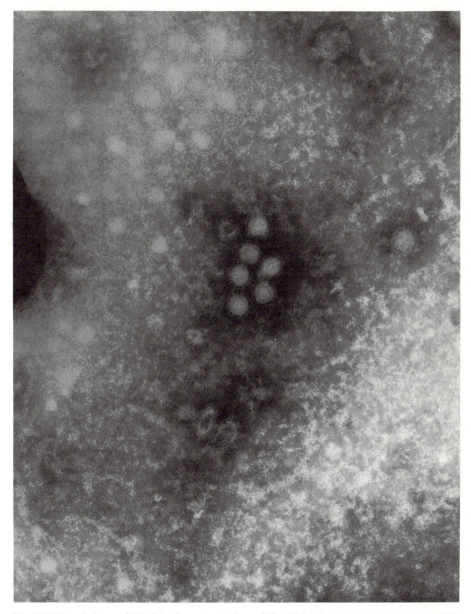

Fig. 22. Morphology of Sindbis virus, a member of the alphavirus group. (MADELEY 1978) × 200,000

The large number of togaviruses does not permit a comprehensive description of all the viruses. Within each genus, the viral infections are relatively similar. A generalized description for each genus will be used to illustrate the features Table 1. All alphaviruses have mosquitoes as vectors. The viruses are maintained in nature by a cycle involving wild birds and the mosquito vector (RUSSELL 1979 a). The infections are transmitted by the bite of the vector, with the virus being deposited directly into the blood or lymph stream (Downs 1976). The infection usually has two phases, the first characterized by replication in nonneural tissue, viremia, usually accompained by fever, chills, and aching. The infection is usually terminated at this point and most infections are subclinical (Downs 1976). The second stage, viral invasion of the central nervous system, may follow the viremic stage and a fulminant form of systemic disease leading to shock and death which may be attributed to the lymphocytolytic properties of the virus (Doherty 1977; Ehrenkranz and Ventura 1974; Gregg 1972). It has recently been shown that the death of mice infected with Sindbis virus is determined by virus genotype and that time of death is determined by the ability of a mutant virus to revert to wild-type (Barrett and Atkins 1979).

The flaviviruses constitute the largest genus of the togaviruses. Approximately 20 have been shown to cause disease in humans. With the exception of dengue virus which requires only a mosquito vector, the flaviviruses have complex cycles of transmission involving arthropods, wild birds, or mammals with humans being accidental hosts (Monath 1979). Dengue hemorrhagic fever is characterized by fever, chills, severe headache, and muscle and joint pain of sudden onset (Rhodes and Van Rooyen 1968). Dengue infection may proceed through the hemorrhagic stage to a shock syndrome (dengue shock syndrome) which is often fatal. One explanation is that the shock syndrome occurs in persons who have had a previous dengue infection and who react to the different dengue subtype with an exaggerated antibody response (Halstead 1970). Recent work supports the hypothesis that severe primary dengue hemorrhagic fever with shock is related to the maternal immune status (Marchette et al. 1979), and has also demonstrated that higher virus titers are present in animals with antisera to virus, again suggesting that severity is regulated by antibody (Halstead 1979). The clinical syndromes associated with St. Louis encephilitis are fever and headache, aseptic meningitis, and encephilitis with increasing severity with advancing age (Monath 1979). Yellow fever virus is viscerotropic, causing primary damage in the liver, kidney, and heart (Strode 1951). In the early stages, yellow fever mimicks dengue but then may manifest the normal syndrome with patients becoming icteric (Elton et al. 1955).

The sole member of the genus rubivirus is rubella virus. Rubella virus is classified as a togavirus on the basis of structural and physical characteristics. It appears to be closely related to the alphaviruses, but no vector is needed for transmission and it is not antigenically related (Andrewes 1970). There appears to be only one antigenic type of rubella virus (Mettler et al. 1968). Primarily, replication is thought to occur in the respiratory epithelium or lymph nodes, viremia follows the virus shedding in the throat (Green et al. 1965). In fetal infection, transmission is by hematogenous spread. Most cases of infection are subclinical but, in patients who do develop symptoms, the adults may have a prodromal phase consisting of malaise, fever, and anorexia for several days (Horstmann 1971). The major symptoms are adenopathy and rash, the rash usually lasting 3–5 days. Fever is usually present only during the first day of the rash (Heggie and Robbins 1969). Complications from rubella virus infection are uncommon but may include arthritis, arthralgia, hemmorhagic manifestations (probably secondary to thrombocytopenia) and encephilitis (Heggie and Robbins 1969).

I. Togaviruses

The Togaviridae are composed of four separate genera, alphavirus, flavivirus, rubivirus, and pestivirus. The first two groups contain viruses transmitted by arthropod vectors and were formerly classified as the group A and B arboviruses. The alphavirus genus includes about 20 viruses including Western, Eastern, and Venezualan encephalitis viruses, Sindbis and Semliki Forest viruses. The flavivirus genus contains more than 40 types, including dengue virus, St. Louis encephalitis virus, and yellow fever virus, the prototype virus for this group (Pfefferkorn and Shapiro 1974). Rubivirus contains only one member, rubella virus, and the pestivirus genus contains agents of animal disease transmitted by contact.

The Togaviruses are small icosahedral viral particles enclosed within a lipid envelope (Fig. 22). The enveloped particles have a diameter of 40–75 nm, the alphaviruses and rubivirus being overall somewhat larger than the flaviviruses and pestiviruses. These viruses were initially classified as togaviruses on the basis of structual similarities; however, classification of the viruses within the different genera is based on antigenic similarities (Casals 1972). All togaviruses are sensitive to detergents and ether, owing to their lipid envelope (Ventura and Scherer 1970) and are relatively heat labile (Purifoy et al. 1968). The lipid envelope which the virus obtains by budding through the host cell plasma membrane contains host cell lipids but only virus-specified proteins. The envelope proteins contain the hemagglutinin and neutralization antigens. Unenveloped virions fail to absorb to susceptible cells, indicating absorption as another function of the envelope (Bose and Sagik 1970). Viral nucleocapsids, unlike those of the picornavirus are susceptible to RNAse attack (Acheson and Tamm 1970; Käärianien and Soderlund 1971). The virion proteins consist of two glycoproteins found in the envelope and one nucleocapsid protein (Schlesinger et al. 1972; Simons et al. 1973). The virion contains a single, linear, infectious RNA molecule, 42 S and about 4×10^6 daltons in molecular weight (Dobos and Faulkner 1970; Boulton and Westaway 1972). Replication of the RNA proceeds through a multistranded intermediate similar to the picornaviruses (Friedman 1968) and the RNA polymerase required to carry out replication is coded for the viral genome (Cardiff et al. 1973). Viral structural proteins are coded for by the 26 S messenger RNA present in infected cells, which represents two thirds of the 3'-end of the virion RNA and produces a polycistronic protein which is cleaved into the structural proteins (Pfefferkorn 1977). The morphogenesis of the viruses includes assembly of nucleocapsid and virion 42 S RNA in the cytoplasm, modification of the cellular plasma membrane, and budding of the nucleocapsid through the modified cellular membrane (Pfefferkorn and Shapiro 1974).

High multiplicity passage of the virus leads to the generation of stocks of virus having a high ratio of physical to infectious particles. Such stocks interfere with the growth of wild-type virus and appear to be defective intefering (DI) particles (Inglot and Chudzio 1972; Schlesinger et al. 1972; Eaton and Faulkner 1973; Shenk and Stollar 1973a). The interference is homotypic (Shenk and Stollar 1973b) and the DI RNA appears to be a deletion mutant of the 42 S RNA (Bruton and Kennedy 1976).

While postnatal rubella is usually a subclinical noncomplicated disease, rubella can be a tragic disease in early gestation causing fetal death, premature birth, and a host of congenital defects. The incidence of rubella varies. The epidemic of 1964 left 30,000 affected infants while a more recent 5-year period (1969–1973) produced only 180 cases of congenital rubella in the United States (MODLIN and BRANDLING-BENNETT 1974; COOPER 1975, GERSHON 1979). The effects of the virus are dependent on the time of infection. In general, the younger the fetus, the more severe the disease, with infection in the first two months having a 40%–60% chance of affecting the fetus (COOPER 1975). The most common congenital defects are deafness, cataracts or glaucoma, congenital heart disease, and mental retardation (COOPER 1975). There is no specific treatment indicated for rubella. A live attenuated vaccine has been available since 1969. The vaccine may cause viremia, and is not recommended for use in pregnant women (GERSHON 1979). It is recommended that women vaccinated against rubella do not become pregnant for 3 months.

All togavirus infections may be diagnosed by virus isolation or through serologic studies. There are no specific treatments other than supportive therapy. Immunity following infection appears to be lifelong.

II. Bunyaviruses

The bunyaviruses are members of the family Bunyaviridae that are arthropod-borne, enveloped, and whose virions contain a single-stranded, segmented, RNA genome (PORTERFIELD et al. 1976). There are approximately 90 bunyaviruses, which have been divided into 11 groups. A member of each group being more related to members of its group than to members of other groups (PORTERFIELD et al. 1976; BERGE 1975; MURPHY et al. 1973b). The 11 groups constitute the Bunyamwera supergroup of viruses (PORTERFIELD et al. 1976; BERGE 1975; MURPHY et al. 1973) and there remain over 80 other bunyaviruses unrelated serologically to the supergroups but which show structural similarities to its members (PORTERFIELD et al. 1976).

The virions of the family Bunyaviridae are spherical, enveloped particles approximately 90–100 nm in diameter. The virions contain three major proteins (OBIJESKI et al. 1976a), two glycoproteins of 120×10^3 and 34×10^3 daltons molecular weight and a nucleocapsid protein of molecular weight 23×10^3 daltons. The virion also contains a RNA-dependent RNA polymerase (BISHOP 1977). The genome of the viruses is composed of three unique RNA species (CLEWLEY et al. 1977; PETTERSSON et al. 1977); the molecular weights of the three species for La Crosse virus are 3×10^6, 1.9×10^6, and 0.5×10^6 daltons. The nucleocapsid is similarly segmented (OBIJESKI et al. 1976a). Complementation and recombination have been shown to occur between temperature-sensitive mutants at a relatively high frequency, suggesting that genome reassortment occurred in mixed infections (GENTSCH and BISHOP 1976). The formation of recombinants also suggests that the genetic information of the virus resides on more than one piece of viral RNA (GENTSCH et al. 1977) while pathogenicity tests of the recombinants indicated they were either no more or less pathogenic than the prototype viruses (GENTSCH et al. 1977). Viral morphogenesis occurs intracellularly, virions mature by budding from Golgi and endoplasmic reticulum vesicles. Virions appear to be released by fusion

Table 1. Spectrum of arboviral infections. (Adapted from Fenner and White 1976)

Virus/disease	Genus	Distribution	Vector	Reservoir
Encephalitis				
Eastern equine encephalitis	Alphavirus	Americas	Mosquito	Birds
Western equine encephalitis	Alphavirus	Americas	Mosquito	Birds, reptiles?
Venezuelan equine encephalitis	Alphavirus	Americas	Mosquito	Rodents
St. Louis encephalitis	Flavivirus	Americas	Mosquito	Birds
Japanese B encephalitis	Flavivirus	East Asia	Mosquito	Birds
Australian encephalitis	Flavivirus	Australia	Mosquito	Birds
West Nile encephalitis	Flavivirus	Africa, Europe	Mosquito	Birds
Tick borne encephalitis	Flavivirus	Eastern Europe	Tick	Mammals
Russian spring-summer encephalitis	Flavivirus	U.S.S.R., Europe	Tick	Rodents
Louping ill	Flavivirus	Britain	Tick	Sheep
Powassan	Flavivirus	North America	Rick	Rodents
California encephalitis	Bunyavirus	North America	Mosquito	Rodents, rabbits
Hemorrhagic fever				
Chikungunya	Alphavirus	Africa, Asia	Mosquito	Monkeys?
Dengue 1–4	Flavivirus	Widespread	Mosquito	Monkeys?
Yellow fever	Flavivirus	Africa, South Africa	Mosquito	Monkeys, man
Kyasanur Forest disease	Flavivirus	India	Tick	Monkeys, rodents
Omsk hemorrhagic fever	Flavivirus	U.S.S.R.	Tick	Mammals
Crimean Congo	Bunayvirus	Central Asia, Africa	Tick	Mammals?
Fever-arthralgia-rash				
Chikungunya	Alphavirus	Asia, Africa	Mosquito	Monkeys?
O'nyong-nyong	Alphavirus	Africa	Mosquito	?
Ross River	Alphavirus	Australia	Mosquito	Mammals?
Sindbis	Alphavirus	Widespread	Mosquito	Birds, mammals
Dengue (types 1–4)	Flavivirus	Widespread, esp. Asia, Pacific, Caribbean	Mosquito	Monkeys?
West Nile	Flavivirus	Africa, Asia	Mosquito	Birds
Sandfly fever	Bunyavirus	Mediterranean	Sandfly	?
Oropouche	Bunyavirus	South America	Mosquito	?
Rift Valley fever	Bunyavirus	Africa	Mosquito	Sheep, cattle
Colorado tick fever	Orbivirus	United States	Tick	Rodents

of vesicle membranes with the plasma membrane or by cell lysis; budding through the plasma membrane is rare (Murphy et al. 1968).

Members of several groups within the Bunyaviridae are of medical importance, Table 1. The California encephalitis group is a major cause of mosquito-borne enchephalitis in the United States, the only group of Bunyaviridae of medical importance in North America (Russell 1979 b). The sandfly fever group causes acute febrile illness in Central and South America, Rift Valley fever virus causes major epidemics in Africa, and Crimean hemorrhagic fever virus causes hemorrhagic fever in the U.S.S.R. and Pakistan (Bishop 1977). Infection of humans by the

California encephalitis group usually results in an asymptomatic infection, but occassionally may present as a severe and sometimes fatal encephalitis. Rift Valley fever virus infection may present as a fever, and arthralgia, and Crimean hemorrhagic fever may present with sudden onset of fever, headache and chills, with hemorrhagic manifestations (FENNER and WHITE 1976; DOWNS 1976). Diagnosis is usually made by demonstration of a rise in antibody to a particular virus (DOWNS 1976) and this immunity is type specific, probably lasting for life.

R. Slow Viruses

Two categories of slow virus disease have been recognized in humans and other animals. First are those caused by known viruses such as subacute sclerosing paraencephalitis (SSPE, paramyxovirus) or progressive multifocal leukoencephalopathy (PML, papovavirus) in which a long incubation period is followed by an inflammatory reaction and serologic symptoms; second are the disease caused by unknown infectious agents such as scrapie, Creutzfeldt–Jakob disease (CJD), and kuru, in which no immunologic signs are apparent and there is no inflammatory response. In both cases, however, the course of the disease leads via degeneration of the central nervous system to death.

Such chronic diseases, although rare, certainly, in humans, are intriguing from several standpoints. First, there is the puzzle of which mechanisms are involved in the slow but inevitable degeneration of tissue, and the possibility that such chronic infection is much more widespread but is either not recognized as an "infectious disease" or is contained by cellular defence mechanisms such that clinical signs may be absent or diffuse. Second, the agent or agents responsible for the subacute spongiform encephalopathies do not behave as any known microorganism, although they seem to be small and infectious. Recent hypotheses that this organism or organisms resembled a plant viroid have not been substantiated.

I. Unconventional Agents

The pathology of these conditions is characteristic: there is no febrile response and no inflammatory response, but an obvious intracellular vacuolation in the gray matter of the brain (astrocytes and neurons). Four diseases have been classically associated with these symptoms, kuru and CJD in humans, and scrapie and mink encephalopathy in other animals: in all cases the responsible agent has been transmitted (via infected brain tissue) experimentally to animals (homologously and heterologously). In these instances, a long incubation period (0.2–8 years) is followed by a 1–6-month period of increasing symptoms and death. Recently, on the basis of such transmision studies, two other human diseases (familial Alzheimer's disease and progressive supranuclear palsy) have been tentatively added to the four original members of the group.

It has been possible to grow in vitro the agents of these diseases by culturing explants of nerve tissue from infected hosts. This procedure establishes a persistent infection in which the agent continues to be present over long periods, but can be detected only by inoculation of the material into an experimental animal: no general cytopathic effect is seen, but some vacuolation of cells in vitro has been reported (Espana et al. 1975–1976). It does not seem possible at present to detect any viral (noncellular) macromolecules in these infected cells, nor to observe unusual structures in the electron microscope. Transmission of infectivity from persistently infected cultures to heterologous cell lines has not been feasible for any length of time (Gibbs and Gadjusek 1978).

Despite the fact that infected nervous tissue from animals with these diseases has high concentrations of infectivity (e.g., kuru-infected brains have more than 10^8 infectious doses/g), density gradient fractionation of the agent (in scrapie) yielded a preparation which resembled smooth vesicular membranes in the electron microscope (Siakotos et al. 1976) with no sign of virus-like material, and freeze-fracture work on infected cells was similarly unrewarding (Dubois-Dalcq et al. 1977).

In many ways these agents are like viruses in that they are small (25–100 nm filtration), transmissible subject to genetic variation in the host (Parry 1960), and can show altered infectious properties upon passage in vivo (Burger and Hartsough 1965). However, they are exceedingly stable to inactivation by procedures which would normally kill conventional viruses (Millison et al. 1976) and this has led to the formulation of several ideas as to their structure, varying, in the case of scrapie, from a replicating polysaccharide (Adams and Caspary 1968) to a conventional virus (Eklund et al. 1967).

As has been discussed, these diseases can be transmitted experimentally into a number of species, including the "normal" host. Scrapie will replicate in the mouse to cause disease, which is a useful model of the natural infection. In this system the agent seems to replicate first in the spleen, then in the brain (and other tissues such as kidney, lymph nodes, spinal cord) without causing obvious "viremia." Also, for some time after experimental inoculation, no infectious agent was detectable anywhere in the animal (Gibbs and Gadjusek 1978).

No antibody against the virus nor any involvement of the immune response in pathogenesis has been seen. Infectivity-neutralizing tests have been negative as have attempts at passive protection with infected animal serum (Porter et al. 1973). Splenectomized and thymectomized mice showed essentially the same pathogenesis as normal animals. Interferon does not seem to play a role in the disease process. It may be, of course, that the agents produce no recognizably antigenic material in the course of their life cycle.

One important feature of the spread of these agents must be their extreme stability to a number of normally inactivating conditions. Gibbs and Gadjusek (1978) have described spread of CJD from electrodes which had been "sterilized" with 70% ethanol and formaldehyde vapor. Also, disease can be spread by oral infection, subcutaneously, intramuscularly, and intracerebrally; in the sheep, contact of the lamb with an infected ewe at birth (infectious placenta) is enough (Pattison et al. 1977). It is also possible for scrapie to be contacted by sheep grazing in infected meadows, but numerous different routes appear possible. In humans, kuru has a fascinating epidemiology, with which most microbiologists are probably familiar owing to the work and pen of Gadjusek and his colleagues (Gadjusek and Gibbs 1973). Transmission by cannibalism of brain material is efficient but no other means of spread has been documented; it will be interesting to see if, with the total eradication of the practice and the death of the practicing generation, the disease disappears entirely. Kuru is confined to a remote corner of the globe, but CJD is worldwide and does not rely on cannibalism for its spread. Its natural transmission route or routes are not clear, but consumption of animal brain has been suggested (BOBOWICK et al. 1973), although some genetic involvement seems a strong possibility (GADJUSEK and GIBBS 1973). These encephalopathies, are caused by a microorganism, with virus dimensions and with virus-like pathogenesis which neither looks like nor behaves immunologically like a virus; it may well be a totally new form of infectious agent.

II. Conventional Agents

Several conventional viruses cause slow disease under a variety of special conditions (e.g., immunosuppression of the host): these include PML and SSPE, and the latter are discussed in the sections dealing with paramyxovirus infection. PML normally occurs (and even then rarely) in patients with reticuloendothelial system problems of some kind, and seems to be due to papovavirus infection (ZU RHEIN 1969). Two human papovaviruses, JC and BK (PADGETT et al. 1971; GARDNER et al. 1971) appear on serologic grounds to be normal and widespread human infectious agents but only JC (of the two) is capable of causing PML. Perhaps surprisingly, SV40, a simian virus, is also a (rarer) cause of PML. After the onset of neurologic degeneration typical of the disease, the patient's death normally occurs within months and it is not clear whether the virus responsible for PML has been inactive (latent) in tissues for some time or if recent infection (in the presence of a predisposed immunocompromised host) is responsible. No doubt the lack of knowledge of the pathogenesis of the disease is directly related to its infrequent occurrence.

Papovaviruses in general are capable of two kinds of interaction with cells – lytic infection and transformation; they may also cause tumors in a particular animal. JC virus can also be oncogenic in hamsters (WALKER et al. 1973) but has proved difficult to grow in cell culture. Recent attempts to obtain infection in cells other than human fetal glial cells using the infectivity of viral DNA proved fruitless, although a reasonable level of infectivity in these cells was obtained (FRISQUE et al. 1979). Interestingly, therefore, failure of certain cells to allow replication of JC virus may not simply be a lack of suitable cell surface receptors, but perhaps a block at some point in the replication cycle.

JC virus DNA is about 5,000 base pairs long (almost identical to SV40) and restriction maps of it have recently become available (MARTIN et al. 1979). There is no consensus yet on the extent of genetic homology between JC virus and SV40, but they do share T and V antigens. Lacking information to the contrary, it is assumed that the replication of JC virus is similar to that of SV40. These viruses have small genomes and employ several interesting means to increase their coding capacity. For example, several coding sequences are read in differant ways to give more than one product and, particularly in the early region of the DNA, polypeptides expressed have more than one function. A good review of this area has been provided by SAMBROOK (1977).

References

Abraham G, Banerjee AK (1976) Sequential transcription of the genes of vesicular stomatitis virus. Proc Nat Acad Sci USA 73:1504–1508

Acheson NH, Tamm I (1970) Ribonuclease sensitivity of Semliki Forest virus nucleocapsids. J Virol 5:714–717

Acres SD, Radsotis OM (1976) The efficacy of a modified live REO-like virus vaccine and E. coli bacterin for prevention of acute undifferentiated neonatal diarrhoea of beef calves. Can Vet J 17:197–212

Acs G, Klett H, Shonberg M, Christman JK, Levin DH, Silverstein SL (1971) Mechanisms of reovirus double-stranded ribonucleic acid synthesis in vivo and in vitro. J Virol 8:684–689

Adam E, Rawls WE, Melnick JL (1974) The association of herpesvirus type 2 infection and cervical carcinoma. Prev Med 3:122–141

Adams DH, Caspary EA (1968) The incorporation of nucleic acid and polysaccharide precursors into a post-ribosomal fraction of scrapie-infected mouse brain. Biochem J 108:38

Albrecht P, Lorenz D, Klutch MJ, Vickers JH, Ennis FA (1980) Fatal measles infection in marmosets: pathogenesis and prophylaxis. Infect Immun 27:969–978

Albrecht T, Rapp F (1973) Malignant transformation of hamster embryo fibroblasts following exposure to ultraviolet-irradiated human cytomegalovirus. Virology 55:53–61

Allaudeen HS, Bertino JR (1978) Isolation of a herpesvirus-specific DNA polymerase from tissues of an American patient with Burkitt lymphoma. Proc Nat Acad Sci USA 75:4504–4508

Almeida JD, Rubenstein D, Stott EJ (1971) New antigen antibody system in Australia antigen positive hepatitis. Lancet 2:1225–1227

Alter JH, Purcell RH, Gerin JL et al. (1977) Transmission of hepatitis B to chimpanzees by hepatitis B surface antigen positive saliva and semen. Infect Immun 16:928–933

Alwine JC, Steinhart WL, Hill CW (1974) Transcription of herpes simplex type 1 DNA in viruses from infected HEp-2 and KB cells. Virology 60:302–307

Ambros V, Baltimore D (1978) Protein is linked to the 5′ end of poliovirus RNA by a phosphodiester link to tyrosine. J Biol Chem 253:5263–5266

Andrewes CH (1970) Generic names of viruses of vertebrates. Virology 40:1070–1080

Appleyard G, Westwood JCN, Zwartouw HT (1962) The toxic effect of rabbitpox virus in tissue culture. Virology 18:159–169

Appleyard G, Hapel A, Boulter EA (1971) An antigenic difference between intracellular and extracellular rabbit pox virus. J Gen Virol 13:9–17

Arens W, Yamashita T, Padmanabban R, Tsumo T, Green W (1977) Adenovirus deoxyribonucleic acid replication. Characterisation of the enzyme activities of a soluble replication system. J Biol Chem 252:7947–7954

Arrand JR, Roberts RJ (1979) The nucleotide sequences at the termini of adenovirus – 2 DNA. J Mol Biol 128:577–594

Aurelian L, Cornish JD, Smith MF (1975) Herpesvirus type 2 induced tumor specific antigen (AG-4) and specific antibody in patients with cervical cancer and controls. IARC Sci Publ 2:79–83

Baer GM, Cleary WF (1972) A model in mice for pathogenesis and treatment of rabies. J Infect Dis 125:520–527

Ball LA, White CN (1976) Order of transcription of genes of vesicular stomatitis virus. Proc Nat Acad Sci 73:442–446

Baltimore D (1970) Viral RNA-dependant DNA polymerase. Nature 226:1209–1211

Baltimore D (1971) Is poliovirus dead? Perspect Virol 7:1–12

Bar, De Lor J, Claussen KP, Hurtubise P, Henle W, Hewetson JF (1974) Fatal infectious mononucleosis. Am J Med 29:43–54

Baringer JR (1975) Herpes simplex virus in sensory ganglia. IARC Sci Publ 2:73–78

Baringer JR, Swoveland P (1973) Persistent herpes simplex infection in rabbit trigeminal ganglia. Lab Invest 30:230–240

Barker LF, Maynard JE, Purcell RH et al. (1975) Hepatitis B infection in chimpanzees: titration of subtypes. J Infect Dis 132:451–458

Barrett PN, Atkins GJ (1979) Virulence of temperature-sensitive mutants of Sindbis virus in neonatal mice. Infect Immun 26:848–852

Bartkoski MJ, Roizman B (1976) RNA synthesis in cells infected with herpes simplex virus. XIII. Differences in methylation patterns of viral RNA during the reproduction cycle. J Virol 20:583–588

Battula N, Temin H (1980) Sites of integration of infectious DNA of avian reticuloendotheliosis viruses in different cellular DNAs. Cell 13:387–398

Becker WB, Kipps A, McKenzie D (1968) Disseminated herpes infection: its pathogenesis based on virological and pathological studies in 33 cases. Am J Dis Child 115:1–8

Beemon K, Hunter T, Sefton BM (1979) Polymorphism of avian sarcoma virus *src* proteins. J Virol 30:190–200

Bégin M, Weber J (1975) Genetic analysis of adenovirus type 2: isolation and genetic characterization of temperature-sensitive mutants. J Virol 15:1–7

Bell JF, Codemell DL, Moore GJ, Raymond GH (1966) Brain neutralization in rabies virus to distinguish recovered animals from previously vaccinated animals. J Immunol 97:747–753

Bellamy AR, Hole LV (1970) Singe-stranded RNA from reovirus type-3. virology 40:808–819

Berge TD (1975) International catalog of arboviruses, 2nd edn. U.S. Department of Health, Education and Welfare Publ. (CDC) 75-8301. Center for Disease Control, Atlanta, Ga

Berk, AJ Sharp PA (1978) Structure of the adenovirus 2 early mRNAs. Cell 14:695–711

Berns KI, Silverman C (1970) Natural occurrence of cross-linked vaccinia virus deoxyribonucleic acid. J Virol 5:299–304

Bishop DH (1977) Virion polymerases. In: Comprehensive virology, vol 10, chap 8. Plenum, New York, pp 117–253

Bishop DHL, Flamand A (1975) The transcription of vesicular tomatitis virus and its mutants in vivo and in vitro. In: Mahy BWJ, Barry RD (eds) Negative strand viruses, vol 1. Academic Press, New York, pp 327–352

Bishop JM (1978) Retroviruses. Ann Rev Biochem 47:35–88

Bishop JM, Varmus H (1975) Molecular biology of RNA tumor viruses. In: Becker FF (ed) Cancer, vol 2. Plenum, New York, pp 3–48

Blumberg BS (1977) Australia antigen and the biology of hepatitis B. Science 197:17

Bose HR, Sagik BP (1970) The virus envelope in cell attachment. J Gen Virol 9:159–161

Bobowick AR, Brodey JA, Matthews MR, Ross R, Gadjusek DD (1973) CJD: a case control study. Am J Epidemiol 98(5):381–394

Both GW, Lavi S, Shatkin AJ (1975) Synthesis of all the gene products of reovirus genome in vivo and in vitro. Cell 4:173–180

Boulton RW, Westaway EG (1972) Comparisons of Togaviruses: Sindbis virus (group A) and Kunjuin virus (group B). Virology 49:283–289

Bradburne AF, Bynoe ML, Tyrrell DA (1967) Effects of a "new" human respiratory virus in volunteers. Br Med J 3:767–769

Bradley DW, Fields HA, McCaustland KA (1978) Biochemical and biophysical characterization of light and heavy density hepatitis A virus particles: evidence that HAV is an RNA virus. J Med Virol 2:175–187

Breshkin AM, Rapp F, Payne FE (1977) Complementation analysis of measles virus temperature-sensitive mutants. J Virol 21:439–441

Brison O, Kedinger C, Clauson P (1979) Adenovirus DNA template for late transcription is not a replicative intermediate. J Virol 32:91–97

Bruton CJ, Kennedy SIAT (1976) Defective interfering particles of Semliki Forest virus: structural differences between standard virus and defective interferring particles. J Gen Virol 31:383–395

Brown F, Newman JFE, Stott J et al. (1974) Poly C in animal viral RNAs. Nature 251:342–344

Brown SM, Subak-Sharpe JH, Warren KG, Wroblewska Z, Koprowski H (1979) Detection by complementation of defective or uninducible HSV-1 virus genomes latent in human ganglia. Proc Nat Acad Sci USA 76:2366–2368

Brugge JS, Erikson RL (1977) Identification of a transformation-specific antigen induced by an avian sarcoma virus. Nature 269:346–348

Buckley SM, Casals J (1970) Lassa fever, a new virus disease of man from West Africa. III. Isolation and characterization of the virus. Am J Trop Med Hyg 19:680–691

Buetti E, Choppin PW (1977) The transcriptase complex of the paramyxovirus SV5. Virology 82:493–508

Burger D, Hartsough GR (1965) Encephalopathy of mink. II. Experimental and natural transmissions. J Infect Dis 115:393–399

Burkitt DP, Wright DH (1966) Geographical and tribal distribution of the African lymphoma in Uganda. Br Med J 5487:569–573

Caliguiri LA (1974) Analysis of RNA associated with the poliovirus RNA replication complex. Virology 58:526–535

Caliguiri LA, Compans RW (1974) Analysis of the in vitro product of an RNA-dependent RNA polymerase isolated from influenza-virus infected cells. J Virol 14:191

Caliguiri LA, Holmes KV (1979) Host dependent restriction of influenza virus maturation. Virology 92:15–30

Cardiff RD, Dalrymple JM, Russell PK (1973) RNA polymerase in group B arbovirus (dengue-2) infected cells. Arch Gesamte Virusforsch 40:392

Carter C (1979) Polyadenylation of proteins in reovirions. Proc Nat Acad Sci USA 3087–3091

Carter CA, Kilbourne ED (1952) Activation of latent herpes simplex by trigeminal sensory root section. N Eng J Med 246:172–176

Carter C, Stoltzfus CM, Banerjee AK, Shatkin AJ (1974a) Origin of reovirus oligo A. J Virol 13:1331–1337

Carter MF, Biswal N, Rawls WE (1973) Characterization of the nucleic acid of Pichinde viruses. J Virol 11:61–68

Carter MF Biswal N, Rawls WE (1974b) Polymerase activity in Pichinde virus. J Virol 13:577–583

Casals J (1972) Antigenic characteristics of Venezuelan equine encephalitis virus: relation to other viruses. In: Venezuelan encephalitis. Proceedings of the Workshop-Symposium on Venezuelan Equine Encephalitis Virus. Pan American Health Organization, Washington, DC, p 77

Center for Disease Control (1977) Reported morbidity and mortality in the United States: MMWR annual summary. Center for Disease Control, Atlanta, Ga

Chanock RM, Parrott RH, Johnson KM, Kapikian AS, Bell JA (1963) Newly recognized myxoviruses from children with respiratory disease. Am Rev Resp Dis 88:152–154

Cheng Y-C, Tsou TY, Hackstadt T, Mallavia LP (1979) Induction of thymidine kinase and DNase in varicella zoster virus infected cells and kinetic properties of the virus-induced thymidine kinase. J Virol 31:172–177

Cherry JD, Feigin RD, Cobes LA Jr et al. (1972) Urban measles in the vaccine era: a clinical epidemiological and serological study. J Pediatr 81:217–230

Chisari FV, Edgington TS, Routenberg JA (1978) Cellular immune reactivity in HBV-induced liver disease. In: Vygas GN, Cohen SN, Schmidt R (eds) Viral hepatitis. Franklin, Philadelphia, pp 245–266

Christie AB (1969) Infectious diseases: epidemiology and clinical practice. Livingstone, Edinburgh, pp 185–237

Clark HF, Koprowski H (1971) Isolation of temperature-sensitive conditional lethal mutants of "fixed" rabies virus. J Virol 7:295–300

Clements JB, Hay J (1977) RNA and protein synthesis in herpesvirus-infected cells. J Gen Virol 35:1–12

Clements JB, Watson R, Wilkie NM (1977) Temporal regulation of herpes simplex virus type 1 transcription: location of transcripts on the viral genome. Cell 12:275–285

Clewley JP, Bishop DHL (1979) Assignment of the large oligonucleotides of vesicular stomatitis virus to the N, NS, M, G, and L genes and oligonucleotide gene ordering within the L gene. J Virol 30:116–123

Clewley J, Gentsch J, Bishop DHL (1977) Three unique viral RNA species of snowshoe hare and La Crosse Bunyaviruses. J Virol 22:459–468

Clough W (1979) Deoxyribonuclease activity found in Epstein-Barr virus producing lymphoblastoid cells. Biochemistry 18:4517–4521

Coffin JM, Billeter MA (1976) A physical map of the Rous sarcoma virus genome. J Mol Biol 100:293–318

Cohen J (1977) Ribonucleic acid polymerase activity associated with purified calf rotavirus. J Gen Virol 36:395–402

Collins BS, Bratt MA (1973) Separation of the mesenger RNAs of Newcastle disease virus by gel electrophoresis. Proc Nat Acad Sci USA 70:2544–2548

Colonno RJ, Stone HO (1976) Isolation of a transcription isoflex from Newcastle disease virions. J Virol 19:1080–1089

Compans RW, Bishop DHL, Meier-Ewert H (1977) Structural components of influenza C virions. J Virol 21:658–665

Conlepis AG, Locarnini SA, Ferris AA, Lehman NI, Gust ID (1978) The polypeptides of hepatitis A virus. Intervirology 10:24–31

Constantine DG (1962) Rabies transmission by nonbite route. Public Health Rep 77:287–289

Cook ML Barstow VB, Stevens JG (1974) Evidence that neurones harbor latent herpes simplex virus. Infect Immun 9:946–951

Cooper LZ (1975) Congenital rubella in the United States. In: Krugman S, Gershon A (eds) Infections of the fetus and the newborn infant. Liss, New York, pp 1–22

Cooper PD (1977) Genetics of picornaviruses. In: Fraenkel-Conrat H, Wagner RR (eds) Comprehensive virology, vol 9. Plenum, New York, pp 133–196

Craig CP, Nahmias AJ (1973) Different patterns of neurological involvement with herpes simplex virus types 1 and 2: isolation of herpes simplex type 2 from the buffy coat of two adults with meningitis. J Infect Dis 127:365–372

Crowell RL (1976) Comparative characteristics of picornavirus receptor interactions. In: Been RF Jr, Barrett EG (eds) Cell membrame receptors for viruses, antigens or antibodies, polypeptide hormones and small molecules. Raven, New York, pp 179–202

Crowell RL, Philipson L (1971) Specific alterations of coxsackievirus B3 eluted from hela cells. J Virol 8:509–518

Crowell RL, Siak J-S (1978) Receptor for group B coxsackieviruses: characterization and extraction from hela cell plasma membranes. Perspect Virol 10:39–55

Cuifo CM, Wayward GS (1980) Tandem repeat defective DNA from the L segment of the herpes simplex virus genome

Dahlberg JE, Sawyer RC, Taylor JM et al. (1974) Transcription of DNA from the 70 S RNA of Rous sarcoma virus. I. Identification of a specific 4 S RNA which serves as primer. J Virol 13:1126–1133

Dal Canto MC, Rabinowitz SG, Johnson TC (1979) Subacute infection with temperature-sensitive vesicular stomatitis virus mutant G41 in the central nervous system of mice. II. Immunofluoresence, morphologic, and immunologic studies. J Infect Dis 139:36–51

Dales S, Gamatos PJ, Hsu KC (1965) The uptake and development of reovirus in strain L cells followed with labeled viral ribonucleic and ferritin-antibody conjugates. Virology 25:193–211

Dalton AJ (1962) Micromorphology of murine tumor virus and of affected cells. Fed Proc 21:936–941

Dambaugh T, Nkrumah FK, Biggar RJ, Kieff E (1979) Epstein-Barr virus RNA in Burkitt tumor tissue. Cell 16:313–322

Dasgupta A, Baron MH, Baltimore D (1979) Poliovirus replicase: a soluble enzyme able to initiate copying of polioviral RNA. Proc Nat Acad Sci USA 76:2679

Datta AK, Feighry RJ, Pagano JS (1980) Induction of Epstein-Barr virus associated DNA polymerase by 12-0-Tetradecanoylphorbol-13-acetate. J Biol Chem 255:5120–5125

Davidson GP, Goller I, Bishop RF, Townley RRW, Holmes IH, Rude BJ (1975) Immunofluoresence in duodenal mucosa of children with acute enteritis due to a new virus. J Clin Pathol 28:263–266

Delius H, Clements JB (1976) A partial denaturation map for herpex simplex type 1 DNA: evidence for inversion of the unique regions. J Gen Virol 33:125–133

Demarchi JM, Kaplan AS (1977) Physiological state of human embryonic lung cells alters their response to human cytomegalovirus. J Virol 23:126–132

Demarchi JM, Blankenship ML, Brown GO, Kaplan AS (1978) Size and complexity of human cytomegalovirus DNA. Virology 89:643–646

De Thé G (1977) Is Burkitt's lymphoma related to a perinatal infection by Epstein-Barr virus? Lancet 1:335–338

De Thé G (1979) The epidemiology of Burkitt's lymphoma; evidence for a causal association with Epstein-Barr virus. Epidemiol Rev 1:32–54

De Thé G, Geser A, Day NE et al. (1978) Epidemiological evidence for a causal relationship between Epstein-Barr virus and Burkitt's lymphoma from Ugandan prospective study. Nature 274:756–761

D'Halluin J-C, Martin GR, Torpier G, Boulanger PA (1978) Adenovirus type 2 assembly analyzed by reversible cross-linking of labile intermediate. J Virol 26:357–363

Dijkema R, Dekker BMM, Feltz VD, Van Der Eb AJ (1979) Transformation of primary rat kidney cells by DNA fragment of weakly oncogenic adenoviruses. J Virol 32:943–950

Dingle J, Langmuir AD (1968) Epidemiology of acute respiratory disease in military recruits. Am Rev Respir Dis 97:1–65

Dobos P, Faulkner P (1970) Molecular weights of Sindbis virus ribonucleic acid as measured by polyacrylamide gel electroporesis. J Virol 6:145–147

Doherty RL (1977) Viral encephalitidies. In: Hoeprich P (ed) Infectious diseases. Harper & Row, Hagerstown, Md, pp 919–927

Douglas RG Jr (1970) Pathogenesis of rhinovirus common colds in human volunteers. Ann Otol Rhinol Laryngol 79:563–571

Downie AW (1970) Infectious agents and host reaction. In: Mudd S (ed). Saunders, Philadelphia, pp 487–518

Downs W (1976) Arboviruses. In: Evans AS (ed) Viral infections of humans. Plenum, New York, p 84

Doyle M, Holland JJ (1973) Persistent noncytocidal vesicular stomatitis virus infections mediated by defective T particles that suppress virion transcriptase. Proc Nat Acad Sci USA 71:2956–2960

Drzeniek R, Billelo P (1972) Dissociation and reassociation of infectious poliovirus particles. Nature New Biol 240:118–122

Dubbs DR, Kit S (1964) Mutant strains of herpes simplex deficient in thymidine kinase-inducing ability. Virology 22:693

Dubois-Dalcg M, Rodriguez M, Reese TS, Gibbs CJ Jr, Gadjusek DC (1977) Search for a specific marker in the neural membranes of scrapie mice. Lab Invest 36:547–553

Dudding BA, Top FH, Winter PE, Buescher EL, Lawson TH, Leibovitz A (1973) Acute respiratory disease in military trainees: the adenovirus surveillance program. Am J Epidemiol 97:187–198

Duesberg PH, Wang L-H, Mellon P, Mason WS, Vogt PK (1976) ICN-UCLA Symp Mol Cell Biol 4:109–125

Duff R, Rapp F (1971) Oncogenic transformation of hamster cells after exposure to herpes simplex virus type 2. Nature New Biol 233:48–50

Dumas AM, Geden JLMC, Maris W, Van der Noordaa J (1980) Infectivity and molecular weight of varicella zoster virus DNA. J Gen Virol 47:233–235

Easterbrook KB (1972) Crystalline aggregates observed in the vicinity of freezeetched poxvirus inclusions. Can J Microbiol 18:403–406

Eaton BT, Faulkner P (1973) Altered pattern of viral RNA synthesis in cells infected with standard and defective Sindbis virus. Virology 51:85–93

Ehrenkranz NJ, Ventura AK (1974) Venezuelan equine encephalitis infection in man. Annu Rev Med 25:9–14

Eisinger M, Kularova O, Sarkar NH, Good RA (1975) Propagation of human wart virus in tissue culture. Nature 256:432–434

Eklund CM, Kennedy RC, Hadlow WJ (1967) Pathogenesis of scrapie virus infection in the mouse. J Infect Dis 117:15–22

Eleftheriou N, Thomas HC, Heathcote J, Sherlock S (1975) Incidence and clinical significance of e antigen and antibody in acute and chronic liver disease. Lancet 2:1171

Ellens DJ, Deleeuw PW (1977) Enzyme-linked immunosorbet assay for diagnosis of rotavirus infections in calves. J Clin Microbiol 6:530–532

Elton NW, Romero A, Trejos A (1955) Clinical pathology of yellow fever. Am J Clin Pathol 25:135–146

Epstein MA, Achong BG (1977) Recent progress in Epstein-Barr virus research. Annu Rev Microbiol 31:421–445

Epstein MA, Achong BA, Barr YM (1964) Virus particles in cultured lymphoblasts from Burkitt's lymphoma. Lancet 1:702–703

Esiri MM, Tomlinson AH (1972) Herpes zoster: demonstration of virus in trigeminal nerve and ganglia by immunofluorescence and electron microscopy. J Neurol Sci 15:35–48

Esparza J, Gil F (1978) A study on the ultrastructure of human rotavirus. Virology 91:141–150

Esposito JJ, Obijeski JF, Nakano JH (1978) Orthopoxvirus DNA: strain differentiation by electrophoresis or restriction endonuclease fragmented virion DNA. Virology 89:53–66

Espana C, Gadjusek DD, Gibbs CJ Jr, Lock K (1976) Transmission of Creutzfeldt-Jakob disease to the Patas monkey *(Erythrocebus patas)* with cytopathological changes in in vitro cultivated brain cells. Intervirology 6:150–155

Essani K, Dales S (1979) Biogenesis of vaccinia: evidence for more than 100 polypeptides in the virion. Virology 95:385–394

Esteban M, Kerr IM (1974) The synthesis of EMC virus polypeptides in infected L-cells and in cell-free systems. Eur J Biochem 45:567–576

Estes MK, Graham DY, Gerba CP, Smith EM (1979) Simian rotavirus SA11 replication in cell cultures. J Virol 31:810–815

Evans AS (1958) Latent adenovirus infections of the human respiratory tract. Am J Hyg 67:256–266

Evans AS (1960) Infectious mononucleosis in University of Wisconsin students: report of a five year investigation. Am J Hyg 71:342–362

Evans AS, Niederman JC (1977) Epstein-Barr virus. In: Evans ASC (ed) Viral infections of humans. Plenum, New York, pp 209–233

Everitt E, Meador SA, Levine AJ (1977) Synthesis and processing of the precursor to the major core protein of adenovirus type 2. J Virol 21:199–219

Farber FE, Rawls WE (1975) Isolation of ribosome-like structures from Pichinde virus. J Gen Virol 26:21–31

Farmer TW, Janeway CA (1942) Infections with the virus of lymphocytic choriomeningitis. Medicine 21:1–63

Fauvel M, Spence L, Babiuk LA, Petro R, Bloch S (1978) Haemagglutination and haemagglutination-inhibition studies with a strain of Nebraska calf diarrhoea virus (bovine rotavirus). Intervirology 9:95–105

Fenner F (1948) The pathogenesis of the acute exanthems. Lancet 2:915

Fenner F (1976) The classification and nomenclature of viruses. Summary of the results of meetings of the international committee on taxonomy of viruses in Madrid, September 1975. Virology 71:371–378

Fenner F, White D (1976) Medical virology, 2nd edn. Academic Press, New York

Fenner FL, Pereira HG, Porterfield JS, Joklik WK, Downie AW (1974) Family and generic names for viruses approved by the international committee on taxonomy of viruses, June 1974. Intervirology 3:193–198

Ferguson M, Murphy MJ (1980) Homotypic and heterotypic interfering activity associated with measles and subacute sclerosing panencephalitis. J Infect Dis 141:414–419

Fialkow P, Klein E, Klein G, Clifford P, Singh S (1973) Immunoglobulin and glucose 6 phosphate dehydrogenase as markers of cellular origin in Burkitt's lymphoma. J Exp Med 138:89–102

Finberg R, Weiner HS, Fields BN, Benacerraf B, Burakoff SJ (1979) Generation of cytolytic T lymphocytes after reovirus infection: role of S1 gene. Proc Nat Acad Sci USA 76:442–446

Fischman HR, Ward FE (1968) Oral transmission of rabies in experimental animals. Am J Epidemiol 88:132–138

Fisher LE, Rapp F (1979) Temperature-dependent expression of measles virus structural proteins in persistently infected cells. Virology 94:55–60

Flamand A, Delagreau JF, Bunerean F (1978) An RNA polymerase activity in purified rabies virions. J Gen Virol 40:233–238

Flanagan JB, Baltimore D (1979) Poliovirus uridylic acid polymerase and RNA replicase have the same viral polypeptide. J Virol 29:352–360

Flewett TH, Bryden A, Davies H (1973) Virus particles in gastroenteritis. Lancet 2:1497

Flint J (1977) The topography and transcription of the adenovirus genome. Cell 10:153–166

Fox JP, Brandt CD, Wassermann RE, Hall CE, Spigland I, Kojan A, Elveback LR (1969) The virus watch program: a continuing surveillance of viral infections in metropolitan New York families. VI. Observations of adenovirus infections: virus excretion patterns, antibody response, efficiency of surveillance, patterns of infection and relation to illness. Am J Epidemiol 89:25–50

Frame JD, Baldwin JM Jr, Gocke DJ, Troup JM (1970) Lassa virus, a new virus disease of man from West Africa. I. Clinical description and pathological findings. Am J Trop Med Hyg 19:670–676

Francis DP, Maynard JE (1979) Transmission and outcome of hepatitis A, B, and non-A, non-B: a review. Epidemiol Rev 1:17–31

Francis T Jr (1940) A new type of virus from epidemic influenza. Science 92:405–408

Francis T, Salk JE, Quilligan JJ (1947) Experience with vaccination against influenza in the spring of 1947. Am J Public Health 37:1013–1016

Frenkel N, Roizman B (1972) Separation of herpesvirus deoxyribonucleic acid duplex into unique fragments and intact strand or alkaline products. J Virol 10:565–572

Frenkel N, Roizman B, Cassai E, Nahmias A (1972) A DNA fragment of herpes simplex 2 and its transcription in human cervical cancer tissue. Proc Nat Acad Sci 69:3784–3789

Frenkel N, Locker H, Batterson W, Hayward GS, Roizman B (1976) Anatomy of herpes simplex virus DNA. VI. Defective DNA originates from the S component. J Virol 20:527–531

Friedman RM (1968) Replicative intermediate of an arbovirus. J Virol 2:547–552

Frisque RJ, Martin JD, Padgett BJ, Walker DL (1979) Infectivity of DNA from four isolates of JC virus. J Virol 32:476–482

Fulgitini VA, Eller JJ, Downie AW, Kempe CH (1967) Altered reactivity to measles virus: atypical measles in children previously immunized with inactivated measles virus vaccine. JAMA 202:1075–1080

Furlong D, Swift J, Roizman B (1972) Arrangement of herpesvirus deoxyribonucleic acid in the core. J Virol 10:1071–1074

Furuichi Y, Muthukrishnan S, Shatkin AJ (1975a) 5′-terminal $M^7G(5′)$ ppp (5′) G_P^m in vivo: identification in rovirus genome. Proc Natl Acad Sci USA 72:742–745

Furuichi Y, Shatkin AJ, Stavnezer E, Bishop JM (1975b) Blocked, methylated 5′-terminal sequence in avian sarcoma virus RNA. Nature 257:618–620

Furukawa T, Tanaka S, Plotkin SA (1975) Stimulation of macromolecular synthesis in guinea pig cells by human CMV. Proc Soc Exp Biol Med 148:211–214

Gadjusek DC, Gibbs CJ Jr (1973) Subacute and chronic diseases caused by atypical infections with unconventional viruses in aberrant hosts. Perspect Virol 8:279–311

Gafford LG, Mitchell EB, Randall CC (1978) Sedimentation characteristics and molecular weights of three poxvirus DNAs. Virology 89:229–239

Gallimore PH, Sharp PA, Sambrook J (1974) Viral DNA in transformed cells. II. A study of the sequence of Ad2 DNA in nine lines of transformed rat cells virus specific fragments of the viral genome. J Mol Biol 89:49–72

Gardner SD, Field AM, Coleman DV, Hulme B (1971) New human papovavirus (BK) isolated from urine of renal transplantation. Lancet 1:1253–1257

Garon CF, Berry KW, Rose JA (1972) A unique form of terminal redundancy in adenovirus DNA molecules. Proc Natl Acad Sci USA 69:2391–2394

Geder L, Lausch R, O'Neill F, Rapp F (1976) Oncogenic transformation of human embryo lung cells by human cytomegalovirus. Science 192:1134–1136

Gentsch J, Bishop DHL (1976) Recombination and complementation between temperature sensitive mutants of a bunyavirus, snowshoe hare virus. J Virol 20:351–354

Gentsch J, Wynne LR, Clewley JP, Shope RE, Bishop DHL (1977) Formation of recombinants between snowshoe hare and La Crosse bunyaviruses. J Virol 24:893–902

Gergely L, Klein G, Ernberg I (1971) The action of DNA antagonists on Epstein-Barr virus (EBV) = associated early antigen (EA) in Burkitt lymphoma lines. Int J Cancer 7:293–302

Gerhart W, Webster RG (1978) Antigenic drift in influenza A viruses. I. Selection and characterization of antigenic variants of A/PR/8/34 [HON1] influenza virus with monoclonal antibodies. J Exp Med 148:383–392

Gershon A (1979) Rubella virus (German measles). In: Mandell GL, Douglas RG, Bennett TE (eds) Principles and practice of infectious disease, part III, chap 112. John Wiley and Sons, New York, pp 1258–1265

Gianni AM, Weinberg RA (1975) Partially single-stranded form of free Maloney viral DNA. Nature 255:646–648

Gibbs CJ Jr, Gadjusek DC (1978) Slow viruses and human disease. Perspect Virol 10:161–198

Gibson W, Roizman B (1971) Compartmentalization of spermine and spermidine in herpes simplex virions. Proc Natl Acad Sci USA 68:2818–2821

Gibson W, Roizman R (1974) Proteins specified by herpes simplex virus. X. Staining and radiolabeling properties of B capsid and virion proteins in polyacrylamide gels. J Virol 13:155–165

Gillespie D, Marshall S, Gallo RC (1972) RNA of RNA tumor viruses contains poly A. Nature New Biol 236:227–231

Gimenez HB, Pringle CR (1978) Seven complementation groups of respiratory syncytial virus temperature-sensitive mutants. J Virol 27:459–464

Ginsberg HS, Young CSH (1977) Genetic of adenovirus. In: Comprehensive virology, vol 9. Plenum, New York, pp 27–88

Gissman C, Pfister H, Zur Hausen H (1977) Human papilloma viruses (HPV): characteristics of four different isolates. Virology 76:569–580

Gissman L, Zur Hausen H (1976) Human papilloma virus DNA: physical mapping and genetic heterogeneity. Proc Natl Acad Sci USA 73:1310–1313

Given D, Kieff ED (1978) DNA of Epstein-Barr virus. IV. Linkage map of restriction enzyme fragments of the B95-8 and W91 strains of EBV. J Virol 28:524–542

Given D, Kieff E (1979) DNA of Epstein-Barr virus. VI. Mapping of the internal tandem reiteration. J Virol 31:315–324

Glazier K, Raglow R, Kingsbury DW (1977) Regulation of sendai virus transcription: evidence for a single promoter in vivo. J Virol 21:863–871

Gold P, Dales S (1968) Localization of nucleotide phosphohydrolase activity within vaccinia. Proc Natl Acad Sci USA 60:845–852

Goldschmidt H, Klingman AM (1958) Experimental inoculation of humans with ectodermotropic viruses. J Invest Dermatol 31:175–182

Golini F, Nomoto A, Wimmer E (1978) The genome-linked protein of picornavirus. IV. Difference in the VP$_g$s of EMC virus and poliovirus as evidence that the genome linked proteins are virus-coded. Virology 89:112–118

Grady LJ, Paoletti E (1977) Molecular complexity of vaccinia DNA and the presence of reiterated sequences in the genome. Virology 337–341

Graessman A, Wolf H, Bornkamm GW (1980) Expression of Epstein-Barr virus genes in different cell types after microinjection of viral DNA. Proc Nat Acad Sci USA 77:433–436

Graf T, Boyer-Pokora B, Beng H (1976) In vitro transformation of specific target cells by avian leukemia viruses. ICN-UCLA Symp Mol Cell Biol 4:321–338

Grafstrom RH, Alwine JC, Steinhart WL, Hill CW (1974) Terminal repetitions in herpes simplex virus type 1 DNA. Cold Spring Harbor Symp Quant Biol 39:679–681

Graham FC, Van der Eb AJ (1973) A new technique for the assay of infectivity of human adenovirus. Virology 52:456–462

Graves MX, Silver SM, Choppin PW (1978) Measles virus polypeptide synthesis in infected cells. Virology 86:254–263

Grayston JF, Yang YF, Johnston PB, Ko LS (1964) Epidemic keratonconjunctivitis on Taiwan: etiological and clinical studies. Am J Trop Med 13:497–498

Green M (1970) Oncogenic viruses. Ann New Biol 39:701–739

Green M, Maskey JK, Wold WSM, Rigden P (1979 a) Thirty one human adenovirus sero-
    types (Ad1-Ad31) from five groups (A-E) based upon genome homologies. Virology
    93:481–492
Green M, Wold WSM, Brackmann KH, Lartas MA (1979 b) Identification of families of
    overlapping polypeptides coded by early "transforming" gene region 1 of human
    adenovirus type 2: Virology 97:275–286
Green M, Wold WS, Mackey JK, Rigden P (1979 c) Analysis of human tonsil and cancer
    DNA, and RNAs for DNA sequences of group C (serotypes 1, 2, 5, & 6) human
    adenoviruses. Proc Natl Acad Sci USA 76:6606–6610
Green RH, Balsamo MR, Giles SP, Krugman S, Mirick GS (1965) Studies on the natural
    history and prevention of rubella. Am J Dis Child 110:348–365
Gregg M (1972) Human disease-USA, In: Venezuelan encephalitis. Proceedings of the
    Workshop-Symposium on Venezuelan Encephalits Virus. Pan American Health Orga-
    nization, Washington, DC, p 225
Gross L (1970) Oncogenic viruses. Pergamon, Oxford
Gross PA, Green RH, Cumen MCM (1973) Persistent infection with parainfluenza type 3
    virus in man. Am Rev Respir Dis 108:894–898
Guntaka RV, Mahy BWJ, Bishop JM, Varmus HE (1975) Ethidium bromide inhibits ap-
    pearance of closed circular viral DNA and integration of viral specific DNA in duck
    cells infected by avian sarcoma virus. Nature 253:507–511
Gutekünst RR, Heggie AD (1961) Viremia and viruria in adenovirus infections: detenction
    in patients with rubella or rubelliform illnes. N Engl J Med 264:374–378
Halbert DN, Spector DJ, Raskas HJ (1979) In vitro translation product specified by the
    transforming region of adenovirus type 2. J Virol 31:621–629
Hall WW, Choppin PW (1979) Evidence for lack of synthesis of the M polypeptide of meas-
    les virus in brain cells in subacute sclerosing panencephalitis. Virology 99:493
Hall WW, Kiessling W, Ter Meulen V (1978) Membrane proteins of subacute sclerosing
    panencephalitis and measles viruses. Nature 272:460–462
Hall WW, Lamb RA, Choppin PW (1979) Measles and subacute sclerosing panencephalitis
    virus proteins: lack of antibodies to the M protein in patients with subacute sclerosing
    panencephalitis. Proc Natl Acad Sci USA 76:2047–2051
Halstead SB (1970) Observations relating to pathogenesis of dengue hemorrhagic fever. VI.
    Hypothesis and discussion. Yale J Biol Med 42:350–362
Halstead SB (1979) In vivo enhancement of dengue virus infection in rhesus monkeys by
    passively transferred antibody. J Infect Dis 140:527–533
Harper L, Bedson HS, Buchan A (1978) Identification of orthopoxviruses by polyacrylam-
    ide gel electrophoresis of intracellular polypeptides. 1. Four major groupings. Virology
    93:435–444
Harris B, Roeder RG (1978) Structure relationships of low molecular weight viral RNAs
    synthesized by RNA polymerase III in nuclei from adenovirus 2-infected cells. J Biol
    Chem 253:4120–4127
Harris T Jr, Brown F (1977) Biochemical analysis of a virulent and avirulent strain of foot
    and mouth disease virus. J Gen Virol 34:75–105
Harter ML, Lewis JB, Anderson CW (1979) Adenovirus type 2 terminal protein: purifica-
    tion and comparison of tryptic peptides with known adenovirus coded proteins. J Virol
    31:823–835
Haseltine WA, Maxam AM, Gilbert W (1977) Rous sarcoma virus genome is terminally re-
    dundant: the 5′ sequence. Proc Natl Acad Sci USA 74:989–993
Hatanaka M, Kakefuda T, Gilden RV, Callan EAD (1971) Cytoplasmic DNA synthesis in-
    duced by RNA tumor viruses. Proc Natl Acad Sci USA 18:1844–1847
Hattwick MAW, Weiss TT, Stechshulte J, Baer GM, Gregg MB (1972) Recovery from ra-
    bies: a case report. Ann Intern Med 76:931–942
Hay AJ, Lomniczi B, Bellamy AR, Skehel JJ (1977) Transcription of influenza virus ge-
    nome. Virology 83:337–355
Hayward GS, Jacob RJ, Wadsworth SC, Roizman B (1975) Anatomy of herpes simplex
    virus DNA: evidence for four populations of molecules that differ in the relative orien-
    tations of their long and short components. Proc Natl Acad Sci 72:4243–4247

Hayward SD, Kieff ED (1976) Epstein-Barr virus specific RNA. I. Analysis of viral RNA in cellular extracts and in the polyribosomal fraction of permissive and non-permissive lymphoblastoid cell lines. J Virol 18:518–525

Hayward SD, Kieff ED (1977) DNA of Epstein-Barr virus. II. Comparison of molecular weights of restriction endonuclease fragments of the DNA of Epstein-Barr virus strains and identification of end fragment of the B95-8 strain. J Virol 23:421–429

Hayward SD, Nogee L, Hayward GS (1980) Organization of repent region within the Epstein-Barr virus DNA molecule. J Virol 33:507–821

Heggie AD, Robbins FC (1969) Natural rubella acquired after birth. Am J Dis Child 118:12–17

Heine JW, Schnaitman CA (1969) Fusion of vesicular stomatitis virus with cytoplasmic membranes of L-cells. J Virol 3:619

Hendley JO, Wenzel RP, Gwaltney JM (1973) Transmission of rhinovirus colds by self-inoculation. N Engl J Med 288:1361–1364

Henle G, Henle W, Diehl V (1968) Relation of Burkitt's tumor-associated herpes type virus to infectious mononucleosis. Proc Natl Acad Sci USA 59:94–101

Henle W, Henle G, Ho HC et al. (1970) Antibodies to Epstein-Barr virus in nasopharyngeal carcinoma, other head, and neck neoplasms and control groups. J Natl Cancer Inst 44:225–231

Heubner RJ (1967) Adenovirus-directed tumor and T antigens. Perspect Virol 5:147–166

Hierholzer JC, Torrence AE, Wright PF (1980) Generalized viral illness caused by an intermediate strain of adenovirus (21/H21 + 35). J Infect Dis 141:281–288

Hinman AR, Frazer DW, Douglas RG (1975) Outbreak of lymphocytic choriomeningitis virus infection in medical center personnel. Am J Epidemiol 101:103–110

Hoagland RJ (1955) The transmission of infectious mononucleosis. Am J Med Sci 229:262–272

Hoagland RJ (1964) The incubation period of infectious mononucleosis 1. Am J Public Health 54:1699–1705

Holmes IH, Ruck BJ, Bishop RF, Davidson GP (1975) Infantile enteritis viruses: morphogenesis and morphology. J Virol 16:937–943

Holmes IH, Rodgers SM, Schnagl RD, Ruck BJ, Gust ID, Bishop RF, Barnes GL (1976) Is lactase the receptor and uncoating enzyme for infantile anteritis (rota) viruses? Lancet 1:1387–1389

Honess RW, Roizman B (1974) Regulation of herpes virus macromolecular synthesis 1. Cascade regulation of the synthesis of three groups of viral proteins. J Virol 14:8–19

Horstmann DM (1971) Rubella: the challenge of its control. J Infect Dis 123:640–654

Hruby DE, Roberts WK (1976) Variations in poly A content and biological activity. J Virol 25:413–415

Hruska JF, Clayton DA, Rubenstein JLR, Robinson WS (1977) Structure of the hepatitis B Dane particle DNA before and after the Dane particle DNA polymerase reaction. J Virol 21:666–672

Huang AS, Baltimore D (1970) Defective viral particles and viral disease processes. Nature 226:325–327

Huang AS, Baltimore D (1977) Defective interfering animal viruses. In: Fraenkel-Conrat H, Wagner RR (eds) Comprehensive virology, vol 10, chap 2. Plenum, New York

Huang E-S (1976) Human cytomegalovirus IV: specific inhibitor of virus-induced DNA polymerase activity and viral DNA replication by phosphonoacetate. J Virol 16:1560–1565

Hughes JV, Johnson TC, Rabinowitz SG, Dal Canto MC (1979) Growth and maturation of a vesicular stomatitis virus temperature-sensitive mutant and its central nervous system isolate. J Virol 29:312–321

Inglot AD, Chudzio T (1972) Incomplete Sindbis virus. In: Melnick HL (ed) Proceedings of the second international congress for virology. Karger, New York

Ishibashi M, Maizel JV (1974) The polypeptides of adenovirus: VI. Early and late glycopeptides. Virology 58:345–361

Jense H, Knauert F, Ehrenfeld E (1978) Two initiation sites for the translation of poliovirus RNA in vitro; comparison of LSC and Mahoney strains. J Virol 28:387–394

Johnson KM (1975) Status of arenavirus vaccines and their application. Bull WHO 52:729–
735
Johnson KM (1977) Epidemic hemorrhagic fevers. In: Hoeprich PD (ed) Infectious diseases,
2nd edn. Harper & Row, Hagerstown, Md, pp 721–725
Joklik WK (1964) Intracellular uncoating of poxvirus DNA. I. The fate of radioactively-
labeled rabbit-pox virus. J Mol Biol 8:263–276
Joklik WK (1974) Reproduction of reoviridae. In: Comprehensive virology, vol 2, Chap 5.
Plenum, New York
Joklik WK, Willett HP, Amos DB (eds) (1980a) Zinsser microbiology, 17th edn. Appleton-
Century-Crofts, New York
Joklik WK, Willett HP, Amos DB (eds) (1980b) Zinsser microbiology, 17th edn, chap 69.
Appleton-Century-Crofts, New York
Jondal M, Klein G (1973) Surface markers on human B and T lymphocytes. II. Presence
of Epstein-Barr virus receptors on B lymphocytes. J Exp Med 138:1365–1378
Jones KW, Kinross J, Maitland N, Norval M (1979) Normal human tissues contain RNA
and antigens related to adenovirus type 2. Nature 277:274–279
Jou WM, Verhoeyen M, Devos R et al. (1980) Complete structure of the hemagglutinin gene
from the human influenza A/Victoria/3/75 (H3N2) strain as determined from cloned
DNA. Cell 19:683–696
Juel-Jensen BE, MacCallum FO (1972) Herpes simplex, varicella and zoster: clinical mani-
festation and treatment. Lippincott, Philadelphia
Kääriainen L, Soderlund H (1971) Properties of Semliki Forest virus nucleocapsid. 1. Sen-
sitivity to pancreatic ribonuclease. Virology 43:291–310
Kalica AH, Sereno MM, Wyatt RG, Mebus CA, Chanock RM, Kapikian AZ (1978) Com-
parison of human and animal rotavirus strains by gel electrophoresis of viral RNA.
Virology 87:247–255
Kang CY, Allen R (1978) Host function-dependent induction of defective interferring particles of vesicular stomatitis virus. J Virol 25:202–206
Kapikian AZ (1969) Coronavirus. In: Diagnostic procedures for viral and rickettsial infection, chap 27. American Public Health Association, pp 941–946
Kapikian AZ, Kim HW, Wyatt RG et al. (1974) Reovirus-like agent in stools: association
with infantile diarrhea and development of serological tests. Science 185:1049–1053
Kapikian AZ, Cline WL, Kim HW et al. (1976) Antigenic relationships among five reovirus-
like (RVL) agents by complement fixation (CF) and development of new substitute (CF)
antigens for the human RVL agents of gastroenteritis. Proc Soc Exp Biol Med 152:535–
539
Kaschka-Dierich C, Adams A, Lindahl R et al. (1976) Intracellular forms of Epstein-Barr
virus DNA in human tumor cells in vivo. Nature 260:302–306
Kawai A (1977) Transcriptase activity associated with rabies virions. J Virol 29:826–835
Keene JD, Shubert M, Lazzarini RA (1980) Intervening sequence between the leader region
and the nucleocapsid gene of vesicular stomatitis virus RNA. J Virol 33:789–794
Keir HM, Gold E (1963) Deoxyribonucleic acid nucleotidyl transferase and deoxyribonuclease from cultured cells infected with herpes simplex virus. Biochim Biophys Acta
72:263–276
Kendall AP (1975) A comparison of "influenza C" with prototype myxoviruses: receptor
destroying activity (neuraminidase) and structural polypeptides. Virology 65:87–99
Kennedy DA, Johnson-Lussenburg CM (1978) Inhibition of coronavirus 229E replication
by actinomycin D. J Virol 29:401–404
Kew OM, Pallansch MA, Omilianowski DR, Reukert RR (1980) Changes in three of the
four coat proteins of oral polio vaccine strain derived from type 1 poliovirus. J Virol
33:256–263
Kieff ED, Bachenheimer SL, Roizman B (1971) Size, composition, and structure of the
deoxyribonucleic acid of subtypes 1 and 2 herpes simplex virus. J Virol 8:125–132
Kilbourne ED (1968) Recombination of influenza A viruses of human and animal origin.
Science 160:74–75
Kolakofsky D, Brutschi A (1975) Antigenomes in Sendai virions and Sendai virusinfected
cells. Virology 66:185–191

Kolakosky D, Boy de la Tour E, Delius H (1975) Molecular weight determinations of parainfluenza virus RNA. In: Mahy BWJ, Barry RD (eds) Negative stand viruses, vol 1. Academic Press, London, pp 243–251

Kozak M, Roizman B (1974) RNA synthesis in cells infected with herpes simplex virus IX. Evidence for accumulation of abundant symmetric transcripts in nuclei. J Virol 15:36–40

Koziorowska J, Wlodarski K, Mazurowa N (1971) Transformation of mouse embryo cells by vaccinia virus. J Natl Cancer Inst 26:225

Kress S, Schluederberg AE, Horrick RB, Morse LJ, Cole JL, Slater EA, McCrumb FR (1961) Studies with live attenuated measles vaccine II. Clinical and immunological response of children in an open community. Am J Dis Child

Krugman S, Giles JP (1973) Viral hepatitis type B (MS-2 strain). Further observations on natural history and prevention. N Engl J Med 288:755–760

Krugman S, Giles JP, Hammond J, (1967) Infectious hepatitis: evidence for two distinct clinical, epidemiological, and immunological types of infection. JAMA 200:365

La Colla P, Weissbach A (1975) Vaccinia virus infection of HeLa cells. I. Synthesis of vaccinia DNA in host cell nuclei. J Virol 15:305–315

Lai MMC, Duesberg PH (1972) Adenylic acid-rich sequence in RNAs of Rous sarcoma virus and Rauscher mouse leukemia virus. Nature 235:383–386

Lai MC, Stohlman SA (1978) RNA of mouse hepatitis virus. J Virol 26:236–242

Lamb RA, Choppin PW (1979) Segment of the influenza virus genome is unique in coding for two polypeptides. Proc Natl Acad Sci USA 76:4908–4912

Lavail JH, Lavail MM (1972) Retrograde axonal transport in the central nervous system. Science 176:146–147

Laver WG (1970) Isolation of an arginine-rich protein from particles of adenovirus type 2. Virology 41:488–496

Laver WG, Downie JL (1976) Influenza virus recombination. I. Matrix protein markers and segregation during mixed infections. Virology 70:105–117

Laver WG, Webster RG (1973) Studies on the origin of pandemic influenza. III. Evidence implicating duck and equine influenza viruses as possible progenitors of the Hong Kong strain of human influenza. Virology 51:383–391

Laver WG, Webster RG (1979) Ecology of influenza viruses in lower mammals and birds. Br Med Bull 35:29–33

Lee YF, Nomoto A, Detjen BM, Wimmer E (1977) A protein covalently linked to the poliovirus genome RNA. Proc Natl Acad Sci USA 74:59–63

Leifer E, Gocke DJ, Bourne H (1970) Lassa fever, a new virus disease of man from West Africa. II. Report of a laboratory-acquired infection treated with plasma from a person recently recovered from the disease. Am J Trop Med Hyg 19:677–679

Lemon SM, Hutt LM, Shaw JE, Li J-LH, Pagano JS (1977) Replication of EBV in epithelial cells during infectious mononucleosis. Nature 268:268–270

Lenard J, Compans RW (1975) Polypeptide composition of incomplete influenza virus grown in MDBK cells. Virology 65:418–426

Levine AJ, Ginsberg HS (1967) Mechanism by which fiber antigen inhibits multiplication of type 5 adenovirus. J Virol 1:747

Levinson AD, Opperman H, Levintow L, Varmus HE, Bishop JM (1978) Evidence that the transforming gene of avian sarcoma virus encodes a protein kinase associated with a phosphoprotein. Cell 15:561–572

Lewis JB, Atkins J, Baum PR, Solem R, Gesteland R, Anderson CW (1976) Location and identification of the genes for adenovirus type 2 early polypeptides. Cell 7:141–151

Lindahl T, Adams A, Bjursell G, Bornkamm GW, Kaschka-Dierich C, Jehn U (1976) Covalently closed circular duplex DNA of Epstein-Barr virus in a human lymphoid cell line. J Mol Biol 102:511–530

Lodmell DL, Niwa A, Hayashi K, Notkins A (1973) Prevention of cell-to-cell spread of herpes simplex virus by leukocytes. J Exp Med 137:706–720

Lomniczi B, Kennedy L (1977) Genome of infectious bronchitis virus. J Virol 24:99–107

Lonsdale DM, Brown SM, Subak-Sharpe JH, Warren KG, Koprowski H (1979) The polypeptide and DNA restriction enzyme profiles of spontaneous isolates of HSV-1 from explants of human trigemial superior cervical and vagus ganglia. J Gen Virol 43:151–171

Lucas A, Coulter M, Anderson R, Dales S, Flintoff W (1978) In vivo and in vitro modes of demyelinating diseases. II. Persistence and host-regulated thermosensitivity in cells of neural derivation infected with mouse hepatitis and measles virus. Virology 88:325–337

Mackenzie RB (1965) Epidemiology of Machupo virus infection. I. Patterns of human infection, San Joaquźn, Bolivia, 1962–1964. Am J Trop Med Hyg 14:808–813

Macnab JCM (1974) Transformation of rat embryo cells by temperature sensitive mutants of HSV. J Gen Virol 24:143–153

MacNaughton MR, Madge MH (1977) The characterization of the virion RNA of avian infectious bronchitis virus. FEBS Lett 77:311–313

Madeley CR (1978) Virus morphology. Churchill Livingstone, Edinburgh London

Maizel JV, White DD, Scharff MD (1968) The polypeptides of adenovirus: evidence for multiple protein components in the virion and a comparison of types 2, 7A, & 12. Virology 36:115–125

Mak I, Ezoe U, Mak S (1979) Structure and function of adenovirus type 12 defective virions. J Virol 32:240–250

Mak S (1971) Defective virions in human adenovirus type 12. J Virol 7:426–433

Malluci L (1965) Observations on the growth of mouse hepatitis virus (MHV-3) in mouse macrophages. Virology 25:30–37

Mandell GL, Douglas RG, Bennett JE (1979) Lymphocytic choriomeningitis virus, Lassa virus, and the Tacarihe group of virus. In: Fraser DW (ed) Principles and practice of infectious disease. John Wiley and Sons, New York, pp 1231–1239

Marchette HJ, Halstead SB, O'Rourke T, Scott R, Bancroft WH, Vanapruks V (1979) Effect of immune status on Dengue 2 virus replication in cultured leukocytes from infants and children. Infact Immun 24:47–50

Marion PL, Salazar FH, Alexander JJ, Robinson WS (1980) State of hepatitis B viral DNA in a human hepatoma cell line. J Virol 38:795–806

Markey JK, Word WSM, Rigden P, Green M (1979) Transforming region of group A, B, & C adenoviruses: DNA hemology studies with twenty-nine human adenovirus serotypes. J Virol 29:1056–1064

Marsden HS, Stow ND, Preston VG, Timbury MC, Wilkie NM (1978) Physical mapping of herpes simplex virus-induced polypeptides. J Virol 28:624–642

Martin JD, Frisque RJ, Padgett BL, Walker DL (1979) Restriction endonuclease cleavage map of the DNA of JC virus. J Virol 29:846–855

Marx PA, Porter A, Kingsbury DW (1974) Sendai virion transcriptase complex: polypeptide composition and inhibition by virion envelope proteins. J Virol 13:107–112

Matsumo S, Inouye S, Kono R (1977) Plaque assay of neonatal calf diarrhoea virus and the neutralizing antibody in human sera. J Clin Microbiol 5:1–4

McGeoch DJ, Kitron N (1975) Influenza virion RNA-dependent RNA polymerase: stimulation by guanosine and related compounds. J Virol 15:686

McGeoch DJ, Fellner P, Newton C (1976) Influenza virus genome consists of eight distinct RNA species. Proc Natl Acad Sci USA 73:3045–3049

McIntosh K (1974) Coronaviruses: a comparative review. Curr Top Microbiol Immunol 63:85–129

McIntosh K (1979) Coronaviruses. In: Principles and practice of infectious disease, part 3, chap 103. John Wiley and Sons, New York, pp 1212–1217

McNulty MS (1978) Review article: rotaviruses. J Gen Virol 40:1–18

McNulty MS, Allan GM, Pearson GR, McFerran JB, Curran WL, McCraken RM (1976) Reovirus-like agent (rotavirus) from lambs. Infect Immun 14:1332–1338

Mebus CA, Wyatt RG, Sharpee RL, Sereno MM, Kalica AR, Kapikian AZ, Twiehaus MJ (1976) Diarrhoea in gnotobiotic calves caused by the reoviruslike agent of human infantile gastroenteritis. Infect Immun 14:471–474

Mebus CA, Wyatt RG, Kapikian AZ (1977) Intestinal lesions induced in gnotobiotic calves by the virus of human infantile gastroenteritis. Vet Pathol 14:273–282

Mebus CA, Underdahl NR, Rhodes MB, Twiehaus MJ (1969) Calf diarrhoea (scours): reproduced with a virus from a field outbreak. Univ Nebraska Agric Exp Stat Res Bull 233

Mellon P, Duesberg PH (1977) Subgenomic, cellular Rous sarcoma virus RNAs contain oligonucleotides from the 3' half and the 5' terminus of virion RNA. Nature 270:631–634

Melnick JL (1976) Enteroviruses. In: Evans AS (ed) Viral infection of humans. Plenum, New York

Mettler NE, Petrelli RI, Casals J (1968) Absence of cross-reactions between rubella virus and arbovirus. Virology 36:503–504

Meyer HM, Hilleman MR, Miesse ML, Crawford IP, Bankhead AS (1957) A new antigenic variant in Far East influenza epidemic, 1957. Proc Soc Exp Biol Med 95:609–616

Meyer J, Lundquist RE, Maizel JV Jr (1978) Structural studies of the RNA component of the poliovirus replication complex: II. Characterization by electron microscopy and autoradiography. Virology 85:445–455

Middleton PJ, Holdaway MD, Petric M, Szymanski MT, Tarn JS (1977) Solidphase radioimmunoassay for the detection of rotavirus. Infect Immun 16:439–446

Miller DA, Miller OJ, Vaithilingham GD, Hashmi S, Tantrauahi R, Medrano L, Green H (1974) Human chromosome 19 carries a poliovirus receptor gene. Cell 1:167–173

Millison GC, Hunter GD, Kimberlin RH (1976) Slow virus disease of animals and man. Front Biol 44:243–264

Mims CA (1976) The pathogenesis of influenza. In: Selby P (ed) Influenza virus vaccines and strategy. Proceedings of a working group on pandemic influenza, Rougernent, 26–28 January 1976. Academic Press, London, pp 95–105

Mims CA, Subrahmanyan TP (1966) Immunoflourescence study of the mechanism of resistance to superinfection in mice carrying the lymphocytic choriomeningitis virus. J Pathol Bacteriol 91:403–415

Modlin JF, Brandling-Bennett AD (1974) Surveillance of the congenital rubella syndrome 1969–1973. J Infect Dis 130:316–318

Monath TP (1975) Lassa fever: review of epidemiology and epizootiology. Bull WHO 52:577–592

Monath TP (1979) Flavivirus (St. Louis encephalitis and dengue). In: Mandell G, Douglas RG, Bennett JE (eds) Principles and practice of infectious disease. John Wiley and Sons, New York, p 1248

Monath TP, Casals J (1975) Diagnosis of Lassa fever and the isolation and management of patients. Bull WHO 52:707

Monto AS (1974) Medical reviews, coronavirus. Yale J Biol Med 47:234

Monto AS (1976) Coronaviruses. In: Evans AS (ed) Viral infections of humans. Plenum, New York

Monto AS, Lim SK (1974) The Tecumseh study of respiratory illness. VI. Frequency of and relationship between outbreaks of coronavirus infection. J Infect Dis 129:271–276

Mocarski ES, Stinski MF (1979) Persistence of the cytomegalovirus genome in human cells. J Virol 31:761–775

Morse LS, Pereira L, Roizman B, Schaffer PA (1978) Anatomy of herpes simplex virus (HSV) DNA. X. Mapping of viral genes by analysis of polypeptides and functions specified by HSV1 X HSV2 recombinants. J Virol 26:389–410

Moss B (1974) Reproduction of poxviruses. In: Frankael-Conrat H, Wagner RR (eds) Comprehensive virology, vol 3. Plenum, New York, pp 405–474

Moss B, Gershowitz A, Wei CM, Boone R (1976) Formation of the guanylated and methylated 5'-terminus of vaccinia virus mRNA. Virology 72:341–351

Munyon W, Kraiselbund E, Davies D, Mann J (1971) Transfer of thymidine kinase to thymidine kinase-less cells by infection with ultraviolet-inactivated herpes simplex virus. J Virol 1:813–820

Murphy BL, Maynard JE, Bradley DW, Ebert JW, Mathiesen LR, Purcell RH (1978) Immunofluorescence of hepatitis A virus antigen in chimpanzies. Infect Immun 21:663–665

Murphy FA, Whitfield SG (1975) Morphology and morphogenesis of arenaviruses. Bull WHO 52:409–419

Murphy FA, Whitfield SG, Coleman PH et al. (1968) California group arboviruses: electron microscopic studies. Exp Mol Pathol 9:44–56

Murphy FA, Harrison AK, Whitfield SG (1973) Bunyaviridae: morphologic and morphogenetic similarities of Bunyamwera serologic supergroup viruses and several other arthropod-borne viruses. Intervirology 1:297–316

Murray V, Holliday R (1979) Mechanism for RNA splicing of gene transcripts. FEBS Lett 106:5–7

Nahmias AJ, Roizman B (1973) Infection with herpes simplex virus 1 & 2. N Engl J Med 289:667–674, 719–726, 781–789

Nahmias AJ, Shore SL, Kohl S, Starr SE, Ashman RB (1976) Immunology of herpes simplex virus infections. Cancer Res 36:836–844

Nakajima K, Ueda M, Sugiura A (1979) Origin of small RNA in Von Magnus particles of influenza virus. J Virol 29:1142–1148

Nayak DP, Tobita K, Jander JM, Davis AR, De BK (1978) Homologous interference mediated by defective interfering influenza virus derived from a temperature-sensitive mutant of influenza virus. J Virol 28:375–386

Nevins JR, Darnell JE Jr (1978) Steps in the processing of Ad2 mRNA: poly (A)+ nuclear sequences are conserved and poly (A) addition precedes splicing. Cell 15:1477–1493

Nevins JR, Winkler JJ (1980) Regulation of early adenovirus transcription: a protein product of early region 2 specifically represses region 4 transcription. Proc Natl Acad Sci USA 77:1893–1897

Nevins JR, Ginsberg HS, Blanchard JM, Wilson MC, Darnell JE (1979) Regulation of the primary expression of the early adenovirus transcription units. J Virol 32:727–733

Newman JFE, Rowlands DJ, Brown F (1973) A physico-chemical subgrouping of the mammalian picornaviruses. J Gen Virol 18:171–180

Nichols JL, Bellamy AR, Joklik WK (1973) Identification of the nucleotide sequences of the oligonucleotides present in reovirions. Virology 49:562–572

Niederman JC, McCollum RW, Henle G, Henle W (1968) Infectious mononucleosis: clinical manifestation in relation to EB virus antibodies. JAMA 203:205–209

Nishoka Y, Silverstein S (1977) Degradation of cellular mRNA during infection by herpes simplex virus. Proc Natl Acad Sci USA 74:2370–2374

Niveleau A, Wild TF (1979) In vitro transcription of measles virus-induced RNA. Virology 96:295–298

Nomoto A, Detjen B, Pozzatti R, Wimmer E (1977) The location of the polio genome protein in viral RNAs and its implication for RNA synthesis. Nature 268:208–213

Nonoyama M, Pagano JS (1973) Homology between Epstein-Barr virus DNA and viral DNA from Burkitt's lymphoma and nasopharyngeal carcinoma determined by DNA-DNA reassociation kinetics. Nature 242:44–47

Norby E (1962) Hemagglutination of measles virus. II. Properties of the hemagglutinin and of the receptors on the erythrocytes. Arch Gesamte Virusforsch 12:164–169

Norby E, Gollmar Y (1975) Identification of measles virus-specific hemolysisinhibiting antibodies separate from hemagglutination-inhibiting antibodies. Infect Immun 11:231–239

Obijeski JF, Bishop DHL, Murphy FA, Palmer EL (1976a) Structural proteins of La Crosse virus. J Virol 19:985–997

Obijeski JF, Bishop DHL, Palmer EL, Murphy FA (1976b) Segmented genome and nucleocapsid of La Crosse virus. J Virol 20:664–675

O'Callaghan DJ, Randall CC (1976) Molecular anatomy of herpesviruses: recent studies. Prog Med Virol 22:152–210

Onodera R, Jenson AB, Won Yoon J, Notkins AL (1978) Virus-induced diabetes mellitus: reovirus infection of pancreatic β cells in mice. Science 201:529–531

O'Rear JJ, Mizutani S, Hoffman G, Fiandt M, Temin HM (1980) Infectious and non-infectious recombinant clones of the provirus of SNV differ in cellular DNA and are apparently the same in viral DNA. Cell 20:423–430

Orellana T, Kieff E Epstein-Barr virus specific RNA. II. Analysis of polyadenylated viral RNA in restringent, abortive, and productive infections. J Virol 22:321–330

Padgett BL, Zu Rhein GM, Walker DL, Eckroade RJ, Dessel BH (1971) Cultivation of papova-like virus from human brain with progressive multifocal leukoencephalopathy. Lancet 1:1257–1260

Pagano JS (1975) Latency and cellular transformation. J Infect Dis 132:209–223

Palese P, Ritchey MB (1977) Live attenuated influenza virus vaccines: strains with temperature-sensitive defects in P3 protein and neuraminidase. Virology 78:183–191

Palese P, Shulman JL (1976) Differences of RNA patterns of influenza A virus. J Virol 17:876–884

Palese P, Tobita K, Ueda M, Compans RW (1974) Characterization of temperaturesensitive influenza virus mutants defective in neuraminidase. Virology 61:397–410

Palese P, Schulman JL, Ritchey MD (1978) Influenza virus genes: characterisation and biologic activity. Perspect Virol 10:57–71

Palmenberg AC, Pallansch MA, Reuckert RR (1979) Protease required for processing picornaviral core protein resides in the viral replicase gene. J Virol 32:770–779

Panem S, Prochonik EV, Reale FR, Kirsten WH (1975) Isolation of type C virions from a normal human fibroblast strain. Science 189:297–299

Paoletti E, Grady LJ (1977) Transcriptional complexity of vaccinia virus in vivo and in vitro. J Virol 23:608–615

Paoletti E, Lipinskas BR, Paricali D (1980) Capped and adenylated low-molecular weight RNA synthesized by vaccinia virus in vitro. J Virol 33:208–219

Parry HH (1960) Scrapie: a transmissible hereditary disease of sheep. Nature 185:441–443

Pasek M, Goto T, Gilbert W et al. (1979) Hepatitis B virus genes and their expression in E. coli. Nature 282:575–579

Pattison IH, Hoan WN, Jebbet JN, Watson WA (1977) Spread of scrapie to sheep and goats by oral dosing with fetal membranes from scrapie-affected sheep. Vet Rec 90:465–468

Payne L (1979) Identification of the vaccinia hemagglutinin polypeptide from a cell system yielding large amounts of extracellular enveloped virus. J Virol 31:147–155

Payne L, Kristensson K (1979) Mechanism of vaccinia virus release and its specific inhibition by N_1-Isoicotinoyl-N_2-3-Methyl-4-chlorobenzoylhydrazine. J Virol 32:614–622

Pearson GR, Orr TW (1976) Antibody-dependent lymphocyte cytotoxicity against cells expressing Epstein-Barr virus antigens. J Natl Cancer Inst 56:485–488

Pennington TH, Follett EAC (1974) Vaccinia virus replication in BSC-I cells: particle production and synthesis of viral DNA and proteins. J Virol 13:488–493

Penttinen K, Cantell K, Soner P, Poikolainen A (1968) Mumps vaccine in the Finnish defense forces. Am J Epidemiol 88:234–299

Pereira HG, Wrigley NG (1974) In vitro reconstruction, hexon bonding, and handedeness of incomplete adenovirus capsid. J Mol Biol 85:617–631

Perez-Bercoff R (1979) Molecular biology of the picornaviruses. Plenum, New York

Perrault J, Leavitt RW (1977) Inverted complementary terminal sequences in singlestranded RNAs and snap-back RNAs from vesicular stomatitis defective interferring particles. J Gen Virol 38:35–50

Petri T, Meier-Ewert T, Crumpton T, Dimmock NJ (1979) RNA of influenza C virus strains. Arch Virol 61:239–243

Pettersson RF, Hewlett MJ, Baltimore D, Coffin JM (1977) The genome of Uukuniemi virus consists of three unique RNA segments. Cell 11:51–63

Pfefferkorn ER (1977) Genetics of togaviruses. In: Fraenkel-Conrat H, Wagner R (eds) Comprehensive virology, vol 9. Plenum, New York, pp 209–238

Pfefferkorn ER, Shapiro D (1974) Reproduction of togaviruses. In: Fraenkel-Conrat H, Wagner RR (eds) Comprehensive virology, vol 2. Plenum, New York, pp 171–230

Philip RN, Reinhard KR, Lackman DB (1959) Observations on a mumps epidemic in a "virgin" population. Am J Hyg 69:91–111

Pierce WE, Rosenbaum MJ, Edwards EA, Perkinpaugh RO, Jackson GG (1968) Outbreak of febrile pharyngitis and conjunctivitis associated with type 3 adenoidal-pharyngeal-conjunctival virus infection. Am J Epidemiol 87:237–246

Pons MW (1976) A re-examination of influenza single- and double-stranded RNAs by gel electrophoresis. Virology 69:789–792

Pons MW, Rochovansky OM (1979) Ultraviolet inactivation of influenza virus RNA in vitro and in vivo. Virology 97:183–189

Porter DD, Porter HG, Cox NA (1973) Failure to demonstrate a humoral immune response to scrapie infection in mice. J Immunol 111:1407–1410

Porter A, Marx PA, Kingsbury DW (1974) Isolation and characterization of Sendai virus temperature sensitive mutants. J Virol 13:298–304

Porterfield JS, Casals J, Chumakov MP et al. (1976) Bunyaviruses and Bunyaviridae. Intervirology 6:12–24

Powell KL, Purifoy DJM, Courtney RJ (1975) The synthesis of herpes simplex virus proteins in the absence of virus DNA synthesis. Biochem Biophys Res Commun 66:262–271

Purifoy DJM, Powell KL (1977) Non-structural proteins of herpes simplex virus 1. Purification of the induced DNA polymerase. J Virol 24:618–626

Preston CM (1979) Abnormal properties of an immediate early polypeptide in cells infected with herpes simplex virus type 1 mutant ts K. J Virol 32:357–369

Preston VG, Davison AJ, Marsden HS, Timbury MC, Subak-Sharpe JH, Wilkie NM (1978) Recombinants between herpes simplex virus types 1 & 2: analyses of genome structures and expression of immediate early polypeptides. J Virol 28:499–517

Prince AM, Szmuness W, Mann MK et al. (1978) Hepatitis B immune globulin: final report of a controlled multicenter trial of efficacy in prevention of dialysis-associated hepatitis. J Infect Dis 137:131–144

Pringle CR (1977) Genetics of rhabdoviruses. In: Fraenkel-Conrat H, Wagner RR (eds) Comprehensive virology, vol 9. Plenum, New York, p 239

Pritchett RF, Hayward SD, Kieff ED (1975) DNA of Epstein-Barr virus. I. Comparative studies of the DNA of Epstein-Barr virus from HR-1 and B95-8 cells: size, structure, and relatedness. J Virol 15:556–569

Purifoy DJM, Purifoy JA, Sagik BP (1968) A mathematical analysis of concomitant virus replication and heat inactivation. J Virol 2:275–280

Purtilo DT (1976) Pathogenesis and phenotypes of an X-linked recessive proliferative syndrome. Lancet 2:882–885

Purtilo DT, De Florio D, Hutt LM, Bhawan J, Yang JPS, Otto R, Edwards W (1977) Variable phenotypic expression of an X-linked recessive lymphoproliferative syndrome. N Engl J Med 297:1077–1081

Rabinowitz SG, Dal Canto MC, Johnson TC (1976) Comparison of central nervous system disease produced by wild-type and temperature-sensitive mutants of vesicular stomatitis virus. Infect Immun 13:1242–1249

Racaniello VR, Palese P (1979) Influenza B virus genome: assignment of viral polypeptides to RNA segments. J Virol 29:361

Ramos BA, Courtney RJ, Rawls WE (1972) Structural proteins of Pichinde virus. J Virol 10:661–667

Reed JS, Boyer JL (1979) Viral hepatitis: epidemiologic, serologic, and clinical manifestations. DM 25:1–61

Rekosh DMK, Russell WC, Bellett ADJ, Robinson AJ (1977) Identification of a protein linked to the ends of adenovirus DNA. Cell 11:283–295

Rhodes AJ, Van Rooyen CE (1968) Textbook of virology, 5th edn, chap 3, sect 6. Williams & Wilkins, Baltimore

Richards JC, Hyman RW, Rapp F (1979) Analysis of DNAs from seven varicellazoster virus isolates. J Virol 32:812–821

Ritchey MB, Palese P (1977) Identification of the defective gene in three mutant groups of influenza virus. J Virol 21:1196–1204

Roa RC, Bose SK (1974) Inhibition by ethidium bromide of the establishment of infection by murine sarcoma virus. J Gen Virol 25:197–205

Rodger SM, Schnagl RD, Holmes IH (1977) Further biochemical characterization including the detection of surface glycoproteins of human, calf and Simian rota viruses. J Virol 29:91–98

Roizman B (1979) The organization of the herpes simplex virus genomes. Annu Rev Genet 13:25–57

Roizman B, Kieff ED (1974) Herpes simplex and Epstein-Barr viruses in human cells and tissues: a study in contrasts. In: Becker FF (ed) Cancer: a comprehensive treatise. Plenum, New York

Roizman B, Hayward G, Jacob R, Wadsworth S, Frenkel N, Honess RW, Kozak M (1975) Human herpesviruses. I. A model for molecular organization and regulation of herpesviruses – a review. IARC Sci Publ 2:3–38

Rosenberg N, Baltimore D (1976) In vitro lymphoid cell transformation by Abelson murine leukemia virus, ICN-UCLA Symp Mol Cell Biol 4:311–320

Ross J, Tronick SR, Scolnick EM (1972) Polyadenylate-rich RNA in the 7OS RNA of murine leukemia-sarcoma virus. Virology 49:230–235

Rübsamen H, Friis RR, Bauer H (1979) "Src" gene product from different strains of avian sarcoma virus: kinetics and possible mechanisms of heat inactivation of protein kinase activity from cell infected by transformation-defective, temperature-sensitive mutants, and wild-type virus. Proc Natl Acad Sci USA 76:967–971

Reuckert RR (1976) On the structure and morphogenesis of picornaviruses. In: Fraenkel-Conrat H, Wagner RR (eds) Comprehensive virology, vol 6. Plenum, New York, pp 131–213

Reuckert RR, Dunker AK, Stoltzfus CM (1969) The structure of the Maus-Elbertcell virus: a model. Proc Natl Acad Sci USA 62:912–919

Russell PK (1979a) Alphavirus (Eastern, Western, and Venezuelan equine encephalitis. In: Mandell A, Douglas RA, Bennett JE (eds) Infectious diseases. John Wiley and Sons, New York, pp 1243–1248

Russell PK (1979b) California encephalitis and other Bunyaviruses. In: Principles and practice of infectious disease, vol 2. John Wiley and Sons, New York, pp 1239–1241

Russell WC, Skehel JJ, Marchado R, Pereira HG (1972) Phosphorylated polypeptides in adenovirus-infected cells. Virology 50:931–934

Rymo L, Forsblum S (1978) Cleavage of Epstein-Barr virus DNA by restriction endonucleases Eco R1, Hind III, Bam. 1. Nucleic Acid Res 5:1387–1402

Sambrook J (1977) The molecular biology of the papovaviruses. In: Nayak P (ed) The molecular biology of animal viruses, vol 2, chap II. Dekker, New York

Sangar DV (1979) Replication of picornaviruses. J Gen Virol 45:1–13

Sangar DV, Rowlands DJ, Cavanagh D, Brown F (1976) Characteristics of the minor polypeptides of foot and mouth disease virus particles. J Gen Virol 31:3546

Sattler F, Robinson WS (1979) Hepatitis B viral DNA molecules have cohesive ends. J Virol 32:226–233

Sawyer RN, Evans AS, Niederman JC, McCollum RW (1971) Prospective studies of a group of Yale University freshmen. I. Occurrence of infectious mononucleosis. J Infect Dis 123:263–269

Scheid A, Choppin PW (1977) Two disulfide-linked polypeptide chains constitute the active F protein of paramyxoviruses. Virology 80:56–66

Schlesinger MJ, Schlesinger S, Burge BW (1972) Identification of a second glycoprotein in Sindbis virus. Virology 47:539–541

Schlesinger S, Schlesinger MJ, Burge BW (1972) Defective virus particles from Sindbis virus. Virology 48:615–617

Schochetman G, Stevens RH, Simpson RW (1977) Presence of infectious polyadenylated RNA in the coronavirus avian infectious bronchitis virus. Virology 77:771–782

Schooley RT, Dolin R (1979) Epstein-Barr virus (infectious mononucleosis). In: Mandell G, Douglas RG, Bennet JE (eds) Principles and practice of infectious diseases. John Wiley and Sons, New York

Scolnick EM, Rands E, Williams D, Parks WP (1973) Studies on the nucleic acid sequences of Kirsten sarcoma virus: A model for formation of a mammalian RNA-containing sarcoma virus. J Virol 12:458–463

Seeff CB, Wright EZ, Zimmerman HK et al. (1980) Type B hepatitis after needle stick exposure. Prevention with hepatitis B immune globulin. Ann Intern Med 88:220–229

Sefton BM, Hunter T, Beemon K (1980) Temperature-sensitive transformation by Rous sarcoma virus and temperature-sensitive protein kinase activity. J Virol 33:220–229

Spencer DJ, Hull HB, Longview AD (1967) Epidemiological basis for eradication of measles in 1967. Public Health Rep 82:1253–1256

Sharp PA, Moore C, Havarty JL (1976) The infectivity of adenovirus 5 DNA-protein complex. Virology 75:442–456

Shatkin AJ (1974) Methylated messenger RNA synthesis in vitro by purified reovirus. Proc Natl Acad Sci USA 71:3204–3207

Shatkin AJ (1976) Capping of eukaryotic mRNAs. Cell 9:645–653

Shatkin AJ, Banerjee AK, Both GW (1977) Translation of animal virus mRNAs in vitro. In: Comprehensive virology, vol 10, chap 1. Plenum, New York

Sheldon PJ, Papamichail M, Hemsted EH, Holborrow EJ (1973) Thymic origin of atypical lymphoid cells in infectious mononucleosis. Lancet 1:1153–1155

Sheldrick P, Berthelot N (1974) Inverted repititions in the chromosome of herpes simplex virus. Cold Spring Harbor Symp Quant Biol 39:667–678

Shenk TE, Stollar V (1973a) Defective interfering particles of Sindbis virus. I. Isolation and some chemical and biological properties. Virology 53:162–173

Shenk TE, Stollar V (1973b) Defective interfering particles of Sindbis virus. II. Homologous interference. Virology 55:530–534

Shi JWK, Gerin JL (1977) Proteins of hepatitis B surface antigen. J Virol 21:347

Shimotohno K, Mizutani S, Temin H (1980) Sequence of retrovirus provirus resembles that of bacterial transposable elements. Nature 285:550–554

Shiroki K, Shimojo H (1974) Analysis of adenovirus 12 temperature-sensitive mutants defective in viral DNA replication. Virology 61:474–479

Siakotos AN, Gadjusek DC, Gibbs CJ Jr, Traub RD, Bucana C (1976) Partial purification of the scrapie agent from mouse brain by pressure disruption and zonal centrifugation in sucrose-sodium chloride gradients. Virology 70:230–237

Siddiqui A, Sattler F, Robinson WS (1979) Restriction endonuclease cleavage map and location of unique features of the DNA of hepatitis B virus, subtype adw$_2$. Proc Natl Acad Sci USA 76:4664–4668

Siegl G, Frosner GG (1978) Characterization and classification of virus particles associated with hepatitis A 11. Type and configuration of nucleic acid. J Virol 26:48–53

Silverstein SC, Dale S (1968) The penetration of reovirus RNA and initiation of its genetic function in L-strain fibroblasts. J Cell Biol 36:197–230

Silverstein SC, Schonberg M, Levin DH, Acs G (1970) The reovirus replicative cycle: conservation of parental RNA and protein. Proc Natl Acad Sci USA 67:275–281

Simons K, Keranen S, Kaariainen L (1973) Identification of a precursor for one of the Semliki Forest virus membrane proteins. FEBS Lett 29:87–91

Simpson RW, Houser RE, Dales S (1969) Viropexis of vesicular stomatitis virus by L cells. Virology 37:285–290

Skehel JJ, Hay AJ (1978) Review article: influenza virus transcription. J Gen Virol 39:1–8

Skehel JJ, Joklik WK (1969) Studies on in vitro transcription of reovirus RNA catalyzed by reovirus cores. Virology 39:822–831

Skup D, Millward M (1980) mRNA capping enzymes are masked in reovirus progeny subviral particles. J Virol 34:490–496

Spear PG (1976) Membrane proteins specified by herpes simplex viruses. 1. Identification of four. J Virol 17:991–1008

Spooner LLR, Barry RD (1977) Participation of DNA-dependent RNA polymerase II in replication of influenza viruses. Nature 268:650–652

Stair EL, Rhodes MB, White RG, Mebus CA (1972) Neonatal calf diarrhea: purification and electron microscopy of a coronavirus-like agent. Am J Vet Res 33:1147–1156

Stallcup K, Wechsler S, Fields B (1979) Purification of measles virus and characterization of subviral components. J Virol 30:166–176

Stanley ED, Jackson GG (1969) Spread of enteric live adenovirus type 4 vaccine in married couples. J Infect Dis 119:51–59

Stannard LM, Schoub BD (1977) Observations on the morphology of two rotaviruses. J Gen Virol 37:435–439

Stanners CP, Goldberg VJ (1975) On the mechanism of neurotropism of vesicular stomatitis virus in newborn hamsters. Studies with temperature sensitive mutants. J Gen Virol 29:281–296

Starr JG, Bart RD, Gold E (1970) Inapparent congenital cytomegalovirus infection: clinical and epidemiological characteristics in early infancy. N Engl J Med 202:1075–1077

Stehelin D, Varmus HE, Bishop JM, Vogt PK (1976) DNA related to transforming genes of avian sarcoma viruses is present in normal avian DNA. Nature 250:170–173

Stern DF, Kennedy SIT (1980) Coronavirus multiplication strategy. I. Identification and characterization of virus-specified RNA. J Virol 34:665–674

Stern H, Tucker SM (1973) Prospective study of cytomegalovirus infection in pregnancy. Br Med J 2:268–270

Sternbergh PH, Moat J, Van Ormandt H, Sussenbach J (1977) The nucleotide sequence at the termini of adenovirus type 5 DNA. Nucleic Acid Res 4:4371–4389

Stevens JG (1972) Latent herpes simplex virus in sensory ganglia. Perspect Virol 8:171–188

Stevens JG, Cook ML (1971) Latent herpes simplex virus in spinal ganglia of mice. Science 173:843–845

Stinski MF (1977) Synthesis of protein and glycoproteins in cells infected with human cytomegalovirus. J Virol 23:751–767

Stinski MF (1978) Sequence of protein synthesis in cells infected by human cytomegalovirus: early and late virus-induced polypeptides. J Virol 26:686–701

Stinski MF, Mocarski ES, Thomsen DR (1979) DNA of human cytomegalovirus: size heterogeneity and defectiveness resulting from serial undiluted passage. J Virol 31:231–239

Stoltzfus CM, Banerjee AK (1972) Two oligonucleotide classes of single-stranded ribopolymers in reovirus A-rich RNA. Arch Biochem Biophys 152:733–743

Stoltzfus CM, Shatkin AJ, Banerjee AK (1973) Absence of polyadenylic acid from reovirus messenger ribonuclei acid. J Biol Chem 248:7993–7998

Straus SE, Aulakh SA, Ruyechan WT, Hay J, Vande Woude GF, Owens J, Smith HA (1981) Structural studies of varicella zoster virus DNA. J Virol

Strode GK (ed) (1951) Yellow fever. McGraw-Hill, New York

Stuart-Harris CH (1965) Influenza and other virus infections of the upper respiratory tract. Williams & Wilkins, Baltimore, pp 8–21

Stuart-Harris CH (1979) The influenza viruses and the human respiratory tract. Rev Infect Dis 1:592–599

Sturman LS (1977) Characterization of a coronavirus. I. Structural protein: effect of preparative conditions on the migration of protein in polyacrylamide gels. Virology 77:637–649

Sturman LS, Holmes KV (1977) Characterization of a coronavirus II. Glycoproteins of the viral envelope: tryptic peptide analysis. Virology 77:650–660

Sturman LS, Holmes KV, Behnke J (1980) Isolation of coronavirus envelope glycoproteins and interaction with the viral nucleocapsid. J Virol 33:449–462

Summers D, Maizel J (1971) Determination of the gene sequence of poliovirus with pactamycin. Proc Natl Acad Sci USA 59:966–971

Summers J, Smolec JM, Snyder R (1978) A virus similar to human hepatitis B virus associated with hepatitis and hepatoma in woodchucks. Proc Natl Acad Sci USA 75:4533–4537

Surina DWR, Bank JL, Ackerman A (1970) Role of measles in skin lesions and koplik spots. N Engl J Med 283:1139–1142

Sussenbach JS (1967) Early events in the infectious process of adenovirus type 5 in Hela cells. Virology 33:567–576

Swanstrom RI, Wagner EK (1974) Regulation of synthesis of herpes simplex type 1 virus mRNA during productive infection. Virology 60:522–533

Sweet C, Smith H (1980) Pathogenicity of influenza virus. Microbiol Rev 44:303–330

Szmuness W (1978) Hepatocellular carcinoma and the hepatitis B virus: evidence for a casual association. Prog Med Virol 29:40–65

Takahaski K, Akahane T, Gotarda T, Mishiro M, Imai Y, Mitakawa Y, Mayumi M (1979) Demonstration of hepatitis B_e antigen in the core of dane particles. J Immunol 122:272–279

Takano T, Hatanaka M (1975) Fate of viral RNA of murine leukemia virus after infection. Proc Natl Acad Sci USA 72:343–347

Tanaka S, Ihara S, Watanabe Y (1978) Human cytomegalovirus induces DNA-dependent RNA polymerases in human diploid cells. Virology 89:179–185

Tannock GA (1973) The nucleic acid of infectious bronchitis virus. Arch Gesamte Virusforsch 43:259–271

Temin HM (1964) The participation of DNA in Rous sarcoma virus production. Virology 20:577–582

Temin HM, Mizutani S (1970) RNA-dependent DNA polymerase in virions of Rous sarcoma virus. Nature 226:1211–1213

Theil WK, Boli EH, Agnes AG (1977) Cell culture propagation of porcine rotavirus (reovirus-like agent). Am J Vet Res 38:1765–1768

Thomas-Powell AL, King W, Kieff E (1979) Epstein-Barr virus specific RNA. III. Mapping of DNA encoding viral RNA in restringent infection. J Virol 29:261–274

Thouless ME, Bryden AS, Flewett TH (1978) Serotypes of human rotavirus. Lancet 1:39

Tibbetts C, Giam C-Z (1979) In vitro association of empty adenovirus capsids with double-stranded DNA. J Virol 32:995–1005

Tighor GH, Shope RE, Gershon RK, Waksman BH (1974) Immunopathologic aspects of infection with Lagos bat virus of the rabies serogroup. J Immunol 112:260–265

Tsipis JE, Bratt MA (1976) Isolation and characterization of temperature sensitive mutants of Newcastle disease virus. J Virol 18:848–855

Thyrrell DAJ, Bynoe ML (1965) Cultivation of a novel type of common cold virus in organ cultures. Br Med J 1:1467–1470

Thyrrell DAJ, Almeida JD, Berry DM et al. (1968a) Coronaviruses. Nature 220:650

Tyrrell DAJ, Bynoe ML, Hoorn B (1968b) Cultivation of "difficult" viruses from patients with common colds. Br Med J 1:606–610

Tyrrell DLJ, Norby E (1978) Structural polypeptides of measles virus. J Gen Virol 39:219–229

Van der Vliet PC, Levine AJ (1973) DNA-binding proteins specific for cells infected with adenovirus. Nature New Biol 246:170–174

Ventura AK, Scherer WF (1970) Different effects of deoxycholate, ether, chloroform, hydrocarbons, acid alcohols on Venezuelan encephalitis viral infection, hemagglutination, and complement fixation. Proc Soc Exp Biol Med 133:711–717

Vezza AC, Bishop DHL (1977) Recombination between temperature-sensitive mutants of the arenavirus pichinde. J Virol 24:712–715

Vezza AC, Clewley JP, Gard GP, Abraham NZ, Compans RW, Bishop DHL (1978) Virion RNA species of the arenaviruses Pichinde, Tacaribe, and Tamiami. J Virol 26:485–497

Von Magnus P (1954) Incomplete forms of influenza virus. Adv Virus Res 2:59–78

Wagner EK, Roizman B (1969a) RNA synthesis in cells infected with herpes simplex virus 11. Evidence that a class of viral mRNA is derived from a high molecular weight precursor synthesized in the nucleus. Proc Natl Acad Sci USA 64:626–633

Wagner EK, Roizman B (1969b) Ribonucleic acid synthesis in cells infected with herpes simplex virus. J Virol 4:36–46

Wagner MJ, Summers WC (1978) Structure of the joint region of termini of the DNA of herpes simplex virus. J Virol 27:379–387

Walker DL, Padgett BL, Zu Rhein GM, Albert AE, Marsh RF (1973) Human papovavirus (JC): induction of brain tumors in hamsters. Science 181:674–676

Wechsler SL, Rustigian R, Stallcup KC, Byers KB, Winston SH, Fields BN (1979) Measles virus – specified polypeptide synthesis in two persistently infected Hela cell lines. J Virol 31:677–684

Wege H, Müller A, Ter Meulen V (1978) Genomic RNA of murine coronavirus JHM. J Gen Virol 41:217–227

Weiner HL, Drayna D, Averill DR Jr, Fields BN (1977) Molecular basis of reovirus virulence: role of the S1 gene. Proc Natl Acad Sci USA 74:5744–5748

Weiner HL, Ramig RF, Mustoe TA, Fields BN (1978) Identification of the gene coding for the hemagglutinin of reovirus. Virology 86:581–584

Weiner HL, Powers ML, Fields BN (1980) Absolute linkage of virulence and central nervous system cell tropism of reoviruses to viral hemagglutinin. J Infect Dis 141:609–616

Welsh RM, Pfau CJ (1972) Determinants of lymphocytic chiriomeningitis interference. J Gen Virol 14:177–187

Welsh RM, O'Connell CM, Pfau CJ (1972) Properties of defective lymphocytic choriomeningitis virus. J Gen Virol 17:355–359

Wetz K, Habermehl K-O (1979) Topographical studies on poliovirus capsid proteins by chemical modification and non-linking with bifunctional agents. J Gen Virol 44:525–534

Wiktor TJ, Koprowski H (1974) Rhabdovirus replication in enucleated host cells. J Virol 14:300–306

Wiktor TJ, Gyorgy E, Schlumberger DH, Sokol F, Koprowski H (1973) Antigenic properties of rabies virus components. J Immunol 110:269–276

Wilcox WC, Ginsberg H (1963) Production of specific neutralizing antibody with soluble antigens of type 5 adenovirus. Proc Soc Exp Biol Med 114:37–42

Wildy P (1967) The progression of herpes simplex virus to the central nervous system of the mouse. J Hyg (Lond) 65:173–192

Wilhelm J, Brison O, Kedinger C, Chambon P (1976) Characterization of adenovirus type 2 transcription complexes isolated from infected Hela cells nuclei. J Virol 19:61–82

Wilkie NM (1973) The synthesis and substructure of herpesvirus DNA: the distribution of alkali-labile single-strand interruptions in HSV-1 DNA. J Gen Virol 21:453–467

Williams JF, Young CSH, Austin P (1974) Genetic analysis of human adenovirus type 5 in permissive and non-permissive cells. Cold Spring Harbor Symp Quant Biol 39:427

Winnaker EL (1978) Adenovirus DNA: structure and function of a novel replicon. Cell 14:761–773

Wolf H, Zur Hausen H, Becker V (1973) Epstein-Barr viral genomes in epithelial nasopharyngeal carcinoma cells. Nature New Biol 244:245–247

Woodward CG, Smith H (1975) Production of defective interfering virus in the brains of mice by an avirulent, in contrast with a virulent, strain of Semliki Forest virus. Br J Exp Pathol 56:363–372

Woode GN, Bridges JC, Jones JM, Flewett TH, Bryden AS, Davies HA, White GBB (1976) Morphological and antigenic relationships between viruses (rotaviruses) from acute gastroenteritis of children, calves, piglets, mice, and foals. Infect Immun 14:804–810

Wright DH (1972) The pathology of Burkitt's lymphoma. IARC Sci Publ 2

Yamanishi K, Rapp F (1979) Induction of host DNA synthesis and DNA polymerase by DNA negative temperature-sensitive mutants of human cytomegalovirus. Virology 94:237–241

Yanagi K, Talavera A, Nishimoto T, Rush MG (1978) Inhibition of herpes simplex virus type 1 replication in temperature-sensitive cell cycle mutants. J Virol 25:42–50

Yogo Y, Wimmer E (1973) Poly A and poly U in poliovirus double stranded RNA. Nature New Biol 242:171–174

Youngner JS, Dubovi EJ, Quagliana DO, Kelly M, Preble OT (1976) Role of temperature-sensitive mutants in persistent infections initiated with vesicular stomatitis virus. J Virol 19:90–101

Zarbl H, Skup D, Millward S (1980) Reovirus progeny subviral particles synthesize uncapped mRNA. J Virol 34:497–505

Zif EB, Evans RM (1978) Coincidence of the promoter and capped 5′-terminus of RNA from the adenovirus type 2 major late transcription unit. Cell 15:1463–1475

Ziola BR, Scraba DG (1974) Structure of the mengovirion 1. Polypeptide and ribonucleotide component of the virus particle. Virology 57:531–542

Zuckerman AJ (1976) Twenty-five centuries of viral hepatitis. Rush Presbyt St Lukes Med Bull 15:57

Zur Hausen H, Schulte-Holthausen H, Klein G, Henle W, Henle G, Clifford P, Santesson L (1970) Epstein-Barr viral DNA in biopsies of Burkitts tumors and anaplastic carcinomas of the nasopharynx. Nature 228:1056–1058

Zur Hausen H, Gissman L, Pfister H, Steiner W, Ojwang S (1978) Papilloma virus and squamous-cell carcinomas in man. Perspect Virol 10

Zu Rhein GM (1969) Association of papova virions with a human demyelinating disease (Progressive multifocal leukoencephalopathy). Prog Med Virol 11:185–247

Zweerink HJ, McDowell MJ, Joklik WK (1971) Essential and non-essential noncapsid reovirus proteins. Virology 45:716–723

Zweerink HJ, Ito Y, Matsuhisa T (1972) Synthesis of reovirus double-stranded RNA within virus-like particles. Virology 50:349–358

Part A

CHAPTER 2

Pyrimidine Nucleosides
with Selective Antiviral Activity

P. H. Fischer and W. H. Prusoff

A. Introduction

A high degree of selectivity has now been achieved in experimental viral chemotherapy in both in vitro and in vivo models. A number of "new generation" agents, of which several are pyrimidine nucleosides, can effectively inhibit the replication of herpes simplex viruses with little or no host cell toxicity (Fig. 1). Although the exact mechanisms of action of those compounds may not be fully elucidated, it is clear that their selectivity is dependent on the exploitation of one or more virally specified enzymes. Thus, despite the fact that viruses are obligate parasites, they do code for proteins which are sufficiently different from their host cell counterparts for selective intervention to be possible. In light of the substantial increases in our understanding of the many virally induced enzymes coded for by numerous viruses (KIT 1979), the development of more highly selective antiviral agents seems quite likely.

Even before the advent of these new drugs, it was clear that virus-induced enzymes were important determinants in antiviral therapy (PRUSOFF and GOZ 1973 a). For example, 5-iodo-2'-deoxyuridine (IdUrd), the first agent shown to be effective in an established viral infection in humans (KAUFMAN 1962; KAUFMAN et al. 1962b), is phosphorylated by the thymidine kinase coded for by herpes simplex viruses. The large increase in activity of this enzyme in virally infected cells and the subsequent intracellular trapping of 5-iodo-2'-deoxyuridine monophosphate (IdUMP) accounts for the selectivity of this drug (PRUSOFF and GOZ 1973 a). Of particular importance, however, is the fact that IdUrd is also a substrate for several host cell enzymes, including thymidine kinase. Thus, metabolic activation and the accompanying cytotoxicity could, and indeed does, occur in normal tissues (CALABRESI et al. 1961). The key difference with respect to the new, highly selective agents is that their interactions with critical virally induced enzymes are highly specific or preferential. They may have little or no interaction with the corresponding host cell enzymes. In some cases, the differences are essentially absolute and the activating reaction is catalyzed only by the virus enzyme (CHEN and PRUSOFF 1979). Thus, an important change in antiviral chemotherapy is that selectivity can now be based on qualitative as well as quantitative exploitation of virus-associated enzymatic activities.

In theory, any virus-specific process could be amenable to chemotherapeutic attack. A number of recent reviews have detailed the potential sites (GOZ and PRUSOFF 1970; MITCHELL 1973; PRUSOFF and WARD 1976; SIDWELL and WITKOWSKI 1979). Depending on the nature of the virus, some or all of the following processes could be susceptible to drug intervention: (1) extracellular inactivation; (2) attachment to the host cell; (3) penetration; (4) uncoating; (5) intracellular biosynthetic events; (6) virus assembly; (7) envelopment; and (8) release of mature virus. However, 2-thiouracil, which inhibits viral absorption (Steele and Black 1967), is the only pyrimidine analog known to act at other than an intracellular site. Thus, the virus-associated and induced enzymes involved in nucleoside and nucleotide metabolism, which are the logical targets for these agents, will be emphasized. Kit (1979) in an excellent review, discussed in detail the many enzymes which are known to be virally induced. Numerous investigators have stressed the importance of focusing on these enzymes in the development of selective antiviral agents (Prusoff 1967; Prusoff and Goz 1973 a; Cheng et al. 1975 b; Cheng 1977; Cohen 1977; Oxford 1977; De Clercq and Torrence 1978 a).

Certain virally induced enzymes catalyze reactions which are unique to the virus-infected cell and are also necessary for viral replication. These enzymes are good targets for selective viral chemotherapy. The RNA transcriptases of influenza and parinfluenza viruses, the RNA replicases of the enteroviruses and rhinoviruses, and the reverse transcriptases of the RNA tumor viruses are examples (see Kit 1979 for review).

Another group of virally induced enzymes catalyze reactions that normally occur in uninfected cells. Often these enzymes are sufficiently different from their host cell counterparts for selective intervention to be possible. As previously mentioned, the thymidine kinase induced by certain of the herpesviruses (Kit and Dubbs 1963) is such an enzyme which has proven susceptible to chemotherapeutic exploitation. The herpes simplex encoded DNA polymerase (Keir and Gold 1963) is also in this group of enzymes. The selective antiherpes actions of the phosphonates appear to be mediated through preferential inhibition of the viral polymerase (Mao and Robishaw 1975). The high degree of selectivity of the unusual purine analog, acycloguanosine, also results, in part, from interference with the herpes-induced DNA polymerase (Elion et al. 1977; see Chap. 3). The deoxycytidine deaminase (Chan 1977), DNase (Keir and Gold 1963), and ribonucleotide diphosphate reductase (Cohen 1972) activities associated with herpes simplex virus infection provided other possible sites of intervention.

The thymidine kinase induced by herpes simplex virus requires special attention because it is critical for the activity of so many pyrimidine nucleoside analogs (De Clercq et al. 1977) and since its multifunctionality and broad substrate specificity have been well characterized. The virus-induced thymidine kinase differs from the host cell enzyme in molecular weight, substrate specificity, electrophoretic mobility, isoelectric point, and immunologic properties (see Kit 1979 for a review). The herpes enzyme has a very broad substrate specificity. It catalyzes the phosphorylation of both deoxythymidine (dThd) and deoxycytidine (dCyd; Jamieson et al. 1974; Jamieson and Subak-Sharpe 1974) and interacts with a host of nucleoside analogs (Cheng 1976, 1977; Cheng et al. 1976; Fyfe et al. 1978; Chen and Prusoff 1979). The multifunctional properties of this protein have been extended to include thymidylate kinase activity (Chen and Prusoff 1978), a property not shared by the host thymidine kinase. These unique biochemical properties make this enzyme chemotherapeutically exploitable, a fact which will be reiterated in the discussions of the individual agents.

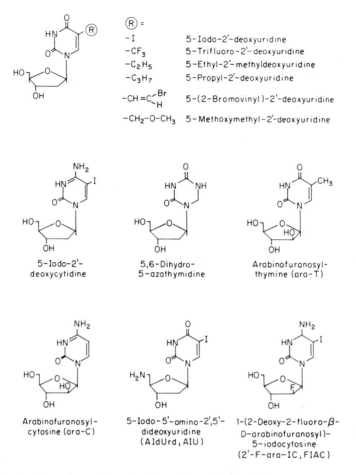

Fig. 1. The structure of several nucleosides with antiviral activity

A number of reviews have recently appeared which deal with various aspects of antiviral chemotherapy (PRUSOFF and WARD 1976; KAUFMAN 1977; DE CLERCQ and TORRANCE 1978; SIDWELL and WITKOWSKI 1979; MÜLLER 1979; DE CLERCQ 1979; PRUSOFF and FISCHER 1979; CHANG and SNYDMAN 1979; SMITH et al. 1980; HERRMANN and HERRMANN 1979). These and other reviews which cover specific agents in more detail will be cited as a further guide to the primary literature.

This discussion will focus on the following aspects of pyrimidine nucleosides which exhibit selective antiviral activity: (1) the biochemical basis of their selectivity; (2) their mechanism of action; and (3) their in vivo effectiveness. The review of the individual agents will be organized according to the position of substitution in the nucleoside. Those analogs with halogen substitutions at the 5 position will be discussed first, followed by other 5-substituted derivatives. Those compounds with an altered pyrimidine ring and those with changes in the carbohydrate moiety will then be presented.

B. 5-Halogenated Pyrimidine 2'-Deoxyribonucleosides

I. 5-Iodo-2'-Deoxyuridine

1. Synthesis

IdUrd was first synthesized by Prusoff (1959) as part of an anticancer program (Welch and Prusoff 1960). The physiochemical and biologic properties of IdUrd have been extensively reviewed (Prusoff 1967; Goz and Prusoff 1970; Sugar and Kaufman 1973; Prusoff and Goz 1975; Langen 1975; Prosoff et al. 1979 a, b). A difference of only 15 pm exists between the van der Waals' radii of iodine and the methyl group, thus the substitution is nearly isosteric. However, the electronic perturbations caused by iodine are significant. The inductive effect of the halogen contributes to a change in the pK_a of dThd from 9.8 to 8.2 for IdUrd (Berens and Shugar 1963).

2. Antiviral Activity

Since IdUrd is a dThd analog, the fact that DNA viruses and those RNA viruses requiring a DNA intermediate are sensitive to its effects is not surprising. Following the initial report of activity against vaccinia virus and herpes simplex virus (Herrmann 1961), the inhibitory effects of IdUrd have been extended to 21 viruses (Prusoff and Goz 1975). Kaufman et al. (1962a) demonstrated the efficacy of IdUrd against herpes keratitis in rabbits and confirmation was soon provided by Perkins et al. (1962). IdUrd has been extensively tested in vivo against many viruses in a number of different hosts. The results have been summarized by Schabel and Montgomery (1972).

IdUrd has been used widely in the treatment of herpes simplex infections of the corneal epithelium in humans. Kaufman (1962) and Kaufman et al. (1962b) first showed that IdUrd was effective in an established virus infection in humans, a breakthrough in antiviral chemotherapy. Reviews of the clinical utility of IdUrd have appeard (Kaufman 1965; Verbov 1979). In addition, Juel-Jenson (1973, 1974) has described the use of IdUrd in a dimethylsulfoxide vehicle for the treatment of numerous viral diseases, including herpetic whitlow, genital herpes, cutaneous herpes, herpes zoster, and vaccinia whitlow. Myelosuppression accompanies the systemic administration of IdUrd (Calabresi et al. 1961) and thus its use in herpes encephalitis is limited (Boston Interhospital Virus Study Group 1975).

3. Effects on Normal Cells

Since IdUrd is metabolized by normal cellular enzymes as well as by virally induced enzymes, it can be toxic to uninfected cells (Prusoff and Goz 1973 a, b). Incorporation of IdUrd into cellular DNA appears to be the critical toxic event (see Goz 1978 for a review). Cells can usually replicate once in the presence of IdUrd, however, there is an associated loss of viability (Mathias et al. 1959). This effect can be prevented by the presence of thymidine in the medium (Mathias and Fischer 1962). Resistance to the 5-halogenated nucleosides can result from a deletion of cellular thymidine kinase activity (Kit et al. 1963). A recent finding indicates that an alteration of the substrate specificity of thymidylate kinase can also account for cellular resistance to IdUrd (KAUFMAN and DAVIDSON 1979). This result suggests that IdUMP is not toxic and that further metabolic activation, presumably to the triphosphate, is required.

4. Mechanism of Action

The metabolism of IdUrd has been extensively detailed by PRUSOFF and GOZ (1975). The metabolic handling of IdUrd and dThd are qualitatively similar in normal and virus-infected cells. However, the induction of thymidine kinase activity by herpes simplex virus increases the phosphorylation of IdUrd and, thereby, traps more metabolites in the virally infected cells. It is this quantitative difference in anabolism which accounts for the antiviral selectivity of IdUrd (PRUSOFF and GOZ 1973a, 1975).

Several of the enzymes involved in the biosynthesis of DNA are inhibited by IdUrd or one of its phosphorylated derivatives. Thymidine kinase, thymidylate kinase, and DNA polymerase are competitively inhibited and utilize the appropriate metabolite as an alternate substrate. Iododeoxyuridine-5′-triphosphate (IdUTP) functions as an allosteric or feedback inhibitor of the regulatory enzymes, thymidine kinase, deoxycytidylate deaminase, and ribonucleoside diphosphate reductase. However, none of these effects accounts for the antiviral activity of IdUrd and it has been proposed that incorporation of the analog into viral DNA was the critical event (PRUSOFF et al. 1965).

Using isolated infectious SV40 DNA, BUETTNER and WERCHAU (1973) showed a relationship between the loss of infectivity and the extent of replacement of thymidine by IdUrd in the viral DNA. Recently, a direct parallelism between the incorporation of IdUrd into viral DNA and the inhibition of herpes simplex virus replication was demonstrated (FISCHER et al. 1980). These results support the importance of the incorporation event, as do the studies of KAPLAN and BEN-PORAT (1966). They found that although pseudorabies viral DNA and viral proteins accumulated in the presence of IdUrd, encapsidation of the DNA did not occur. Their data suggest that biologically inactive proteins were synthesized as a result of IdUrd incorporation into viral DNA. IdUrd inhibited the rate of synthesis of late proteins but not early proteins in adenovirus-2-infected cells (KAN-MITCHELL and PRUSOFF 1979). In this system, the early proteins are translated from mRNA transcribed off parental DNA whereas the mRNA for late proteins is transcribed from progeny DNA which is synthesized in the presence of IdUrd. WIGAND and KLEIN (1974) did not, however, detect IdUrd-induced differences in the physiologic or immunologic characteristics of adenovirus capsid proteins. A marked decrease in the formation of virus-specific SV40 antigens was caused by the presence of IdUrd during virus replication (MAASS and HAAS 1966). These data, taken together with studies on the time course of drug action, strongly implicate the incorporation of IdUrd into viral DNA as the critical event. IdUrd does not appear to inhibit the absorption of herpesviruses to cells or to prevent the release of mature virus particles from infected cells (SMITH 1963; SMITH and DUKES 1964). If the exposure of IdUrd to cells infected with herpes simplex virus is limited to the first 2 h after infection, no inhibitory effects are seen. A 2–4-h exposure causes a dThd-reversible effect, whereas treatment with IdUrd after 4 h results in irreversible inhibition (ROIZMAN et al. 1963).

Thus,although several lines of evidence support the importance of analog incorporation into viral DNA as the most important effect, the molecular mechanism or mechanisms which subsequently lead to the inhibition of viral replication remain to be elucidated. Considerable effort has been directed at this problem and numerous investigations have dealt with a variety of topics,ranging from halogen-induced changes in the stacking energy found in DNA (STERNGLANZ and BUGG 1975) to increases in the binding affinity of the lac repressor to DNA which contained 5-bromo-2′-deoxyuridine (BrdUrd) (LIN and RIGGS 1972). Detailed discussions of the possible molecular mechanisms involved have recently appeared (PRUSOFF and GOZ 1975; GOZ 1978; PRUSOFF et al. 1979 a, b).

II. 5-Trifluoromethyl- 2′-Deoxyuridine

1. Synthesis

5-Trifluoromethyl-2′-deoxyuridine (CF_3dUrd) was synthesized by HEIDELBERGER et al. (1964) as a thymidine analog. The compound, while stable under acidic conditions, undergoes hydrolysis in mildly alkaline conditions to generate the 5-carboxy derivative (HEIDELBERGER et al. 1964). The synthesis, development, and biologic properties of CF_3dUrd and other fluorinated pyrimidines and their nucleosides have recently been reviewed (HEIDELBERGER 1975a, b; HEIDELBERGER and KING 1979).

2. Antiviral Activity

The replication of a number of DNA viruses, including herpes simplex, vaccinia, and adenoviruses, is inhibited by CF_3dUrd in vitro. The compound is quite potent, inhibiting the replication of vaccinia virus in HeLa cells at 10^{-7} M (UMEDA and HEIDELBERGER 1969). The efficacy of CF_3dUrd in the treatment of herpes keratitis in rabbits was demonstrated by KAUFMAN and HEIDELBERGER (1964). In addition, CF_3dUrd was shown to inhibit IdUrd-resistant strains of the virus. It appears that CF_3dUrd is superior to IdUrd and arabinosyladenine for treatment of this disease (SUGAR et al. 1973; PAVAN-LANGSTON 1979). Under conditions of topical administration, which are similar to those used in the treatment of ocular herpes, IdUrd was reported to be teratogenic in pregnant rabbits whereas CF_3dUrd was not (ITOI et al. 1975). CLOUGH and PARKHURST (1977) have shown that CF_3dUrd increases the life span of mice with herpes encephalitis.

In a recent review HEIDELBERGER and KING (1979) concluded that in humans, CF_3dUrd may be the best available drug for the treatment of superficial infections of the eye caused by herpes simplex viruses. Recent studies suggest that CF_3dUrd is quite useful in patients who have previously failed to respond to IdUrd (McGILL et al. 1974; JONES et al. 1975) or to arabinosyladenine (JONES et al. 1975). CF_3dUrd appears equal to or better than arabinosyladenine (McKINNON et al. 1975; COSTER et al. 1976; TRAVERS and PATTERSON 1978) and better than IdUrd (WELLINGS et al. 1972; LAIBSON et al. 1977; PAVAN-LANGSTON and FOSTER 1977) in treatment of superficial herpes infections.

3. Effects on Normal Cells

Although the antiviral effects of CF_3dUrd are of the utmost clinical significance, the compound also possesses anticancer activity (HEIDELBERGER and ANDERSON 1964). A logical consequence of this fact is the likelihood of toxicity upon systemic administration. Since CF_3dUrd is a thymidine analog, its phosphorylation to CF_3dUMP by thymidine kinase (BRESNICK and WILLIAMS 1967) and subsequent incorporation into mammalian cellular DNA was not unexpected (HEIDELBERGER et al. 1965; FUJIWARA and HEIDELBERGER 1970). However, it is inhibition of thymidylate synthetase by CF_3dUMP (REYES and HEIDELBERGER 1965) rather than its incorporation into DNA which appears to account for the cytotoxicity of CF_3dUrd (UMEDA and HEIDELBERGER 1968).

4. Mechanism of Action

Studies on the mechanism of action of the antiviral effect of CF_3dUrd, primarily against vaccinia virus, have been reviewed (HEIDELBERGER 1975a, b; HEIDELBERGER and KING 1979). The metabolism of CF_3dUrd in the virally infected and the host cell appears similar, however, the mechanisms of toxicity are probably different. Preferential incorporation of CF_3dUrd into viral DNA appears to account for its selective antiviral activity (TONE and HEIDELBERGER 1973). The biochemical basis for this difference, at least for vaccinia virus, is at the level of the DNA polymerases. Although both the cellular DNA polymerases were inhibited by 5-trifluoromethyl-2'-deoxyuridine triphosphate (CF_3dUTP), the viral enzyme utilized the nucleotide as an alternative substrate much more efficiently (TONE and HEIDELBERGER 1973).

Several lines of evidence support the idea that incorporation of the analog into viral DNA is the critical event. CF_3dUrd inhibits virus replication most effectively if it is added 1–2 h postinfection (PARKHURST et al. 1976), and dThd can prevent this effect only if it is added before progeny DNA synthesis occurs (UMEDA and HEIDELBERGER 1969). In the presence of CF_3dUrd, noninfectious, morphologically defective vaccinia virions with fragmented viral DNA are produced (FUJIWARA and HEIDELBERGER 1970). The synthesis of late mRNA, but not early mRNA, in cells infected with vaccinia virus is altered by CF_3dUrd (OKI and HEIDELBERGER 1971). The late mRNA, while still synthesized, has about 30% fewer sequences than the late mRNA which is normally transcribed (DEXTER et al. 1973). Although the mechanism of action of CF_3dUrd-induced inhibition of herpes simplex virus has not been elucidated, phosphorylation of the analog by the virally induced thymidine kinase appears necessary (DE CLERCQ et al. 1977).

III. 5-Iodo-2'-Deoxycytidine

1. Synthesis

CHANG and WELCH (1961) synthesized 5-iodo-2'-deoxycytidine (IdCyd) in an effort to decrease the catabolism and increase the stability and solubility of IdUrd. Although this was achieved, IdCyd proved to be less effective than IdUrd as an anticancer agent (CRAMER et al. 1962). The development, biologic properties, and clinical effectiveness of IdCyd have recently been reviewed (PRUSOFF et al. 1979b; MARTENET 1979).

2. Antiviral Activity

IdCyd has been shown to inhibit the replication of herpes simplex virus (Herr-mann 1961; Renis and Buthala 1965; Roux and Mandin 1969), cytomegalovirus (Sidwell et al. 1970), and pseudorabies virus (Renis 1970) in tissue culture. The efficacy of IdCyd in the treatment of herpes keratitis in rabbits (Perkins et al. 1962; Mendez et al. 1971) and its usefulness in deep stromal infections have been report-ed (Mendez and Martenet 1972; Martenet 1975). Greer et al. (1975) were able to show an increased survival rate in mice treated with 5-bromo-2'-deoxycytidine and tetrahydrouridine after intracranial inoculation with herpes simplex virus. Martenet (1979) has reported some clinical success in treating disciform keratitis with IdCyd.

3. Effects on Normal Cells

IdCyd was synthesized as an anticancer agent and, as such, it shows limited activity (Cramer et al. 1962). The fact that IdCyd is a poor substrate for cellular deoxy-cytidine(dCyd) kinase (Cooper and Greer 1973b) and dThd kinase (Bresnick and Thompson 1965) contributes to its relative ineffectiveness. The toxic effects of Id-Cyd are similar to those of IdUrd; alopecia, stomatitis, and hematologic effects (Calabresi et al. 1963), and its metabolism accounts for this similarity. The effects of IdCyd are, in fact, due to IdUrd as a result of the action of cytidine deaminase. Thus, cells which do not have this enzyme activity are resistant to the toxicity of IdCyd whereas cell growth is inhibited by IdCyd when deamination occurs (Schildkraut et al. 1975).

4. Mechanism of Action

Whereas the antiviral activity of IdCyd depends on its metabolic conversion to IdUTP and subsequent incorporation into viral DNA, its selectivity against repli-cating herpes simplex and varicella zoster viruses depends on the induction of a viral pyrimidine nucleoside kinase. As previously mentioned, IdCyd is not a good substrate for cellular deoxycytidine kinase or deoxythymidine kinase. The thy-midine kinases induced by herpes simplex and varicella zoster viruses are, however, capable of efficiently phosphorylating 5-halogenated-2'-deoxycytidine analogs (Cooper 1973; Dobersen et al. 1976; Jerkofsky et al. 1977; Dobersen and Greer 1978; Summers and Summers 1977). In cells infected with these viruses IdCyd is phosphorylated to iododeoxycytidine-5'-monophosphate (IdCMP) and then con-verted to IdUMP by the action of deoxycytidine-5'-monophosphate (dCMP) dea-minase (Maley 1967). After phosphorylation to the di- and triphosphates, IdUMP can be incorporated into DNA. Thus, selective activation of IdCyd can occur, but only if deamination to IdUrd does not occur first. It is this reaction, catalyzed by cytidine deaminase, which can lead to toxicity in uninfected cells. Clinical and phar-macologic studies in humans with IdCyd found that about 85%–95% of an intra-venous dose was deaminated (Calabresi et al. 1963) and similar findings were made by Kriss et al. (1963). Tetrahydrouridine, an inhibitor of cytidine deaminase has been used to reduce the toxicity of deoxycytidine analogs in cells that contain high levels of this enzyme (Cooper and Greer 1973a; Schildkraut et al. 1975).

C. Other 5-Substituted 2′-Deoxyuridine Derivatives

I. 5-Ethyl-2′-Deoxyuridine

1. Antiviral Activity

The synthesis of 5-ethyl-2′-deoxyuridine (EtdUrd), described by GAURI and MALORNY (1967) and by SWIERKOWSKI and SHUGAR (1969), has been shown to inhibit the replication of herpesvirus (GAURI and MALORNY 1967; DE CLERCQ and SHUGAR 1975; CHENG et al. 1976) and vaccinia virus (DE CLERCQ and SHUGAR 1975) in cell culture. This nucleoside is effective in the treatment of herpetic keratitis in rabbits (GAURI and MALORNY 1967; GAURI 1968) and also in deep ocular herpes infections (MARTENET 1975). The mortality associated with herpes simplex encephalitis in mice can be reduced with EtdUrd if the animals are not immunosuppressed (DAVIS et al. 1978, 1979). EtdUrd does not appear to be immunosuppressive (GAURI et al. 1969). Topical application of EtdUrd as a 1% water-soluble ointment did not significantly increase the survival time of athymic hairless mice inoculated intracutaneously with herpes simplex virus type 1 (HSV-1; DESCAMPS et al. 1979). GAURI and ELZE (1977) and ELZE (1979) have reported that EtdUrd is of value in the treatment of herpes keratitis in humans.

2. Effects on Normal Cells

EtdUrd is not very cytotoxic, although it is incorporated into the DNA of mouse (SILAGI et al. 1977) and human (SINGH et al. 1974; SWIERKOWSKI et al. 1973) cells. Chromosome damage was not apparent after such incorporation (SWIERKOWSKI et al. 1973; SINGH et al. 1974) and the analog was not mutagenic (PIETRZYKOWSKA and SHUGAR 1966; SWIERKOWSKI and SHUGAR 1969).

3. Mechanism of Action

The basis of the antiviral activity of EtdUrd has not been worked out; however, its selectivity may be due to higher levels of thymidine kinase activity in the virally infected cells. Induction of the viral enzyme appears to be necessary for the antiviral activity of EtdUrd (CHENG et al. 1976; DE CLERCQ et al. 1977). HeLa cells which are thymidine kinase deficient are not inhibited by EtdUrd at 25 μM whereas 1 μM of the compound inhibits HSV-1 transformed variants of these cells (CHENG et al. 1976). These data suggest an important activation role for the viral thymidine kinase. The monophosphate of EtdUrd has been reported to inhibit thymidylate synthetase isolated from *Escherichia coli* (WALTER and GAURI 1975).

II. 5-Propyl-2′-Deoxyuridine

1. Antiviral Activity

The activity of 5-propyl-2′-deoxyuridine (PrdUrd) against herpes simplex virus was first reported by GAURI and MALORNY (1967). It has subsequently been shown to be selective in its inhibition of herpes simplex virus types 1 and 2 (CHENG et al. 1976) and to show little activity toward vaccinia virus (DE CLERCQ et al. 1978). At effective antiviral concentrations, PrdUrd does not inhibit host cell growth (CHENG et al. 1976; DE CLERCQ et al. 1978). In a recent study (DESCAMPS et al. 1979) PrdUrd did not increase the life span of athymic hairless mice inoculated intradermally with herpes simplex virus type 1.

2. Mechanism of Action

Although the biochemical basis for the antiviral action of PrdUrd remains to be elucidated, the compound does appear to interact preferentially with the nucleoside kinase induced by herpes simplex virus (CHENG et al. 1976). PrdUrd is a weak inhibitor of mitochondrial or cytoplasmic thymidine kinase (LEE and CHENG 1976) and the herpes enzyme is required for antiviral activity (CHENG et al. 1976). HeLa cells deficient in thymidine kinase are insensitive to PrdUrd, whereas variants transformed by herpes simplex virus are susceptible to inhibition of growth (CHENG et al. 1976). Herpes simplex virus replication is most sensitive to the effects of PrdUrd 3–6 h postinfection, a time when viral DNA synthesis is not maximal. Thus, although PrdUrd is incorporated into viral DNA, this may not be the critical biochemical effect (CHENG et al. 1979).

III. E-5-(2-Bromovinyl)-2′-Deoxyuridine (BVdUrd)

The synthesis of a promising new antiviral agent, E-5-(2-bromovinyl)-2′-deoxyuridine (BVdUrd), was recently reported (JONES et al. 1979; DE CLERCQ et al. 1979). BVdUrd is a very potent inhibitor of HSV-1 replication in tissue culture (DE CLERCQ et al. 1979). In addition, it is effective against experimental herpes simplex keratitis in rabbits (MAUDGAL et al. 1980). BVdUrd suppresses the development of cutaneous lesions and the associated mortality in athymic hairless mice inoculated intradermally with herpes simplex virus (DE CLERCQ et al. 1979; DESCAMPS et al. 1979). These effects were achieved with no detectable toxicity to the host.

Using a bioassay for the determination of BVdUrd levels, DE CLERCQ et al. (1979 b) studied the pharmacokinetics of this analog in mice. Biologically active blood levels (1.0 µg/ml) persisted up to 320 min following oral administration of BVdUrd. Although detectable brain levels were achieved, the concentrations were about ten-fold lower than serum drug levels. The basis of the selectivity and antiviral action of BVdUrd is unknown.

IV. 5-Methoxymethyl-2′-Deoxyuridine

5-Methoxymethyl-2′-deoxyuridine (MMdUrd) was synthesized by BUBBAR and GUPTA (1970). The compound selectively inhibits the replication of infectious bovine rhinotracheitis (MELDRUM et al. 1974) and herpes simplex virus (BABIUK et al. 1975) in vitro. At 100 times the antiviral concentration, MMdUrd did not cause host cell toxicity (BABIUK et al. 1975).The analog was ineffective against vaccinia virus, murine cytomegalovirus, equine rhinopneumonitis, and feline pneumonitis viruses as well (BABIUK et al. 1975). MMdUrd does not appear to be immunosuppressive (BABIUK and ROUSE 1975; ROUSE et al. 1977) and the basis for its selectivity and its mechanism of action are unknown.

V. Miscellaneous 5-Substituted 2'-Deoxyuridine Derivatives

Many other 5-substituted 2'-deoxyuridine derivatives have been synthesized which have antiviral activity. A number of recent reviews provide the apropriate references (SCHABEL and MONTGOMERY 1972; DE CLERCQ and TORRENCE 1978; SIDWELL and WITKOWSKI 1979; PRUSOFF and FISCHER 1979; DE CLERCQ 1979). Generally, these compounds have either not shown a high degree of antiviral selectivity or they have not yet been extensively studied and will not be further discussed.

D. Pyrimidine Nucleosides with an Altered Ring Structure

Among the nucleosides of this class, 5,6-dihydro-5-azathymidine (DHAdT), appears to be the most selective in its antiviral action. DHAdT is a nucleoside antibiotic which inhibits the replication of herpes simplex viruses primarily and, to a lesser extent, varicella zoster and vaccinia viruses (RENIS 1978). The compound is mildly cytotoxic (RENIS 1978). The severity of lesions in cutaneous herpes simplex infections in hairless mice was decreased and the life span of such animals was increased after treatment with DHAdT (UNDERWOOD and WEED 1977). Under conditions in which DHAdT was not toxic, its administration protected mice inoculated intravenously with herpes simplex virus and reduced the appearance of virus in the central nervous system (RENIS and EIDSON 1979). The basis for the selectivity of DHAdT and its mechanism of action are unknown.

E. Pyrimidine Nucleosides with an Altered Carbohydrate Moiety

I. Arabinofuranosylthymine

1. Antiviral Activity

Arabinofuranosylthymine (ara-T) was isolated from a sponge, *Cryptotechya crypta* (BERGMANN and FEENEY 1951) and later identified as a D-arabinosyl nucleoside by BERGMANN and BURKE (1955). The activity of ara-T against herpes simplex virus keratitis in rabbits was reported by UNDERWOOD et al. (1964). Inhibition of herpes simplex virus replication in culture was soon documented (DERUDDER and PRIVAT-DEGARILHE 1965–1966, RENIS and BUTHALA 1965). Effects of ara-T on equine herpes infections of hamsters have been described (ASWELL et al. 1977) and reviewed (GENTRY et al. 1979). Ara-T selectively inhibits the replication of herpes simplex virus in baby hamster kidney cells (GENTRY and ASWELL 1975) and of varicella zoster virus in human embryo fibroblasts (MILLER et al. 1977). The antiviral activity of the aranucleosides and aranucleotides has been recently reviewed (NORTH and COHEN 1979).

2. Effects on Normal Cells

Despite the selectivity exerted by ara-T in some systems, the growth of certain cell types is inhibited appreciably. MÜLLER et al. (1978 b) have shown ara-T to be a potent inhibitor of mouse L5178y cell replication ($ED_{50} = 9.8 \, \mu M$). Intracellular phosphorylation to arabinofuranosylthymine-5'-triphosphate (ara-TTP) occurred rapidly in these cells and there was some incorporation of arabinofuranosylthymine-5'-monophosphate (ara-TMP) into DNA (MÜLLER et al. 1978 b). Inhibition of DNA polymerases α and β by ara-TTP has been reported (MÜLLER et al. 1978 a; MATSUKAGE et al. 1978) but the relative sensitivity of the two polymerases to inhibition varied with the cell type. Inhibition of DNA synthesis at the level of DNA polymerase may account for the cytotoxicity of ara-T.

3. Mechanism of Action

Studies by ASWELL et al. (1977) indicate that the selectivity which ara-T exerts against herpes simplex virus is dependent on phosphorylation by the virally induced thymidine kinase. Their conclusion was based on the following evidence: (1) the formation ara-T nucleotides occurred in BHK cells infected with herpes simplex, but not in uninfected cells; (2) ara-T inhibited the growth of LM cells transformed to a pyrimidine deoxyribonucleoside kinase positive phenotype by ultraviolet-inactivated herpes simplex virus, but not that of wild-type LM cells; and (3) mutant strains of HSV-1 and HSV-2 which lack pyrimidine deoxyribonucleoside kinase activity were not sensitive to ara-T (ASWELL et al. 1977). MILLER et al. (1977) similarly found that mutants of herpes simplex virus deficient in pyrimidine deoxyribonucleoside kinase were quite insensitive to the effects of ara-T. In addition, these investigators found that the growth of CV-1 cells was inhibited by ara-T. Taken together with the data of MÜLLER et al. (1978 b),these results suggest that the preferential effects of ara-T against virus replication depend on the host cell type. Recently, however, FALKE et al. (1979 a, b) found ara-T to inhibit the replication of a mutant of herpes simplex virus deficient in thymidine kinase, whether the virus was grown in primary rabbit kidney or baby hamster kidney cells. Thus, an alternate form of activation of ara-T may be important. MÜLLER et al. (1979) found that cells infected with a thymidine kinase minus strain of herpes simplex virus have a ten-fold higher phosphorylating capacity than uninfected cells, suggesting the induction of the host cell thymidine kinase or a pyrimidine nucleoside phosphotransferase. In addition, incorporation of ara-T into host DNA, but not into viral DNA, was detected. Inhibition of the herpes simplex virus-induced DNA polymerase by ara-TTP was also found, an effect which may account for the antiviral activity of ara-T (MÜLLER et al. 1979).

II. Arabinofuranosylcytosine

Arabinofuranosylcytosine (ara-C) is a potent inhibitor of the replication of DNA viruses (see CH'IEN et al. 1973; NORTH and COHEN 1979 for reviews). The compound appears to act by inhibiting DNA synthesis (LEVITT and BECKER 1967; BEN-PORAT et al. 1968), but the effects are not selective. Thus, although ara-C is effective against herpes simplex keratitis in both rabbits (UNDERWOOD 1962) and humans (KAUFMAN and MALONEY 1963), it is too toxic to be of clinical use (KAUFMAN et al. 1964).

III. 5-Iodo-5′-Amino-2′,5′-Dideoxyuridine

1. Synthesis

The synthesis of 5-iodo-5′-amino-2′,5′-dideoxyuridine (AIdUrd) was first reported by LIN et al. (1976) and a second procedure, affording the preparation of large quantities, was then developed (LIN and PRUSOFF 1978 a). The rationale for the synthesis of AIdUrd was based in part, on the findings of LANGEN and KOWOLLIK (1968) and LANGEN et al. (1969, 1972). These investigators showed that thymidine analogs with 5′-halogen substitutions are inhibitors of thymidylate kinase but are not incorporated into DNA. Since the toxicity of many antiviral agents is a consequence of their incorporation into DNA, it seemed that the development of new compounds which would not be phosphorylated constituted a useful approach. The synthesis and development of AIdUrd has recently been reviewed in detail (PRUSOFF et al. 1979 b).

2. Antiviral Activity

The highly selective nature of the actions of AIdUrd was first reported by CHENG et al. (1975 a). AIdUrd was shown to inhibit herpes simplex virus replication in Vero cells in the absence of detectable host cell toxicity. This lack of cytotoxicity has been extended to many cell types (PRUSOFF et al. 1977). AIdUrd has been shown to inhibit the replication of the following herpesviruses: (a) HSV-1 and HSV-2 (PRUSOFF et al. 1977); (b) guinea pig herpes-like virus (PRUSOFF et al. 1977); (c) varicella zoster virus (ILTIS et al. 1979); Epstein–Barr virus (HENDERSON et al. 1979); and the RNA leukemia viruses (PRUSOFF et al. 1977).

AIdUrd is not toxic to newborn or suckling mice, even when it is administered intraperitoneally at doses up to 450 mg/kg for 5 days (ALBERT et al. 1979). Its effectiveness in the treatment of herpes simplex keratitis in rabbits as a solution (ALBERT et al. 1976) or an ointment (PULIAFITO et al. 1977) has been established. Topical AIdUrd and acycloguanosine both had significant therapeutic efficacy in oral HSV-2 infection in mice, however, the latter agent was more effective (PARK et al. 1979).

3. Mechanism of Action

Although AIdUrd was synthesized in order to develop an agent that would not be phosphorylated, the biochemical basis of its selectivity is in fact, selective phosphorylation. AIdUrd is phosphorylated to AIdUDP by the herpes simplex virus-encoded multifunctional thymidine kinase (CHEN and PRUSOFF 1979). In uninfected cells no phosphorylation of AIdUrd occurs, whereas, in herpes simplex virus-infected cells the triphosphate of AIdUrd is readily detectable (CHEN et al. 1976 a). CHEN et al. (1976 a) clearly documented that AIdUrd is internally incorporated into host cell and viral DNA, but only in herpes simplex virus-infected cells. The synthesis and chemical properties of AIdUTP have also been reported (CHEN et al. 1976 b).

In herpes simplex virus-infected cells AIdUrd decreased the incorporation of thymidine into DNA, but did not inhibit the incorporation of uridine into RNA or of amino acids into protein (M. S. Chen et al., unpublished work 1976). The expansion of the 5′-triphosphate pools of deoxyadenosine, deoxyguanosine, and deoxycitidine in these cells is consistent with an effect on DNA synthesis. It appears, however, that incorporation of AIdUrd into viral DNA correlates most closely with its antiherpes simplex virus activity (Fischer et al. 1980). The incorporation of this amino nucleoside into viral DNA induced fragmentation, particularly single-stranded breakage, as judged by the behavior of the DNA on neutral and alkaline sucrose gradients. This damage does not, however, appear to be necessary for the antiviral activity of 5-iodo-substituted deoxyuridines (Fischer et al. 1980). The 5′-amino derivative of thymidine (5′-AdThd) appears to share the selective antiviral properties of AIdUrd (Lin et al. 1976; Lin and Prusoff 1978 b). In an effort to reduce the toxicity of IdUrd and yet retain its high degree of efficacy, IdUrd and 5′-AdThd were used in combination against herpes simplex virus (Fischer et al. 1979). Therapeutic synergism, resulting from selective inhibition of host cell toxicity and additive antiviral effects, was obtained.

IV. 1-(2-Deoxy-2-Fluoro-β-D-Arabinofuranosyl)-5-Iodocytosine

An interesting series of 2′-fluoro derivatives of 2′-deoxyarabinofuranosyl-pyrimidine nucleosides has recently been synthesized (Watanabe et al. 1979). One compound in particular, 1-(2-deoxy-2-fluoro-β-D-arabinofuranosyl)-5-iodo-cytosine (2′-F-Ara-IC), showed excellent antiviral activity against herpes simplex virus. In addition, the cytotoxicity of this analog was low, indicating that these novel derivatives may act selectively.

References*

Albert DM, Lahav M, Bhatt PN et al. (1976) Successful therapy of herpes hominis keratitis in rabbits by 5-iodo-5′-amino-2′,5′-dideoxyuridine (AIU): a novel analog of thymidine. Invest Opthalmol 15:470–478

Albert DM, Percy DH, Puliafito CA, Fritsch E, Lin T-S, Ward DC, Prusoff WH (1979) Postnatal treatment of mice with the antiviral nucleosides AIU or IdUrd. Adv Ophthalmol 38:89–98

Aswell JF, Gentry GA (1977) Cell dependent antiherpesviral activity of 5-methylarabino-furanosylcytosine. Ann NY Acad Sci 284:342–350

Aswell JF, Allen GP, Jamieson AT, Campbell DE, Gentry GA (1977) Antiviral activity of arabinosylthymine in herpesviral replication: mechanism of action in vivo and in vitro. Antimicrob Agents Chemother 12:243–254

Babiuk LA, Rouse BT (1975) Effect of anti-herpesvirus drugs on human and bovine lymphoid function in vitro. Infect Immun 12:1281–1289

Babiuk LA, Meldrum B, Gupta VS, Rouse BT (1975) Comparison of the antiviral effects of 5-methoxymethyl-deoxyuridine with 5-iododeoxyuridine, cytosine arabinoside, and adenine arabinoside. Antimicrob Agents Chemother 8:643–650

Ben-Porat T, Brown M, Kaplan AS (1968) Effect of 1-β-D-arabinofuranosylcytosine on DNA synthesis. II. In rabbit kidney cells infected with herpes viruses. Mol Pharmacol 4:139–146

Berens K, Shugar D (1963) Ultraviolet absorption spectra and structure of halogenated uracils and their glycosides. Acta Biochim Pol 10:25–47

---

* The literature reviewed includes papers published through 1979

Bergmann W, Burke DC (1955) Contributions to the study of marine products. XXXIX. Nucleosides of sponges. III. Spongothymidine and spongouridine. J Org Chem 20:1501–1507

Bergmann W, Feeney R (1951) Contributions to the study of marine products. XXXII. The nucleosides of sponges. J Org Chem 16:981–987

Boston Interhospital Virus Study Group and the NIAID-Sponsored Cooperative Antiviral Clinical Study (1970) Failure of high dose 5-iodo-2′-deoxyuridine in the therapy of herpes simplex virus encephalitis. N Engl J Med 292:599–603

Bresnick E, Thompson UB (1965) Properties of deoxythymidine kinase partially purified from animal tumors. J Biol Chem 240:3967–3974

Bresnick E, Williams SS (1967) Effects of 5-trifluoromethyldeoxyuridine on deoxythymidine kinase. Biochem Pharmacol 16:503–507

Bubbar GL, Gupta VS (1970) Synthesis of 5-substituted ether derivatives of 5-hydroxymethyldeoxyuridine and their α-isomers. Can J Chem 48:3147–3153

Buettner W, Werchau H (1973) Incorporation of 5-iodo-2′-deoxyuridine (IUdR) into SV40 DNA. Virology 52:553–561

Calabresi P, Cardoso Finch SC, Kligerman MM, Von Essen CF, Chu NY, Welch AD (1961) Initial clinical studies with 5-iodo-2′-deoxyuridine. Cancer Res 21:550–554

Calabresi P, Creasey WA, Prusoff WH, Welch AD (1963) Clinical and pharmacological studies with 5-iodo-2′-deoxycytidine. Cancer Res 23:583–592

Chan T-S (1977) Induction of deoxycytidine deaminase activity in mammalian cell lines by infection with herpes simplex virus type 1. Proc Natl Acad Sci USA 74:1734–1738

Chang PK, Welch AD (1961) Preparation of 5-iodo-2′-deoxycytidine. Biochem Pharmacol 8:327–328

Chang T-W, Snydman DR (1979) Antiviral agents: action and clinical use. Drugs 18:354–376

Chen MS, Prusoff WH (1978) Association of thymidylate kinase activity with pyrimidine deoxyribonucleoside kinase induced by herpes simplex virus. J Biol Chem 253:1325–1327

Chen MS, Prusoff WH (1979) Phosphorylation of 5-iodo-5′-amino-2′,5′-dideoxyuridine by herpes simplex virus type 1 encoded thymidine kinase. J Biol Chem 254:10449–10452

Chen MS, Ward DC, Prusoff WH (1976 a) Specific herpes simplex virus-induced incorporation of 5-iodo-5′-amino-2′,5′-dideoxyuridine into deoxyribonucleic acid. J Biol Chem 251:4833–4838

Chen MS, Ward DC, Prusoff WH (1976 b) 5′-amino-2′,5′-dideoxyuridine-5′-N′-triphosphate synthesis, chemical properties, and effect on Escherichia coli thymidine kinase activity. J Biol Chem 251:4839–4842

Cheng Y-C (1976) Deoxythymidine kinase induced in HeLa TK⁻ cells by herpes simplex virus type I and type II. Substrate specificity and kinetic behavior. Biochim Biophys Acta 452:370–381

Cheng Y-C (1977) A rational approach to the development of antiviral chemotherapy. Alternate substrates of herpes simplex virus type 1 (HSV-1) and type 2 (HSV-2) thymidine kinase. Ann NY Acad Sci 284:594–598

Cheng Y-C, Goz B, Neenan JP, Ward DC, Prusoff WH (1975 a) Selective inhibition of herpes simplex virus by 5′-amino-2′,5′-dideoxy-5-iodouridine. J Virol 15:1284–1285

Cheng Y-C, Goz B, Prusoff WH (1975 b) Deoxyribonucleotide metabolism in herpes simplex virus infected cells. Biochim Biophys Acta 390:253–263

Cheng Y-C, Domin BA, Sharma RA, Bobek M (1976) Antiviral action and cellular toxicity of four thymidine analogues: 5-ethyl-, 5-vinyl-, 5-propyl-, and 5-allyl-2′-deoxyuridine. Antimicrob Agents Chemother 10:119–122

Cheng Y-C, Grill S, Dutschman G (1979) Time-dependent action of 5-propyldeoxyuridine as antiherpes simplex virus type 1 and type 2 agents. Biochem Pharmacol 28:3529–3532

Ch'ien LT, Schabel FM Jr, Alford CA (1973) Arabinosyl nucleosides and nucleotides. In: Carter WA (ed) Selective inhibitors of viral functions. CRC Press, Cleveland, Ohio, pp 227–256

Clough DW, Parkhurst JR (1977) Experimental herpes simplex virus type 1 encephalitis: treatment with trifluoromethyl-2′-deoxyuridine. Antimicrob Agents Chemother 11:307–311

Cohen GH (1972) Ribonucleotide reductase activity of synchronized KB cells infected with
    herpes simplex virus. J Virol 9:408–418

Cohen SS (1977) A strategy for the chemotherapy of infectious disease. Science 197:431–432

Cooper GM (1973) Phosphorylation of 5-bromodeoxycytidine in cells infected with herpes
    simplex virus. Proc Natl Acad Sci USA 70:3788–3792

Cooper GM, Greer S (1973 a) The effect of inhibition of cytidine deaminase by tetrahy-
    drouridine on the utilization of deoxycytidine and 5-bromodeoxycytidine for deoxy-
    cytidine acid synthesis. Mol Pharmacol 9:698–703

Cooper GM, Greer S (1973 b) Phosphorylation of 5-halogenated deoxycytidine analogues
    by deoxycytidine kinase. Mol Pharmacol 9:704–710

Coster DJ, McKinnon JR, McGill JI, Jones BR, Fraunfelder FT (1976) Clinical evaluation
    of adenine arabinoside and trifluorothymidine in the treatment of corneal ulcers caused
    by herpes simplex virus. J Infect Dis S-133:A173–A177

Cramer JW, Prusoff WH, Welch AD, Sartorelli AC, Delamore IW, Von Essen CF, Chang
    PD (1962) Studies on the biochemical pharmacology of 5-iodo-2′-deoxycytidine *in vitro*
    and *in vivo*. Biochem Pharmacol 11:761–768

Davis WB, Oakes JE, Taylor JA (1978) Effects of treatment with 5-ethyl-2′-desoxyuridine
    on herpes simplex virus encephalitis in normal and immunosuppressed mice. Anti-
    microb Agents Chemother 14:743–748

Davis WB, Oakes JE, Vacik JP, Rebert RR, Taylor JA (1979) 5-ethyl-2′-deoxyuridine as
    a systemic agent for treatment of herpes simplex virus encephalitis. Adv Ophthalmol
    38:140–150

De Clercq E (1979) New trends in antiviral chemotherapy. Arch Int Physiol Biochim
    81:353–395

De Clercq E, Shugar D (1975) Antiviral activity of 5-ethyl pyrimidine deoxyribonucleosides.
    Biochem Pharmacol 24:1073–1078

De Clercq E, Torrence PE (1978) Nucleoside analogs with selective antiviral activity. J Car-
    bohydr Nucleosides Nucleotides 5:187–224

De Clercq E, Krajewska E, Descamps J, Torrence PF (1977) Antiherpes activity of
    deoxythymidine analogues: specific dependence on virus-induced deoxythymidine
    kinase. Mol Pharmacol 13:980–984

De Clercq E, Descamps J, Shugar D (1978) 5-Propyl-2′-deoxyuridine: specific anti-herpes
    agent. Antimicrob Agents Chemother 13:545–547

De Clercq E, Descamps J, Desomer P, Barr PJ, Jones AS, Walker TR (1979 a) E-5-(2-
    bromo-vinyl)-2′-deoxyuridine: a potent and selective antiherpes agent. Proc Natl Acad
    Sci USA 76:2947–2951

De Clercq E, Descamps J, Desomer P, Barr PJ, Jones AS, Walker RT (1979 b) Pharma-
    cokinetics of E-5-(2-bromo-vinyl)-2′-deoxyuridine in mice. Antimicrob Agents
    Chemother 16:234–236

Derudder J, Privat-Degarilhe M (1965/1966) Inhibitory effect of some nucleosides on the
    growth of various human viruses in tissue culture. Antimicrob Agents Chemother 1965/
    1966:578–584

Descamps J, De Clercq E, Barr PJ, Jones AS, Walker RT, Torrence PF, Shugar D (1979)
    Relative potencies of different anti-herpes agents in the topical treatment of cutaneous
    herpes simplex infection of athymic nude mice. Antimicrob Agents Chemother 16:680–
    682

Dexter DL, Oki T, Heidelberger C (1973) Fluorinated pyrimidines. XLII. Effect of 5-
    trifluoromethyl-2′-deoxyuridine on transcription of vaccinia viral messenger ribonucleic
    acid. Mol Pharmacol 9:283–292

Dobersen MJ, Greer S (1978) Herpes simplex virus type 2 induced pyrimidine nucleoside
    kinase: enzymatic basis for the selective antiherpetic effect of 5′-halogenated analogues
    of deoxycytidine. Biochemistry 17:920–928

Dobersen MJ, Jerkofsky M, Greer S (1976) Enzymatic basis for the selective inhibition of
    varicella-zoster virus by 5-halogenated analogues of deoxycytidine. J Virol 20:478–486

Elion GB, Furman PA, Fyfe JA, De Miranda P, Beauchamp L, Schaeffer HJ (1977) Selec-
    tivity of action of an antiherpetic agent, 9-(2-hydroxyethoxymethyl) guanine. Proc Natl
    Acad Sci USA 74:5716–5720

Elze K-L (1979) Ten years of clinical experiences with ethyldeoxyuridine. Adv Ophthalmol 38:134–139

Falke D, Moser H, Link D, Müller WEG (1979a) The effects of α- and β-D-arabino-furanosylthymine on the growth of herpes simplex virus types 1 and 2. J Gen Virol 42:435–438

Falke D, Moser H, Lind D, Müller WEG (1979b) The effects of α- and β-D-arabinosyl-ladenosine and β-D-arabinosylthymine on the synthesis of HSV types 1- and 2-infected cells. Adv Opthalmol 38:197–203

Fischer PH, Lee JJ, Chen MS, Lin T-S, Prusoff WH (1979) Synergistic effect of 5′-amino-5′-deoxythymidine and 5-iodo-2′-deoxyuridine against herpes simplex virus infections in vitro. Biochem Pharmacol 28:3483–3486

Fischer PH, Chen MS, Prusoff WH (1980) The incorporation of 5-iodo-5′-amino-2′,5′-dideoxyuridine and 5-iodo-2′-deoxyuridine into herpes simplex virus DNA: a relationship to their antiviral activity and effects on DNA structure. Biochim Biophys Acta 606:236–245

Fujiwara Y, Heidelberger C (1970) Fluorinated pyrimidines. XXXVIII. The incorporation of 5-trifluoromethyl-2′-deoxyuridine into the deoxyribonucleic acid of vaccinia virus. Mol Pharmacol 6:281–291

Fyfe JA, Keller PM, Furman PA, Miller RL, Elion GB (1978) Thymidine kinase from herpes simplex virus phosphorylates the new antiviral compound, 9-(2-hydroxyethoxy-methyl) guanine. J Biol Chem 253:8721–8727

Gauri KK (1968) Subconjunctival application of 5-ethyl-2′-deoxyuridine in the chemotherapy of experimental keratitis in rabbits. Klin Monatsbl Augenheilkd 153:837–841

Gauri KK, Elze KL (1977) Concentration dependent effectiveness of 5-ethyl-2′-deoxyuridine in animal experiments and in the clinic. Klin Monatsbl Augenheilkd 171:459–463

Gauri KK, Malorny G (1967) Chemotherapie der Herpes-Infektion mit neuen 5-alkylura-cildesoxyribosiden. Naunyn Schmiedebergs Arch Pharmacol 257:21–22

Gauri KK, Malorny G, Schiff W (1969) Immunobiological studies with the virostatics 5-ethyl-2′-deoxyuridine and 1-allyl-3,5-diethyl-6-chlorouracil. Chemotherapy 14:129–132

Gentry GA, Aswell JF (1975) Inhibition of herpes simplex virus replication by Ara-T. Virology 65:294–296

Gentry GA, McGowan J, Barnett J, Nevine R, Allen G (1979) Arabinosylthymine, a selective inhibitor of herpes virus replication: current status of in vivo studies. Adv Ophthalmol 38:164–172

Goz B (1978) The effects of incorporation of 5-halogenated deoxyuridines into the DNA of eukaryotic cells. Pharmacol Rev 29:249–272

Goz B, Prusoff WH (1970) Pharmacology of viruses. Annu Rev Pharmacol 10:143–170

Greer S, Schildkraut I, Zimmerman T, Kaufman H (1975) 5-Halogenated analogs of deoxy-cytidine as selective inhibitors of the replication of herpes simplex viruses in cell culture and related studies of intracranial herpes simplex virus infections in mice. Ann NY Acad Sci 255:359–365

Heidelberger C (1975a) On the molecular mechanism of the antiviral activity of trifluorothymidine. Ann NY Acad Sci 255:317–325

Heidelberger C (1975b) Fluorinated pyrimidines and their nucleosides. In: Sartorelli AC, Johns DG (eds) Antineoplastic and immunosuppressive agents. Springer, Berlin Heidelberg New York (Handbook of experimental pharmacology, vol 38/2, pp 193–231)

Heidelberger C, Anderson SW (1964) Fluorinated pyrimidines. XXI. The tumorinhibitory activity of 5-trifluoromethyl-2′-deoxyuridine. Cancer Res 24:1979–1985

Heidelberger C, King DH (1979) Trifluorothymidine. Pharmacol Ther 6:427–442

Heidelberger C, Parsons DG, Remy DC (1964) Synthesis of 5-trifluoromethyluracil and 5-trifluoromethyl-2′-deoxyuridine. J Med Chem 7:1–5

Heidelberger C, Boohar J, Kampschroer B (1965) Fluorinated pyrimidines. XXIV. In vivo metabolism of 5-trifluoromethyluracil-2-^{14}C and 5-trifluoromethyl-2′-deoxyuridine-2-[14]C. Cancer Res 25:377–381

Henderson EE, Long WK, Ribeck R (1979) Effects of nucleoside analogs on Epstein-Barr virus-induced transformation of human umbilical cord leukocytes and Epstein-Barr virus-expressions in transformed cells. Antimicrob Agents Chemother 15:101–110

Herrmann EC Jr (1961) Plaque inhibition test for detection of specific inhibitors of DNA containing viruses. Proc Soc Exp Biol Med 107:142–145

Herrmann EC Jr, Herrman JA (1979) Diagnosis of viral disease and the advent of antiviral drugs. Pharmacol Ther 7:35–69

Iltis JP, Lin T-S, Prusoff WH, Rapp F (1979) Effect of 5-iodo-5'-amino-2',5'-dideoxyuridine on varicella zoster virus *in vitro*. Antimicrob Agents Chemother 16:92–97

Itoi M, Gefter JW, Kaneko N, Ishii Y, Ramer RM, Gassert S (1975) Teratogenicities of ophthalmic drugs. I. Antiviral ophthalmic drugs. Arch Ophthalmol 93:46–51

Jamieson AT, Subak-Sharpe JH (1974) Biochemical studies on the herpes simplex virus-specified deoxypyrimidine kinase activity. J Gen Virol 24:481–492

Jamieson AT, Gentry GA, Subak-Sharpe JH (1974) Induction of both thymidine and deoxycytidine kinase activity by herpes viruses. J Gen Virol 24:465–480

Jerkofsky MA, Dobersen MJ, Greer S (1977) Selective inhibition of the replication of varicella-zoster virus by 5-halogenated analogs of deoxycytidine. Ann NY Acad Sci 284:389–395

Jones AS, Verhelst G, Walker RT (1979) The synthesis of the potent anti-herpes virus agent E-(5)-(2-bromovinyl)-2'-deoxyuridine and related compounds. Tetrahedron Lett 45:4415–4418

Jones BR, McGill JI, McKinnon JR, Holt-Wilson AD, Williams HP (1975) Preliminary experience with adenine arabinoside in comparison with idoxuridine and trifluorothymidine in the management of herpestic keratitis. In: Pavan-Langston D, Buchannan RA, Alford CA Jr (eds) Adenine arabinoside: an antiviral agent. Raven, New York, pp 411–416

Juel-Jensen BE (1973) Herpes simplex and zoster. Br Med J 1:406–410

Juel-Jensen BE (1974) Virus diseases. Practitioner 213:508–518

Kan-Mitchell J, Prusoff WH (1979) Studies of the effects of 5-iodo-2'-deoxyuridine on the formation of adenovirus type 2 virions and the synthesis of virus induced polypeptides. Biochem Pharmacol 28:1819–1829

Kaplan AS, Ben-Porat T (1966) Mode of antiviral action of 5-iodouracil deoxyriboside. J Mol Biol 19:320–332

Kaufman ER, Davidson RL (1979) Altered thymidylate kinase substrate specificity in mammalian cells selected for resistance to iododeoxyuridine. Exp Cell Res 123:355–363

Kaufman HE (1962) Clinical cure of herpes simplex keratitis by 5-iodo-2'-deoxyuridine. Proc Soc Exp Biol Med 109:251–252

Kaufman HE (1965) Problems in virus chemotherapy. Prog Med Virol 7:116–159

Kaufman HE (1977) Antiviral drugs. Int J Dermatol 16:464–475

Kaufman HE, Heidelberger C (1964) Therapeutic antiviral action of 5-trifluoromethyl-2'-deoxyuridine in *herpes simplex* keratitis. Science 145:585–586

Kaufman HE, Maloney ED (1963) IDU and cytosine arabinoside in experimental keratitis. Arch Ophthalmol 69:262–629

Kaufman HE, Maloney ED, Nesburn AB (1962a) Comparison of specific antiviral agents in herpes simplex keratitis. Invest Ophthalmol 1:686–692

Kaufman HE, Martola E, Dohlman L (1962b) Use of 5-iodo-2'-deoxyuridine (IDU) in treatment of herpes simplex keratitis. Arch Ophthalmol 68:235–239

Kaufman HE, Capella JA, Maloney ED, Robbins JE, Cooper GM, Utolila MH (1964) Corneal toxicity of cytosine arabinoside. Arch Ophthalmol 72:535–540

Keir HM, Gold E (1963) Deoxyribonucleic acid nucleotidyltransferase and deoxyribonuclease from cultured cells infected with herpes simplex virus. Biochim Biophys Acta 72:263–276

Kit S (1979) Viral-associated and induced enzymes. Pharmacol Ther 4:501–585

Kit S, Dubbs DR (1963) Acquisition of thymidine kinase activity by herpes simplex-infected mouse fibroblast cells. Biochem Biophys Res Commun 11:55–59

Kriss JP, Maruyama Y, Tung LA, Bond GB, Revesz L (1963) Fate of 5-bromodeoxyuridine, 5-bromodeoxycytidine and 5-iododeoxycytidine in man. Cancer Res 23:260–268

Laibson PR, Arentsen JJ, Mazzanti WD, Eiferman RA (1977) Double-controlled comparison of IDU and trifluorothymidine in thirty-three patients with superficial herpetic keratitis. Trans Am Ophthalmol Soc 75:316–324

Langen P (1975) Antimetabolites of nucleic acid metabolism. Gordon & Breach, New York

Langen P, Kowollik G (1968) 5′-Deoxy-5′-fluorothymidine, a biochemical analogue of thymidine-5′-monophosphate selectively inhibiting DNA synthesis. Eur J Biochem 6:344–351

Langen P, Kowollik G, Schütt M, Etzold G (1969) Thymidylate kinase as target enzyme for 5′-deoxythymidine and various 5′-deoxy-5′-halogeno pyrimidine nucleosides. Acta Biol Med Ger 23:K19–K22

Langen P, Etzold G, Kowollik G (1972) Inhibition of DNA synthesis and thymidylate kinase by halogeno derivatives of 3′,5′-dideoxythymidine. Acta Biol Med Ger 28:K5–K10

Lee L-S, Cheng Y-C (1976) Human deoxythymidine kinase. II. Substrate specificity and kinetic behavior of the cytoplasmic and mitochondrial isozymes derived from blast cells of acute myelocytic leukemia. Biochemistry 15:3686–3690

Levitt J, Becker Y (1967) The effect of cytosine arabinoside on the replication of herpes simplex virus. Virology 31:129–134

Lin SY, Riggs AD (1972) *Lac* operator analogues: bromodeoxyuridine substitution in the *lac* operator affects the rate of association of the *lac* repressor. Proc Natl Acad Sci USA 69:2574–2576

Lin T-S, Prusoff WH (1978a) A novel synthesis and biological activity of several 5-halo-5′-amino analogues of deoxyribopyrimidine nucleosides. J Med Chem 21:106–109

Lin T-S Prusoff WH (1978b) Synthesis and biological activity of several amino analogues of thymidine. J Med Chem 21:109–112

Lin T-S, Neenan JP, Cheng Y-C, Prusoff WH, Ward DC (1976) Synthesis and antiviral activity of 5- and 5′-substituted thymidine analogs. J Med Chem 19:495–498

Maass G, Haas R (1966) Über die Bildung von virusspezifischem SV-40 Antigen in Gegenwart von 5-iodo-2′-desoxyuridine. Arch Gesamte Virusforsch 18:253–256

Maley F (1967) Deoxycytidylate deaminase. Methods Enzymol 12A:170–182

Mao JC-H, Robishaw EE (1975) Mode of inhibition of herpes simplex virus DNA polymerase by phosphonoacetate. Biochemistry 14:5475–5479

Martenet A-C (1975) The treatment of experimental deep herpes simplex keratitis with 5-ethyldeoxyuridine and iodo-deoxycytidine. Ophthalmol Res 7:170–180

Martenet A-C (1979) Experiences with iododeoxycytidine in the treatment of ocular herpes simplex infections. Adv Ophthalmol 38:105–109

Mathias AP, Fischer GA (1962) The metabolism of thymidine by murine leukemia lymphoblasts (L5178Y). Biochem Pharmacol 11:57–68

Mathias AP, Fischer GA, Prusoff WH (1959) Inhibition of the growth of mouse leukemia cells in culture by 5-iodo-deoxyuridine. Biochim Biophys Acta 36:560–561

Matsukage A, Ono K, Ohashi A, Takahashi T, Nakayama C, Saneyoshi M (1978) Inhibitory effect of 1-β-D-arabinofuranosylthymine 5′-triphosphate and 1β-D-arabinofuranosylcytosine 5′-triphosphate on DNA polymerases from murine cells and oncornavirus. Cancer Res 38:3076–3079

Maudgal PC, De Clercq E, Descamps J et al. (1980) (E)-5-(bromovinyl)-2′-deoxyuridine in the treatment of experimental herpes simplex keratitis. Antimicrob Agents Chemother 17:8–12

McGill J, Holt-Wilson AP, McKinnon JR (1974) Some aspects of the clinical use of trifluorothymidine in the treatment of herpetic ulceration of the cornea. Trans Ophthalmol Soc UK 94:342–352

McKinnon JR, McGill JI, Jones BR (1975) A coded clinical evaluation of adenine arabinoside and trifluorothymidine in the treatment of ulcerative herpetic keratitis. In: Pavan-Langston D, Buchanan RA, Alford CA (eds) Adenine arabinoside-an antiviral agent. Raven, New York, p 401

Meldrum JB, Gupta VS, Saunders JR (1974) Cell culture studies on the antiviral activity of ether derivatives of 5-hydroxy-methyldeoxyuridine. Antimicrob Agents Chemother 6:393–396

Mendez MS, Martenet A-C (1972) Activité de l'iodo-desoxycytidine (IDC) sur la kératite herpétique expérimentale profonde. Annls. Oculist 205:199–206

Mendez M, Martenet AC, Steinbrunner W (1971) L'iododesoxycytidine nouveau virostatique contre la kératique herpétique. Ann Ocul 204:1219–1228

Miller RL, Iltis JP, Rapp F (1977) Differential effect of arabinofuranosylthymine on the replication of human herpes viruses. J Virol 23:679–684

Mitchell WM (1973) Active sites of the animal viruses: potential sites of specific chemotherapeutic attack. In: Carter WA (ed) Selective inhibitors of viral functions. CRC Press, Cleveland, Ohio, pp 51–80

Müller WEG (1979) Mechanisms of action and pharmacology: chemical agents. In: Galasso GJ (ed) Antiviral agents and viral diseases of man. Raven, New York, pp 77–149

Müller WEG, Zahn RK, Arendes J (1978 a) Arabinosyl nucleosides. XIII. Influence of arabinofuranosylthymine on DNA-, RNA-, and protein-synthesizing systems in vitro. Chem Biol Interact 23:151–158

Müller WEG, Zahn RK, Maidhof A, Beyer R, Arendes J (1978 b) Arabinosyl nucleosides. XII. Influence of arabinofuranosylthymine on growth of L5178Y cells. Chem Biol Interact 23:141–150

Müller WEG, Zahn RK, Arendes J, Falke D (1979) Phosphorylation of arabinofuranosylthymine in non-infected and herpesvirus (TK$^+$ and TK$^-$)-infected cells. J Gen Virol 43:261–271

North TW, Cohen SS (1979) Aranucleosides and aranucleotides in viral chemotherapy. Pharmacol Ther 4:81–108

Oki T, Heidelberger C (1971) Fluorinated pyrimidines. XXXIV. Effects of 5-trifluoromethyl-2′-deoxyuridine on the replication of vaccinia viral messenger RNA and proteins. Mol Pharmacol 7:653–662

Oxford JS (1977) Specific inhibitors of influenza related to the molecular biology of virus replication. In: Oxford JS (ed) Chemoprophylaxis and virus infections of the respiratory tract. CRC Press, Cleveland, Ohio, pp 139–186

Park N-H, Pavan-Langston D, Hettinger ME, McLean SL, Albert DM, Lin T-S, Prusoff WH (1979) Topical therapeutic efficacy of 9-(2-hydroxethoxymethyl) guanine and 5-Iodo-5′-amino-2′,5′-dideoxyuridine on oral HSV-2 infection in mice. J Infect Dis 141:575–579

Parkhurst JR, Dannenberg PV, Heidelberger C (1976) Growth inhibition of cells in culture and of vaccinia virus infected HeLa cells by derivatives of trifluorothymidine. Chemotherapy 22:221–232

Pavan-Langston D (1979) Current trends in therapy of ocular herpes simplex: experimental and clinical studies. Adv Opthalmol 38:82–88

Pavan-Langston D, Foster CS (1977) Trifluorothymidine and iododeoxyuridine therapy of ocular herpes. Am J Ophthalmol 84:818–825

Perkins ES, Wood RM, Sears ML, Prusoff WH, Welch AD (1962) Antiviral activities of several iodinated pyrimidine deoxyribonucleosides. Nature 194:985–986

Pietryzkowska I, Shugar D (1966) Replacement of thymine by 5-ethyluracil in bacteriophage DNA. Biochem Biophys Res Commun 25:567–572

Prusoff WH (1959) Synthesis and biological activities of iododeoxyuridine an analog of the thymidine. Biochim Biophys Acta 32:295–296

Prusoff WH (1967) Recent advances in chemotherapy of viral diseases. Pharmacol Rev 19:209–250

Prusoff WH, Fischer PH (1979) Basis for the selective antiviral and antitumor activity of pyrimidine nucleoside analogs. In: Walker RT, De Clercq E, Eckstein F (eds) Nucleoside analogs. Plenum, New York, pp 281–318

Prusoff WH, Goz B (1973 a) Potential mechanisms of action of antiviral agents. Fed Proc 32:1679–1687

Prusoff WH, Goz B (1973 b) Chemotherapy-molecular aspects. In: Kaplan AS (ed) The herpes viruses. Academic Press, New York, p 641

Prusoff WH, Goz B (1975) Halogenated pyrimidine deoxyribonucleosides. In: Sartorelli AC, Johns DG (eds) Antineoplastic and immunosuppressive Agents. Springer, Berlin Heidelberg New York (Handbook of experimental pharmacology, vol 38/2, pp 272–347)

Prusoff WH, Ward DC (1976) Nucleosides with antiviral activity. Biochem Pharmacol 25:1233–1239

Prusoff WH, Bakhle YS, Sekely L (1965) Cellular and antiviral effects of halogenated deoxyribonucleosides. Ann NY Acad Sci 130:135–150

Prusoff WH, Ward DC, Lin T-S et al. (1977) Recent studies on the antiviral and biochemical properties of 5-halo-5'-amino-deoxyribonucleosides. Ann NY Acad Sci 284:335–341

Prusoff WH, Chen MS, Fischer PH, Lin T-S, Shiau GT (1979 a) 5-iodo-2'-deoxyuridine. In: Hahn FE (ed) Mechanism of action of antieukaryotic and antiviral compounds. Springer, Berlin Heidelberg New York (Antibiotics, vol 5/2, pp 236–261)

Prusoff WH, Chen MS, Fischer PH, Lin T-S, Shiau GT, Schinazi RF, Walker J (1979 b) Antiviral iodinated pyrimidine deoxyribonucleosides: 5-iodo-2'-deoxyuridine; 5-iodo-2'-deoxycytidine; 5-iodo-5'-amino-2',5'-dideoxyuridine. Pharmacol Ther 7:1–34

Puliafito CA, Robinson NL, Albert DH, Pavan-Langston D, Lin T-S, Ward DC, Prusoff WH (1977) Therapy of experimental herpes simplex keratitis in rabbits with 5-iodo-5'amino-2',5'-dideoxyuridine. Proc Soc Exp Biol Med 156:92–96

Renis HE (1970) Comparison of cytotoxicity and antiviral activity of 1-β-D-arabino-furanosyl-5-iodocytosine with related compounds. Cancer Res 30:189–194

Renis HE (1978) 5,6-Dihydro-5-azathymidine: in vitro antiviral properties against human herpes viruses. Antimicrob Agents Chemother 13:613–617

Renis HE, Buthala DA (1965) Development of resistance to antiviral drugs. Ann NY Acad Sci 130:345–354

Renis HE, Eidson EE (1979) Activities of 5,6-dihydro-5-azathymidine against herpes simplex virus infections in mice. Antimicrob Agents Chemother 15:213–219

Reyes P, Heidelberger L (1965) Fluorinated pyrimidines. XXVI. Mammalian thymidylate synthetase, its mechanism of action and inhibition by flurorinated nucleotides. Mol Pharmacol 1:14–30

Roizman G, Aurelian L, Roane PR Jr (1963) The multiplication of herpes simplex virus. I. The programming of viral DNA duplication in HEp-2 cells. Virology 21:482–498

Rouse BT, Babiuk LA, Gupta VS (1977) The effect of the antiherpes drug 5-methoxy-methyl-2'-deoxyuridine on the humoral immune response in vivo. Can J Microbiol 23:1059–1061

Roux J, Mandin J (1969) Action sur le virus herpétique de la 5-iodo-2'-deoxyuridine et de la 5-iodo-2'-deoxycytidine. Doc Chavin-Blache

Schabel FM Jr, Montgomery JA (1972) Purines and pyrimidines. In: Bauer DJ (ed) Chemotherapy of virus diseases. Pergamon, Oxford, pp 231–363

Schildkraut I, Cooper GM, Greer S (1975) Selective inhibition of the replication of herpes simplex virus by 5-halogenated analogues of deoxycytidine. Mol Pharmacol 11:153–158

Sidwell RW, Witkowski JT (1979) Antiviral agents. In: Wolf ME (ed) Burger's medicinal chemistry, 4 th edn. part II. John Wiley and Sons, New York, pp 543–593

Sidwell RW, Arnett G, Brockman RW (1970) Comparison of the anticytomegalovirus activity of a group of pyrimidine analogs. Ann NY Acad Sci 173:592–602

Silagi S, Balint RF, Gauri KK (1977) Comparative effects on growth and tumorigenicity of mouse melanoma cells by thymidine and its analogs, 5-ethyl- and 5-bromo-deoxyuridine. Cancer Res 37:3367–3373

Singh S, Willers I, Goedde HW, Gauri KK (1974) 5-Ethyl-2'-deoxyuridine: absence of effect on the chromosomes of human lymphocytes and fibroblasts in culture. Humangenetik 24:135–139

Smith KO (1963) Some biologic aspects of herpesvirus-cell interactions in the presence of 5-iodo-2'-desoxyuridine (DU). J Immunol 91:582–590

Smith KO, Dukes CD (1964) Effects of 5-iodo-2'-desoxyuridine (IDU) on herpes virus synthesis and survival in infected cells. J Immunol 92:550–554

Smith RA, Sidwell RW, Robins RK (1980) Antiviral mechanisms of action. Annu Rev Pharmacol Toxicol 20:259–281

Steele FM, Black FL (1967) Inactivation and heat stabilization of poliovirus by 2-thiouracil. J Virol 1:653–658

Sternglanz H, Bugg CE (1975) Relationship between mutagenic and base-stacking properties of halogenated uracil derivatives. The crystal structures of 5-chloro and 5-bromouracil. Biochim Biophys Acta 378:1–11

Sugar J, Kaufman HE (1973) Halogenated pyrimidines in antiviral therapy. In: Carter WA (ed) Selective inhibitors of viral functions. CRC Press, Cleveland, Ohio, p 377

Sugar J, Varnell E, Centiafanto Y, Kaufman HE (1973) Trifluorothymidine treatment of herpetic iritis in rabbits and ocular penetration. Invest Ophthalmol 12:532–534

Summers WC, Summers WP (1977) [^{121}I]-deoxycytidine used in rapid, sensitive, and specific assay for herpes simplex virus type 1 thymidine kinase. J Virol 24:314–318

Swierkowski KM, Jasinska JK, Steffen JA (1973) 5-Ethyl-2′-deoxyuridine: evidence for incorporation into DNA and evaluation of biological properties in lymphocyte cultures grown under conditions of amethopterine-imposed thymidine deficiency. Biochem harmacol 22:85–93

Swierkowski KM, Shugar D (1969) A nonmutagenic thymidine analog with antiviral activity. 5-Ethyldeoxyuridine. J Med Chem 12:533–534

Tone H, Heidelberger C (1973) Interaction of 5-trifluoromethyl-2′-deoxyuridine-5′-triphosphate with deoxyribonucleic acid polymerases. Mol Pharmacol 9:783–791

Travers JP, Patterson A (1978) A controlled trial of adenine arabinoside and trifluorothymidine in herpetic keratitis. J Int Med Res 6:102–104

Umeda M, Heidelberger C (1968) Fluorinated pyrimidines. XXX. Comparative studies of fluorinated pyrimidines with various cell lines. Cancer Res 28:2529–2538

Umeda M, Heidelberger C (1969) Fluorinated pyrimidines. XXXI. Mechanism of inhibition of vaccinia virus replication in HeLa cells by pyrimidine nucleosides. Proc Soc Exp Biol Med 130:24–29

Underwood GE (1962) Activity of 1-β-D-arabinofuranosylcytosine hydrochloride against herpes simplex keratitis. Proc Soc Exp Biol Med 111:660–664

Underwood GE, Weed SD (1977) Efficacy of 5,6-β-dihydro-5-azathymidine against cutaneous herpes simplex virus in hairless mice. Antimicrob Agents Chemother 11:565–567

Underwood GE, Wisner CA, Weed SD (1964) Cytosine arabinoside (CA) and other nucleosides in herpes virus infections. Arch Ophthalmol 72:505–512

Verbov J (1979) Local idoxuridine treatment of herpes simplex and zoster. J Antimicrob Chemother 5:126–128

Walter RD, Gauri KK (1975) 5-Ethyl-2′-deoxyuridine-5′-monophosphate inhibition of the thymidylate synthetase from *Escherichia coli*. Biochem Pharmacol 24:1025–1027

Watanabe KA, Reichman U, Hirota K, Lopez C, Fox JJ (1979) Nucleosides 110. Synthesis and antiherpes virus activity of some 2′-fluoro-2′-deoxyarabinofuranosylpyrimidine nucleosides. J Med Chem 22:21–24

Welch AD, Prusoff WH (1960) A synopsis of recent investigations of 5-iodo-2′-deoxyuridine. Cancer Chemother Rep 6:29–36

Wellings PC, Audry PN, Bors FH, Jones BR, Brown DC, Kaufman HE (1972) Clinical evaluation of trifluorothymidine in the treatment of herpes simplex corneal ulcers. Am J Ophthalmol 23:932–942

Wigand R, Klein W (1974) Properties of adenovirus substituted with iodo-deoxyuridine. Arch Gesamte Virusforsch 45:298–300

CHAPTER 3

Purines

N. H. PARK and D. PAVAN-LANGSTON

A. Introduction

Of the hundreds of potential anticancer and antiviral agents synthesized over the past three decades, certain nucleosides have proved to be the most effective as antiviral agents, and are the only class of antiviral drugs which have ultimately reached the hands of practicing physicians for widespread clinical use against herpesvirus. Although the pyrimidine nucleoside, 5-iodo-2′-deoxyuridine (idoxuridine, IdUrd), was the first of these to do so, the purine nucleosides have not been far behind and are now rapidly moving to the fore. Of special interest is 9-β-D-arabinofuranosyladenine (vidarabine, ara-A, vira-A®), known to scientists since 1960, and its many analogs described in this chapter. Ara-A was the first and is still the only antimetabolite to be approved by the U.S. Food and Drug Administration (FDA), both for topical use against ocular herpes and for systemic use in herpetic encephalitis. While ara-A is not without certain toxic side effects, these are negligible when compared with those of previous antiviral nucleosides, particularly when the compound is given systemically. The approval of this drug for clinical use marked a great stride forward in antiviral chemotherapy.

But another more specific and less toxic purine nucleoside is now capturing the attention of many of the clinical and basic research virologists: 9-(2-hydroxyethoxymethyl)guanine (acyclovir). As greater understanding of the mechanisms of viral cell–enzyme interaction evolved, the molecular configuration of new antiviral agents changed from a "shotgun" approach to one of highly specific and intentional structuring, aimed at blocking specific enzymes necessary for the replication of the herpesviruses. The results, thus far, are the synthesis of the purine nucleoside, acyclovir, and the pyrimidine nucleoside, (E)-5(2-bromovinyl)-2′-deoxyuridine. With the new and vastly superior technology involved in antiviral chemotherapy, many new frontiers have opened within the past few years and the promise for the future is bright, not least among these new antiviral agents being the purine nucleosides.

B. 9-β-D-Arabinofuranosyladenine

I. Introduction and History

Since naturally occuring arabinosyl nucleosides, i.e., 1-β-D-arabinofuranosylthymine and 1-β-arabinofuranosyluracil, were isolated from the Caribbean sponge, *Cryptotechya crypta* by BERGMANN and FEENEY (1950, 1951), considerable effort

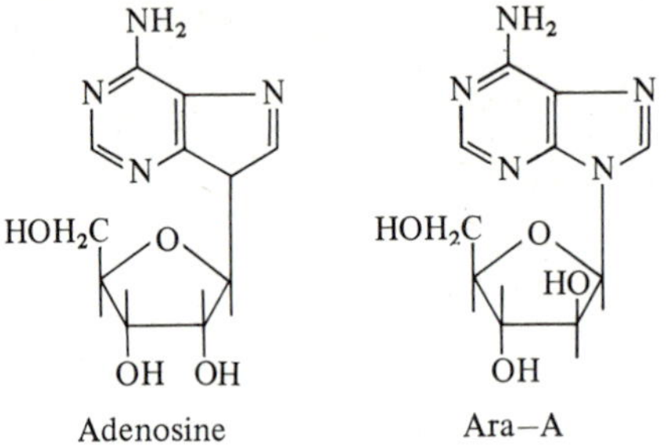

Fig. 1. Chemical structures of adenosine and ara-A

has been expended by many investigators in the search for other anticancer and antiviral nucleosides. Ara-A was originally synthesized by LEE et al. (1960) as a potential anticancer agent, and later isolated from culture filtrates of *Streptomyces antibioticus* by Parke, Davis and Co.

II. Chemistry

Ara-A is structurally different from adenosine in its sugar moiety. The 2'-OH group and 2'-H atom are interchanged in ara-A to form D-arabinose, whereas adenosine has D-ribose as its sugar moiety (Fig. 1). Proton magnetic resonance spectroscopy shows that ara-A and adenosine have closely similar solid-state conformations. This may account for their similar behavior in some biochemical reactions. In aqueous medium, however, the conformations on the sugar rings of the natural forms are apparently different (REMIN et al. 1976). Moreover, unlike adenosine, which has a local minimum in the high *anti* conformation, ara-A is highly unstable in high *anti* conformation (MILES et al. 1977). Since high *anti* glycosidic conformation is the prerequisite for ara-A and adenosine as substrates of adenosine kinase, they may show somewhat different metabolic effects in animal cells (MILES et al. 1977). Ara-A is colorless, stable in distilled water, and has relatively low water solubility (maximum 1.8 mg/ml at 37 °C; MÜLLER 1979).

III. Antiviral Spectrum

In vitro, ara-A has shown broad spectrum activity against many DNA viruses, i.e., herpesviruses [herpes simplex types 1 and 2 (HSV-1 and HSV-2), herpes marmoset (T), herpes simiae (B), herpes saimiri, varicella zoster, cytomegalovirus, pseudorabies, infectious bovine rhinotracheitis, feline herpes, bovine herpes, and catfish herpes viruses], and poxviruses (vaccinia, monkeypox, tanapox, Yaba, and myxoma viruses). Ara-A also has variable, but clinically poor activity against adenoviruses and papovaviruses. Most nononcogenic RNA viruses, i.e., picornaviruses, orthomyxoviruses, paramyxoviruses, and arboviruses are, however, resistant to ara-A, while oncogenic RNA viruses (oncornaviruses) are somewhat susceptible to ara-A (SHANNON 1975). In vivo, both topical and systemic ara-A administration have shown a significant therapeutic efficacy in experimental animals and humans.

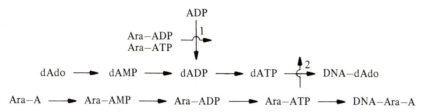

Fig. 2. Pathway for biosynthesis of DNA-deoxyadenosine and DNA-Ara-A, and sites of inhibition by ara-A and its phosphorylated derivatives. (1) Ara-ADP and ara-ATP inhibit ribonucleotide reductase activity. (2) Ara-ATP inhibits the activity of DNA polymerase, α and β, and terminal deoxynucleotidyl transferase

IV. Mechanism of Action

A number of review articles have appeared recently, which describe the mechanism of action of ara-A (CH'IEN et al. 1973; PRUSOFF and GOZ 1973; SHANNON 1975; DE CLERCQ and TORRENCE 1978; MÜLLER 1979). Although the exact mechanism of action of ara-A has not yet been fully elucidated, current studies indicate that the biologic activity of ara-A is attributed to a phosphorylation of ara-A: ara-A is phosphorylated to its monophosphate form, ara-AMP, and ara-AMP is further phosphorylated to form ara-ADP and ara-ATP (BRINK and LE PAGE 1964 a; ILAN et al. 1970; LE PAGE 1970). Ara-ATP inhibits DNA synthesis of culture cells, tumor cells, and virus, either by incorporation into DNA (WAGAR et al. 1971; MÜLLER et al. 1977), or by inhibition of DNA polymerase (FURTH and COHEN 1968; YORK and LE PAGE 1966; MÜLLER et al. 1977; DICIOCCIO and SRIVASTAVA 1977; FALKE et al. 1979). Ara-ADP and ara-ATP also inhibit the activity of ribonucleotide reductase (YORK and LE PAGE 1966; MOORE and COHEN 1967; Fig. 2).

Since ara-A has not been shown to be an active substrate of adenosine kinase in human laryngeal tumor cells (HEp-2) (SCHNEBLI et al. 1967) and the biologic activity of ara-A is antagonized by deoxyadenosine, not by adenosine (SMITH et al. 1976), deoxyadenosine kinase is believed to be the enzyme responsible for the phosphorylation of ara-A to ara-AMP. The enzyme efficiency in conversion of ara-A to its phosphate forms is variable among the host cells. In *Plasmodium berghei*, approximately 93% of ara-A is converted to ara-ATP (ILAN et al. 1979). In contrast to such a prokaryote, eukaryotes have low capacity to phosphorylate ara-A. Biotransformation studies of ara-A conducted by DRACH et al. (1974) have shown that only 2%–5% of ara-A converted to nucleotides after 2 h incubation (Fig. 3 a). After 18 h incubation, 40% of ara-A converted to nucleotides, but about 90% of the nucleotide fraction was identified as inosine monophosphate (IMP) as can be seen in Fig. 3 b. BENNETT et al. (1975) also demonstrated that the major metabolites of ara-A in both herpesvirus-infected and uninfected HEp-2 cells were arabinofuranosylhypoxanthine (ara-Hx) and nucleotides of adenine.

The mode of action of ara-A has been extensively studied in numerous animal tumor cells. BRINK and LE PAGE (1964a, b, 1965) demonstrated that ara-A inhibited the growth of TA3 or 6C3HED cells by inhibiting DNA biosynthesis of these cells. They also showed that ara-A was readily phosphorylated to its triphos-

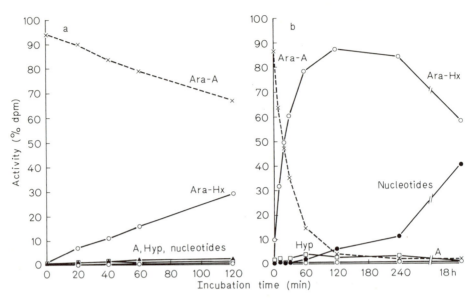

Fig. 3a, b. Metabolism of ara-A by erythrocyte lysates. Lysates from rat **a** and human **b** erythrocytes were incubated with 19 μM ara-A ^{3}H, 2.5 mM Mg^{2+} and 2.5 mM ATP. Aliquots were removed at the indicated times, deproteinized, and analyzed by TLC. Silica gel layers were spotted with 40,000–80,000 dpm for nucleoside determinations; PEI-cellulose layers were spotted with 60,000–100,000 dpm for nucleotide quantitation. A = adenine; Hyp = hypoxanthine. (Drach et al. 1974)

phate level and incorporated into the adenylic and guanylic components of animal tumor cells. Later, York and Le Page (1966), Furth and Cohen (1967, 1968), and Müller et al. (1977) reported that ara-ATP inhibited DNA synthesis by inhibiting DNA polymerase activity of mammalian cells. Moreover, Dicioccio and Srivastava (1977) presented evidence that ara-ATP inhibits terminal deoxynucleotidyl transferase and DNA polymerase, α and β, by biologic competition mechanisms (Fig. 4). Wagar et al. (1971) demonstrated that ara-A incorporates into DNA and acts as a chain terminator in mammalian cells.

In herpesvirus-infected cells, Miller et al. (1968) first observed that ara-A neither possesses virucidal activity nor prevents viral attachment or penetration into cells. Shipman and Drach (1974) reported that ara-A at low concentration (2 μg/ml), which does not effect the cellular DNA synthesis, reduced viral DNA synthesis by 43%. Bennett et al. (1975) also reported that ara-AMP and ara-ATP significantly inhibited DNA-dependent DNA polymerase activity in both herpesvirus-infected and uninfected HEp-2 cells. In herpesvirus-infected, synchronized cultures of KB cells, Shipman et al. (1976) showed that ara-A, at a concentration (3.2 μg/ml) which does not change the total cellular DNA synthesis, reduced viral DNA synthesis by 74%. They inferred that the selective inhibition of viral DNA synthesis by ara-A was probably due to the preferential inhibition of the nucleotide metabolism catalyzed by a virus-specific enzyme. Müller et al. (1977) presented evidence that ara-A incorporates into viral DNA and acts as a DNA chain terminator. Ara-

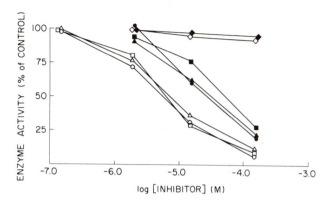

Fig. 4. Inhibition of terminal transferase and DNA polymerase α, β, and γ activities of T-lymphocyte (Molt-4) cells by adenine arabinoside triphosphate (aATP) or cytosine arabinoside triphosphate (aCTP). Standard reaction mixtures containing either aATP *(open symbols)* or aCTP *(full symbols)* were incubated with either 0.1 unit terminal transferase *(squares)*, 0.2 unit DNA polymerase α *(circles)*, 0.2 unit DNA polymerase β *(triangles)*, or 0.02 unit DNA polymerase γ *(diamonds)*. Controls without aATP and aCTP incorporated: 103 and 85 pmol dAMP for DNA polymerase α and β *(open symbol* controls), 48 and 51 pmol dCMP for DNA polymerases α and β *(full symbol* controls), 36 pmol dGMP for terminal transferase, and 11 pmol dTMP for DNA polymerase γ. (DICIOCCIO and SRIVASTAVA 1977)

A incorporates into viral DNA and presents at the end of 3′-OH position of the DNA chain. The HSV DNA pieces, containing incorporated ara-A, are of low molecular weight ($<2.6 \times 10^6$ daltons) and are not found in high molecular weight aggregates.

V. Metabolism, Distribution, and Excretion

In addition to the low level of phosphorylation of ara-A, which yields the metabolically active form in mammalian cells, ara-A is rapidly metabolized to ara-hypoxanthine (ara-Hx) in animal cells (BRINK and LE PAGE 1964 a, b), *Escherichia coli* (HUBERT-HABART and COHEN 1962; COHEN 1966) and crude, cell-free preparations of mammalian cells (LE PAGE and JUNGA 1965; KOSHIURA and LE PAGE 1968). Adenosine deaminase was found and isolated as the enzyme which converts ara-A to ara-Hx (CORY and SUHADOLNIK 1965; FREDERIKSEN 1966; BLOCH et al. 1967). DRACH et al. (1977) also demonstrated that ara-A significantly inhibited cellular growth and DNA synthesis in adenosine deaminase-negative cell lines (B-mix K-44/6). They also showed that when adenosine deaminase-containing calf serum was added to the media, the cytotoxic effect of ara-A was almost reversed. In equimolar concentrations, ara-Hx is only one-tenth as active as ara-A against HSV (MILLER et al. 1968; SHIPMAN et al. 1976).

Considerable efforts have been devoted to the search for potent inhibitors of adenosine deaminase in order to prevent the rapid deamination of ara-A and to increase the antiviral chemotherapeutic efficacy of ara-A. SAWA et al. (1967), SCHAEFFER and SCHWENDER (1974), and WOO et al. (1974) have isolated adenosine

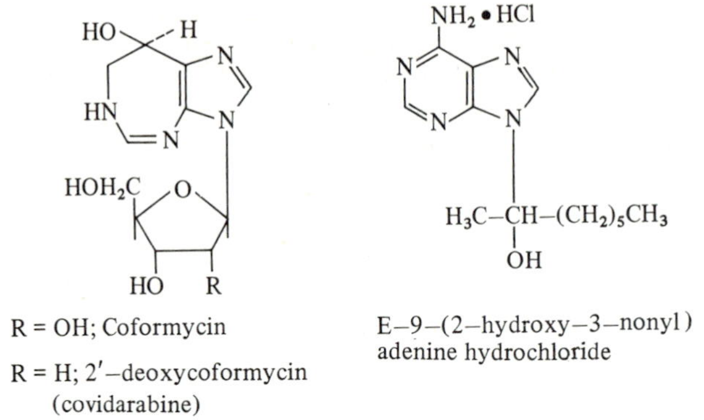

R = OH; Coformycin

R = H; 2′–deoxycoformycin
(covidarabine)

E–9–(2–hydroxy–3–nonyl)
adenine hydrochloride

Fig. 5. Chemical structures of adenosine deaminase inhibitors: coformycin, deoxycoformy-cins, and E-9(2-hydroxy-3-nonyl)adenine hydrochloride

deaminase inhibitors, i.e., coformycin, 2′-deoxycoformycin (covidarabine) and erythro-9-(2-hydroxy-3-3-nonyl)adenine hydrochloride (Fig. 5). CASS and AU-YEUNG (1976) presented evidence that 2′-deoxycoformycin, which alone had no activity, significantly enhanced cytopathic and cytotoxic activities of ara-A in L1210 cells. Tumor cell lines resistant to ara-A have been shown to be responsive to ara-A, when an effective inhibitor of the adenosine deaminase, 2′-deoxycoformycin, was combined with ara-A (LE PAGE et al. 1976). BORONDY et al. (1977) reported ara-A easily converted to ara-Hx in human blood in the absence of adenosine deaminase inhibitor, and the major metabolite was identified as ara-Hx monophosphate (ara-HxMP). With deaminase inhibitors, ara-HxMP was not found to any significant extent, but high levels of ara-A nucleotides were identified as the major metabolite of ara-A in human blood. Erythro-9-(2-hydroxy-3-nonyl) adenine has also been reported to reduce the deamination of ara-A in mouse fibroblasts. Cellular ara-ATP concentration was sharply increased when ara-A was added with erythro-9-(2-hydroxy-3-nonyl)adenine into mouse fibroblasts (PLUNKETT and CO-HEN 1975). SCHWARTZ et al. (1976) reported that the antiviral activity of ara-A against HSV-1 was increased approximately 20-fold by coformycin. The combination of ara-A and coformycin was 90 times more potent in blocking HSV replication than was ara-Hx (SCHWARTZ et al. 1976). SLOAN et al. (1977) also demonstrated a ten-fold increase of the antiviral activity by ara-A and covidarabine combined treatment in comparison with the treatment of ara-A alone against in vivo and in vitro herpesvirus and vaccinia viruses infection. They indicated that the combined treatment of ara-A and covidarabine might be considered as future therapy for systemic virus infections in humans, including herpes encephalitis.

    There is limited information on the metabolism and excretion of ara-A in humans. However, ara-A has been reported to be well distributed into tissue and rapidly metabolized to ara-Hx when administered by intravenous infusion. The daily intravenous (i.v.) infusion of ara-A yields plasma levels of ara-Hx, which reflect the rate of infusion. The elimination half-life is 3.5 h, and the red blood cell level of ara-Hx equal to the plasma level, whereas the cerebrospinal fluid levels are approximately 35% of the plasma levels (GLAZKO et al. 1975).

VI. Clinical and Experimental Therapeutic Aspects

Topical ara-A treatment has been reported to be effective in herpetic keratitis and keratouveitis in both experimental animals (SIDWELL et al. 1968; KAUFMAN et al. 1970) and humans (PAVAN-LANGSTON and DOHLMAN 1972; PAVAN-LANGSTON 1975; PAVAN-LONGSTON and BUCHANAN 1976; JONES 1975; ABEL et al. 1975). Moreover, ara-A was reported to be effective against idoxuridine(IdUrd)-resistant herpes keratitis in rabbits (NESBURN et al. 1974; Hyndiuk et al. 1975).

Systemic administration of ara-A has also been shown to have significant therapeutic activity against herpesviral infectious diseases. Systemic ara-A is effective against HSV encephalitis in hamsters (SCHARDEIN and SIDWELL 1969), mice (SLOAN et al. 1968, 1973; GRIFFITH et al. 1975; PARK et al. 1979a), and humans (CH'IEN et al. 1975; TABER et al. 1977; WHITLEY et al. 1977). A pilot study by CH'IEN et al. (1975) indicated a therapeutic effect of ara-A in neonatal herpes encephalitis if it were administered early, within 3 days after the onset of neurologic signs. TABER et al. (1977) and WHITLEY et al. (1977) have, furthermore, reported the successful control of biopsy-proven HSV encephalitis with systemic vidarabine treatment. Also, the drug has been demonstrated to be effective against herpes zoster in the immunosuppressed patient (CH'IEN et al. 1976; WHITLEY et al. 1976) and ara-A does not appear to depress host cellular immune responses (STEELE et al. 1975). Even though a number of reports have indicated the positive therapeutic efficacy of ara-A for the management of cutaneous herpes infections (LIEBERMAN et al. 1973; SLOAN 1975; KLEIN et al. 1974), topical therapy of ara-A for human herpes labialis (ROWE et al. 1979) or herpes genitalis (ADAMS et al. 1976; HILTON et al. 1978) has been reported to have no significant therapeutic effect.

VII. Untoward Effects

The acute single parenteral median lethal dose (LD_{50}) of ara-A in rodents exceeds 5,000 mg/kg. When ara-A is injected intramuscularly as a 20% suspension, rats tolerate at least 150 mg/kg, and dogs tolerate 50 mg/kg without significant clinical, laboratory, or pathologic manifestations of toxicity (KURTZ 1975). Ara-A has been shown to possess teratogenic effects in rats and rabbits, but not in rhesus monkeys. A single 5 mg/kg ara-A injection or topical application of 10% ara-A ointment to pregnant rabbits produced malformed fetuses (KURTZ 1975). Although no serious acute toxicity has been reported in humans, anorexia, nausea, vomiting, weight loss, weakness, magaloblastic changes in erythroid elements of bone marrow, tremors, and thrombophlebitis have been encountered with systemic application of vidarabine in daily doses of 20 mg/kg (Ross et al. 1976). RAMOS et al. (1979) reported a syndrome of inappropriate secretion of antidiuretic hormone following ara-A systemic therapy in a herpes zoster patient.

VIII. Analogs of Ara-A

Even though ara-A appears to be an effective and relatively nontoxic antiviral agent for the management of some infections caused by HSV, it has several disadvantages as an antiviral agent. First, the water solubility is extremely low. Second, in vivo, ara-A is rapidly metabolized to the less effective ara-Hx or ineffective metabolites, such as adenine (PAVAN-LANGSTON et al. 1974; BENNETT et al. 1975). Third, ara-A must be metabolized to ara-AMP, the 5′-phosphorylated form of ara-A, which is the substrate for the formation of ara-ADP and ara-ATP, the active metabolites for antiviral action (BENNETT et al. 1975; MÜLLER 1979). In order to remedy these disadvantages, several analogs of ara-A were synthesized and tested. Ara-AMP (9-β-D-arabinofuranosyladenine 5′-monophosphate) was synthesized to overcome the poor water solubility of ara-A.

PLUNKETT et al. (1974) reported that in exponentially growing L cells, a small amount of ara-AMP penetrated the cells as an intact nucleotide, was further phosphorylated to the di- and triphosphates and subsequently incorporated by phosphodiester bond linkage into DNA. LE PAGE et al. (1972) reported on the metabolism and excretion of ara-AMP in cancer patients. High doses of ara-AMP by intravenous push resulted in sustained tissue levels of ara-AMP, ara-A, and ara-Hx. BAKER and HASKELL (1977) presented evidence that ara-AMP is metabolically very stable. Also, KURTZ et al. (1977) reported that ara-AMP is nor more toxic, and, in some aspects, less toxic than its parent compound, ara-A. Ancillary studies suggested that the diminished toxicity of the 5′-monophosphate, where it exists, is probably due to its high solubility, which results in enhancement of its metabolism and excretion (KURTZ et al. 1977).

There are many reports on the chemotherapeutic efficacy of ara-AMP. SIDWELL et al. (1973) demonstrated that ara-AMP administered intraperitoneally, intracerebrally, or perorally prevented the HSV-1 encephalitis death or prolonged the mean survival time of mice. PAVAN-LANGSTON et al. (1976) have shown that ara-AMP had a significant therapeutic effect in the treatment of HSV-2 keratoconjunctivitis and prevented the development of encephalitis from HSV-2 corneal infection. TROBE et al. (1976) presented evidence that 2% ara-AMP had equal efficiency to 3% ara-A ointment in HSV-1 epithelial keratitis in rabbits and that 20% ara-AMP was superior to 3% ara-A. No toxicity was observed in the rabbits receiving a 20% solution of ara-AMP. More recently, SPRUANCE et al. (1979) have, however, reported the failure of treatment of recurrent herpes labialis with 10% ara-AMP ointment. They concluded that the failure may be due to the poor penetrability of ara-AMP into cutaneous lesions, because the therapeutic efficacy of ara-AMP is markedly enhanced by increasing the skin penetration of topical ara-AMP by iontophoresis in the hairless mouse model of HSV skin infection (PARK et al. 1978). In addition to ara-AMP, numerous derivatives of ara-A have been described. For example: (1) ara-Hx, which is the metabolic product of ara-A; (2) arabinosyl-N^6-hydroxyadenine, in which the amino group at C-6 is replaced by an hydroxylamino group; (3) 5′-O-esters of ara-A such as ara-A 5′-palmitate and 5′-benzoate; (4) O′-methyl esters of ara-A. However, none of these compounds are found to be superior to the parent compound, ara-A, in their antiviral efficacy (DE CLERCQ and TORRENCE 1978).

IX. Perspectives

Today, ara-A is used primarily as a highly effective 3% topical ointment for the treatment of primary and recurrent herpetic infections of the human cornea, and as prophylaxis against enhancement of spontaneous recurrence when topical ocular steroids are in use for herpetic immune keratitis or uveitis. It is also effective, but not FDA approved, for therapy of ocular vaccinia (PAVAN-LANGSTON and DOHLMAN 1972; HYNDIUK et al. 1976). As a systemic agent, the drug will successfully control herpes simplex encephalitis in humans if given early in the course of disease, and it is effective against herpes zoster (varicella) infections in immunosuppressed patients.

There are problems, however, with either route of administration. Topically, prolonged use may result in less severe, but nontheless the same side effects as those seen with topical idoxuridine: punctate keratopathy, clinical resistance, lacrimal punctal occlusion, and interference with stromal wound healing. As 3% drops, ara-A is significantly less effective than guttate idoxuridine and is, therefore, not used in this form (PAVAN-LANGSTON et al. 1979a).

As a parenteral agent, its low solubility necessitates the administration of a significant volume of fluid, which may tax the cardiovascular system of some patients and, as previously mentioned, nausea, vomiting, bone marrow suppression, and thrombophlebitis have been reported in some patients. All of these side effects were reversible upon withdrawal of the drug after the appropriate therapeutic dose had been given. Potential teratogenicity and mutagenicity, however, precludes its use in pregnant women.

Because of these side effects, work continues on analogs of ara-A, the most promising of which is currently ara-AMP. Because of its total solubility, this drug may be delivered in very small fluid volumes, thus obviating cardiovascular stress and the nausea and vomiting which, in part, are due to the large fluid load. As a topical agent, this drug has proven very effective but too toxic for frequent delivery in therapy of ocular infections (FOSTER and PAVAN-LANGSTON 1977). Further advances in this area, then, as well as in therapy of dermal or genital herpes must come with the development of effective, but less toxic or less readily metabolized, analogs of ara-A.

C. 9-(2-Hydroxyethoxymethyl)guanine

I. Introduction and History

9-(2-Hydroxyethoxymethyl)guanine (acyclovir, acycloguanosine, BW-248U, Zovirax®) is a product of research revolving around synthetic chemical compounds designed to mimic substrates for a known model enzyme, adenosine deaminase, which is essential to nucleic acid synthesis. SCHAEFFER et al. (1971) had found that the 2'- and 3'-OH groups of adenosine do not play a critical role in substrate activity. Various acyclic analogs of adenosine, containing several functional groups, have been shown to be substrates for adenosine deaminase (SCHAEFFER et al. 1971). Among them, the 2,6-disubstituted purines with 9-(2-hydroxyethoxymethyl) chains were the compounds which proved to be the most effective antivirals in vitro (Personal communication with R. E. Keeney, 1980). On the basis of these observations, acyclovir was synthesized and found to possess a potent antiviral activity in vitro and in vivo (ELION et al. 1977; SCHAEFFER et al. 1978).

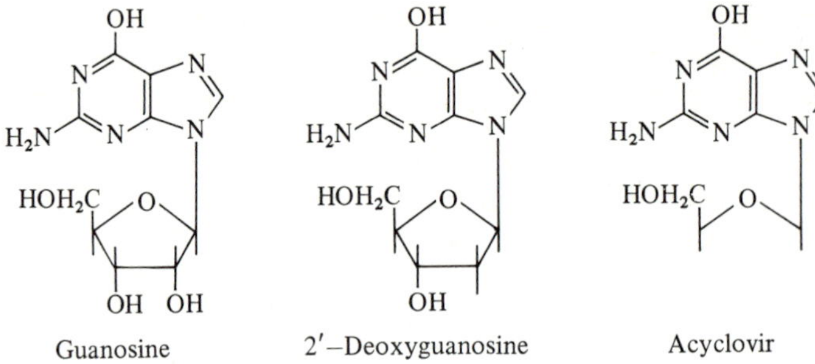

| Guanosine | 2'−Deoxyguanosine | Acyclovir |

Fig. 6. Chemical structures of guanosine, 2'-deoxyguanosine, and acyclovir

Table 1. Relative potencies of acyclovir and some standard antiherpes compounds. (Schaeffer et al. 1978)

Compounds	$ID_{50}(\mu M)$ [a]	Potency (relative to idoxuridine = 100)
Phosphonoacetic acid	57.5	1.7
Vidarabine	16	6
Trifluorothymidine	1.5	67
Idoxuridine	1	100
Cytarabine	0.2	500
Acyclovir	0.1	1,000

[a] Concentration inhibiting plaque formation by 50%

II. Chemistry

Acyclovir is an anlog of guanosine or deoxyguanosine in which the 2' and 3' carbon atoms are missing (Fig. 6). This compound is a white, crystalline substance with a solubility of 0.12% in water at 25 °C (Pavan-Langston et al. 1978). Acyclovir is known as a very stable compound. At 5°, 25°, or 37 °C, acyclovir is stable for 12 months (Personal communication with R. E. Keeney, 1980).

III. Antiviral Spectrum

In vitro, acyclovir has been shown to be effective against DNA viruses, especially the herpesvirus family, i.e., HSV-1, HSV-2, varicella zoster virus and murine cytomegalovirus. Human cytomegalovirus and herpes virus B are also sensitive, but require higher drug concentrations (Schaeffer et al. 1978). Adenovirus and poxvirus do not appear to be affected by acyclovir. Table 1 shows the relative potencies of acyclovir and other antivirals in comparison with idoxuridine, the compound most frequently used in clinical practice. Acyclovir has strong antiviral potency; 160 times more potent than vidarabine and 10 times more potent than idoxuridine.

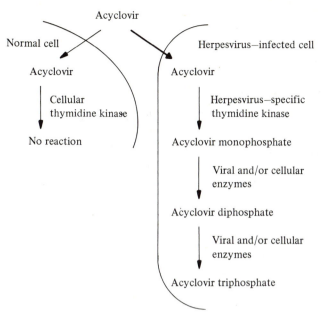

Fig. 7. Selective phosphorylation of acyclovir by herpesvirus-specific thymidine kinase

IV. Mechanism of Action

Acyclovir is an effective and selective inhibitor of herpesvirus replication. This compound is specifically phosphorylated to form acyclovir monophosphate by herpesvirus-coded thymidine kinase and further phosphorylated to acyclovir di- and triphosphates. In the noninfected host cell, the phosphorylation of acyclovir occurs to a very limited extent (Fig. 7). ELION et al. (1977) have presented evidence that specific phosphorylation of acyclovir occurs in HSV-infected cells, but not in uninfected cells: ^{3}H-labeled or ^{14}C-labeled acyclovir was specifically phosphorylated to form mono-, di-, and triphosphates in HSV-1-infected Vero cells, but was not phosphorylated in uninfected Vero cells (Fig. 8). Furthermore, FYFE et al. (1978) have presented evidence that the enzyme responsible for the phosphorylation of acyclovir was identified as the herpesvirus-coded thymidine kinase. The evidence included: (1) the proportional increase in the rates of phosphorylation of thymidine and acyclovir after infection of Vero cells; (2) the loss of phosphorylation of thymidine and acyclovir with the infection of viruses deficient in thymidine kinase; (3) comigration and copurification of thymidine and acyclovir kinase activities on polyacrylamide gel electrophoresis and with an affinity chromatography procedure, respectively; (4) the similar inhibitor specificities of thymidine and acyclovir.

Acyclovir triphosphate acts to inhibit the viral DNA polymerase and to terminate the elongation of the viral DNA chain by incorporation into DNA (ELION et al. 1977; FURMAN et al. 1979). In their preliminary experiments, ELION et al. (1977) have demonstrated that acyclovir triphosphate inhibits HSV DNA polymerase (DNA nucleotidyl transferase) 10–30 times more effectively than cellular DNA

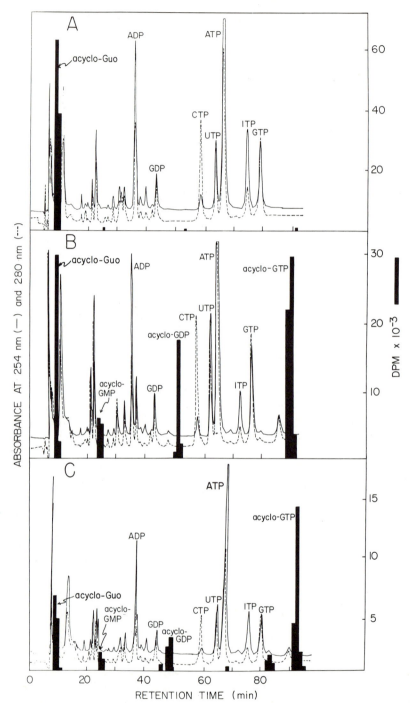

Fig. 8, A–C. High pressure liquid chromatography profiles of extracts of uninfected and HSV-1 (H29 strain)-infected Vero cells incubated with acyclovir for 6 h. **A** uninfected cells treated with acyclovir ^{3}H (1.0 mM); **B** infected cells treated with acyclovir ^{3}H (0.5 mM); **C** infected cells treated with acyclovir 8-^{14}C (0.5 mM). (Elion et al. 1977)

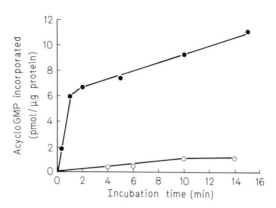

Fig. 9. Incorporation of acyclo GMP ^{14}C into calf thymus DNA, using Vero cell and HSV-1 (H29 strain) DNA polymerase. The contents of the reaction mixture were identical to those described in the text except that dGTP was replaced with acyclo GTP ^{14}C (24 μm, 14 dpm/pmol). *Full circles*, HSV-1 DNA polymerase (1.7 U/ml reaction mixture) with a specific activity of 0.7 pmol/min per μg protein; *open circles*, Vero cell DNA polymerase α (2.0 U/ml reaction mixture) with a specific activity of 1.0 pmol/min per μg protein. (FURMAN et al. 1979)

polymerase. They have also shown that one needs an approximately 3,000-fold higher concentration of acyclovir to inhibit the host cell growth than that needed to inhibit the viral replication. Actually, FURMAN et al. (1979) have presented evidence that acyclovir triphosphate can serve as a substrate for HSV-1 DNA polymerase and, to a much smaller extent, for the DNA polymerase α of cells. They have observed the incorporation of monophosphate ^{14}C acyclovir into calf thymus DNA, using Vero cell and HSV-1 DNA polymerases (Fig. 9). Because of the lack of the 3′-OH group on the sugar moiety of acyclovir, the incorporation of acyclovir monophosphate into DNA would be expected to terminate the DNA chain elongation.

V. Metabolism, Distribution, and Excretion

The absorption of acyclovir through oral administration is variable among different animal species. Approximately 50% of orally administered acyclovir is absorbed in mice, and poorer absorbance has been noticed in rats. The maximal plasma drug level usually occurs at about 2–4 h after oral administration in mice and rats. When the drug is injected intravenously, the plasma levels of acyclovir were dose dependent and were consistent with a half-life of 3–4 h in dogs (Personal communication with R. E. KEENEY, 1980). RECENTLY, SPECTOR et al. (1979) have reported that the plasma elimination half-life was 1.6–3.25 h following the single i.v. injection of acyclovir in cancer patients. DE MIRANDA et al. (1979) have also shown that the half-life of acyclovir in the slow disposition phase ranged from 2.2 to 5 h after 1 h i.v. infusion in humans.

Acyclovir is metabolically stable in mice, rats, dogs, and humans and there is no evidence of increased metabolism on chronic administration. Acyclovir is distributed into all tissues and, with poor binding, to plasma protein in mice and dogs

(Personal communication with R. E. Keeney, 1980). In humans, acyclovir is known to be excreted through glomerular filtration and tubular secretion (De Miranda et al. 1979).

VI. Clinical and Experimental Therapeutic Aspects

Schaeffer et al. (1978) showed that acyclovir in ointment concentrations from 0.3% to 3% was effective against established HSV epithelial keratitis in rabbits and was well tolerated. Several controlled studies of the activities of 3% acyclovir against experimental HSV keratitis in rabbits have been reported (Pavan-Langston et al. 1978; Shiota et al. 1979; Falcon and Jones 1979). Acyclovir was significantly more active than IdUrd, ara-A, ara-AMP, or F_3dThd (trifluorothymidine, 5-trifluoromethyl-2'-deoxyuridine, CF_3dUrd), producing more rapid healing and showing no significant toxicity. Furthermore systemic acyclovir treatment was effective in treating established herpes keratitis and iritis in rabbits and prevented death from encephalitis (Kaufman et al. 1978; Bauer et al. 1979). Recently, the excellent therapeutic effect of systemic acyclovir treatment on experimental HSV encephalitis in mice was reported by the authors (Park et al. 1979a). The therapeutic accomplishments of nontoxic doses of acyclovir were comparable to those of maximally tolerated doses of ara-A. Topical acyclovir treatment was effective for cutaneous HSV infections in guinea pigs (Schaeffer et al. 1978; Park et al. 1980a), hairless mice (Klein et al. 1979; Park et al. 1980b) and mice (Park et al. 1979b). Moreover, topical or systemic acyclovir treatments, when initiated early, significantly reduced or completely prevented the establishment of ganglionic latent infection of HSV in mice (Field et al. 1979; Park et al. 1979b) and in hairless mice (Klein et al. 1979; Park et al. 1980b). Pavan-Langston et al. (1979b) have reported that systemic acyclovir treatment given during the latent HSV-1 infection period resulted in a significant reduction of latent infection in trigeminal ganglia of mice. However, Field et al. (1979) and Klein et al. (1979) have reported that acyclovir could not eliminate the established latent HSV infection in mice. In these studies, however, the animal species, strain of virus, sites of infection, doses of drug, isolation method of latent virus, and the duration of treatment were different. A clinical human study by Jones et al. (1979) has indicated that acyclovir is a clinically effective antiviral drug against herpes simplex keratitis in humans without any evident side effects.

VII. Untoward Effects

Since acyclovir is activated specifically by herpesvirus-coded thymidine kinase, this drug is considered as a very safe substance. In our laboratory, we have recently demonstrated the lack of toxicity of acyclovir in corneal wound healing of rabbits (Lass et al. 1979). Masked controlled rabbit studies were done to determine the toxic effect on corneal wound healing of 3% acyclovir and 0.5% idoxuridine ointments in therapeutically effective concentrations. Acyclovir was found to have no notable detrimental effect in comparison with controls on the quality of regenerating epithelium or the reepithelization of epithelial wounds. Idoxuridine treatment caused significant toxic changes in the regenerating epithelium clinically and histologically with a significant delay in epithelial wound healing in comparison with control or acyclovir-treated eyes. Acyclovir had no significant effect on the collagen content of stromal wounds as measured by hydroxyproline assay. Idoxuridine caused a reduction in collagen content not significantly different from controls, but significantly lower than acyclovir. Systemic administration of acyclovir by 1 h i.v. infusion to 14 human volunteers did not induce any toxicity either clinically or from laboratory findings in any of the volunteers (DE MIRANDA et al. 1979).

VIII. Perspectives

Although not yet FDA approved for general release, acyclovir has shown great promise both as a topical agent for infectious ocular, dermal, and venereal herpes simplex and as a parenteral drug for disseminated and encephalitic disease, all caused by members of the herpesvirus group. Clinical studies in England on ocular infection (JONES et al. 1979) have been particularly successful. A similar multicenter investigation using the 3% ointment is currently under way in the United States as is an herpetic dermatitis study using 5% acyclovir in polyethylene glycol gel. Topical therapy of venereal infections will soon be initiated. Animal studies on models of all of the previously mentioned forms of herpetic infection hold great promise for the outcome of this clinical work.

Perhaps the most significant breakthrough with acyclovir, however, has been in the study of its potential as a parenteral agent for eliminating the source of recurrent disease – herpesvirus lying latent in the neuronal ganglia. Work on this has, of course, not yet reached clinical levels and, in all likelihood, will not do so until the safety of systemically administered drug has been well established. Of all nucleosides now under study, however, this appears to be the one drug which is extremely effective against both HSV-1 and HSV-2 as well as all other members of the herpesvirus group. It has an extremely high therapeutic index due to its specificity for activation only by herpetic thymidine kinase, is not metabolized to a less or inactive form, and is absorbed orally and through the skin as well as by the usual ocular and parenteral routes. The next few years will show the full and highly promising potential of this new and exciting purine nucleoside.

References

Abel R, Kaufman HE, Sugar J (1975) Intravenous adenine arabinoside against herpes simplex keratouveitis in humans. Am J Ophthalmol 79:659–664

Adams HG, Bensen EA, Alexander ER, Vontver LA, Remington MA, Holmes KK (1976) Genital herpetic infection in men and women: clinical course and effect of topical application of adenine arabinoside. J Infect Dis 133:A151–A159

Baker DC, Haskell TH (1977) A labelled 9-β-D-arabinofuranosyladenine 5′-monophosphate having increased metabolic stability. Ann NY Acad Sci 284:30–33

Bauer DJ, Collins P, Tucker WE Jr, Macklin AW (1979) Treatment of experimental herpes simplex with acycloguanosine. Br J Ophthalmol 63:429–435

Bennett LL, Shannon WM, Allen PW, Arnett G (1975) Studies on the biochemical basis for the antiviral activities of some nucleoside analogs. Ann NY Acad Sci 255:342–358

Bergmann W, Feeney RJ (1950) The isolation of a new thymidine pentoside from sponges. J Am Chem Soc 72:2809–2810

Bergmann W, Feeney RJ (1951) Contribution to the study of marine products. XXXII. The nucleosides of sponges. J Org Chem 16:981–987

Bloch A, Robins MJ, McCarthy JR (1967) The role of the 5′-hydroxyl group of adenosine in determining substrate specificity for adenosine deaminase. J Med Chem 10:908–912

Borondy PE, Chang T, Maschewske E, Glazko AJ (1977) Inhibition of adenosine deaminase by co-vidarabine and its effects on metabolic disposition of adenine-arabinoside (vidarabine). Ann NY Acad Sci 284:9–20

Brink JJ, Le Page GA (1964a) Metabolism and distribution of 9-β-D-arabinofuranosyladenine in mouse tissue. Cancer Res 24:1042–1049

Brink JJ, Le Page GA (1964b) Metabolic effects of 9-D-arabinosylpurines in ascites tumor cells. Cancer Res 24:312–318

Brink JJ, Le Page GA (1965) 9-β-D-Arabinofuranosyladenine as an inhibitor of metabolism in normal and neoplastic cells. Can J Biochem 43:1–15

Cass CE, Au-Yeung TH (1976) Enhancement of 9-β-D-arabinofuranosyladenine cytotoxicity to mouse leukemia L1210 in vitro by 2′-deoxycoformycin. Cancer Res 36:1486–1491

Ch'ien LT, Schabel FM Jr, Alford CA Jr (1973) Arabinosylnucleosides and nucleotides. In: Carter WA (ed) Selective inhibitors of viral functions. Chemical Rubber Company Press, Cleveland, Ohio, pp 227–265

Ch'ien LT, Whitley RJ, Nahmias AJ et al. (1975) Antiviral chemotherapy and neonatal herpes simplex virus infection: a pilot study-experience with adenine arabinoside (ara-A). Pediatrics 55:678–685

Ch'ien LT, Whitley RJ, Alford CA Jr, Galasso GL, Collaboratory Study Group (1976) Adenine arabinoside for therapy of herpes zoster in immunosuppressed patients: preliminary results of a collaboratory study. J Infect Dis 133:A184–A191

Cohen SS (1966) Introduction to the biochemistry of D-arabinosylnucleosides. Prog Nucleic Acid Res Mol Biol 5:1–88

Cory JG, Suhadolnik RJ (1965) Structural requirements of nucleosides for binding by adenosine deaminase. Biochemistry 4:1729–1732

De Clercq E, Torrence PF (1978) Nucleoside analogs with selective antiviral activity. J Carbohydr Nucleosides Nucleotides 5:187–224

De Miranda P, Whitley RJ, Blum MR, Keeney RE (1979) Pharmacokinetics of the antiviral drug acyclovir (Zovirax™) in man (Abstr 255). Presented in 11th International Congress of Chemotherapy, Boston. American Society of Microbiology

Dicioccio RA, Srivastava BIS (1977) Kinetic inhibition of deoxynucleotide-polymerizing enzyme activities from normal and leukemic human cells by 9-β-D-arabinofuranosyladenine 5′-triphosphate and 1-β-D-arabinofuranosylcytosine 5′-triphosphate. Eur J Biochem 79:411–418

Drach JC, Bus JS, Schultz SK, Sandberg JN (1974) Biotransformation of 9-β-D-arabinofuranosyladenine by rat and human erythrocytes. Biochem Pharmacol 23:2761–2767

Drach JC, Sandberg JN, Shipman C Jr (1977) Antiproliferative effects of 9-β-D-arabinofuranosyladenine in a mammalian cell line devoid of adenosine deaminase activity. J Dent Res 56:275–288

Elion GB, Furman PA, Fyfe JA, De Miranda P, Beauchamp J, Schaeffer HJ (1977) Selectivity of action of an antiherpetic agent, 9-(2-hydroxyethoxymethyl)guanine. Proc Natl Acad Sci USA 74:5716–5720

Falcon MG, Jones BR (1979) Acycloguanosine: antiviral activity in the rabbit cornea. Br J Ophthalmol 63:422–424

Falke D, Ronge K, Arendes J, Müller WEG (1979) Differential and selective inhibition of cellular and herpes simplex virus DNA synthesis by arabinofuranosyladenine. Biochim Biophys Acta 563:36–45

Field HJ, Bell SE, Elion GB, Nash AA, Wildy P (1979) Effect of acycloguanosine treatment on acute and latent herpes simplex infections in mice. Antimicrob Agents Chemother 15:554–561

Foster CS, Pavan-Langston D (1977) Corneal wound healing and antiviral medication. Arch Ophthalmol 95:2062–2067

Frederiksen S (1969) Specificity of adenosine and 2′-deoxyadenosine analogues. Arch Biochem Biophys 113:383–388

Furman PA, St Clair MH, Fyfe JA, Rideout JL, Keller PM, Elion GB (1979) Inhibition of herpes simplex virus-induced DNA polymerase activity and viral DNA replication by 9-(2-hydroxyethoxymethyl)guanine and its triphosphate. J Virol 32:72–79

Furth JJ, Cohen SS (1967) Inhibition of mammalian DNA polymerase by the 5′-triphosphate of 9-β-D-arabinofuranosyladenine. Cancer Res 27:1528–1533

Fyfe JA, Keller PM, Furman PA, Miller RL, Elion GB (1978) Thymidine kinase from herpes simlex virus phosphorylates the new antiviral compound, 9-(2-hydroxyethoxymethyl)guanine. J Biol Chem 253:8721–8727

Glazko AJ, Chang T, Drach JC et al. (1975) Species differences in the metabolic disposition of ara-A. In: Pavan-Langston D, Buchanan RA, Alford CA Jr (eds) Adenine arabinoside: an antiviral agent. Raven, New York, pp 111–113

Griffith JF, Fitzwilliam JF, Casagrande S, Butler SR (1975) Experimental herpes simplex virus encephalitis: comparative effects of treatment with cytosine arabinoside and adenine arabinoside. J Infect Dis 132:506–510

Furth JJ, Cohen SS (1968) Inhibition of mammalian DNA polymerase by the 5′-triphosphate of 1-β-D-arabinofuranosylcytosine and 5′-phosphate of 9-β-D-arabinofuranosyladenine. Cancer Res 21:1528–1533

Hilton AL, Bushell TEC, Waller D, Blight J (1978) A trial of adenine arabinoside in genitalis herpes. Br J Vener Dis 54:50–52

Hubert-Habart M, Cohen SS (1962) The toxicity of 9-β-D-arabinofuranosyladenine to purine-requiring Escherichia coli. Biochim Biophys Acta 59:468–471

Hyndiuk RA, Hull DS, Schultz RO, Chin GN, Laibson PR, Drachmer JH (1975) Adenine arabinoside in idoxuridine unresponsive and intolerent herpetic keratitis. Am J Ophthalmol 79:655–658

Hyndiuk RA, Okumoto M, Damiano RA, Valenton M, Smolin G (1976) Treatment of vaccinal keratitis with vidarabine. Arch Ophthalmol 94:1363–1364

Ilan J, Tokuyasu K, Ilan J (1970) Phosphorylation of D-arabinosyladenine by *Plasmodium berghei* and its partial protection of mice against malaria. Nature 228:1300–1301

Jones DB (1975) Adenine arabinoside in herpes simplex keratitis treatment of idoxuridine-failure epithelial disease and combined corticosteroid therapy in stromal keratitis. In: Pavan-Langston D, Buchanan RA, Alford CA Jr (eds) Adenine arabinoside: an antiviral agent. Raven, New York, pp 371–380

Jones BR, Coster DJ, Fison PN, Thompson GM, Cobo LM, Falcon MG (1979) Efficacy of acycloguanosine (Wellcome 248U) against herpes-simplex corneal ulcers. Lancet 1:243–244

Kaufman HE, Ellison BS, Townsend WM (1970) The chemotherapy of herpes iritis with adenine arabinoside and cytarabine. Arch Ophthalmol 84:783–787

Kaufman HE, Varnell ED, Centifanto TM, Rheinstrom SD (1978) Effect of 9-(2-hydroxyethoxymethyl)guanine on herpes virusinduced keratitis and iritis in rabbits. Antimicrob Agents Chemother 14:842–845

Klein RJ, Friedman-Kien AE, Brady E (1974) Herpes simplex virus skin infections in hairless mice: treatment with antiviral compounds. Antimicrob Agents Chemother 5:318–322

Klein RJ, Friedman-Kien AE, De Stefano E (1979) Latent herpes simplex virus infections in sensory ganglia of hairless mice prevented by acycloguanosine. Antimicrob Agents Chemother 15:723–729

Koshiura R, Le Page GA (1968) Some inhibitors of deamination of 9-β-D-arabinofuranosyladenine and 9-β-D-xylofuranosyladenine by blood and neoplasms of experimental animals and humans. Cancer Res 28:1014–1020

Kurtz SM (1975) Toxicology of adenine arabinoside. In: Pavan-Langston D, Buchanan RA, Alford CA Jr (eds) Adenine arabinoside: an antiviral agent. Raven, New York, pp 145–157

Kurtz SM, Fitzgerald JE, Schardein JL (1977) Comparative animal toxicology of vidarabine and its 5′-monophosphate. Ann NY Acad Sci 284:6–8

Lass J, Pavan-Langston D, Park NH (1979) Medication of acyclic antimetabolite and corneal wound healing. Am J Ophthalmol 88:102–108

Lee WW, Benitez A, Goodman L, Baker BR (1960) Potential anticancer agents. XI. Synthesis of the β-anomer of 9-(D-arabinofuranosyl)-adenine. J Am Chem Soc 82:2648–2649

Le Page GA (1970) Arabinosyladenine and arabinosylhypoxanthine metabolism in murine tumor cells. Can J Biochem 48:75–78

Le Page GA, Junga IG (1965) Metabolism of purine nucleoside analogs. Cancer Res 25:46–52

Le Page GA, Lin YT, Orth RE, Gottlieb JA (1972) 5'-Nucleotides as potential formulators for administering nucleoside analogs in man. Cancer Res 32:2441–2444

Le Page GA, Worth LS, Kimball AP (1976) Enhancement of the antitumor activity of arabinofuranosyladenine by 2'-deoxycoformycin. Cancer Res 36:1481–1485

Lieberman M, Schafer TW, Came PE (1973) Chemotherapy of cutaneous herpesvirus infection of hairless mice. J Invest Dermatol 60:203–206

Miles DL, Miles DW, Redington P, Eyring H (1977) A conformational basis for the selective action of ara-adenine. J Theor Biol 67:499–514

Miller FA, Dixon GJ, Ehrlich J, Sloan BJ, McLean IW Jr (1968) The antiviral activity of 9-β-D-arabinofuranosyladenine (ara-A). I. Cell culture studies. Antimicrob Agents Chemother 1968:136–147

Moore EC, Cohen SS (1976) Effect of arabinomononucleotides on ribonucleotides reduction by an enzyme system from rat tumor. J Biol Chem 242:2116–2118

Müller WEG (1979) Mechanisms of action and pharmacology: chemical agents. In: Galasso GJ, Merigan TC, Buchanan RA (eds) Antiviral agents and viral diseases of man. Raven, New York, pp 77–149

Müller WEG, Maidhof A, Zahn RK, Shannon WN (1977) Effect of 9-β-D-arabinofuranosyladenine on DNA synthesis in vitro. Cancer Res 37:2282–2290

Nesburn AB, Robinson C, Dickinson R (1974) Adenine arabinoside effect on experimental idoxuridine-resistant herpes simplex infection. Invest Ophthalmol 13:302–304

Park NH, Gangarosa LP, Kwon BS, Hill JM (1978) Iontophoresis of adenine arabinoside monophosphate (ara-AMP) to HSV-1 infected hairless mice skin. Antimicrob Agents Chemother 14:605–608

Park NH, Pavan-Langston D, McLean SL, Albert DM (1979 a) Therapy of experimental herpes simplex encephalitis with acyclovir in mice. Antimicrob Agents Chemother 15:775–779

Park NH, Pavan-Langston D, McLean SL, Lass J (1980 a) Topical acyclovir therapy of cutaneous herpes simplex virus infection in guinea pigs. Arch Dermatol 116:672–675

Park NH, Pavan-Langston D, McLean (1979 b) Acyclovir in oral and ganglionic herpes simplex. J Infect Dis 140:802–806

Park NH, Pavan-Langston D, Hettinger ME (1980 b) Acyclovir therapy for the orofacial and ganglionic HSV infection in hairless mice. J Dent Res 59:2080–2086

Pavan-Langston D (1975) Clinical evaluation of ara A and IDU in treatment of ocular herpes. Am J Ophthalmol 80:495–502

Pavan-Langston D, Buchanan RA (1976) Vidarabine therapy of simple and IDU-complicated herpetic keratitis. Trans Am Acad Ophthalmol Otol 81:813–825

Pavan-Langston D, Dohlman CH (1972) Adenine arabinoside therapy of viral keratoconjunctivitis – a clinical study. Am J Ophthalmol 74:81–90

Pavan-Langston D, Langston RHS, Geary PA (1974) Prophylaxis and therapy of experimental ocular herpes simplex. Comparison of idoxuridine, adenine arabinoside and hypoxanthine arabinoside. Arch Ophthalmol 92:417–421

Pavan-Langston D, Campbell R, Lass J (1978) Acyclic antimetabolite therapy of experimental herpes simplex keratitis. Am J Ophthalmol 86:618–623

Pavan-Langston D, Lass J, Campbell R (1979 a) Antiviral drops. Comparative therapy of experimental herpes simplex keratouveitis. Arch Ophthalmol 97:1132–1135

Pavan-Langston D, North RD, Geary PA, Kinkel K (1976) Intra-ocular penetration of the soluble antiviral, ara-AMP. Arch Ophthalmol 94:1585–1588

Pavan-Langston D, Park NH, Lass J (1979 b) Herpetic ganglionic latency. Aciclovir and vidarabine therapy. Arch Ophthalmol 97:1508-1510

Plunkett W, Cohen SS (1975) Two approaches that increase the activity of analogs of adenine nucleosides in animal cells. Cancer Res 35:1547–1554

Plunkett W, Lapi L, Ortiz PJ, Cohen SS (1974) Penetration of mouse fibroblasts by the 5′-phosphate of 9-β-D-arabinofuranosyladenine and incorporation of the nucleotide into DNA. Proc Natl Acad Sci USA 71:73–77

Prusoff WH, Goz B (1973) Potential mechanisms of action of antiviral agents. Fed Proc 32:1679–1689

Ramos E, Timmons RF, Schimpff SC (1979) Inappropriate antidiuretic hormone following adenine arabinoside administration. Antimicrob Agents Chemother 15:142–144

Remin M, Darzymkiewicz E, Ekiel I, Shugar D (1976) Conformation in aqueous medium of the neutral, protonated, and anionic forms of 9-β-D-arabinofuranosyladenine. Biochim Biophys Acta 435:405–416

Ross AH, Julia A, Balakrishnan C (1976) Toxicity of adenine arabinoside in humans. J Infect Dis [Suppl I] 133:A192–A198

Rowe NH, Brooks SL, Young SK et al. (1979) A clinical trial of topically applied 3 percent vidarabine against recurrent herpes labialis. Oral Surg 47:142–147

Sawa T, Fukagawa Y, Homma I, Takeuchi T, Umezawa H (1967) Mode of inhibition of coformycin on adenosine deaminase. J Antibiot (Tokyo) 20A:227–231

Schaeffer HJ, Schwender DF (1974) Enzyme inhibitors. J Med Chem 17:6–8

Schaeffer HJ, Gurwara S, Vince R, Bittner S (1971) Novel substrate of adenosine deaminase. J Med Chem 14:367–369

Schaeffer HJ, Beauchamp L, De Miranda P, Elion GB, Bauer DJ, Collins P (1978) 9-(2-Hydroxyethoxymethyl)guanine activity against viruses of the herpes group. Nature 272:583–585

Schardein JL, Sidwell RW (1969) Antiviral activity of 9-β-D-arabinofuranosyladenine. III. Reduction in evidence of encephalitis in treated herpes simplex-infected hamsters. Antimicrob Agents Chemother 1968:155–160

Schnebli HP, Hill DL, Bennett LL Jr (1967) Purification and properties of adenosine kinase from human tumor cells of type HEp-2. J Biol Chem 242:1997–2004

Schwartz PM, Shipman C, Drach JC (1976) Antiviral activity of arabinosyladenine and arabinosylhypoxanthine in herpes simplex virus-infected KB cells: selective inhibiton of deoxyribonucleic acid synthesis in the presence of an adenosine deaminase inhibitor. Antimicrob Agents Chemother 10:64–74

Shannon WM (1975) Adenine arabinoside: antiviral activity in vitro. In: Pavan-Langston D, Buchanan RA, Alford CA (eds) Adenine arabinoside: an antiviral agent. Raven, New York, pp 1–43

Shiota H, Inove S, Yamane S (1979) Efficacy of acycloguanosine against herpetic ulcers in rabbit cornea. Br J Ophthalmol 63:425–428

Shipman C Jr, Drach JC (1974) Effect of arabinosyladenine on cellular and viral DNA synthesis in herpes simplex virusinfected synchronized KB cells (Abstr Annu Meet). Am Soc Microbiol 1974:97

Shipman C, Smith SH, Carlson RH, Drach JC (1976) Antiviral activity of arabinosyladenine and arabinosylhypoxanthine in herpes simplex virus-infected KB cells: selective inhibition of viral deoxyribonucleic acid synthesis in synchronized suspension cultures. Antimicrob Agents Chemother 9:120–127

Sidwell RW, Dixon GJ, Shabel FM Jr, Kaump DH (1968) Antiviral activity of 9-β-D-arabinofuranosyladenine II. Activity against herpes simplex keratitis in hamsters. Antimicrob Agents Chemother 1968:148–154

Sidwell RW, Allen LB, Huffman HJ, Khwaja TA, Tolman RL, Robins RK (1973) Anti-DNA virus activity of 5-nucleotide and 3′,5′cyclic nucleotide of 9-β-D-arabinofuranosyladenine. Chemotherapy 19:325–340

Sloan BJ (1975) Adenine arabinoside: chemotherapy studies in animals. In: Pavan-Langston D, Buchanan RA, Alford CA (eds) Adenine arabinoside: an antiviral agent. Raven, New York, pp 45–94

Sloan BJ, Miller FA, Ehrlich J, McLean IW, Machamer HE (1968) Antiviral activity of 9-β-D-arabinofuranosyladenine. IV. Activity against intracerebral herpes simplex virus infections in mice. Antimicrob Agents Chemother 1968:161–171

Sloan BJ, Miller FA, McLean IW Jr (1973) Treatment of herpes simplex virus type 1 and 2 encephalitis in mice with 9-β-D-arabinofuranosyladenine. Antimicrob Agents Chemother 3:74–80

Sloan BJ, Kielty JK, Miller FA (1977) Effect of a novel adenosine deaminase inhibitor (Covidarabine, Co-V) upon antiviral activity *in vitro* and *in vivo* of vidarabine (Vira-A) for DNA virus replication. Ann NY Acad Sci 284:60–80

Smith SH, Shipman C Jr, Brach JC (1976) Deoxyadenosine reversal of the antiviral activity of arabinosyladenine (Abstr 101). In: Program and abstracts, 16th intersciene conference on antimicrobial agents and chemotherapy, Chicago

Spector SA, Hintz M, Quinn RP, Keeney RE, Connor JD (1979) Single dose pharmacokinetic and toxic properties of acyclovir (Acv) (Abstr 256). 11th international congress of chemotherapy, Boston

Spruance SL, Crumpacker CS, Haines H et al. (1979) Ineffectiveness of topical adenine arabinoside 5'-monophosphate in the treatment of recurrent herpes simplex labialis. N Engl J Med 300:1180–1184

Steele RW, Chapa IV, Vincent MM, Hensen SA, Keeney RE (1975) Effects of adenine arabinoside on cellular immune mechanisms in humans. Antimicrob Agents Chemother 7:203–207

Taber LH, Greenberg SB, Perez FI, Couch RB (1977) Herpes simplex encephalitis treated with vidarabine (adenine arabinoside). Arch Neurol 34:608–610

Trobe JO, Centifanto Y, Zam ZS, Varnell E, Kaufman HE (1976) Antiherpes activity of adenine arabinoside monophosphate. Invest Ophthalmol 15:196–199

Wagar MA, Burgoyne LA, Atkinson MR (1971) Deoxyribonucleic acid synthesis in mammalian nuclei: incorporation of deoxyribonucleotides and chain-terminating nucleotide analogues. Biochem J 121:803–809

Whitley RJ, Ch'ien LT, Dolin R, Galasso GJ, Alford CA, Collaborative Study Group (1976) Adenine arabinoside therapy of herpes zoster in the immunosuppressed. N Engl J Med 294:1193–1199

Whitley RJ, Soong SJ, Dolin R, Galasso GJ, Ch'ien LT, Alford CA, Cooperative Study Group (1977) Adenine arabinoside therapy of biopsy-proved herpes simplex encephalitis. N Engl J Med 297:289–294

Woo PWK, Dion HW, Lange SM, Dahl LT, Surham LJA (1974) A novel adenosine and ara-A deaminase inhibitor. J Heterocycl Chem 11:641–643

York JL, Le Page GA (1966) A proposed mechanism for the action of 9-β-D-arabinofuranosyladenine as an inhibitor of the growth of some ascites cells. Can J Biochem 44:19–26

CHAPTER 4

Amantadine and Its Derivatives

J. L. Schulman

A. Introduction and History

Amantadine hydrochloride (1-adamantanamine hydrochloride) was the first antiviral chemotherapeutic agent (1966) to be licensed for general use in the United States. However, despite the demonstrated efficacy of this compound in the prophylaxis (and more recently in the treatment) of influenza A virus infections, it has never been widely employed and its recommended use remains the subject of considerable controversy (Sabin 1978).

B. Chemical Structure

Amantadine hydrochloride (Fig. 1) is a synthetic symmetrical C_{10} primary amine. The compound is soluble in water and alcohol, has a pK of 9.0 and remains stable upon heating. A number of derivatives have been tested experimentally, but among these, only α-methyladamantanethylamine hydrochloride (rimantadine hydrochloride) has been used extensively in clinical trials.

C. Spectrum of Antiviral Activity

Initial studies of the antiviral effects of amantadine in cell culture provided evidence of inhibition of replication of different strains of influenza A virus, influenza C virus, Sendai virus, and pseudorabies virus (Davies et al. 1964; Neumayer et al. 1965; Hoffman et al. 1965; Schild and Sutton 1965). In contrast, no inhibition was observed with influenza B virus, parainfluenza virus types 1–3, mumps virus, Newcastle disease virus, or with a variety of other viruses. Subsequently, inhibitory effects on the replication of rubella virus in cell culture were described (Maassab and Cochran 1964; Plotkin 1965; Oxford and Schild 1967). However, attempts

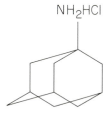

NH₂HCl

Fig. 1. Structure of 1-adamantanamine hydrochloride (amantadine hydrochloride)

to demonstrate an effect of amantadine in rhesus monkeys infected with rubella virus were not successful. Treated animals developed viremia and shed virus from the pharynx as readily as untreated controls (STEPHENSON et al. 1965). In other studies OXFORD and SCHILD (1967) observed that amantadine had no antiviral effect against rubella virus in hamsters and rabbits.

In concentrations of 10–50 μg/ml, amantadine has been reported to inhibit the replication of arenaviruses in cell culture (WELSH et al. 1971; PFAU et al. 1972). In addition, it has been reported that amantadine inhibits the formation of foci of tumor cells by chick embryo fibroblasts infected with Rous sarcoma virus (WALL-BANK et al. 1966).

The inhibitory effects of amantadine on the replication of influenza A virus in cell culture are in part dependent on the test system employed. Maximum inhibition is observed when cell cultures are infected with low doses of virus. With larger inocula of challenge virus, higher concentrations of drug are required and the inhibitory effects may be reflected in a longer interval before peak virus titers are reached rather than in reductions of final virus yields (OXFORD 1977).

Considerable variation in sensitivity among different influenza A viruses has been observed repeatedly (reviewed in OXFORD 1977). In general "laboratory" strains which have been adapted to embryonated eggs are less sensitive to the inhibitory effects of amantadine than low passage virus isolates. It is noteworthy that recent H1N1 and H3N2 isolates are relatively susceptible, i.e., reduction of virus yields are comparable to those observed with earlier H3N2 and H2N2 strains. In contrast, recent influenza B virus isolates continue to be resistant to the inhibitory effects of amantadine.

The amantadine sensitivities of different strains of influenza A virus have also been compared in a plaque reduction assay in which the concentration of drug required to reduce the plaque numbers by 50% is determined. By this method laboratory strains such as influenza A/PR/8/34 (H0N1) and A/WSN/33 (H0N1) viruses were approximately 100-fold less sensitive than influenza A/Hong Kong/68 (H3N2) and A/Ned/68 (H2N2) viruses (50% reduction in plaque number at amantadine concentrations of 25 μg/ml compared with concentrations of 0.2 μg/ml). Avian, equine, and porcine influenza A viruses have not been studies as systematically, but those which have been examined appear to be relatively sensitive (OXFORD 1977).

D. Mechanism of Action

The mechanism by which amantadine inhibits virus replication has not been unequivocally determined. It is clear that amantadine has no direct effect on the virus, as demonstrated by intact infectivity titers of virus suspensions incubated with the drug prior to infection of cell monolayers. Similarly, infection of cells in the presence of amantadine followed by removal of the drug is not associated with decreased virus yields, indicating that amantadine does not inhibit attachment of the virus to cell receptors. Addition of amantadine to cell cultures 30 min after infection has no effect on replication, indicating that amantadine exerts its effect on an early step in virus replication (HOFFMAN et al. 1965). It has been suggested that amantadine may block penetration of virus into the cell (HOFFMAN et al. 1965). However, electron micrographs of cells infected in the presence of amantadine provided no evidence that the drug blocks virus penetration (DOURMASHKIN and TYRRELL 1974).

KATO and EGGERS (1969) found that following infection in the presence of amantadine, intracellular virus particles (replicated previously in the presence of neutral red) remained photosensitive, whereas in the absence of the drug photosensitivity was rapidly lost. On the basis of these observations these investigators proposed that amantadine blocks virus uncoating. More recently KOFF and KNIGHT (1979) came to a similar conclusion on the basis of observations of prolonged RNase resistance of radiolabeled influenza virus RNA in cells infected in the presence of rimantadine. In another recent study ZVONARJEV and GHENDON (1980) demonstrated that transcriptase activity of influenza A virus ribonuclear protein (RNP) complexes is reduced by the addition of M protein and that further inhibition of transcriptase activity of RNP–M protein complexes is observed in the presence of amantadine. From these observations they concluded that rimantadine indirectly inhibits primary transcription by virtue of its effects on M protein. Although it has been reported that amantadine derivatives may directly inhibit virus transcriptase activity in vitro (KALNINYA and INDULEN 1976), other investigators have observed no inhibitory effects (OXFORD 1977; SKEHEL et al. 1977).

In summary, the available data indicate that amantadine acts on an early step in virus replication, after attachment of virus to cell receptors. Genetic evidence (see Sect. H) suggests the possibility that amantadine may interact with M protein within infected cells and inhibit or delay the uncoating process that precedes primary transcription.

E. Pharmacology

I. Absorption

Amantadine hydrochloride is a water-soluble drug which is absorbed rapidly from the gastrointestinal tract. In humans, after oral administration of 2.5 mg/kg, peak serum levels of 0.3 µg/ml, and nasal secretion levels of 0.02–0.08 µg/ml are reached within 2–4 h and, after administration of 4.0 mg/kg, serum levels of 0.6 µg/ml are observed.

II. Metabolism

Although amantadine is actively metabolized in some species, such as rabbits, there is no evidence of metabolic alteration of the compound in human subjects. Approximately 90% of the administered dose can be recovered in the urine. The excretion rate varies slightly from subject to subject and can be increased by acidification of the urine (BLEIDNER et al. 1965).

III. Side Effects

Studies of toxic effects of amantadine in animals indicate that extremely large doses are required before toxic levels are achieved. Evidence of central nervous system

(CNS) stimulation including occasional convulsions were observed in rats, dogs, and rhesus monkeys given doses of 100 mg/kg for up to 2 years, but these effects were completely reversible upon discontinuing administration of the drug. No evidence of histologic abnormality was observed in brain sections of these animals (Vernier et al. 1969).

In different studies, side effects have been recorded in 3%–30% of human subjects given the usual dose of 100 mg twice daily. In general, these reactions have been referable to the CNS, consisting of nervousness, drowsiness, difficulty in concentration, insomnia, and depression. These symptoms usually appear within 48 h and disappear rapidly when drug administration is discontinued. A slight, but statistically significant difference in the incidence of side effects has been observed among amantadine recipients in double-blind studies with placebo controls (Monto et al. 1979). However, in another double-blind study of a college population, temporary decreased performance in tests of maximal and sustained attention were clearly observed in amantadine-treated subjects (Bryson et al. 1980). Taken together, the available data suggest that amantadine therapy may be associated in a minority of subjects with significant CNS-related side effects, which in all instances have been found to be readily reversible upon cessation of drug administration.

F. Animal Studies

I. Prophylaxis

Early studies provided evidence that administration of amantadine to mice prior to or very shortly after challenge with influenza A viruses results in decreased virus replication in the lungs, decreased pneumonia, and increased survival (Davies et al. 1964; Grunert et al. 1965). Comparison of amantadine and rimantadine in mice indicated that rimantadine was much more effective in inhibiting virus replication and reducing pneumonia. Furthermore, these latter studies demonstrated that rimantadine-treated infector mice transmitted infection to uninfected contact mice less readily than untreated infectors, and that rimantadine-treated contact mice were less susceptible to the acquisition of infection (Schulman 1968).

Studies in ferrets have produced different results, depending on the virus used in challenge. Cochran et al. (1965) treated ferrets with amantadine for 12 days, beginning at the time of infection with PR8 virus (a relatively insensitive strain) and found that disease was somewhat more severe in treated animals. Likewise, Squires (1970) found that prophylactic administration of amantadine had no effect in ferrets infected with A/Singapore/57 (H2N2) virus. On the other hand, Fenton et al. (1977) found that amantadine treatment begun 1 day before infection and continued until 7 days after infection had antiviral activity in ferrets infected with Port Chalmers (H3N2) virus. Treated animals had lower titers of virus in nasal washings and less fever than controls, but treatment had no effect on the local inflammatory response to infection, as measured by increased concentrations of protein in nasal secretions. Bryans et al. (1966) observed a prophylactic effect of amantadine in horses experimentally challenged with Heq2Neq2 virus.

The variability of effectiveness of amantadine in prophylaxis of influenza virus infection in experimental animals may in part be due to the experimental design which is generally employed. As a rule, animals are challenged with relatively large doses of virus adapted to replicate to high titer in these animals. Studies in tissue culture, on the other hand, suggest that amantadine has a more significant inhibitory effect during multicycle replication with relatively low levels of input virus.

II. Treatment

Limited data are available which indicate that amantadine, and its derivatives may have some therapeutic value in influenza A virus infection of experimental animals when therapy is initiated after infection. GRUNERT et al. (1965) observed increased survival of mice infected with influenza A/AA/60 (H2N2) virus when oral amantadine therapy was initiated 48 h after infection. WALKER et al. (1976) found that aerosal therapy, either with amantadine or rimantadine, initiated as late as 72 h after infection of mice with mouse-adapted A/Aichi/2/68 (H3N2) virus had a significant effect in increasing survival. In contrast, intraperitoneal amantadine therapy begun as early as 6 h after infection had no effect on survival. Paradoxically, although aerosal administration of these drugs resulted in increased survival, these therapeutic effects were not correlated with more rapid decline in virus titers or less extensive pneumonia 7 days after infection.

G. Clinical Trials

I. Prophylaxis

Numerous clinical trials involving thousands of subjects have been conducted over the past 15 years to test the efficacy of prophylactic administration of amantadine in the prevention of influenza A virus infection in a variety of experimental settings, including challenge studies with volunteer and studies of naturally occurring epidemics of different strains of influenza virus. Although results varied somewhat from one study to another, in general these trials provided evidence that amantadine prophylaxis (usually 100 mg twice daily) reduced infection rates by approximately 50% and illness rates by approximately 60% (reviewed in COUCH and JACKSON 1976).

In one double-blind study, GALBRAITH et al. (1969) administered amantadine to family contacts for 10 days after the onset of clinical influenza in a family member. Clinical influenza was reduced by 80% and subclinical influenza, as assessed by serum antibody rises, was reduced by 60% in amantadine-treated contacts. In another study in a hospital, O'DONAHUE et al. (1973) compared the incidence of influenza in amantadine-treated and placebo-treated patients admitted to a hospital during a nosocomial influenza epidemic. Clinical influenza was completely prevented and subclinical infection was reduced by 80% in the amantadine-treated group. More recently, MONTO et al. (1979) in another double-blind study, found that amantadine prophylaxis reduced the incidence of influenza due to A/USSR-like (H1N1) viruses by 70.7%.

Thus, the prophylactic effectiveness of amantadine has been demonstrated repeatedly in carefully controlled clinical trials during naturally occurring epidemics of H2N2, H3N2, and H1N1 viruses. In addition it should be emphasized that, in instances in which studies were conducted during combined influenza A and influenza B virus epidemics, amantadine was effective in reducing the incidence of influenza A, but not influenza B virus disease.

II. Treatment

The available evidence regarding the beneficial effects of amantadine therapy begun after the onset of influenza is not comprehensive nor as convincing as that related to its prophylactic effects. Nevertheless, placebo-controlled, double-blind studies of the therapeutic effects of oral administration of amantadine or rimantadine (100 mg twice daily) after infection of volunteers or after the onset of influenza-like symptoms during natural epidemics have repeatedly shown at least marginal effects. These therapeutic effects have been manifested by a less intense and slightly shorter-lasting fever and illness (WINGFIELD et al. 1969; TOGO et al. 1970; KNIGHT et al. 1970; GALBRAITH et al. 1971; KITAMOTO et al. 1971), and by reduced abnormalities of pulmonary function (LITTLE et al. 1976; LITTLE et al. 1977). In addition, in two trials in which virus shedding was studied by quantitation of virus titers in respiratory secretions, lower titers of virus and more rapid cessation of virus shedding were observed in drug-treated groups (KNIGHT et al. 1970; VAN VORIS et al., to be published). The finding that more rapid recovery from disease is associated with drug effects on virus shedding provides some evidence that the therapeutic effects of amantadine are mediated by its antiviral action. In addition, in one study of the therapeutic effects of amantadine during simultaneous epidemics due to influenza A and influenza B viruses, retrospective analysis indicated that the drug was of some benefit in subjects infected with influenza A virus, but had no effect on symptoms in persons with influenza B virus infection (GALBRAITH et al. 1973).

More recently, attempts have been made to employ aerosol mists of amantadine or rimantadine in the treatment of influenza, on the assumption that by this method higher local concentrations of drug in the respiratory tract can be achieved. In one such study, college students infected with H3N2 or H1N1 viruses during a natural mixed epidemic were exposed three times daily for 20 min each to mists of amantadine or to distilled water for 4 days after the onset of treatment. Respiratory symptoms abated more quickly in the drug-treated group than in controls but no effects on fever, other constitutional symptoms, or pulmonary function were observed. Although virus titers in respiratory secretions tended to be lower in the treated groups, the differences were not statistically significant (HAYDEN et al. 1980). Unfortunately, insufficient data are available at present to determine whether amantadine therapy has any effect in the treatment of primary influenza virus pneumonia, an uncommon but usually fatal complication of influenza.

H. Resistant Variants

As discussed in Sect. C, different strains of influenza A virus vary considerably (more than 50-fold) in their sensitivity to the inhibitory effects of amantadine, both in cell culture and in experimental animals. Studies involving the analysis of susceptibility of genetically defined recombinant viruses derived from relatively resistant and susceptible parental strains indicated that the gene coding for M protein influences resistance. Recombinants which derived the gene for M protein from an amantadine-resistant parent were resistant and all amantadine-sensitive recombinants were found to derive the gene for M protein from a sensitive parent. These data were interpreted as being consistent with the hypothesis that amantadine interacts with M protein, leading to inhibition of virus penetration or virus uncoating (LUBECK et al. 1978). However, in those studies, exceptions were found in the form of amantadine-resistant recombinants which derived the M gene from the sensitive parent. Subsequent analysis of cloned stocks of the parental sensitive Hong Kong virus strain revealed a frequency of amantadine-resistant variants of 4×10^{-4} which was in accord with the earlier findings of APPLEYARD (1977) who observed amantadine-resistant mutants at a frequency of 1×10^{-3} in a population of amantadine-sensitive A/Bel/42 (H0N1) virus.

In other studies, amantadine-resistant mutants have been isolated after passage of virus in cell culture, embryonated eggs, or mice treated with amantadine (COCHRAN et al. 1965; OXFORD et al. 1970), but thus far isolation of amantadine-resistant variants from human subjects receiving the drug have not been reported. Nevertheless, the ease with which resistant variants can be obtained in the laboratory and the relatively high frequency of resistant mutants in cloned virus populations are disquieting, and the possibility that amantadine-resistant mutants might emerge to predominance following use of the drug in large populations cannot be ignored.

J. Conclusions and Perspectives

The data available from clinical trials involving thousands of subjects strongly suggest that amantadine may be of value in prophylaxis of influenza. Nevertheless, controversy continues regarding its recommended use (SABIN 1978). Some of this controversy can be attributed to the fact that, in many epidemics, influenza A virus infection may be responsible for only a portion of the viral (and nonviral) respiratory infections leading to an influenza-like syndrome. The specificity of the antiviral effects of amantadine in inhibiting the replication of influenza A virus infection has been clearly established and it is predictable that chemoprophylaxis with amantadine will have no effect on disease due to influenza B virus or to other respiratory viruses. Hence, beneficial effects from the prophylactic use of amantadine may be expected only in those epidemics in which disease is preponderantly due to infection with influenza A virus. Second, variability of the immune status of individual members of a population may be expected to have a significant impact on chemoprophylactic trials, i.e., the protective effects of amantadine against epidemic influenza may not be evident in a population in which a significant proportion of its members possess protective levels of antibody.

On the other hand, amantadine could prove to be an extremely useful chemoprophylactic agent, particularly in those circumstances in which novel antigenic variants appear and suitable vaccines are not yet available. In particular, persons considered to be at high risk might be provided temporary protection until vaccines have become available and immunization programs have been implemented. Other circumstances in which chemoprophylaxis might be recommended include laboratory-confirmed nosocomial epidemics or outbreaks of confirmed influenza A virus infection in closed unimmunized populations in nursing homes. The routine administration of amantadine to family contacts of index cases would be of questionable value unless laboratory confirmation of the nature of the illness in the index case is available.

The therapeutic value of amantadine is even more controversial. Although the existing data indicate that treated subjects recover more rapidly, the benefits appear to be marginal at best and not sufficient to justify routine chemotherapy of patients with influenza-like disease. On the other hand, the poor prognosis associated with influenza virus pneumonia justifies continued attempts at chemotherapy of that complication, despite the absence of data demonstrating efficacy. In particular, the possibility that aerosol therapy will prove to be beneficial deserves further exploration.

Restraint in the routine use of amantadine can be justified on other grounds. Although toxic side effects of amantadine occur in low incidence and are readily reversible, these effects are largely limited to the CNS and routine use of the drug in large population groups could create unacceptable public health problems. In addition there is the potential problem of emergence of drug-resistant variants which could prevent effective use of the drug in circumscribed situations where its employment could otherwise have been of great value.

Attempts to synthesize additional analogs of amantadine are continuing and the possibility that a more effective compound can be made cannot be excluded. Although early studies in cell culture and experimental animals indicated that rimantadine is more effective than amantadine, controlled side-by-side-comparisons of the two drugs in human subjects thus far have failed to reveal any consistent difference.

References

Appleyard G (1977) Amantadine resistance as a genetic marker for influenza viruses. J Gen Virol 36:249–255

Bleidner WE, Harmon JB, Hewes WE, Lynes TE, Herman EC (1965) Absorbtion distribution and excretion of amantadine hydrochloride. J Pharmacol Exp Ther 150:484–490

Bryans JT, Zent WW, Grunert RR, Boughton DC (1966) 1-Adamantanamine prophylaxis for experimentally induced A/equine 2 influenza virus infection. Nature 212:1542–1544

Bryson YJ, Monahan C, Pollack M, Shields WD (1980) A prospective double-blind study of side effects associated with the administration of amantadine for influenza A prophylaxis. J Infect Dis 141:543–547

Cochran KW, Maassab HF, Tsunoda A, Berlin BS (1965) Studies on the antiviral activity of amantadine hydrochloride. Ann NY Acad Sci 130:432–439

Couch RB, Jackson GG (1976) Antiviral agents in influenza. Summary of Influenza Workshop VIII. J Infect Dis 134:516–527

Davies WL, Grunert RR, Haff RF et al. (1964) Antiviral activity of 1-adamantanamine (amantadine). Science 144:862–863

Dourmashkin RR, Tyrrell DJ (1974) Electron microscope evidence of the entry of influenza virus into susceptible cells. J Gen Virol 24:129–141

Fenton RJ, Bessell C, Spilling CR, Potter CW (1977) The effects of peroral or local aerosal administration of 1-aminoadamantane hydrochloride (amantadine hydrochloride) on influenza infection of the ferret. J Antimicrob Chemother 3:463–472

Galbraith AW, Oxford JS, Schild GC, Watson GL (1969) Protective effects of 1-adaman-
tanamine hydrochloride on influenza A2 infections in the family environment. Lancet
2:1026–1028

Galbraith AW, Oxford JS, Schild GC, Potter CW, Watson GI (1971) Therapeutic effect of
1-adamantanamine hydrochloride in naturally occurring influenza A2/Hong Kong infection. A controlled double-blind study. Lancet 2:113–115

Gailbraith AW, Schild GC, Potter CW, Watson GI (1973) The therapeutic effect of amantadine in influenza occurring during the winter of 1971–72 assessed by double-blind study.
J Coll Gen Pract 23:34–37

Grunert RR, McGahen JW, Davies WL (1965) The in vitro activity of 1-adamantanamine
(amantadine). Prophylactic and therapeutic value against influenza viruses. Virology
26:262–269

Hayden FG, Hall WJ, Doublas RG (1980) Therapeutic effects of aerosolized amantadine
in naturally acquired infection due to influenza virus. J Infect Dis 141:535–542

Hoffman CE, Neumayer EM, Haff RF, Goldsby RA (1965) Mode of action of the antiviral
activity amantadine in tissue culture. J Bacteriol 90:623–628

Kalninya VA, Indulen MK (1976) Effect of amantadine derivatives on the activity of orthomyxovirus RNA-dependent RNA polymerase. Acta Virol (Praha) (Engl ed) 20:343–
346

Kato N, Eggers HJ (1969) Inhibition of uncoating of fowl plague virus by 1-adamantan-
amine hydrochloride. Virology 37:632–641

Kitamato O (1971) Therapeutic effectiveness of amantadine hydrochloride in naturally occurring Hong Kong influenza double-blind studies. Jpn J Tuberc 17:1–7

Knight V, Fedson D, Baldini J, Douglas RG, Couch RB (1970) Amantadine therapy of epidemic influenza A2 (Hong Kong). Infect Immun 1:200–204

Koff WC, Knight V (1979) Effect of amantadine on influenza virus replication. Proc Soc
Exp Biol Med 160:246–253

Little JW, Hall WJ, Douglas RG Jr, Hyde RW, Speers DM (1976) Amantadine effect on
peripheral airways abnormalities in influenza – a study in 15 students with natural influenza infection. Ann Intern Med 85:177–182

Little JW, Hall WJ, Douglas RG Jr (1977) Small airways dysfunction in influenza virus infection. Therapeutic role and potential mode of action of amantadine. Ann NY Acad
Sci 284:106–117

Lubeck MD, Schulman JL, Palese P (1978) Susceptibility of influenza A viruses to amantadine is influenced by the gene coding for M protein. J Virol 28:710–716

Maassab HF, Cochran KW (1964) Rubella virus inhibition in vitro by amantadine hydrochloride. Science 145:1443–1444

Monto AS, Gunn RA, Bandyk MG, King CL (1979) Prevention of Russian influenza by
amantadine. JAMA 241:1003–1007

Neumayer EM, Haff RF, Hoffman CE (1965) Antiviral activity of amantadine hydrochloride in tissue culture and in ovo. Proc Soc Exp Biol Med 119:393–396

O'Donahue JM, Ray CG, Terry DW Jr, Beatty HN (1973) Prevention of nasocomial influenza infections with amantadine. Am J Epidemiol 97:276–282

Oxford JS (1977) Specific inhibitors of influenza related to the molecular biology of virus
replication. In: Oxford JS (ed) Chemoprophylaxis and virus infections of the respiratory
tract, vol I. CRC Press, Cleveland, Ohio, pp 140–187

Oxford JS, Schild GC (1967) The evaluation of antiviral compounds for rubella virus using
organ cultures. Arch Ges Virusforsch 22:349–356

Oxford JS, Logan IS, Potter CW (1970) Passage of influenza strains in the presence of
aminoadamantane. Ann NY Acad Sci 173:300–313

Pfau CV, Trowbridge RS, Welsh RM, Staneck LD, O'Connell CM (1972) Arenaviruses: inhibition by amantadine hydrochloride. J Gen Virol 14:209–211

Plotkin SA (1965) Inhibition of rubella virus by amantadine. Arch Ges Virusforsch 16:438–
442

Sabin AB (1978) Amantadine and influenza: evaluation of conflicting reports. J Infect Dis
138:557–566

Schild GC, Sutton RN (1965) Inhibition of influenza viruses in vitro and in vivo by 1-ada-
mantanamine hydrochloride. Br J Exp Pathol 46:263–273

Schulman JL (1968) Effect of 1-amantanamine hydrochloride (amantadine CHl) on transmission of influenza virus infection in mice. Proc Soc Exp Biol Med 128:1173–1178

Skehel JJ, Hay AJ, Armstrong JA (1977) On the mechanism of inhibition of influenza virus replication by amantadine hydrochloride. J Gen Virol 38:97–110

Squires SL (1970) The evaluation of compounds against influenza viruses. Ann NY Acad Sci 173:229–248

Stephenson JA, Artenstein MS, Parkman PD, Buescher EL, Druzd AD (1965) Effect of amantadine hydrochloride on rubella virus infection in the rhesus monkey. Antimicrob Agents Chemother 548–552

Togo Y, Hornick RB, Felitti VG, Kaufman ML, Dawkins AT, Kilpe VE, Claghorn JL (1970) Evaluation of therapeutic efficacy of amantadine in patients with naturally occurring A2 influenza. JAMA 211:1149–1156

Van Voris LP, Betts RF, Hayden FG, Christmas WA, Douglas RG Jr (to be published) Oral amantadine and rimantadine therapy of naturally occurring influenza A/USSR/77 H1N1. JAMA

Vernier VG, Harmon JB, Stump JM, Lynes TE, Marvel JP, Smith DH (1969) The toxicologic and pharmacologic properties of amantadine hydrochloride. Toxicol Appl Pharmacol 15:642–665

Wallbank AM, Matter RE, Klinkowski RG (1966) 1-Adamantanamine hydrochloride: inhibition of Rous and Esh sarcoma viruses in cell culture. Science 152:1760–1761

Walker JS, Stephen ES, Spertzel RO (1976) Small particle aerosols of antiviral compounds in treatment of type A influenza in pneumonia in mice. J Infect Dis [Suppl A] 133:140–A144

Welsh RM, Trowbridge RS, Kowalski JB, O'Connell CM, Pfau CJ (1971) Amantadine hydrochloride inhibition of early and late stages lymphocytic choriomeningitis virus-cell interactions. Virology 45:679–686

Wingfield WL, Pollack D, Grunert RP (1969) Therapeutic efficacy of amantadine HCl and rimantadine HCl in naturally occurring influenza A2 respiratory illness in man. N Engl J Med 281:579–584

Zvonarjev AY, Ghendon YZ (1980) Influence of membrane (M) protein of influenza A virus virion transcriptase activity *in vitro* and its susceptibility to amantadine. J Virol 33:583–586

CHAPTER 5

The Thiosemicarbazones

C. J. Pfau

A. Introduction

The thiosemicarbazones stand as milestones in the emerging era of the specific treatment of viral diseases. They were the first true antiviral substances to be synthesized; although a number of random events had to take place before their potential was realized. The thiosemicarbazones were the first compounds to be found active in virus-infected animals. They were also the focus of the first systematic studies on the relationship between chemical structure and antiviral activity. Furthermore, these compounds were the first to be effective in humans and placed in clinical medicine. Finally, there are no other compounds known which appear able to block the genetic expression of such a wide variety of viruses.

There is an impressive literature on the antitumor activity of the thiosemicarbazones (SARTORELLI et al. 1977; AGRAWAL and SARTORELLI 1978; PETERING 1980). Even though a well-established link exists between viruses and malignancy, this area will not be included here. Two excellent reviews on the antiviral activity of the thiosemicarbazones are available (BAUER 1972; LEVINSON 1973). I will largely avoid an in-depth coverage of the same material, but will stress literature published in the last 10 years.

B. History

The first publication about an effective antiviral agent virtually escaped attention. In 1950, HAMRE et al. reported that p-aminobenzaldehyde-3-thiosemicarbazone (Fig. 1, $R_1 = NH_2$, $R_2 = H$, $R_3 = H$) caused a significant delay in death, as well as survival of a small percentage, of chick embryos and mice infected with vaccinia virus. At that time there was a general atmosphere of pessimism about the discovery of antiviral agents. This mood was enhanced by the unfortunate false start made with the discovery that antibacterial agents were effective against the rickettsia and lymphogranuloma–psittacosis groups, considered for many years to be viruses. However, it was the sensitivity of the tuberculosis bacillus to the thiosemicarbazones that led HAMRE and colleagues to test these compounds against viruses.

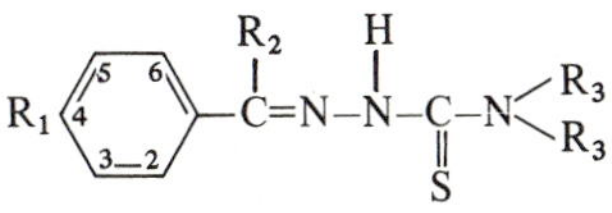

Fig. 1

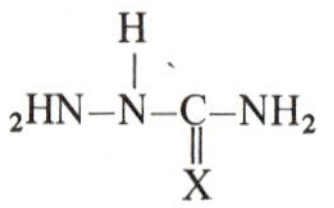

$$\underset{\underset{X}{\|}}{_2HN-N-C-NH_2}$$

with H above the first N.

Fig. 2

The antibacterial activity of thiosemicarbazones appears to have been revealed by chance. Domagk (the discoverer of the first sulfa drugs), when engaged in structure–activity studies with Behnisch, found that sulfathiazoles were potent inhibitors of *Mycobacterium tuberculosis* (Domagk et al. 1946). Further structure–activity studies led to the synthesis of sulfathiadiazoles. Essential intermediates in the latter's preparation were 2-aminothiadiazoles which were formed from the corresponding thiosemicarbazones by oxidative ring closure with ferric chloride. One of the thiosemicarbazones synthesized, and tested for biologic activity, was benzaldehyde thiosemicarbazone (Fig. 1, R_1 = H, R_2 = H, R_3 = H). It has been claimed (Bock 1957) that at the time of this discovery the investigators at I.G. Farben also found that benzaldehyde thiosemicarbazone had no activity against a variety of pathogenic microorganisms. These included, pneumonia virus of mice, influenza virus, lymphocytic choriomeningitis virus, and two members of the poxvirus family – ectromelia and canarypox. Many years later, in the same laboratories, the murine antipox activity of thiosemicarbazones was confirmed (Bock 1957) and shown to be quite dependent on the strain of virus used.

Benzaldehyde thiosemicarbazone was first synthesized by Freund and Schander 44 years prior to the discovery of its biologic potential. In that era, semicarbazide (Fig. 2, X = O) was standardly used as a derivatizing agent for aldehydes and ketones. Freund and Schander (1902) suggested, apparently without historical impact, that thiosemicarbazide (Fig. 2, X = S) should be used instead, because the presence of the sulfur atom could be easily detected in the precipitates (thiosemicarbazones) formed in the presence of aldehydes or ketones in a reaction mixture.

C. Chemistry

This part of the review is centered on studies of the introduction of substituents into various thiosemicarbazones and the subsequent effect on the compounds' antiviral properties. Many of the key structure–activity relationships were established in mice infected with poxviruses, and were subsequently shown to hold true in studies with other virus families. However, as shown in many of the following sections, antiviral agents with in vitro activity have been found or tested much more frequently than those with in vivo effectiveness. The structure–activity relationships found in any one of these systems should not necessarily be taken to hold true for the other, even though the same virus was used. The investigations discussed here will be divided into sections dealing with specific types of thiosemicarbazones. The radical nomenclature is that which is currently accepted (Rigaudy and Klesney 1979).

I. Aryl Thiosemicarbazones

The thiosemicarbazone (TSC) first chosen for antiviral studies by investigators at the Squibb Institute for Medical Reseach was p-aminobenzaldehyde-TSC (Fig. 1, $R_1 = NH_2$, $R_2 = H$, $R_3 = H$), because it was the most water-soluble compound in their collection (HAMRE et al. 1950). One of the initial reliable methods for testing antiviral agents had just been developed there (BROWNLEE and HAMRE 1951) with vaccinia as the model virus. The compound was indeed shown to have chemotherapeutic activity in vaccinia-infected eggs and mice. It was most fortunate that this virus was used because it would be another 10 years before other thiosemicarbazones were found that had activity against nonpox viruses (O'SULLIVAN and SADLER 1961; see Sects. C.IV, D.IV). This initial investigation also included one other thiosemicarbazone: p-acetamidobenzaldehyde-TSC (Fig. 1, $R_1 = CH_3$-C-NH-, R_2
$$\overset{\|}{O}$$
$= H$, $R_3 = H$). It was somewhat less active than the primary compound, but significantly more toxic (the 10% aqueous triethylene glycol necessary for solubilization was innocuous).

A wider series of benzaldehyde thiosemicarbazones was then studied for antiviral activity. HAMRE et al. (1951) found that substitution of glucose or cyclohexane for the benzene ring resulted in almost complete loss of activity. The substitution of oxygen for sulfur in the thiosemicarbazone moiety also caused loss of activity (greatly reduced activity of semicarbazones would be repeatedly shown in future investigations with related compounds). Furthermore, thiosemicarbazide (Fig. 2, $X = S$) had little, if any, activity (another result that would be confirmed in most later investigations). The effect of substitutions in the benzaldehyde moiety (other than the p-amino and p-acetamido groups) on chemotherapeutic activity was examined next. Nine compounds were substituted in the 4 position (Fig. 1), two were disubstituted in the 3 and 4 positions, and the last was unsubstituted. The disubstituted compounds (4-hydroxy-3-methoxy and 4-hydroxy-3-sulfo) had no activity. All monosubstitutions led to either decreased or unchanged activity compared with the unsubstituted compound or the two 4-substituted compounds tested initially. The groups producing little, or no, change in activity at the 4 position were methoxy (CH_3O), propoxy (CH_3CH_2-CH_2O), and ethylsulfonyl ($C_2H_5SO_2$). In further experiments, butyl groups were substituted for both hydrogen atoms at the end of the thiosemicarbazone side chain [Fig. 1, $R_2 = H$, $R_3 =$ -$(CH_2)_3$-CH_3]. All compounds altered in this way (the unsubstituted benzaldehyde thiosemicarbazone and the p-amino- and p-acetamido derivatives) retained activity against vaccinia virus. This behavior is in marked contrast to such dialkyl substitutions at the terminal amino group of isatin-β-thiosemicarbazone (BAUER and SADLER 1960a; Sect. C.III).

The chemotherapeutic activity of benzaldehyde-TSC was confirmed by THOMPSON et al. (1951) both in minced chick embryo culture (Maitland culture) and in mice infected with vaccinia virus. Unlike HAMRE et al., they found that all substitutions at the 4 position of the benzaldehyde moiety (except for NO_2), or at the terminal amino position in the thiosemicarbazone side chain (Fig. 1) reduced activity in both test systems. This cannot be taken as a true contradiction, even though both groups used essentially the same substitutions. Whereas HAMRE et al. used

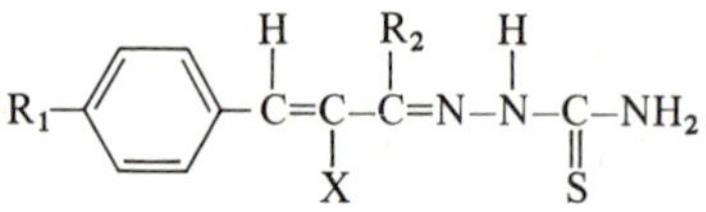

$$R_1 - \underset{X}{\underset{|}{C}} = \overset{H}{\underset{|}{C}} - \overset{R_2}{\underset{|}{C}} = N - N - \overset{H}{\underset{|}{N}} - \overset{}{\underset{\parallel}{C}} - NH_2$$

Fig. 3

concentrations close to the toxic dose of each compound, THOMPSON et al. tested all compounds at about the same concentration. Thus, certain mono- and disubstituted compounds were found effective at more than ten times the concentration found to be ineffective by the THOMPSON group. However, the same group (THOMPSON et al. 1953b) went on to confirm that benzaldehyde semicarbazone and thiosemicarbazide were lacking in activity. They also established that addition of methylene or vinyl groups between the benzaldehyde and thiosemicarbazone portions of the molecule decreased activity.

Integrity of the thiosemicarbazone side chain was found to be critical. Loss of the sulfur atom, as well as substitution of a methyl (CH_3), ethyl (C_2H_5), carbethoxy ($C_2H_5CO_2$), or benzyl ($C_6H_5CH_2$) group at the aldehyde carbon atom (R_2 in Fig. 1) abolished or reduced activity. Except as noted in the following paragraphs, studies on the antiviral properties of benzaldehyde-TSCs virtually ceased in 1953 when attention was focused on the heterocyclic thiosemicarbazones.

That substitution of a methyl group at the aldehyde carbon atom reduced activity against vaccinia virus was confirmed many years later by RUNTI et al. (1968). They carried out more extensive investigations of these acetophenone-TSCs (Fig. 1, $R_2 = CH_3$, $R_3 = H$) particularly with regard to synthesis of lipophilic compounds with substitutions in the benzene ring. Thirteen of these compounds were used in a virus plaque reduction test (the drug is placed in a center well of an agar plaque assay plate; as the drug diffuses the highest concentrations lead to a clearly visible cell toxicity zone, but beyond that there may be a zone of specific inhibition of plaque development) against eight different viruses. The authors concluded that the acetophenone-TSCs had a different antiviral spectrum from the benzaldehyde or isatin (Sect. C.III) series of TSCs. Specifically, p-nitro-, p-bromo-, and p-methoxyacetophenone-TSCs were moderately active against influenza and parainfluenza viruses. Activity could not be demonstrated when the sulfur atom was replaced by oxygen in the TSC side chain, nor was there activity against any of the other viruses, including vaccinia. However, 2,4-dimethoxyacetophenone-TSC was active against vaccinia, but not against any of the other viruses.

Three other reports, all appearing prior to that of RUNTI et al. (1968) claimed that aryl-TSCs were effective against influenza viruses. IWASAKI et al. (1955) tested 26 compounds of benzaldehyde- (Fig. 1, $R_2 = H$, $R_3 = H$), acetophenone- (Fig. 1, $R_2 = CH_3$, $R_3 = H$), cinnamaldehyde- (Fig. 3, X = H, $R_1,R_2 = H$), and benzalacetone- (Fig. 3, X = H, $R_1 = H$, $R_2 = CH_3$) TSCs against influenza A and B viruses as well as Newcastle disease virus. All four types of unsubstituted TSCs were examined, as well as nitro, dimethylamino [$(CH_3)_2N$], amino, and acetamido para substituents (R_1 in Fig. 3) in each of the four categories. In addition, a bromine substituent (X in Fig. 3) was added to the cinnamaldehyde and benzalacetone series of compounds. From their results the following generalities can be made for the influenza viruses:

a) The unsubstituted TSCs were the most active; these were, in increasing order of effectiveness, benzaldehyde, acetophenone, cinnamaldehyde, and benzalacetone
b) Most of the *para*-substituted compounds were reduced in activity; the order of the greatest to the least reductions was: acetamido, amino, dimethylamino, and nitro substituents
c) In general, the bromo substitutents had little, or no, effect on antiviral activity

With regard to Newcastle disease virus, benzalacetone-TSC was the only active unsubstituted compound. The three other active compounds were the *p*-nitro derivatives of benzalacetone-, cinnamaldehyde-, and benzaldehyde-TSCs. LUM and SMITH (1957), apparently unaware of the paper by IWASAKI et al. (1955), showed that *p*-nitrobenzaldehyde-TSC, *p*-hydroxybenzaldehyde-TSC, anisaldehyde-TSC (Fig. 1, R_1 = NO_2, HO, and CH_3O, respectively) and α-pentylcinnamaldehyde-TSC [Fig. 3, X = H, R_1 = $CH_3(CH_2)_4$, R_2 = H] inhibited influenza A and B viruses in chick chorioallantoic Maitland cultures and also spared 50% of the mice inoculated with these viruses. ZAK (1959) noted that isopropylbenzaldehyde-TSC (Fig. 1, R_1 = $isoC_3H_7$) caused a slight reduction in the febrile period of patients with influenza virus infections.

In connection with studying cyanothiophene-TSCs (Sect. C.II) WINKELMANN and ROLLY (1972) synthesized a number of corresponding cyanobenzaldehyde-TSCs. Replacement of the cyano group (N≡C) in both series of compounds by carboxylic acid, carboxamide, ester, or imidate groups produced less active or inactive products when tested in vaccinia-infected mice. In the benzaldehyde series, when the cyano group was introduced at the 2,3, or 4 positions (Fig. 1) of the aromatic ring, the 4-isomer was found to be most active.

II. Quinoline, Pyridine, and Thiophene Thiosemicarbazones

In 1953 a second major advance was made that would eventually lead to clinical application (Sect. H). It was the discovery that heterocyclic TSCs could possess antiviral activity (THOMPSON et al. 1953b). Compounds containing pyridine (Fig. 4), quinoline (see Fig. 5), thiophene (see Fig. 7), and isatin (see Fig. 8) groups protected mice to a degree equal to, or greater than, that obtained with the benzaldehyde-TSCs. The bulk of the structure–activity relationship studies would be carried out with the isatin-TSCs (Sect. C.III), but it should be noted that this initial study with pyridine- and quinoline-TSCs established an important feature of these compounds – the thiosemicarbazone moiety affixed to the heterocyclic ring in a position α to the ring nitrogen atom, as in 2-formylpyridine-TSC (Fig. 4), had no activity in mice infected with vaccinia virus. When the TSC side chain was placed in another position, as in 4-formylpyridine- or 4-formylquinoline-TSC (Fig. 5), the

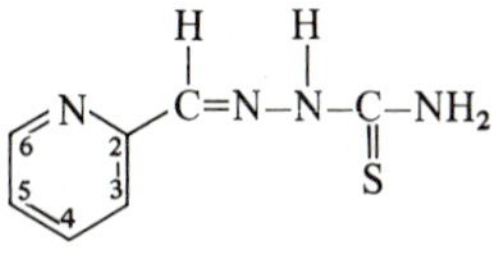

Fig. 4

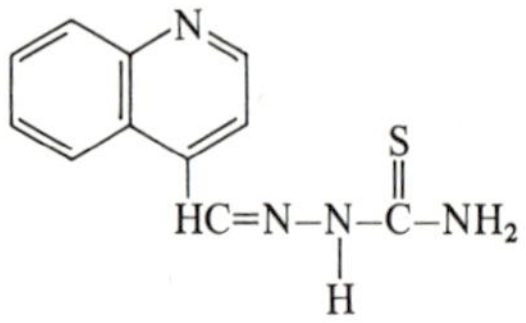

Fig. 5

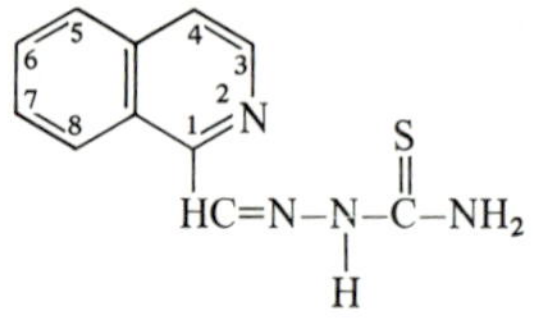

Fig. 6

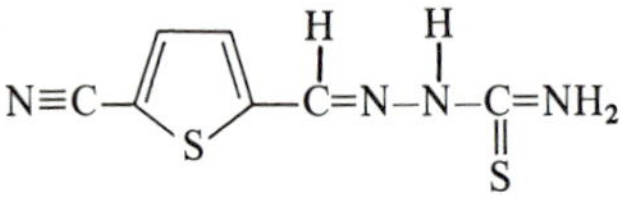

Fig. 7

compound would protect against lethal infection (THOMPSON et al. 1953 b). Further studies indicate that the β position was optimal (Sects. C.III, VI). However, in tissue culture studies using vaccinia as well as other viruses, the opposite appeared to be true. BROCKMAN et al. (1970) found that pyridine- and quinoline-TSCs would prevent herpes-induced cytopathology in tissue culture only if the TSC was α to the ring nitrogen atom. 2-Formylpyridine-TSC was active but the 3- and 4- formyl isomers were not (Fig. 4). Furthermore, 1-formylisoquinoline-TSC (Fig. 6), and its 5-hydroxy derivative, were active (as was 6-formylpurine-TSC), but no protection was noted with isatin-β-TSC or 1-methylisatin-β-TSC (Fig. 8, R_1 = H or CH_3, R_2 = H, R_3 = H_2, X = S). KATZ et al. (1974) found that 5-hydroxy-2-formyl-pyridine-TSC (Fig. 4) and 1-formylisoquinoline-TSC (Fig. 6) would prevent vaccinia plaque formation in tissue culture. However, the mode of action of these compounds was unique compared with four other active TSCs where the side chain was not α to the ring nitrogen atom (Sect. F.II). More recently LEVINSON et al. (1977 b) found that 1-formylisoquinoline-TSC (Fig. 6) and 2-pyridine-TSC would inhibit the production of Rous sarcoma virus. Further extension of these studies with 2- and 4-formylpyridine-TSC (Fig. 4) showed that the former was much more active than the latter (KASKA et al. 1978). Parenthetically, one notes that the minimum requirement for antitumor activity of pyridine- and isoquinoline-TSCs is that the TSC side chain must be attached α to an unencumbered ring nitrogen atom (AGRAWAL and SARTORELLI 1978).

Although the thiophene-TSCs have received little attention (KATZ et al. 1974), 5-cyanothiophene-2-formylthiosemicarbazone (Fig. 7) has been reported (ROLLY and WINKELMANN 1972) to be superior to 1-methylisatin-β-thiosemicarbazone in its in vivo antivaccinia activity in several animal species (Sects. C.III, D.II). Structure–activity studies indicated that substitutions in the side chain or thiophene moiety, as well as lengthening of the side chain, produced compounds of diminished activity (WINKELMANN and ROLLY 1972).

III. Isatin-β-Thiosemicarbazones

Unlike the thiosemicarbazones discussed previously, long-lasting interest in the isatin series of compounds was maintained because of their potency and potential

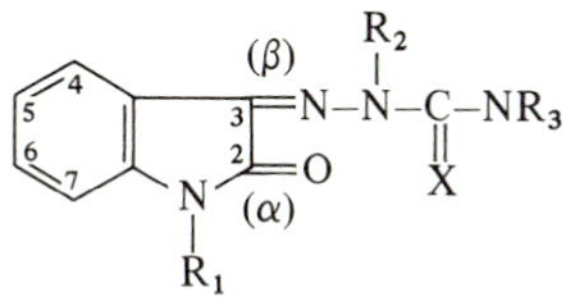

Fig. 8

for clinical application. In 1953 MINTON et al. discovered that isatin-β-thiosemicar-bazone (IBT; Fig. 8, R_1, R_2 = H, R_3 = H_2, X = S) was effective when given in-traperitoneally in only a single dose. This would protect mice against lethal infec-tion with a poxvirus isolated from a patient presenting the clinical picture of mild smallpox (a finding that would be exploited later by D. J. BAUER at the Wellcome Laboratories and by his colleagues). Initial structural studies with IBT showed that bromo and nitro (MINTON et al. 1953), as well as methyl (THOMPSON et al. 1953 b) substitutions at the 5 position of the aromatic ring (Fig. 8) substantially reduced, or abolished, activity. It was also shown that the semicarbazone had no effect on vaccinia infection in the mouse.

Two years later BAUER (1955) presented results indicating that IBT was even more potent against mouse-adapted neurovaccinia virus than had been previously reported. Using the mouse model, BAUER and SADLER (1960 a) then went on to study the relationship between structure and activity in much greater detail than the initial steps taken by the THOMPSON group.

1. Substitution in the Aromatic Ring

Fourteen derivatives were prepared with single substitutions at the 4, 5, 6, or 7 po-sitions (Fig. 8). Methyl, methoxy, iodo, chloro, or bromo substituents were mostly used. These groups commonly led to reduction or total loss of activity of the com-pound. Substituents at the 5 position had a particularly marked effect in eliminat-ing biologic activity; except for substituents, such as fluorine, with small atomic or group radii. The interaction between the size of the halogen atom substituted at this position and the degree of antiviral activity was confirmed recently (BORYSIE-WICZ and LUCKA-SOBSTEL 1978) using Mannich base derivatives of IBT. BAUER and SADLER (1960 a) found that activity was reduced to a lesser extent in the 4 or 6 positions, and some of the 7-substituted compounds still retained high activity. The importance of the steric effects was further supported by the finding that larger fused ring systems, such as naphthisatins, in which the additional benzene ring is fused to the 4,5, or 5,6, or 6,7 positions, were inactive (BAUER and SADLER 1960 a; SADLER 1965).

2. N-Substitution in the Pyrrolidine Ring

Studies were then undertaken on the effect of N-substitution in the pyrrolidine ring (BAUER and SADLER 1960 a). Alkylation at this position (R_1 in Fig. 8) produced a conspicuous rise in activity, reaching a maximum with 1-ethylisatin-TSC. This compound had almost three times the activity of the parent compound; although

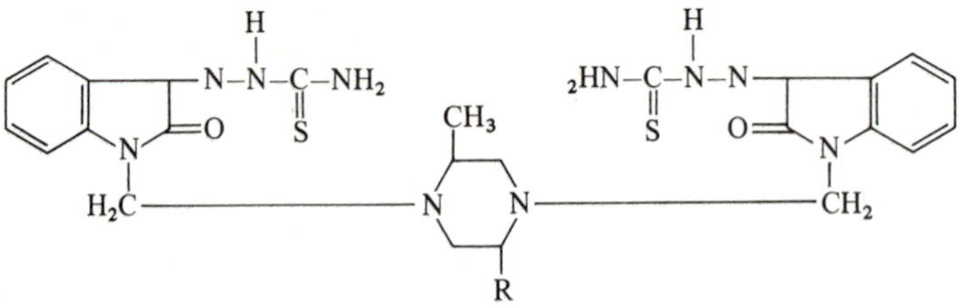

Fig. 9

the N-methyl derivative (MIBT) would be used in almost all further studies because of the ease and low cost of production. Activity fell off rapidly with further lengthening of the side chain; the 1-pentyl derivative was practically inactive. More recent attempts to increase activity by substitution at this position have led to the synthesis of N-methylthiomorpholine- (CH$_2$-N⟨ ⟩S)-IBT (SMEJKAL et al. 1972). It manifested practically the same activity against vaccinia-infected mice as the N-methyl derivative. Also examined were a series of 17 mono- and 9 bis-piperazine derivatives of IBT. Studies were carried out in both vaccinia-infected tissue culture systems (BORYSIEWICZ et al. 1973; BORYSIEWICZ and LUCKA-SOBSTEL 1978; ZGORNIAK-NOWOSIELSKA et al. 1973) and mice (ZGORNIAK-NOWOSIELSKA et al. 1976). Both in vivo and in vitro experiments indicated that three bis-piperazine derivatives were the most active (Fig. 9, R = H, CH$_3$ cis, or CH$_3$ trans). In the mouse system, the N,N'-bis-(β-thiosemicarbazonemethylisatin)-2-methylpiperazine (Fig. 9, R = H) was more active than the cis or trans dimethylpiperazine derivatives, but it was slightly less active than MIBT. However, in tissue culture (BORYSIEWICZ and LUCKA-SOBSTEL 1978), MIBT was less active than the Mannich base compounds, with the difference in activity between the three Mannich derivatives being much more pronounced than observed in mice. As stressed in Sect. C, one cannot project in vitro structure–activity relationships to those likely to hold in vivo, or vice versa.

3. Modification of the Pyrrolidine Ring

This showed that the α-carbonyl group (Fig. 8) was essential: 1-acetylindoxyl-TSC (Fig. 10) was inactive, as was isatin-α-TSC (BAUER and SADLER 1960 a). Extension of the side chain, as in 1-methyloxindole-3-formyl-TSC (Fig. 11, R$_1$ = CH$_3$, R$_2$ = H, X = =O) resulted in loss of activity. However, indole-3-acetyl-TSC (Fig. 11, R$_1$, X=H, R$_2$=CH$_3$) was found to inhibit vaccinia virus in tissue culture (BUU-HOI et al. 1968) although no animal experiments were reported. Studies on the for-

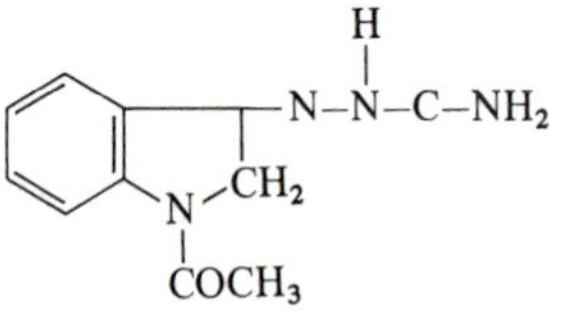

Fig. 10

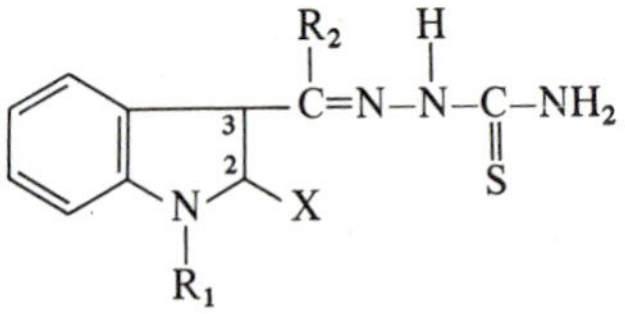

Fig. 11

myl-TSCs were pursued further by ANDREANI et al. (1975, 1978). Their approach was to restore and extend the antiviral activity and spectrum of these compounds by changing the oxygen atom at position 2 (Fig. 11) to another electronegative substituent, and by changing the substituent at position 1 because it was so critical for heightened activity in the isatin series. Of 28 compounds synthesized (ANDREANI et al. 1975), 11 inhibited the growth of vaccinia virus in tissue culture (two of these compounds also inhibited parainfluenza type 3). Under their test conditions, three compounds were even more active against vaccinia than MIBT. These were 1-(o, m, or p-chlorobenzoyl)-2-chloroindole-3-formyl-TSC (Fig. 11, R_1 = CO—⟨⟩—Cl, R_2 = H, X = Cl). Extending these findings with the synthesis of 11 more compounds ANDREANI et al. (1978) concluded that: (a) bromo instead of chloro substitution at position 2 decreased toxicity while retaining antipox activity; and (b) antipox activity was retained with methyl, chloro, and bromobenzoyl substituents at position 1. In this case, as in the initial studies with the chlorobenzoyl substituent, the *meta* positioning of the halogen or methyl group was most active.

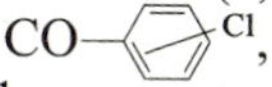

4. Modification of the TSC Side Chain

BAUER and SADLER (1960a) showed that modification in any of a number of ways of the TSC side chain led to loss of activity. That methylation at the sulfur atom abolished antipox activity was confirmed in later (TONEW et al. 1974b), more extensive studies on isothiosemicarbazones (see Fig. 13). Further lengthening of this alkyl side chain (Sects. C.V, D.V) led to the emergence of activity in vaccinia-infected mice as well as against the unrelated RNA-containing Mengo virus (VECKENSTEDT and ZGORNIAK-NOWOSIELSKA 1979). After the antiviral spectrum of MIBT was extended to influenza virus (BAUER et al. 1970; Sect. D.III), studies were undertaken by SMEJKAL et al. (1972) to determine if there was potentiation with the well-known anti-influenza drug, amantadine (see Chap. 4). This tricyclic C_{10} primary amine with a very symmetrical structure was combined with MIBT as a single molecule (Fig. 12), but was found to be only moderately more active than amantadine alone. However, MIBT by itself, under the test conditions employed, was even more active against influenza virus.

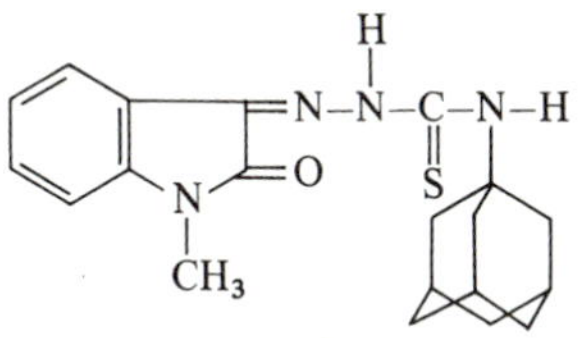

Fig. 12

5. Other Compounds

A number of miscellaneous compounds, including isatin and thiosemicarbazide, were also tested by BAUER and SADLER (1960a) and found to be devoid of activity.

Structural studies on a much smaller scale were also carried out in a poxvirus-infected tissue culture system (SHEFFIELD et al. 1960), as well as in mice infected with various types of poxviruses (BAUER et al. 1962). These confirmed that substitution in the aromatic ring, as well as in the side chain led to loss of activity.

IV. Isatin-β-4′,4′-Dialkylthiosemicarbazones

When BAUER (1955) confirmed the antipox acivity of IBT he showed that the compound was not effective against a number of other murine viruses, including what he believed to be lymphocytic choriomeningitis virus. What was actually tested was pseudolymphocytic choriomeningitis, or ectromelia – a poxvirus (D. J. BAUER personal communication 1975). In 1957 BOCK reported that mice infected with either ectromelia or canarypox were not protected by IBT under conditions which spared neurovaccinia-infected mice. With the realization that ectromelia-infected mice were insensitive to IBT (in tissue culture the compound had very low activity at the limit of detectability; SHEFFIELD et al. 1960), BAUER and SADLER (1960a) tested this virus along with vaccinia virus against a number of compounds synthesized in their comprehensive studies on structural modification of IBT.

The initial studies showed that monoalkyl substitution at the terminal nitrogen atom of the TSC side chain (R_3 in Fig. 8) resulted in compounds with no activity against either vaccinia or ectromelia viruses. However, further studies on modification of the molecule (BAUER and SADLER 1961) showed that dialkyl substitution (dimethyl, diethyl, dibutyl) at the side chain terminal nitrogen atom (R_3 in Fig. 8) led to high activity against ectromelia and little or no activity against vaccinia. All three derivatives retained activity when methyl or ethyl groups were added to the pyrrolidine nitrogen atom (R_1 in Fig. 8). More detailed studies with the 4′,4′-dialkylthiosemicarbazones (BAUER 1963; O'SULLIVAN et al. 1963) showed that alkylation of the pyrrolidine nitrogen (R_1 in Fig. 8) steadily lowered activity as the carbon chain was lengthened – the exact opposite effect was seen with IBT (Sect. C.III). In a like manner, lengthening of the dialkyl substituents at the terminal nitrogen atom of the thiosemicarbazone moiety decreased activity: the relative effectiveness of the 4′,4′-di-n-butyl compound was six-fold lower than the 4′,4′-dimethyl derivative. Another difference in the effectiveness of the two types of compounds was that with the dialkyl derivatives, mono substitution in the aromatic ring, irrespective of position, produced only small reductions in activity against ectromelia. However, in both series of compounds, disubstitution in the benzene ring abolished activity. These dialkyl compounds were also tested against poliovirus types 1 and 2. Most compounds were inactive against poliovirus type 1, but they were highly effective against poliovirus type 2 (O'SULLIVAN and SADLER 1961). The dibutyl derivative, supposedly because of optimal activity, was chosen for further study (Sects. D.IV, F.IV).

V. Isatin-β-Isothiosemicarbazones

Viral specificity of isatin-β-thiosemicarbazone was markedly changed by dialkyl substitution at the side chain terminal nitrogen atom (R_3 in Fig. 8; see Sect. C.IV). Although initial investigations (BAUER and SADLER 1960a) showed that methylation at the sulfur atom (a methyl-substituted isothiosemicarbazone, Fig. 13, $R_1 = $ H, $R_2 = CH_3$, $R_3 = H_2$) was without activity, more extensive alkylation studies of this type were undertaken with the aim of producing compounds with new virostatic action (TONEW et al. 1974b; Franke et al. 1975). Confirming previous observations with the benzaldehyde and isatin thiosemicarbazones (Sects. C.I, III),

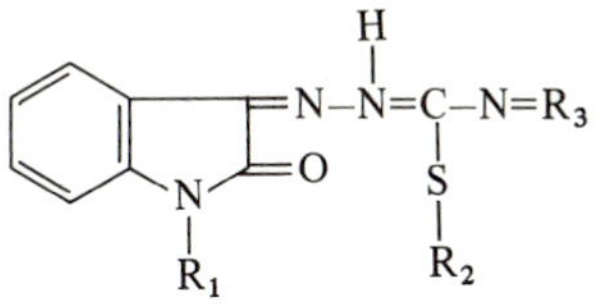

Fig. 13

compounds without sulfur were inactive. Of 24 substituted isothiosemicarbazones synthesized (HEINISCH and KRAMARCZYK 1972) 11 had antiviral activity in tissue culture systems (TONEW et al. 1974b). Of 6 compounds active against vaccinia virus, 5 were also effective against Mengo virus. Derivatives showing this dual activity shared the following structural features:

a. N-Propyl, isopropyl, or n-butyl substituents were present on the sulfur atom (R_2 in Fig. 13)

b. While ethyl substitution at the pyrrolidine nitrogen atom (R_1 in Fig. 13) was more effective than the unsubstituted or methyl-substituted compounds, no activity was found with higher alkylation.

Compounds active only against Mengo virus maintained these structural relationships at the pyrrolidine ring, but methyl, ethyl, or benzyl ($CH_2C_6H_5$) substituents at the sulfur atom also produced active compounds. Furthermore, cyclohexyl substitution at the side chain terminal nitrogen (Fig. 13, $R_1 = C_2H_5$,

$$R_3 = \begin{array}{c} CH_2-CH_2 \\ \diagup \qquad \diagdown \\ \qquad\qquad CH_2 \\ \diagdown \qquad \diagup \\ CH_2-CH_2 \end{array}$$) resulted in biologic activity against Mengo virus but not

vaccinia virus. Of the 11 compounds active against Mengo virus in tissue culture, 3 (Fig. 13, $R_1 = CH_3$ or C_2H_5, $R_2 = C_2H_5$, $R_3 = H_2$, $R_1 = C_2H_5$, $R_2 = C_4H_9$, $R_3 = H_2$) have been claimed to protect mice against encephalitis induced by Mengo virus (VECKENSTEDT and HORN 1974; VECKENSTEDT and ZGORNIAK-NOWOSIELSKA 1979).

VI. Thiazole Thiosemicarbazones

Antipox activity of thiosemicarbazones was extended to an isothiazolecarbonyl series of compounds (Fig. 14); one of which would be used in clinical trials against smallpox (Sect. H). The most active compound against neurovaccinia-infected mice, of over 40 synthesized (CATON et al. 1965), was 3 methyl-4-bromo-5-formyl-isothiazole-TSC (Fig. 14, $R_1 = CH_3$, $R_2 = Br$, $R_3 = CH = NNHCSNH_2$). Antiviral activity was markedly dependent on the position of the TSC moiety in the isothiazole ring: the 4-formylisothiazole (Fig. 14, $R_1 = CH_3$, $R_2 = CH = NNHCSNH_2$, $R_3 = H$) was marginally active whereas the 3-formyl compound (Fig. 14, $R_1 = CH = NNHCSNH_2$, $R_2 = H$, $R_3 = H$) was totally inactive. In the

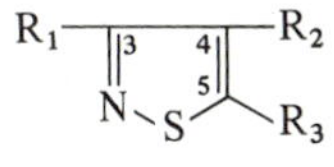

Fig. 14

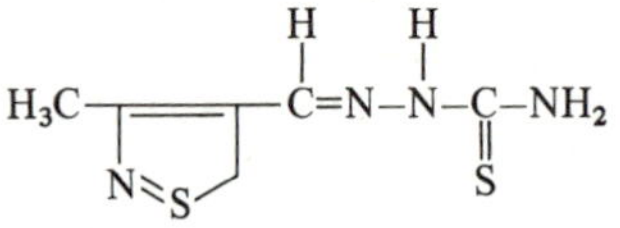

$$H_3C\text{---}C=N\text{--}N\text{--}C\text{--}NH_2$$

Fig. 15

5-formylisothiazole series, substitution by halogen (Cl, Br, I) in the 4 position increased activity with a decrease in toxicity. The 4-bromo substituent was particularly effective. A 3-methyl substituent decreased toxicity slightly without decreasing activity, and when combined with the 4-bromo substitutent led to the most active compound of the series. Nitro and methyl substituents at the 4 position had little effet on activity, but a carboxy group at this position completely abolished activity. As in the isatin-TSC series, compounds substituted in the side chain were, in general, inactive. Cyclizing the side chain of active formylisothiazoles to mercaptotriazoles or aminothiadiazoles greatly reduced or eliminated activity. A closely related compound (Fig. 15) which was reported to have antipox activity in mice, was 4-methyl-5-formylthiazole-TSC (CAMPAIGNE et al. 1959). This observation has been confirmed in tissue culture using 5-formylthiazole-TSC (KATZ et al. 1974). Little information is available on structure–activity relationships aside from the finding that placing the TSC side chain in the 4 position (α to the ring nitrogen atom; see Sects. C.II, III) resulted in total loss of activity, and that 4-methyl-2-methylthio-5-formylthiazole-TSC was only moderately active (CAMPAIGNE et al. 1959).

VII. Pyrrolidine and Pyrazolone Thiosemicarbazones

Two reports appear to indicate the potential antiviral activity of some pyrrolidine thiosemicarbazones, but the brief nature of the presentations prevents a critical evaluation of the findings. Two TSCs derived from substituted 2,3-dioxypyrrolidines were found to be active against influenza infections in mice (GERZON 1965). These were 1-ethylpyrrolidine-2,3-dione-TSC (Fig. 16, R = C_2H_5) and its β-hydroxyethyl congener (Fig. 16, R = CH_2CH_2OH). The latter was the more effective antiviral agent, a result that was the opposite of the corresponding substitution studies in the antivaccinia isatin series (BAUER and SADLER 1960a). Unlike the isatin compounds, these pyrrolidines had no activity against vaccinia virus.

A series of 13 thiosemicarbazones was synthesized from substituted 3-arylidene-4,5-dioxypyrrolidine nuclei (Fig. 17). Some of these compounds, all of which were tested in tissue culture, were active against vaccinia virus, parainfluenza virus,

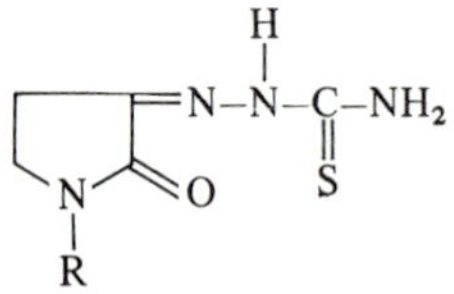

Fig. 16

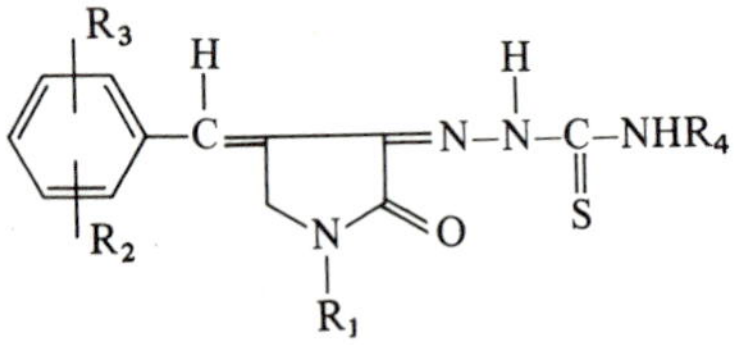

Fig. 17

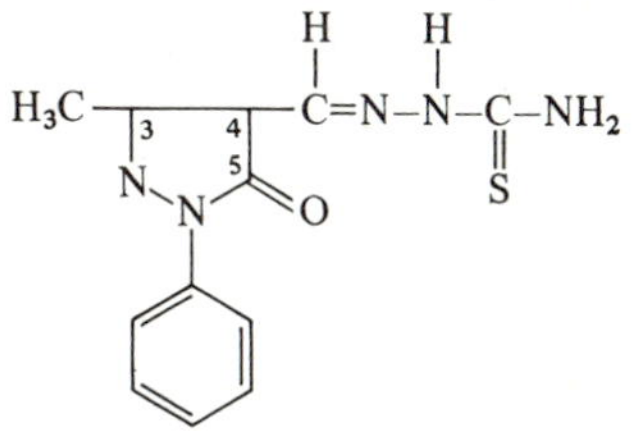

Fig. 18

rhinovirus, coxsackievirus, and influenzavirus (SINGH and SUGDEN 1971). The authors claimed that: none of the compounds was as effective against vaccinia as N-methylisatin-β-thiosemicarbazone (Sect. C.III); phenethyl or benzyl substitution at the pyrrolidine nitrogen atom (R_1 in Fig. 17), was necessary for maximal activity while methyl substitution abolished antiviral properties; the nature of the R_2 and R_3 groups (hydroxy, methoxy, halogen) attached to the arylidine ring appeared to have little effect on activity; and substitution of the primary amine group (R_4 in Fig. 17) of the TSC side chain greatly reduced activity. Although no systematic structure–activity studies were carried out on 4-formyl-3-methyl-1-phenyl-5-pyrazolone-TSC (Fig. 18), it was reported to inhibit rhinovirus growth in tissue culture (BUU-HOI et al. 1968).

VIII. Noncyclic Thiosemicarbazones

Cyclic thiosemicarbazones have generally been found essential for antiviral activity. However, there are at least three known exceptions. The first two came to light at the time of intensive investigation of benzaldehyde-TSCs (Sect. C.I). It was found that thiosemicarbazones with an aliphatic oxime nucleus possessed the capacity to protect mice against vaccinia virus (THOMPSON et al. 1953a). Of six compounds tested, five had antiviral properties. The most effective was butane-2,3-dione-oxime-TSC (Fig. 19, R = H) and the corresponding methoxime (R = CH_3). The structure–activity relationships were not examined in detail but appeared to be similar to the isatin series, in that both oxime and methoxime semicarbazones were inactive. The methoxime was the more active of the two when given intraperitoneally (instead of in the diet). Another observation that the cyclic structure was not essential for antiviral activity was the finding of LEVINSON et al. (1977a). They showed that kethoxal-bis-(thiosemicarbazone) inhibited the replication of vesicular stomatitis virus in chick embryo culture (Fig. 20). Neither MIBT (Fig. 8) nor 2-

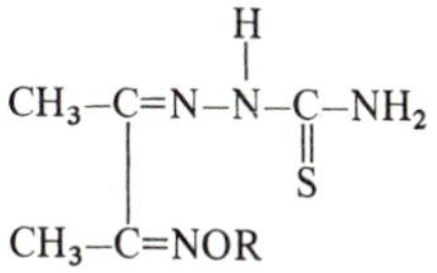

Fig. 19

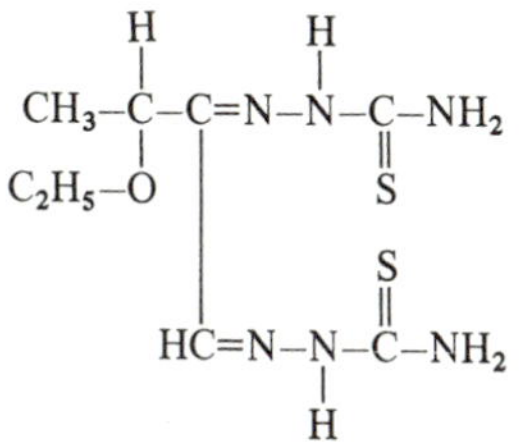

Fig. 20

formylpyridine-TSC (Fig. 4) had any effect on this virus. However, all three compounds were able to inhibit the cell-transforming ability of Rous sarcoma virus (Kaska et al. 1978).

IX. Miscellaneous Thiosemicarbazones

In the isatin series of compounds (Sect. C.III) the carbonyl group at the C-2 position of the pyrrolidine ring was considered essential for biologic activity. However, a series of γ-thiochromanone-4-thiosemicarbazones (Fig. 21) was found to be active against vaccina virus (Tsunoda et al. 1971). Methyl or chloro substitution at the 6 position of the aromatic ring did not alter activity. γ-Thiochromanone-4-thiosemicarbazone appeared to be about as active as 1-methyl-isatin-β-thiosemicarbazone (Sect. C.III) in tissue culture as well as in mice. No additive effect of the two compounds was observed in the animal tests. The thiochromanone-TSC activity in tissue culture has been confirmed (Katz et al. 1974, 1975).

A single report (Buu-Hoi et al. 1968) exists indicating that 3,9-diethyl-6-formylcarbazole-TSC (Fig. 22) inhibits the growth of rhinoviruses in tissue culture, but not influenza or vaccinia viruses.

Varma and Nobles (1967) screened indanedione-TSCs for activity in tissue culture against poliovirus type 2, herpes simplex, measles, and influenza viruses. Of six compounds synthesized, two inhibited poliovirus. These were 1,3-indanedione-4'-n-butyl-TSC [Fig. 23, R_1 = =O, R_2 = H, R_3 = n-$(CH_2)_3CH_3$] and 1,3-indanedione-4'-methyldithiosemicarbazone (Fig. 23, R_1 = $NNHCSNHCH_3$, R_2 = H, R_3 = CH_3). The antiviral potential of indanedione dithiosemicarbazones was confirmed by Giannella and Gualtieri (1970) and by Gianella et al. (1973) who synthesized a large number of carbamates, thiosemicarbazones, semicarbazones, and γ-hydroxyiminoketones. Only the dithiosemicarbazone of 2-hydroxyimino-1,3-indanedione (Fig. 23, R_1 = =$NNHCSNH_2$, R_2 = =NOH, R_3 = H) showed in vitro activity against vaccinia virus. The corresponding semicarbazone was not active. Furthermore, all compounds were ineffective in vitro against herpes simplex and influenza viruses. However, 2-hydroxyimino-1,3-indanedione dithiosemicarbazone was shown to prolong the life of mice lethally infected with influenza A viruses.

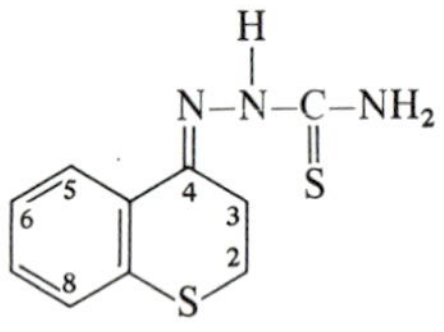

Fig. 21

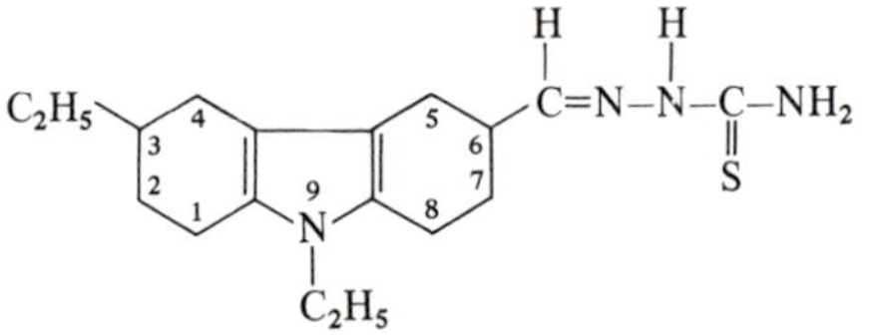

Fig. 22

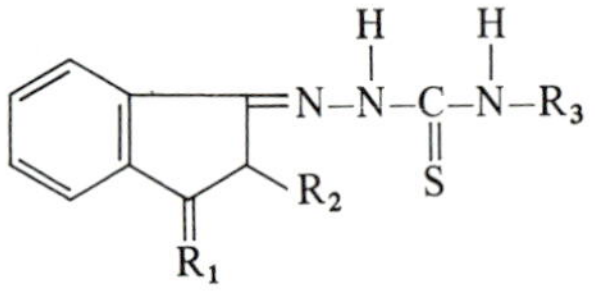

Fig. 23

D. Virus-Inhibitory Spectrum

The ability of thiosemicarbazones to inhibit viruses will be discussed in the order of their general structures as categorized in Sect. C. With few exceptions the effects of specific substituents in a parent compound will not be emphasized. This information can be determined by referring to the appropriate parts of the preceding section.

I. Aryl Thiosemicarbazones

Mice, embryonated chicken eggs, and Maitland cultures derived from them, were found to be protected by specific benzaldehyde-TSCs infected with any of the tested strains of vaccinia virus (Table 1). It was noted (THOMPSON et al. 1953 b) that while benzaldehyde-TSCs having activity in mice usually possessed some capacity to inhibit virus replication in vitro, compounds had been synthesized that were totally inactive in vivo although highly active in vitro. The effect of benzaldehyde-TSCs in rabbits infected intradermally with the IHD strain of vaccinia virus was marginal. THOMPSON et al. (1953 b) reported that, although the number of observations was too small to draw definite conclusions, the impression was gained that treatment did not prevent formation of lesions at the sites of inoculation of virus, although generalization of the infection and development of necrosis at the site of the lesions was prevented.

LUM and SMITH (1957) reported that p-nitro-, p-hydroxy-, or p-methoxybenzaldehyde-TSCs would prevent death in mice infected with influenza A and B viruses. However, HAMRE et al. (1950) could find no murine activity against swine influenza using p-aminobenzaldehyde-TSC. Furthermore, BOCK (1957) stated that unpublished data by G. DOMAGK et al. showed that mice infected with an influenza virus were not spared by treatment with an unspecified benzaldehyde-TSC. These discrepancies have remained unresolved and could possibly be explained by chemical, viral, or murine specificities. Mice infected with two members of the Togaviridae family (PORTERFIELD et al. 1978) Semliki Forest (in the genus *Alphavirus*) and

Table 1. Antiviral spectrum of aryl thiosemicarbazones

Compound[a]	Virus	Strain	Host[b]	Primary citation
Bd	Vaccinia	NYBH	Chicken egg, mouse	HAMRE et al. (1951)
		CV II	Chick Mec	THOMPSON et al. (1951)
		IHD	Mouse	THOMPSON et al. (1951)
			Mouse Mec	THOMPSON et al. (1953b)
		WR	Mouse	BOCK (1957)
Bd, C	Influenca	A, B	Mouse	LUM and SMITH (1957)
A, Bc, Bd, C	Influenza	A, B	Chick Cmc	IWASAKI et al. (1955)
Bc, Bd, C	Newcastle disease	Miyadera	Chick Cmc	IWASAKI et al. (1955)
A	Parainfluenza	1	Tissue culture	RUNTI et al. (1968)

[a] Acetophenone (A), benzalacetone (Bc), benzaldehyde (Bd), cinnamaldehyde (C) thiosemicarbazones
[b] Maitland embryo culture (Mec); chorioallantoic membrane culture (Cmc)

St. Louis encephalitis (in the genus *Flavivirus*) were not protected by treatment with benzaldehyde-TSCs (MINTON et al. 1953). Mice infected with these and a number of other arthropod-transmitted viruses have not responded to treatment with other types of TSCs (Sects. D.II, III).

BOCK (1957) noted that preliminary screening of benzaldehyde-TSCs, done at the time of DOMAGK's discovery of their antibacterial properties, failed to detect activity against two poxviruses; ectromelia and canarypox. Later studies with the isatin series of TSCs would show that ectromelia was insensitive to TSCs that inhibited all other poxvirus murine infections (Sect. D.III). BOCK also reported that in the same studies the disease in mice caused by either lymphocytic choriomeningitis virus or pneumonia virus was not altered by benzaldehyde-TSCs.

II. Quinoline, Pyridine, and Thiophene Thiosemicarbazones

Certain of these heterocyclic compounds were effective against two strains of vaccinia virus and two members of the herpesvirus family (Table 2). Furthermore, isoquinoline- and pyridine-TSCs can inactivate on contact extracellular herpesvirus and Rous sarcoma virus (Table 2; Sect. F.II). While 5-cyanothiophene-2-formyl-TSC (Fig. 7) was unique in its effectiveness against vaccinia virus in rabbits and rats, as well as in mice, it was not active against ectromelia or canarypox viruses (see also Sects. D.I, III for the insensitivity of other TSCs against these viruses). Although active in mice, 4-formylquinoline-TSC (Fig. 5) had limited effectiveness in vaccinia-infected rabbits (THOMPSON et al. 1953 b). Poliovirus synthesis in tissue culture has been found to proceed normally (KATZ et al. 1974) in the presence of 1-formylisoquinoline-TSC (Fig. 6) and 5-hydroxy-2-formylpyridine (Fig. 4). In a report dealing with these three types of compounds (MINTON et al. 1953) the general statement was made that thiosemicarbazones were not found to protect mice against St. Louis encephalitis or Semliki Forest virus (Togaviridae, see Sect. D.I).

Table 2. Antiviral spectrum of quinoline, pyridine, and thiophene thiosemicarbazones

Compound[a]	Virus	Strain	Host	Primary citation
P, Q	Cytomegalovirus	NIH	WI-38 cells	BROCKMAN et al. (1970)
P, Q	Herpesvirus	Simplex-HF	HEP-2 cells	BROCKMAN et al. (1970)
I, P		Simplex type 1	[c]	LEVINSON et al. (1974)
I, P	Rous sarcoma	B-77	[c]	LEVINSON et al. (1977b)
				KASKA et al. (1978)
P, Q, T	Vaccinia	IHD	Mouse	THOMPSON et al. (1953b)
			Mouse mec[b]	
		WR	BSC-1 cells	KATZ et al. (1974)
T	Vaccinia	?	Mouse	ROLLY and WINKELMAN
			Rabbit	(1972)
			Rat	

[a] Isoquinoline (I), pyridine (P), quinoline (Q), thiophene (T) thiosemicarbazones
[b] Maitland embryo culture
[c] Contact inactivation of extracellular virus

III. Isatin-β-Thiosemicarbazones

The most extensive studies on the antiviral spectrum of these compounds have been carried out with isatin-β-thiosemicarbazone and its N_1-methyl derivative. Mice infected with all tested poxviruses, with the exception of canarypox, monkeypox, and ectromelia, will survive when given these drugs (Table 3). As yet, no other in vivo infections with other types of viruses have been convincingly shown to respond strongly to these compounds. Furthermore, as will be shown, many conflicting reports exist concerning the activity of these TSCs against in vitro infection with various viruses.

In 1966 BAUER and APOSTOLOV reported that MIBT at concentrations from 5 to 40 μM could inhibit the replication of adenovirus types 3, 7, 9, 11, 14, 16, 17, 21, and 28 in a HeLa cell tissue culture system. A preliminary study of structure–activity relations of MIBT against these viruses showed that the compound followed the same pattern as that of the poxviruses (Sect. C.III). Replacement of the sulfur with oxygen, substituting two alkyl groups at the terminal amino sequence of the side chain, and changing the methyl group from the N-1 to the C-5 position (Fig. 8) led to loss of activity. Yet, neither HARFORD et al. (1972) nor HERRMANN (1968) could confirm this antiviral activity. Both reports were based on observations in HeLa cells treated with MIBT. In the former case, a 40 μM concentration was used against adenovirus types 2 and 7, while in the latter case, a plaque inhibition test (the drug diffusing from a central disc) was used with adenovirus types 1, 2, 5, and 7. As proposed later (Sect. F), the presence or absence of critical concentrations of divalent cations of first transition series metals should be considered as a possible determining factor in the outcome of these experiments. Isatin-β-thiosemicarbazone has afforded no protection to mice infected with various ar-

Table 3. Response of murine poxvirus infections to isatin-β-thiosemicarbazone and its N_1-methyl derivative

Virus	Strain	Primary citation
Therapeutic		
Variola-vaccinia	Williamsport	MINTON et al. (1953)
Vaccinia	IHD	THOMPSON et al. (1953b)
	WR	BOCK (1957)
Rabbitpox	Utrecht	BAUER and SHEFFIELD (1959)
Cowpox	WCP	BAUER (1961)
	CP	
Alastrim	Schofield	BAUER and SADLER (1960b)
Variola major	Harvey	BAUER et al. (1962)
Noncurative		
Canarypox	Kikuth–Golubschen	BOCK (1957)
Ectromelia	Be	BOCK (1957)
	Sandom	BAUER (1955)[a]
Monkeypox	Copenhagen	CHO et al. (1970)

[a] Ectromelia or pseudolymphocytic choriomeningitis was incorrectly identified in this report as lymphocytic choriomeningitis

Table 4. Studies on herpesvirus sensitivities to isatin or N-methylisatin-β-thiosemicarbazones

Virus	Strain	Host[a]	Protection	Primary citation
In vivo				
Cytomegalovirus	Smith	Mouse	No	SCHMIDT-RUPPIN (1971)
Herpesvirus	Simplex	Mouse	No	BAUER and SADLER (1960a)
	Simplex type 1	Rabbit	Marginal[b]	LEVINSON et al. (1974)
Marek's disease	3 K	Chick	Marginal	KUDRIAVTSEV et al. (1977)
In vitro				
Cytomegalovirus	NIH	WI-38	No	BROCKMAN et al. (1970)
Herpesvirus	Simplex	Primary RKF	No	RAPP (1964)
		Primary HTC	Yes	CAUNT (1967)
		HeLa cells	No	HERRMANN (1968)
		HEP-2 cells	No	BROCKMAN et al. (1970)
Infectious bovine rhinotracheitis	Brown	MDBK cells	Yes	Munro and Sabina (1970)
Varicella	Zoster	HeLa cells	No	RAPP (1964)
		Primary HTC	Yes	CAUNT (1967)

[a] RKF = rabbit kidney fibroblast; HTC = human thyroid cells
[b] Thiosemicarbazide used because no suitable vehicle was found for M IBT

thropod-transmitted viruses (BAUER 1955; BAUER and SADLER 1960a). Six viruses from the family Togaviridae (PORTERFIELD et al. 1978) were screened: one from the genus *Alphavirus* (Semliki Forest) and the others from the genus *Flavivirus* (dengue, Ilheus, Nytoya, yellow fever, and Zika). The remaining viruses were in the family Bunyaviridae or were Bunyavirus-like (BISHOP and SHOPE 1979). In the former category were Anopheles A, California, and Wyeomyia; and in the latter category were Anopheles B and Rift Valley fever viruses. The median lethal dose (LD_{50}) of a stock of Rift Valley fever virus was 0.5 log units higher in mice treated with IBT, and this represents the only possible example of slight protection by the drug. BAUER et al. (1970) have reported that the yield of Semliki Forest and Bunyamwera virus in HeLa or monkey kidney tissue culture was reduced by MIBT in a dose-related fashion. The specificity of the antiviral effect was shown by the finding that under similar conditions the yield of another alphavirus (Sindbis) was unchanged in the presence of the drug.

There are conflicting reports concerning the responses of various herpesvirus infections to IBT and MIBT (Table 4). They are too few in number and superficial to enable one confidently to suggest the possible cause of the discrepancies (see the paragraph on adenoviruses in this section). While murine infections with cytomegalovirus and herpesvirus appear to proceed normally in the presence of these compounds, there was marginal activity in rabbits and chicks infected with herpesvirus and Marek's disease virus, respectively. Because they could not find a pharmacologically acceptable vehicle to dissolve IBT or MIBT, LEVINSON et al. (1974) tested the ability of thiosemicarbazide to ameliorate the course of herpes keratitis in rabbits. While there was a statistically significant decrease in the number and severity of dendritic lesions, the effect was much less than that observed with either iododeoxyuridine or proflavine with exposure to light. With these encouraging results,

Table 5. Studies on orthomyxovirus and paramyxovirus sensitivities to isatin or *N*-methylisatin-
β-thiosemicarbazones

Virus	Strain	Host	Protection	Primary citation
Influenza	A/NWS	Mouse	No	BAUER (1955)
	A/Singapore	Mouse	Marginal[a]	SMEJKAL et al. (1972)
	A/Hong Kong	Mouse	No[b]	SMEJKAL et al. (1972)
	A/England	Calf kidney cells	Yes	BAUER et al. (1970)
Parainfluenza	1	Calf kidney cells	Yes	BAUER et al. (1970)
Newcastle disease	?	ERK cells[c]	No	SHEFFIELD (1962)

[a] Survival time increased two-fold
[b] A modest reduction in infectious virus was noted
[c] Derived from embryonic rabbit kidney

it would be of interest to repeat the experiments with isatin-β-thiosemicarbazones. In limited studies we have found that these drugs will dissolve in a nonirritating solution composed of 50% polyethylene glycol 400, 40% polypropylene glycol, and 10% ethanol. Using single, or preferably multiple, injections of IBT or MIBT, KUDRIAVTSEV et al. (1977) found retardation of the growth of Marek's disease virus in chicks infected when 1 day old. The morbidity, as measured by the presence of tumors in internal organs, was over two-fold lower in MIBT-treated chicks, but no difference was seen with IBT. Only MIBT lowered mortality, although no data were presented. Furthermore, it appeared that both drugs delayed, but did not eliminate the virus infection. This may have been partially due to the immunosuppressive properties of these compounds (Sect. G), since virus was no longer detectable in most control chickens 40 days after infection.

Tissue culture studies with the herpesviruses using the isatin-β-thiosemicarbazones were initiated by RAPP (1964). Using 4 μ*M* MIBT in a semisolid overlayer (higher concentrations of the drug precipitated), no reduction in plaque number was noted with either herpes simplex or herpes zoster viruses. This observation was confirmed by HERRMANN (1968), using a plaque reduction method relying on diffusion of either IBT or MIBT from an impregnated antibiotic disc. Both CAUNT (1967) and MUNRO and SABINA (1970), using 20 μ*M* MIBT in liquid tissue culture overlayers, found that the yield of herpes simplex and infectious bovine rhinotracheitis were significantly reduced. Unlike most other studies, IBT appeared to be more effective than MIBT against infectious bovine rhinotracheitis (MUNRO and SABINA 1970).

The number of reports (and their brevity) are too small to evaluate critically the lack of effect of the isatin-β-thiosemicarbazones in influenza-infected mice (Table 5). However, BAUER et al. (1970) found that MIBT was effective against influenzavirus and parainfluenzavirus, as shown by a decrease in the ability of virus-infected tissue cultures to hemadsorb red blood cells. The isatin-β-thiosemicarbazones have shown no activity in mice infected with picornaviruses (Table 6). However, in tissue culture, at about 40 μ*M*, MIBT has reduced the yield of a variety of different picornaviruses in a number of cell lines. Perplexingly, two of the four reports dealing with poliovirus indicate that IBT and its N_1-alkyl derivatives, in concentrations as high as 100 μ*M* were without effect on virus synthesis. Again one

Table 6. Studies on the sensitivity of picornaviruses to isatin or N-methylisatin-β-thiosemicarbazones

Virus	Strain	Host	Protection	Primary citation
Encephalo-myocarditis	MM	Mouse	No	Bauer (1955)
Foot-and-mouth disease	A 119	Bovine kidney cells	Yes	Polatnick (1965)
Poliovirus	MEF 1	Mouse	No	Bauer and Sadler (1960a)
	1, 2	Tissue culture	No	O'Sullivan and Sadler (1961)
	1, 2, 3	HeLa cells	No	Pearson and Zimmerman (1969)
	1, 2, 3	HeLa cells	Yes	Bauer et al. (1970)
	1	KB cells	Yes	Lwoff and Lwoff (1964)
Rhinovirus	1059-H	WI-26 cells	Yes	Gladych et al. (1969)
	3242-H	WI-38 cells		
	HGP-M			

could suggest that critical concentrations of divalent cations might have been all-important in the outcome of the experiments.

Returning to the poxviruses, MIBT was not effective when administered (by intubation) to rabbits infected subcutaneously with vaccinia virus (Herrlich et al. 1965; Kackell et al. 1966). However, the drug had marginal activity if injected intracutaneously at the site of vaccination (Kackell et al. 1966). Whereas MIBT did not spare mice infected with ectromelia virus (Table 3), the drug in an aqueous overlayer had borderline activity in suppressing cytopathic effects in HeLa cells infected with the virus (Sheffield et al. 1960). Furthermore, when the drug was in a semisolid overlayer, plaque formation by ectromelia virus was almost completely prevented (Bauer 1972). A similar pattern appeared with monkeypox virus. While MIBT was equally effective inhibiting plaque formation by vaccinia and monkeypox viruses in monkey kidney tissue culture cells, it had marginal or nor activity in chicken eggs, mice, and monkeys (Cho et al. 1970). With the exception of the replication of molluscum contagiosum virus in human amnion (FL) cells (Francis and Bradford 1976) the growth of all other poxviruses in tissue culture appears to be inhibited by IBT or MIBT. Virtually all vertebrate viruses can be inactivated on contact with N_1-ethyl- or N_1-methylisatin-β-thiosemicarbazone and divalent cations of first transition series metals (Table 7). Of the first transition series metals (Mn, Fe, Ni, Cu, Zn), copper appears to be the most effective (Levinson et al. 1971, 1974; Logan et al. 1975). Varying amounts of divalent cations are needed for the reaction to proceed. Even though leukoviruses can be inactivated by addition of IBTs only, interaction with metals appears to be required, since chelating agents abrogate the phenomenon in all systems thus far examined (Levinson et al. 1973b; Logan et al. 1975), and deliberate addition of divalent cations results in a strong synergistic effect (Levinson et al. 1973b). While metal "contaminants" are all that are required to interact with IBTs to inactivate leukoviruses, all other viruses require more than trace amounts. Such chelating agents as Tris buffer or histidine (in tissue culture media), when present with IBTs, will prevent inactivation of her-

Table 7. Viruses inactivated on contact with isatin-β-thiosemicarbazones and first transition series metals

Genus	Virus	Reference
Alphavirus	Sindbis	Fox et al. (1977)
	Semliki Forest	Hanson (1977)
Flavivirus	Dengue	Fox et al. (1977)
Arenavirus	LCM	Logan et al. (1975)
	Latino	J. Kubis and C.J. Pfau (unpublished work 1975)
	Parana	
	Pichinde	
	Tacaribe	
Enterovirus	Poliovirus type 1	Fox et al. (1977)
	Poliovirus type 2	
Herpesvirus	Herpes simplex type 1	Levinson et al. (1974)
	Herpes simplex type 2	
	Herpesvirus saimiri	
Leukovirus	Rous sarcoma	Levinson et al. (1971)
	Murine leukemia	Levinson et al. (1973a)
	Murine sarcoma	Levy et al. (1976)
	Visna	Haase and Levinson (1973)
	Maedi	
	Progressive pneumonia	
	Feline sarcoma	Levinson et al. (1973b)
Orthomyxovirus	Influenza	Fox et al. (1977)
Paramyxovirus	Newcastle disease	Fox et al. (1977)
Orthopoxvirus	Vaccinia, rabbitpox	Fox et al. (1977)
Reovirus	Reovirus type 3	Hanson (1977)
Rhabdovirus	Vesicular stomatitis,	Fox et al. (1977)
	Rabies	
Bacteriophage	Lambda	Levinson and Helling (1976)

pesvirus (Levinson et al. 1974). The remaining viruses that have been examined (Logan et al. 1975; Fox et al. 1977) are inactivated by IBTs very slowly unless exogenous $CuSO_4$ is supplied. Invariably, inactivation proceeds faster in phosphate-buffered saline than in tissue culture medium. The reaction is also dependent on pH and temperature (Pfau 1977). Even though in vitro the IBTs in the presence of divalent copper can inactivate all viruses thus far used in murine infections treated with the drug (see Tables 3–6; also Pfau 1975; Levy et al. 1976; Bauer and Sadler 1960a for data on LCM, murine leukemia, and rabies viruses), therapeutic activity has only been demonstrated against the poxviruses. This may be due to their unique content of copper (Sect. F). Enhancement of the murine leukemia infection seen with MIBT treatment may be due to the immunosuppressive potential of the drug (Sect. G).

IV. Isatin-β-4′,4′-Dialkylthiosemicarbazones

None of the compounds in the isatin series with unsubstituted thiosemicarbazone side chains were found to be effective against ectromelia or canarypox viruses (Sect. D.III). However, both isatin-β-4′,4′dimethylthiosemicarbazone and its N_1-

methyl derivative (BAUER and SADLER 1961) protected mice against lethal infection with ectromelia (the only other compound claimed to be effective is 5-cyanofuran-2-formylthiosemicarbazone; WINKELMANN and ROLLY 1972). N_1-methylisatin-β-4',4'-dibutylthiosemicarbazone (Busatin) has been found to inhibit the replication of poliovirus types 1, 2, and 3 (PEARSON and ZIMMERMAN 1969) and inactivate on contact influenza A viruses (BOPP 1976; M. P. FOX and C. J. PFAU unpublished work 1976).

V. Isatin-β-Isothiosemicarbazones

Various isothiosemicarbazones have been found to be active in tissue culture (TONEW et al. 1974 b) and mice (VECKENSTEDT and ZGORNIAK-NOWOSIELSKA 1979) against vaccinia and Mengo virus infections.

VI. Thiazole Thiosemicarbazones

No studies other than on poxviruses have been reported for these compounds.

VII. Pyrrolidine and Pyrazolone Thiosemicarbazones

Pyrrolidine-TSCs have been reported to protect mice against influenza A infections (GERZON 1965). SINGH and SUGDEN (1971) claimed that certain pyrrolidine-TSCs were active in tissue culture against influenza A virus, parainfluenza (type 1), coxsackievirus, and rhinovirus (types 1 and II). Inhibition of rhinovirus in tissue culture has also been reported for a pyrazolone-TSC (BUU-HOI et al. 1968).

VIII. Noncyclic Thiosemicarbazones

THOMPSON et al. (1953 a) found that oxime- and methoxime-TSCs would spare mice lethally infected with vaccinia virus. Ketoxal-bis-TSC has been shown to inhibit the replication of vesicular stomatitis virus in chick embryo cells (LEVINSON et al. 1977 a), and inactivate on contact Rous sarcoma virus (KASKA et al. 1978).

IX. Miscellaneous Thiosemicarbazones

γ-Thiochromanone-4-TSC has been shown to inhibit mouse tail lesion formation by the IHD strain of vaccinia virus (TSUNODA et al. 1971), and to prevent the cytopathic effects in chick embryo cells infected with that strain of virus as well as in HeLa cells infected with the WR strain of vaccinia (KATZ et al. 1974). 6-Formyl-3,9-diethylcarbazole-TSC was active against the HPG strain of rhinovirus when grown in tissue culture (BUU-HOI et al. 1968). Indanedione-TSCs have been found to be inhibitory in tissue culture to poliovirus type 2 (VARMA and NOBLES 1967) and vaccinia virus (GIANNELLA and GUALTIERI 1970). These compounds have also been shown to prolong the life span of mice infected with either the PR8 strain of influenza A or the Lee strain of influenza B (GIANNELLA et al. 1973).

E. Effects on Normal Cells

In the early 1950s, the beginnings of antiviral chemotherapy as we know it today, relatively little attention was paid to the effect of a drug on normal cells. There were a variety of reasons for this. Some of these were: (a) tissue culture model systems were not readily available; (b) appropriate molecular biology technology was not standardly used or developed; (c) such studies were not considered worthwhile until a drug was found to be effective in primates; and (d) there was less intervention by government regulatory agencies than exists today. Thus, in this context, the amount of literature available depends on when the thiosemicarbazone was discovered, how intensively it was investigated, and during what time period this interest was maintained. The various thiosemicarbazones will be discussed in the order established in Sect. C.

I. Aryl Thiosemicarbazones

No qualitative data is available for the effect these compounds have on normal cells. The only measurements to be found are maximum tolerated doses of drug per egg, mouse, or Maitland culture as measured, respectively, by survival time, weight gain, or ability of cells to divide.

II. Quinoline, Pyridine, and Thiophene Thiosemicarbazones

With the exception of two reports to be cited, the same comments as given in Sect. E.I apply here. BROCKMAN et al. (1970) found a correlation between inhibition of ribonucleotide reductase in uninfected tissue culture cells of epidermoid carcinoma origin and inhibition of herpesvirus growth in these cells. Two inhibitors with this dual function, 1-formylisoquinoline-TSC and 2-formylpyridine-TSC, caused no visible cytotoxicity in control cultures over the time period prior to virus harvest. 1-Formylisoquinoline-TSC has recently been found to induce the synthesis of four new proteins in chick embryo cells (LEVINSON et al. 1979). The details of these studies are given in Sect. E.VIII.

III. Isatin-β-Thiosemicarbazones

As stated in Sects. E.I and II, the early work with eggs and mice was rather uninformative with regard to the specific effect of drugs on normal cells. With the first tissue culture studies on IBT (SHEFFIELD et al. 1960), toxicity was determined by following growth of HeLa cells for 7 days in the presence of drug. The maximum tolerated dose was determined as that concentration that would cause minimal morphological changes in the cells when examined under low power (54 ×) magnification in the light microscope. That concentration was established as 40 μM, eight-fold more than was necessary to decrease vaccinia virus yields by 90% at 18 h after infection. Even though 5 μM IBT had no effect on cell morphology, SHEFFIELD (1962) investigated the metabolism and growth rate of cells in the presence of the compound. The growth rate was determined by counting cells in a hemocytometer after dispersal with trypsin. Total protein content of the cells was also determined as well as their rate of utilization of glucose. At 40 μM IBT there was no detectable inhibition of cell growth, protein synthesis, or glucose utilization during the first 24-h period. By extending the duration of the experiment to 5 days, very small differences in growth rates became measurable. BACH and MAGEE (1962) noted that the incorporation of tritiated thymidine into uninfected HeLa cells over the course of 12 h was the same in the presence or absence of 10 μM IBT. MIBT has recently been found to induce the synthesis of four new proteins in chick embryo cells (LEVINSON et al. 1979). The details of these studies are given in Sect. E.VIII.

IV. Isatin-β-4′,4′-Dialkylthiosemicarbazones

Although the IBTs had no discernible inhibitory effect on HeLa cells at concentrations well above those necessary to inhibit vaccinia virus (Sect. E.III), this was not the case with the dialkylthiosemicarbazones. At 10 μM MAGEE and BACH (1965) found that N_1-methylisatin-β-4′,4′-dimethylthiosemicarbazone reduced vaccinia virus yield in HeLa cells by 90%, but also reduced tritiated thymidine incorporation into uninfected cells by about the same amount. While studying the inhibitory effect of N_1-methylisatin-β-4′,4′-dibutylthiosemicarbazone on poliovirus synthesis (which does not depend on DNA template function), PEARSON and ZIMMERMAN (1969) found that at 20 μM the compound completely suppressed DNA synthesis within 60 min in HeLa cells. At this time RNA and protein synthesis were little affected, although RNA synthesis became more impaired with time. These inhibitory effects were reversible, for up to 3 h, by washing the cells twice with fresh medium.

V. Isatin-β-Isothiosemicarbazones

TONEW and TONEW (1974) found that tritiated uridine incorporation into the RNA of normal human amnion (FL) cells was reduced by 80% within 6 h after addition of any one of three isothiosemicarbazones (Fig. 13) at concentrations that would almost completely block Mengo virus synthesis in these cells. The isothiosemicarbazones were N_1-ethyl (or methyl)isatin-S-ethylisothiosemicarbazone, and N_1-ethylisatin-S-n-butylisothiosemicarbazone. Since uridine is not a direct precursor of RNA, i.e., it has to enter the cell and then be phosphorylated to uridine-5′-triphosphate, they set out to determine if the effect was due to inhibition of transport or incorporation into RNA. They utilized the previous finding that at low temperatures uridine can be taken up by cells and phosphorylated to the mono-, di-, or triphosphate forms without significant incorporation into RNA. Prelabeling the cells at 16 °C prior to drug addition revealed no diminution, or only a small diminution, of cellular RNA synthesis. This technique was used to show that the compounds had a selective effect on Mengo virus RNA synthesis (Sect. F.V).

VI. Thiazole Thiosemicarbazones

No information is available for the effect of these compounds on normal cells.

VII. Pyrrolidine and Pyrazolone Thiosemicarbazones

No information is available for the effect of these compounds on normal cells.

VIII. Noncyclic Thiosemicarbazones

Kethoxal-bis-thiosemicarbazone (Fig. 20, KTS) has been the only compound in this category to receive attention concerning its effect on normal cells. There is a large literature on the antitumor activity of the compound and in this context its effect on normal cells can be traced through the references cited here. When studying the inhibition of vesicular stomatitis virus (VSV) polypeptides by KTS, LEVINSON et al. (1977a) noted that the drug induced the synthesis of four proteins in uninfected as well as infected chick embryo cells (Sect. F.VIII). Two of these migrated between the L and G viral peptides and two migrated close to the M viral peptide (Sect. F.VIII). Although actinomycin D inhibited their induction, implying the requirement for DNA-dependent RNA synthesis, it blocked neither the synthesis of VSV nor the antiviral effect of KTS. In further studies LEVINSON et al. (1978b) followed the kinetics of synthesis of these proteins and established their molecular weights as 100,000, 70,000, 35,000, and 25,000 daltons. Furthermore, it was clear from their gel analysis that overall protein synthesis was normal, and that under $\times 30$ or $\times 500$ phase contrast microscopy no alteration in the cells could be observed. KTS was also found to induce three or four new proteins of the expected molecular weight classes in human foreskin fibroblasts as well as in mouse and duck embryo cells. Pulse-chase experiments in chick embryo cells revealed neither precursors nor products of these proteins. Since KTS or its copper complex had previously been shown to inhibit nuclear DNA synthesis and also respiration in mitochondria, the authors unsuccessfully tried to induce these proteins, which might have been products to circumvent a blocked metabolic pathway or enzymes with a catabolic function, using cytosine arabinoside, fluorodeoxyuridine, sodium cyanide, or dinitrophenol. The authors next speculated that these four proteins might be drug-detoxifying enzymes (LEVINSON et al. 1978b). Since microsomal mixed-function oxidases are known for their detoxification functions, they tried, again unsuccessfully, to induce the four proteins with sodium phenobarbital and ethyl alcohol – known inducers of cytochrome microsomal oxidase enzymes. They also considered the possibility that these four proteins were those of endogenous RNA viruses. Although this possibility seemed unlikely since the molecular weights of the induced proteins did not correspond to those of a purified prototype endogenous virus of chicken cells (Rous associated virus) they attempted to determine whether uridine[3]H-labeled particles with a density of 1.16 were produced in drug-treated cells. No indication of this was found in treated or untreated cells. Another possibility was that the drug–copper complex became bound to DNA and these proteins were induced as a result. This hypothesis was based on their previous observations (MIKELENS et al. 1976) that drug–copper complexes, but not drug alone, were bound to DNA and RNA in vitro. Indeed, LEVINSON et al. (1979) found that a number of chelating agents including 1-formylisoquinoline-TSC (Sects. C.II, D.II), N_1-methylisatin-β-TSC (Sects. C.III, D.III), pyruvaldehyde-TSC, glyoxal-bis-thiosemicarbazone, and a number of other nonthiosemicarbazones would induce these four proteins in chick embryo cells. However, not all chelating agents tested would induce proteins. The determining factor for effectiveness was that the agent be an ionophore for ^{64}Cu. Without coming to any definite conclusions they speculated about the mechanism of induction by copper. Levinson et al. (1979) suggested that: (a) copper could interact with sulfhydryl groups in enzymes, and by inactivating them cause their induction (the interaction between copper and thiosemicarbazones, but not semicarbazones, has been described in Sects. D and F; (b) copper could interact with sulfhydryl groups in repressors that become altered sufficiently to allow mRNA transcription for the four proteins; (c) copper could be a cofactor for four metalloenzymes whose synthesis increases when copper concentration increases; and (d) copper could damage DNA sufficiently to induce repair enzymes.

IX. Miscellaneous Thiosemicarbazones

γ-Thiochromanone-1-thiosemicarbazone (Fig. 21; TCT) has been the only compound in this category to receive even superficial attention concerning its effect on normal cells. Tsunoda et al. (1971) noted that 8.4 μM TST showed definte toxicity to chick embryo cells during the first 24 h. No toxicity was observed at 4.2 μM, a concentration that inhibited vaccinia yield by 3 log units 24 h after infection.

F. Mechanism of Action

Most studies have centered on the inhibition of vaccinia virus by isatin-β-thiosemicarbazones. As the molecular strategy of poxvirus infections has been unraveled (Moss 1974; Cooper et al. 1979), many of the possible modes of action have been eliminated. At this writing we do not know the specific mode of action of any of the thiosemicarbazones. Furthermore, one must keep in mind in the forthcoming discussions that what is found in cultured cells may not reflect what is happening in vivo. This is especially true with the isatin series of compounds which have been repeatedly shown to suppress the immune response (Sect. G). The various thiosemicarbazones will be discussed in the order established in Sect. C.

I. Aryl Thiosemicarbazones

The earliest studies on the mode of antiviral action of the thiosemicarbazones were carried out over 30 years ago with the benzaldehyde series of compounds. Then, only the most basic questions were asked about virus–cell interactions in the presence of these compounds. Hamre et al. (1950) first suggested that the sparing ability of p-aminobenzaldehyde-TSC (Fig. 1) on vaccinia-infected eggs could not be due to a virucidal effect. They found that the same result was obtained when injection of the drug was delayed until 4 h after infection, compared with the usual 30-min interval. This would also indicate that the compound did not interfere with adsorption of virus to cells. They went on to show (Hamre et al. 1951) that even when the virus was mixed with 100 times the concentration of drug needed to inhibit vaccinia growth in the chorioallantoic membrane of eggs and held for 2 h at room temperature, there was still no direct inactivating effect. Using benzaldehyde-TSC

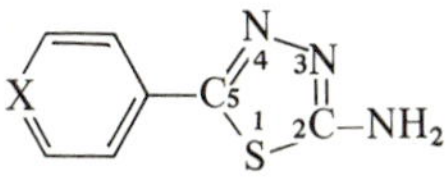

Fig. 24

(Fig. 1) to confirm the sparing ability of this series of compounds in vaccinia-infected mice, THOMPSON et al. (1951) found that there was slightly more inactivation of extracellular virus in the presence than in the absence of the compound. The same result was obtained with the p-acetamido analog, but in both cases the authors appeared to consider the differences insignificant. The same group (MINTON et al. 1953) found that the virus titers in the brains of mice spared by benzaldehyde-TSC were no different from the controls. These results may indicate that the immunopathologic disease pattern was altered (Sect. G), but they suggest strongly that direct inactivation of virus did not occur. Using cinnamaldehyde- or benzalacetone-TSC (Fig. 3), IWASAKI et al. (1955) found that either compound could be added as late as 6 h postinfection to influenza-infected chick embryo Maitland cultures with no decrease in effectiveness. If added at 24 h postinfection (the experiment being terminated after 48 h) the hemagglutination titers were one-half those of the controls. Both cinnamaldehyde- and benzalacetone-TSCs and their p-dimethylamino derivatives had a direct inactivating effect on influenza virus. The virus was suspended in allantoic fluid and the compounds were added at a concentration that would reduce by 80% the hemagglutination titer from infected Maitland cultures. After 24 h at 37 °C the unsubstituted compounds reduced titers by about 2 log units, whereas the dimethylamino derivatives caused about a 1 log unit drop in infectivity. On the other hand LUM and SMITH (1957) found that neither benzaldehyde- nor cinnamaldehyde-TSCs, at maximum nontoxic concentrations, would inactivate influenza viruses. They also observed that the compounds slightly inhibited adsorption of virus to chick chorioallantoic membrane cells, and that there was no noticeable effect on release of newly synthesized virus from cells.

BAUER (1965a) raised the question as to whether the benzaldehyde-TSCs exerted their antiviral activity in the same way as the isatin series of compounds. He focused on the structure of the two groups. The aldehyde-TSCs differ in one marked respect from the TSCs of isatin, which are diketones, in that the side chain contains an extra hydrogen atom. This atom can be cyclized by oxidation with ferric chloride to form a thiadiazole, a reaction that cannot take place with the isatin-β-TSCs. BAUER considered that the cyclization could occur in vivo and that these were the acive compounds. To test this point, benzaldehyde-TSC (Fig. 1) was cyclized to 2-amino-5-phenyl-1,3,4-thiadiazole (Fig. 24, X = C). The compound had antipox activity, but it was somewhat lower than that of benzaldehyde-TSC. The cyclized derivative of 4-formylpyridine, 2-amino-5-(4′pyridyl)-1,3,4-thiadiazole (Fig. 24, X = N), was also active, but again the results did not demonstrate a requirement for cyclization.

II. Quinoline, Pyridine, and Thiophene Thiosemicarbazones

MINTON et al. (1953) found that 5-bromothiophene-2-TSC and 4-formylquinoline-TSC spared mice from lethal infection with vaccinia virus, yet none of the compounds tested was found to reduce the viral content of the brains of these animals consistently. ROLLY and WINKELMANN (1972) confirmed these findings using cyanothiophene-TSCs. These results may indicate that the immunopathologic disease pattern was altered (Sect. G). However, KATZ et al. (1974) found that in HeLa cells there was virtually no replication of vaccinia virus in the presence of 2-formylpyridine-TSC or 1-formylisoquinoline-TSC. The inhibition occurred prior to the synthesis of virus-specific DNA since none could be found in the cells. Vaccinia virus replicates in the cytoplasm (see Sect. F.III for a detailed account of the poxvirus infectious cycle) and thus virus-specific DNA synthesis is relatively easy to follow. This was done by determining the amount of radioactively labeled DNA precursor (thymidine) that was incorporated into cells which had been lysed and centrifuged to remove nuclei. The specificity of the inhibition was shown by the fact that the RNA-containing poliovirus was able to grow normally in cells treated with concentrations of compounds inhibitory to DNA virus replication (KATZ et al. 1974). Furthermore, these findings were well correlated with previously reported observations (BROCKMAN et al. 1970) that these compounds were inhibitors of DNA synthesis.

BROCKMAN et al. (1970), using pyridine- and isoquinoline-TSCs, noted a correlation between antiherpesvirus activity and inhibition of ribonucleotide reductase in the uninfected host cells. Only those compounds examined in which the thiosemicarbazone side chain was affixed α to the heterocyclic ring nitrogen were active in inhibiting both reductase and the herpesviruses. They suggested, and to date there is no support for this, that the activity of ribonucleotide reductase may be the limiting factor in the replication of these viruses. LEVINSON et al. (1974) also studied the effect of these compounds on various herpesviruses. They found that pyridine- and isoquinoline-TSCs could inactivate extracellular herpesvirus on contact as long as the suspending medium was free of agents, such as histidine, capable of chelating divalent cations of the first transition series metals (Sect. F.III). Thus, contact inactivation is an unlikely explanation for the results of BROCKMAN et al. (1970), since these studies were carried out in tissue culture medium containing the blocking amino acids. The same group (HAASE and LEVINSON 1973; LEVINSON et al. 1971, 1973a, b) had found a striking correlation between the ability of various isatin-TSCs to inactivate the infectivity, and reduce virus-particle-associated reverse transcriptase of Rous sarcoma virus and of three slow RNA viruses of sheep. Since MIBT, as well as isoquinoline- and pyridine-TSCs, could inactivate herpesviruses (LEVINSON et al. 1974) a virion-associated RNA or DNA polymerase was sought. Because none was found the site of action was considered to be the nucleic acid template and not the enzyme function since it was shown that MIBT and cupric ions form stable complexes with which nucleic acids associate firmly (MIKELENS et al. 1976). The same binding experiments were carried out with the isoquinoline- and pyridine-TSCs, but no good correlation was found. Although 2-formylpyridine-TSC had the most antiviral activity and complexed well with DNA in the presence of $CuSO_4$, the other TSCs of 5-hydroxy-2-formylpyridine and 1-formylisoquinoline having moderate antiviral activity hardly complexed at all with DNA (LEVINSON et al. 1974; MIKELENS et al. 1976). One could speculate that other metals are involved in the action of these compounds (LEVINSON et al. 1977b). When studying various TSC–metal complexes for their ability to inibit the transforming activity of Rous sarcoma virus and its RNA-dependent DNA polymerase, LEVINSON et al. (1977b) and KASKA et al. (1978) found that 2-formylpyridine-TSC in the presence of cupric ions was as active as any of the isatin series of compounds that had previously been investigated for these properties. In further studies 2-pyridine-TSC was found to possess these antiviral properties (LEVINSON et al. 1977b), but its ability to bind to DNA with or without added copper was minimal LEVINSON et al. 1978a). However, in this regard it was more effective than any of the other thiosemicarbazones when tested in the presence of cobalt (LEVINSON et al. 1978a). In studying a wide variety of compounds (LEVINSON et al. 1978a), it became apparent that not all agents active against Rous sarcoma virus bound to nucleic acids and not all ligands that bound to nucleic acids were active against Rous sarcoma virus. Furthermore, some copper-binding ligands were neither active against Rous sarcoma virus, nor were they bound to nucleic acids. At this time there appears to be no simple relationship between the antiviral activity of copper-binding ligands and their nucleic acid-binding ability.

III. Isatin-β-Thiosemicarbazones

Because some of the IBTs spare both mice and humans against smallpox infection, a great deal of attention has been focused on the mode of action of these compounds against poxviruses. All studies have been carried out in tissue culture systems where virus–cell interactions in the presence or absence of drug can be more easily analyzed. The following represents the small amount of data that has led to the generally accepted conclusion that these compounds inhibit virus replication in vivo. MINTON et al. (1953) initially found that while IBT spared mice infected with the Williamsport strain of vaccinia virus, it failed to prevent virus replication as measured in the brain homogenates from these animals. Furthermore, the greatest concentration of virus was present in the brains of treated animals at approximately the same time as those of the untreated mice and the titers were similar. However, in later experiments the same group (THOMPSON et al. 1953a) showed that serial passage of vaccinia virus in IBT-treated mice led to a gradual decrease in the amount of virus demonstrable in their brains. Specifically, after the fourth serial transfer, virus recovered from untreated mice was comparable in titer to that found in the beginning of the experiment; whereas in treated mice there was a drop of 2.3 log units. In confirming the therapeutic antipox activity of IBT, BAUER (1955) found that under his experimental conditions the drug was much more potent than previously realized. One aspect of this was his finding that on initial exposure to IBT the titers of the IHD strain of vaccinia virus in the brains of treated mice were usually 1 log unit lower than the controls. BAUER and SADLER (1960a) found that as the chloroform solubility of simple N_1-alkyl derivatives of IBT (see Sect. C.III) increased, decreasing amounts of the compounds were needed to protect vaccinia-infected mice. They speculated that this increased activity could result entirely from their improved lipid solubility, which might enable them to more readily pass the blood–brain barrier and so reach the neurotropic strain of vaccinia (this would also account for the inactivity of compounds bearing strongly polar substituents). Using N_1-ethylisatin-β-thiosemicarbazone, POLLIKOFF et al. (1965) found that vaccinia titers in the brains of treated mice were almost 2 log units lower than in the controls. The same observation was made by Kaptsova and Maren-nikova (1967) using N_1-methylisatin-β-thiosemicarbazone and smallpox virus (variola major). Furthermore, histopathologic studies by Pollikoff et al. (1965) revealed few recognizable vaccinia virus particles or inclusion bodies (using hematoxylin–eosin or Feulgen reagent staining) in the brains of treated mice.

When the IBTs were found to prevent cytopathic effects in vaccinia-infected tissue culture, studies were begun on the mode of action of these compounds. The initial investigations were carried out by Bauer and his associates (Sheffield et al. 1960). They first established that IBT had no effect on the virus itself. The inactivation kinetics of neurovaccinia and rabbitpox over a 10-h period at 37 °C in the presence of 40 µM IBT (a ten-fold lower concentration would inhibit poxvirus growth by over 90% in cells derived from embryonic rabbit kidney; Sheffield 1962) were identical. This type of result has been repeatedly confirmed (Easterbrook 1962; Zgorniak-Nowosielska et al. 1973; Fox et al. 1977), even though contact inactivation of vaccinia and rabbitpox virus by MIBT occurs in the presence of exogenously added $CuSO_4$ (Fox et al. 1977). The latter is a provocative finding because vaccinia contains copper; at least, it has not been eliminated from virus preparations as purification techniques have improved (Hoagland et al. 1941; Joklik 1962; Zwartouw 1964). Although more will be said later in this section about the possible significance of copper in the intracellular inhibition of poxvirus replication by the IBTs, copper associated with the intact virus may be inaccessible to IBT or held in a chelate of higher stability constant.

I will discuss the remaining mode of action studies, not necessarily in the chronology of their publication, but in the chronology of the sequential stages in the poxvirus–cell interaction. These stages will be divided into five general categories essential for virus replication: (1) adsorption, penetration, and uncoating; (2) transcription of the genome into messenger RNA (mRNA); (3) translation of the messages into virus-specific proteins; (4) replication of the genome; and (5) structural proteins and viral assembly.

1. Adsorption, Penetration, and Uncoating

Sheffield et al. (1960) demonstrated that IBT did not interfere with the adsorption of rabbitpox virus to cells. Their protocol was to infect a number of rabbit kidney cell monolayers with a uniform dilution of virus that would yield a high, but countable, number of plaques after incubation for 40 h at 37 °C. In one-half of the plates the virus inoculum contained 80 µM IBT. The virus was then removed from individual monolayers (with or without drug) at 0.5, 1, 2, and 4 h after infection. The plates were exhaustively washed and incubation continued in the absence of drug. The kinetics of adsorption could be established by following the increasing number of plaques that eventually developed as the time interval was increased between inoculum addition and removal. In more extensive studies of the mode of action of IBT, Easterbrook (1962) showed that such cells were able to adsorb a second virus challenge. He found that 22 h after infection of KB (human epidermoid carcinoma) cells with vaccinia virus, initiation of the infectious cycle with rabbitpox virus proceeded equally well as in cells never exposed to the drug. Gladych et al. (1969), when investigating the inhibition of rhinoviruses by IBT and

MIBT, also concluded that these compounds did not interfere with virus adsorption to human embryonic lung cells.

Poxviruses enter cells by phagocytosis or by fusion with the cell membrane. Constitutive enzymes of these cells carry out the early stages of the uncoating process which involves release of all the phospholipids in the virion as well as one-half of the viral protein. The resulting essentially noninfectious "core" structures at this stage become a transcription factory for the mRNAs encoding the enzymes (among many others) responsible for degrading the cores and completing the uncoating process. These stages in the poxvirus–cell interaction were shown by EASTERBROOK (1962) to proceed normally in the presence of IBT. He found that the rapid decrease in KB-cell-associated virus during the first 7 h after infection (the eclipse phase) was the same with or without drug. This loss in cell-associated infectivity was also apparent even after a second challenge virus infection. Indirect confirmation of this type of result has come from experiments showing that IBT can be added as late as 3–4 h after infection of ERK (human epitheloid carcinoma) cells without any decrease in antipox activity (APPLEYARD et al. 1965). Furthermore, ZGORNIAK-NOWOSIELSKA et al. (1973), using bis-piperazine derivatives of IBT (Fig. 9), observed that these compounds were as effective in L-132 (human embryonic lung) cells whether added 1 or 4 h after the vaccinia virus adsorption period. Employing electron microscopy, LOVAS and HOLLOS (1969) found that the morphology of vaccinia virus during adsorption, penetration, and uncoating was the same in both MIBT-treated and untreated chick chorionic cells.

2. Transcription

The existence of a DNA-dependent RNA polymerase in poxviruses and the clear separation between host and viral transcriptions sites (these viruses multiply in the cytoplasm) has made the study of vaccinia virus-specific mRNAs particularly illuminating. The overall production of poxvirus mRNAs is clearly biphasic. The initial small burst of mRNA synthesis resulting from transcription of cores is followed by a second wave, representing mostly late mRNA sequences the synthesis of which is dependent on viral DNA replication. About 14% of the viral genome is transcribed from cores and extruded by a mechanism which specifically requires ATP. Early and late mRNA sequences can be distinguished by molecular hybridization competition and by differences in sedimentation rates. The early messenger RNAs appear to have a very long half-life compared with late mRNAs. WOODSON and JOKLIK (1965) established that neither the extent of synthesis of vaccinia-specific mRNA (early as well as late), nor its time course, was affected in HeLa cells exposed to IBT. Their methods depended on the fact that in uninfected HeLa cells all RNAs were synthesized in the nucleus. They found that in the cytoplasm of virus-infected cells, rapidly labeled (with uridine ^{14}C) RNAs were synthesized within 1 h having sedimentation coefficients of 10–14 S. The sedimentation coefficients of the rapidly labeled RNA formed 3 h after infection were 16–23 S. Both types of RNAs, and not 4 S transfer RNAs also found in the cytoplasm, were found to hybridize with DNA from purified vaccinia. KATZ et al. (1978 b) have confirmed that IBT did not cause a significant change in the sedimentation profile of the early (1 h) and late (5 h) viral mRNA. WOODSON and JOKLIK (1965) also determined that the mRNAs made prior to genome replication were functional in the sense that they could be incorporated into polyribosomes (packets of ribosomes simultaneously translating an mRNA molecule). Polyribosomes obtained from IBT-treated cells were analyzed by sucrose density gradient centrifugation. For the first 2 h after infection, the distribution of these polyribosomes, as determined by optical density and radioactivity of the mRNAs, was similar to that from the drug-free infected cells.

3. Translation

Primary transcription of approximately 14% of the parental DNA by the virion polymerase leads to the synthesis, not only of early enzymes that function in the biosynthesis of progeny poxvirus genomes, but also of a few of the 30 different polypeptides found in the mature virus particle. The early enzymes induced in vaccinia-infected cells include: thymidine kinase, polynucleotide ligase, DNA polymerase, polyadenylic acid-dependent polymerase, a double-stranded-specific exoDNase, and a single-stranded-specific endoDNase. By combining quantitative immunoprecipitation with autoradiography of gel diffusion plates, it has been established that at least two core polypeptides and one surface polypeptide are made prior to viral DNA synthesis. Temporal studies on viral protein synthesis have been carried out by pulse labeling infected cells with radioactive amino acids, followed by analysis using either immunodiffusion or polyacrylamide gels.

In 1965 MAGEE and BACH found that all of the early enzymatic changes that they could measure in vaccinia-infected cells (thymidine kinase and DNA polymerase) proceeded at normal, or nearly normal, rates in the presence of IBT. MAGEE and BACH (1965), and later BABLANIAN (1968), also noted that IBT had no effect on the early cytopathic effect that had been observed by various investigators in different cell lines within 1 h after infection with vaccinia. All future findings would indicate that this rounding of cells was the result of the synthesis of one or more virus-induced early proteins (BABLANIAN 1968). APPLEYARD et al. (1965) observed antigen–antibody precipitation reactions in gels by the method of Ouchterlony (double diffusion in two directions). They found that IBT had no effect on the incorporation of short pulses of ^{14}C-labeled amino acids into whole cells during the first 2.5–3 h. Using the same approach with additional analysis of solubilized radioactively labeled proteins by polyacrylamide gel electrophoresis, KATZ et al. (1973 b) established that IBT had no effect on the gradual transition from the synthesis of host proteins to early viral proteins. Polyacrylamide gel analysis of early vaccinia proteins formed in IBT-treated cells has repeatedly shown the normally expected pattern (PENNINGTON 1977; COOPER et al. 1979). As will be shown later, IBT profoundly effects viral protein synthesis that occurs after replication of the genome. COOPER et al. (1979) addressed themselves to the possibility that the inhibition of protein synthesis was obtained so late in the infection because IBT took many hours to exert its effect. To rule out this trivial explanation fluorodeoxyuridine (FUDR), an inhibitor of DNA replication, was added to infected cultures to prevent late protein synthesis. In normally infected cells, early protein synthesis is inhibited at the translational level, i.e., a product (possibly a protein) of late mRNA (synthesized from progeny DNA template) is necessary for turnoff of early protein synthesis. Even after 8 h FUDR treatment IBT did not block early protein synthesis.

4. Replication

The synthesis of viral DNA, which requires continuous protein synthesis, takes place in discrete regions of the cytoplasm not intermingled with the usual cytoplasmic organelles. The number of such foci is proportional to the multiplicity of infection (m.o.i.) and at a low m.o.i. only one focus is evident for each cell. Vaccinia DNA synthesis takes place between 1.5 and 6 h after infection, and maturation of the DNA into virions requires a further period of up to 10 h. A convenient way to determine this DNA synthesis quantitatively is to measure incorporation of thymidine ^3H with time into cytoplasmic acid-insoluble material after separating the infected cells into nuclear and cytoplasmic fractions.

In 1962 EASTERBROOK, as well as BACH and MAGEE, concluded that IBT had no effect on vaccinia DNA synthesis. Using tritiated thymidine and autoradiographic techniques, they counted the number of DNA-synthesizing "factories" in the cytoplasm of infected cells. These findings were confirmed by APPLEYARD et al. (1965) who counted cytoplasmic "factories" by using the nucleic acid-binding dye, acridine orange. BACH and MAGEE also followed the temporal uptake of tritiated thymidine into perchloric acid solubilized DNA from the cytoplasm of infected cells. Unimpeded uptake of thymidine into cytoplasmic DNA of vaccinia-infected cells in the presence of IBT has been repeatedly confirmed (WOODSON and JOKLIK 1965; KATZ et al. 1973 a, b). Several investigators considered the possibility that DNA made in the presence of IBT was defective in some way. MAGEE and BACH (1965) first considered that IBT might be bound to DNA. They observed that IBT gave a 3 °C stabilization of the melting temperature of calf thymus DNA, and a very slight shift to higher wavelengths in the DNA absorption spectrum (in the 260–300 nm range). They concluded that direct interaction between IBT and DNA was not likely to be the primary mode of action of this agent. As shown later in this section, IBT in the presence of divalent copper can change the physical configuration of DNA (MIKELENS et al. 1976). Furthermore, later work would confirm a slight change in the adsorption spectrum of DNA (PILLAI et al. 1977) but a profound change in the adsorption spectrum of MIBT (λ_{max}= 356 nm) in the presence of DNA (or bovine serum albumin) and divalent copper (ROHDE et al. 1979). MAGEE and BACH (1965) next considered if IBT effected the "reading" of DNA. They found that the turnoff of early protein synthesis (specifically thymidine kinase), which depends on translation of late mRNA, occurs normally in the presence of drug. The same investigators (BACH and MAGEE 1962; MAGEE and BACH 1965) also determined that the progeny DNA made in the presence of IBT could be packaged into mature virions. They incubated vaccinia-infected cells in the presence of IBT and tritiated thymidine for the first 4 h after infection. The cells were then washed and normal medium was replaced to allow a partial virus yield. After purification, the specific activity (radioactivity/infectious units) of the virus was determined. This, combined with the appearance of the virus in the electrom microscope, led MAGEE and BACH (1965) to conclude that DNA made in the presence of drug could be incorporated into functional particles. WOODSON and JOKLIK

(1965) also questioned if vaccinia DNA made in the presence of IBT could be coated. They defined coating by the loss of susceptibility to DNase. If IBT was allowed to remain for the entire time of the normal growth cycle no more than 15% of the DNA became insusceptible to enzymatic digestion. Katz et al. (1973 b) confirmed these findings but also noted, as did Magee and Bach (1965), that IBT withdrawal during the early part of the growth cycle allowed DNA to be converted to a DNase-resistant form.

5. Proteins and Viral Assembly

Several observations reported in 1962 indicated that IBT affected a late stage in the poxvirus–cell interaction. Bach and Magee found that IBT was effective even when added to cells after cessation of a viral DNA synthesis. Easterbrook showed that virus-specific antigens responsible for complement fixation and reaction with fluorescein-labeled antibody were produced in IBT-treated cells. He also followed the development of virus by electron microscopy. The first difference between virus-infected and normal cells as seen in the electron microscope is the appearance of "factory" areas in the cytoplasm 2–3 h after infection. They appear as areas of dense granules and randomly oriented threads devoid of mitochondria and other cytoplasmic organelles. The dense material of the "factory" then aggregates into clumps of compact filaments within and around which membranes form. These membranes appear to develop as arc-like fragments at one edge of the condensate and gradually grow to form a spherical surface which eventually completely surrounds the "immature" particle. Subsequently, small foci appear eccentrically within the "immature" particle. These foci probably contain DNA and are thought to the precursors of the prominent dumbbell-shaped core within each mature virus particle. Final maturation leads to a particle which is smaller or more condensed than the "immature" form, but much more complex structurally, with large lateral bodies and an outer double membrane on either side of the core. Easterbrook (1962) was the first to note that, in the presence of IBT, vaccinia-infected cells contained few, if any, mature particles. However, these cells contained a large number of immature forms, most of which appeared to have complete membranes. All subsequent electron microscopic studies showed that IBT or MIBT would both delay virion morphogenesis and block it at the "immature" particle stage (Harford et al. 1972; Lovas and Hollos 1969; O'Sullivan et al. 1964). It has been stated (Zgnoriak-Nowosielska et al. 1978) that a derivative of MIBT [N,N'-bis(β-thiosemicarbazone-methylisatin) -2-methylpiperazine, Sect. C.III] allows formation of mature vaccinia virus particles, not differing morphologically from virions observed in drug-free infected HeLa cells.

Katz et al. (1978 a) purified immature particles by sucrose density gradient techniques and compared these high density DNA–protein complexes arising in IBT-treated cells to those found under normal conditions. Using methionine ^{35}S labeled protein they found that both types of immature particles sedimented at approximately the same rate. However, tritiated thymidine labeling (Katz et al. 1978 a) revealed that the immature particles made in the presence of IBT contained very little DNA. Furthermore, using polyacrylamide gel electrophoresis techniques, these investigators also established that there were profound differences in the polypeptide composition of both types of immature particles. Up to 30 polypeptides can be resolved from detergent-dissociated mature virus by polyacrylamide gel electrophoresis. The sum of the molecular weights of these peptides (ranging from 10,000 to 200,000 daltons) is 2×10^6 daltons or about 20% of the coding capacity of the genome. Three polypeptides account for 35% of the total protein, 8 peptides for an additional 50%, and 19 for the remaining 15%. At least three major late proteins (4a, 4b, and 10) comprising more than one-third of the protein mass of vaccinia virions are formed by cleavage of higher molecular weight precursors.

KATZ et al. (1978a) found that the immature particles formed in the presence of IBT lacked two of the main core polypeptides: 4a and 4b. The KATZ group had previously established by pulse-chase experiments that, while precursors P4a and P4b were cleaved in the presence of IBT to produce the structural polypeptides 4a and 4b (KATZ et al. 1973b), the amounts made were only about 50% of those found in the total cytoplasmic fraction (obtained after boiling with detergent and mercaptoethanol) of cells in the absence of drug (KATZ and FELIX 1977). Furthermore, using quantitative immunoprecipitation and polyacrylamide gel electrophoresis techniques, they found an overall quantitative slowdown in late viral protein synthesis (KATZ and FELIX 1977); a conclusion also reached by PENNINGTON in 1977 (the failure of APPLEYARD et al. 1962, 1965 to observe many late antigens in rabbitpox-infected cells may have been due to the low sensitivity of the immunoprecipitation in agar technique that was used or the inability to detect "insoluble" antigens such as P4a and 4a). Thus, IBT appeared to block the integration of 4a and 4b into the immature particles. This block in core polypeptide integration must be a reflection of the inhibition of either messenger RNA synthesis, the translation process, or interference with processing of precursor. Synthesis of late virus-specific proteins with either enzymatic or structural functions is paralleled by an increase in RNA synthesis and the appearance of mRNA that was not present in the early phase of virus growth. The late mRNA appears to have a very short half-life compared with the early mRNAs. WOODSON and JOKLIK (1965) were the first to examine late mRNAs in vaccinia-infected cells treated with IBT. Under these conditions they found that mRNAs of normal size (16 S) and quantity were synthesized and that these mRNAs could be incorporated into polyribosomes. However, these 16 S RNAs could only be demonstrated after short labeling periods (3.5 min) with tritiated uridine. Longer labeling periods of 8–13 min produced RNAs with median sedimentation coefficients considerably smaller than 16 S, in the neighborhood of 8 S. These results fit in with their observations that few polyribosomes were present in cells 4 h after infection in the presence of IBT. WOODSON and JOKLIK questioned whether this was due to lack of formation, or rapid breakdown, of polyribosomes. To explore the latter possibility, cells infected 4 h previsously with vaccinia were exposed to varying concentrations of IBT for 30 and 60 min. Indeed, it was found that polyribosomes were unstable in the presence of the compound (as measured by an increase with time in the number of single ribosomes) in a dose-dependent fashion. KATZ et al. (1978b) confirmed that in the presence of IBT there was a significant decrease of heavy polyribosomes late in infection. Furthermore, using 12-min labeling periods with tritiated uridine they found that late mRNAs synthesized in the presence of IBT appeared smaller or degraded (COOPER et al. 1979).

Utilizing the then recent understanding that eukaryotic mRNAs contain 3′ terminal polyadenylic acid, poly (A), sequences, Cooper et al. (1979) passed the cytoplasmic RNAs through a polyuridylic acid–sepharose column which would retain the mRNAs with poly (A) sequences. In this way it was found that although the total uridine incorporation into the cytoplasmic RNA was unchanged in the presence of IBT (as originally reported by Woodson and Joklik), incorporation into the poly (A) messenger RNA was reduced by about 50%. This mRNA hybridized with vaccinia DNA but some of it appeared smaller or more degraded than that of the control. This group then determined if virus-specific mRNA made in the presence of IBT was methylated. Eukaryotic mRNAs contain 5′ terminal methylated caps and the cap in vaccinia mRNA appears to be required for ribosome binding and efficient translation. Cells 6–8 h after infection were doubly labeled, in the presence or absence of IBT, with uridine ^{14}C and methyl ^{3}H methionine. The RNA was purified by cesium chloride centrifugation and poly (U)–sepharose chromatography, and hybridized to vaccinia DNA. Virus-specific RNA was indeed found to be methylated in the presence of IBT. Since the cells contained considerable amounts of apparently intact virus-specific mRNA, yet late protein synthesis was inhibited by 95% (under their experimental conditions), the authors (Cooper et al. 1979) considered that the mRNA was not translated for some unknown reason. To test this hypothesis a message-dependent, cell-free, protein-synthesizing system was prepared using rabbit reticulocytes. They had previously shown that this system could accurately translate early and late vaccinia virus mRNAs. Using total cytoplasmic RNA obtained from cells at various times late in the infection cycle, they found as much as a 50% reduction in the amount of methionine ^{35}S incorporated into newly synthesized peptides; a figure consistent with the relative amount of intact virus-specific mRNA obtained from the IBT-treated cells. They then determined if the mRNAs isolated from the IBT-treated cells coded for the full spectrum of late virus-specific peptides. Even though total incorporation was reduced by 50%, all polypeptides which could be resolved by the separation methods used were synthesized. However, the synthesis of large polypeptides was reduced more than that of the small polypeptides. They also added IBT directly to the reticulocyte cell-free system containing normal virus-specific mRNA. Even adjusting for the intracellular five-fold increase in concentration of IBT over the extracellular concentration, as found by Woodson and Joklik (1965), translation was not inhibited. As suggested later in this section, copper may possible play a key role in the ability of IBT to inhibit poxvirus synthesis. Thus it would be of interest if these cell-free protein-synthesizing systems could function in the absence of chelating agents so that copper could be deliberately added to the system. Cooper et al. (1979) concluded that further work was necessary to define the mechanism of inhibition of protein synthesis since, in the presence of IBT, approximately one-half of the expected amount of mRNA was capped, properly methylated, polyadenylated, and translatable in a cell-free protein-synthesizing system, yet polypeptide synthesis was inhibited by 95%.

The realization that IBTs could complex with virtually any nucleic acid (Mikelens et al. 1976) evolved from observations initially made by Levinson et al. (1971). While determining if IBTs had any effect on oncogenic viruses they observed that EIBT (the N_1-ethyl derivative) apparently inhibited synthesis of Rous sarcoma virus in virus-transformed cells. However, sucrose density gradient analysis revealed that particles of Rous sarcoma virus labeled with tritiated uridine were being produced. This paradox was resolved by subsequent experiments in which Rous sarcoma virus was exposed to EIBT prior to infection of cells. These experiments demonstrated that EIBT inactivated the virus on contact. Furthermore, LEVINSON et al. (1973 b) established that either MIBT or $CuSO_4$ could inactivate the virus, and when combined they could inactivate at concentrations where either alone had no activity. In fact, with no deliberate addition of $CuSO_4$ the action of MIBT could be blocked by ethylenediaminetetracetic acid (EDTA), as well as other chelating agents. Thus, LEVINSON et al. (1973 b) considered that MIBT acted as a scavenger (for trace contamination from glassware or media) and vehicle to transport copper to an appropriate site. Parenthetically, $CuSO_4$ alone (or elemental copper in the case of influenza virus) has been found to inactivate on contact herpesvirus (LEVINSON et al. 1974), rabies virus (Fox et al. 1977), Sindbis virus (Fox et al. 1977), and influenza virus (ONG 1958). After inactivation, Rous sarcoma virus was shown still to retain its ability to adsorb to cells (LEVINSON et al. 1973 a).

A striking correlation was found between the ability of various thiosemicarbazones to inactivate the infectivity as well as the virus-particle-associated reverse transcriptase of Rous sarcoma (LEVINSON et al. 1973 b) and visna viruses (HAASE and LEVINSON 1973). For a while it was considered that the contact inactivation of these viruses was a reflection of the thiosemicarbazones and copper to inactivate these enzymes, yet herpesviruses which were lacking this enzyme were still susceptible to the complex (LEVINSON et al. 1974). Further work showed that the Rous sarcoma virus-particle-associated enzymes, lactic dehydrogenase and tRNA nucleotidyl transferase, which do not require template, as well as ribonuclease H which is located on the RNA-dependent DNA polymerase itself, were not sensitive to MIBT (LEVINSON et al. 1973 a; WANG and LEVINSON 1978). This group (MIKELENS et al. 1976; LEVINSON et al. 1977 b) has hypothesized that the mode of inhibition of MIBT on the enzyme activity of the leukoviruses was due to binding of a ligand–metal complex to nucleic acid rather than to enzyme. This was based on their finding that MIBT and $CuSO_4$ formed stable complexes with which any type of nucleic acid of at least 25,000 daltons would firmly associate. This could be quantitatively measured by retention of radioactively labeled nucleic acid on 0.45 µm nitrocellulose filters. Either histidine (at a concentration similar to that in tisue culture medium, see Sect. D.III, or EDTA in a mixture containing MIBT, $CuSO_4$, and nucleic acid would prevent the latter from being retained on these filters. Furthermore, $CuSO_4$ alone (even 1,000 times its effective concentration when combined with MIBT) had no ability to cause trapping of nucleic acid. Other results (Fox et al. 1977) with Sindbis virus and poliovirus also indicated that the possession of virion-associated enzymes was not a prerequisite for contact inactivation and would lend support to the Levinson hypothesis.

When LEVINSON et al. found that nucleic acids bound to MIBT–copper complexes in vitro it was of obvious interest to determine whether the interaction in the test-tube with purified nucleic acids was biologically pertitent. It seemed to be in this sense that MIBT–copper complexes inhibited the transfection of λ phage DNA in *Escherichia coli* (LEVINSON and HELLING 1976). Furthermore, they (LEVINson et al. 1978a) also attempted to determine whether a nucleic acid–MIBT–copper complex was formed within Rous sarcoma virions when they were exposed under conditions similar to those used to inactivate the biologic activities of the virus. Purified tritiated uridine-labeled Rous sarcoma virus was exposed to $CuSO_4$, MIBT, or a combination of the two. After incubation, the virus was disrupted and excess calf thymus DNA was added to react with any originally unbound MIBT–copper complexes. The samples were then centrifuged in a sucrose density gradient. As in the nitrocellulose filter technique, these experiments demonstrated that MIBT–copper complexes changed the configuration of virus nucleic acid. While $CuSO_4$ had little effect on the sedimentation of Rous sarcoma virus RNA, MIBT treatment resulted in the loss of approximately 50% of the RNA in the normally expected profile. Treatment with both compounds resulted in the complete loss of the RNA. Presumably the RNA was pelleted, rather than degraded, since none of the radioactivity was at the top of the gradient. Furthermore, EDTA added directly to the virus after exposure to MIBT and $CuSO_4$ completely prevented the loss of RNA in the gradient.

Since IBT and its N_1-alkyl derivatives in the presence of divalent copper directly interact with virtually all viruses and nucleic acids, it appears that a good deal of significance should be attached to the ability of the IBTs to be effective in vertebrates against only one family of viruses, the poxviruses. No other viruses but the poxviruses have been reported to contain copper (Hoagland et al. 1941; Joklik 1962; Zwartouw 1964) and this may be what sets them apart in their in vivo sensitivity to the IBTs. Thompson et al. (1953a) were aware that thiosemicarbazones were chelating agents and they attempted to determine, not if metals would enhance the antipox activity of these compounds, but rather if they would inhibit their activity in mice. A number of substances, including monovalent cuprous chloride, were found to have no influence on the activity of various thiosemicarbazones. When Bauer (1955) first confirmed the antipox activity of IBT in mice he noted that the maximum degree of protection was obtainable with a quite small dose, and that the effect could not be substantially increased by greatly increasing the dose (or by daily dosage; Pollikoff et al. 1965). He felt that the possible limitation of the therapeutic effet was brought about by the presence in the brain (where virus was injected) of a fixed concentration of some substance essential for the activity of IBT. He speculated that a *host* factor, possibly copper or some other metal, might form chelate complexes with IBT and this might be the active compound.

Recognizing that a single report existed (Hoagland et al. 1941) concerning the copper content of vaccinia, Bauer (1958) proposed that copper from the virus might somehow play a role in the inhibition of cellular function. He felt that copper salts or compounds, deliberately added to the diet of vaccinia-infected mice might have antiviral activity by competing with the copper from the virus. Indeed he found that copper in the divalent, but not the monovalent, state would prolong the survival time of vaccinia-infected mice by 20%–50%. Divalent copper had no effect on 23 other murine viruses. When Bauer and Sadler (1960a) established that sulfur in the side chain of IBT was necessary for antipox activity, they felt that its ability to chelate metals was a key factor. They suggested that since vaccinia was thought to contain copper it was this circumstance that brought about the selective therapeutic effect of IBT on neurovaccinia. The present author's hypothesis is that IBTs interfere with late mRNA stability or function because it is only late in the infection when copper is brought into the "factory" or "virosome" areas of the cytoplasm to be incorporated into maturing virions. To support or refute this hypothesis the copper content of mature vaccinia virions could be reestablished using better virus purification and analytical chemistry techniques than were available 15 years ago. The copper content of virus at various stages in the maturation process could also be determined. One wonders whether IBT-resistant mutants of poxviruses (see Sect. H) contain copper. In this regard it is of interst to note that IBT-resistant mutants of both vaccinia and rabbitpox virus lose their resistance to the drug when grown in the presence of the wild-type virus (APPLEYARD and WAY 1966; KATZ et al. 1973c).

IV. Isatin-β-4′,4′-Dialkylthiosemicarbazones

Unlike the monoalkyl or unsubstituted thiosemicarbazones, these compounds are able to protect mice against lethal infection with ectromelia viruses. Isatin-β-4′,4′-dimethylthiosemicarbazone has been clearly shown to block virus replication as measured in the brains of treated mice (O'SULLIVAN et al. 1963). Under the same conditions isatin-β-4′,4′-tetra- or pentamethylenethiosemicarbazone has been found to arrest virus synthesis (BAUER 1963). Although only one published report deals with the mode of action of these dialkylthiosemicarbazones, all interpretations would be clouded because the exquisite poxvirus specificities of the IBTs and dialkylthiosemicarbazones demonstrable in mice (Sect. C.IV) break down in tissue culture (Sect. D.III). MAGEE and BACH (1965) found that, unlike the IBTs, N-methylisatin-β-4′,4′-dimethylthiosemicarbazone inhibited both vaccinia and cellular DNA synthesis, the former being more sensitive than the latter.

In tissue culture studies, N-methylisatin-β-4′,4′-dibutylthiosemicarbazone was shown by PEARSON and ZIMMERMAN (1969) to be equally effective in inhibiting the replication of poliovirus types 1, 2, and 3. It did not appear to block virus adsorption or penetration, because it could be added to cells 30 min after infection. In fact, the compound could be added at any time during the growth cycle of the virus and would rapidly prevent further virus replication without inactivating previously synthesized virus. Using actinomycin D to unmask virus specific RNA synthesis in HeLa cells, PEARSON and ZIMMERMAN (1969) found viral RNA to be completely blocked within 1 h after addition of the compound, even when viral RNA was being synthesized at a maximal rate. This inhibition occurred before viral polyribosomes were degraded and protein synthesis slowed. Using an in vitro cell-free poliovirus polymerase reaction, they showed that the compund could inhibit the incorporation of uridine ^{3}H 5′triphosphate into acid-precipitable material.

N-methylisatin-β-4′-4′-dibutylthiosemicarbazone has been found to inactivate on contact influenza A (strains WSN and PR8) and B (strain Lee) viruses (BOPP 1976; M.P.FOX and C.J.PFAU, unpublished work 1976). These viruses fully retained their hemagglutination activity. Neuraminidase activity, tested only for the A viruses, was also found to be unchanged (PFAU 1977). In view of the data presented in Sect. F.III (and the poliovirus results) this may indicate that these dialkylthiosemicarbazones also effect nucleic acid function.

V. Isatin-β-Isothiosemicarbazones

A series of studies by E. and M. TONEW and co-workers centered around the mode of action of these compounds against Mengo virus replication in human amnion (FL) cells. The initial studies (TONEW et al. 1974b) using N_1-ethylisatin-S-ethyliso-thiosemicarbazone (Fig. 13) showed that the compound had no virucidal effect on this RNA-containing virus. Furthermore, it did not intefere with the adsorption or penetration of the virus. The former was measured by the amount of virus that could be washed from the cells after the virus adsorption period. The latter was measured by the loss of ability of virus-specific antibody to neutralize cell-adsorbed virus. Extending these studies to include N_1-methyl-isatin-S-ethylisothiosemicarbazone and N_1-ethylisatin-S-n-butylisothiosemicarbazone TONEW and TONEW (1974) found that these compounds inhibited uridine transport in uninfected FL cells (Sect. E.V). If a nucleotide pool was established in FL cells by allowing uptake of tritiated uridine to occur at 16 °C for 1 h prior to drug addition, incorporation of radioactivity into RNA proceeded normally for a period long enough to follow viral synthesis. Using this technique with Mengo virus-infected cells, along with actinomycin D treatment to unmask virus-specific RNA, they found that the isothiosemicarbazones prevented viral RNA synthesis. These investigators then examined Mengo virus-specific RNA-dependent RNA polymerase activity in FL cells as well as in a cell-free system. No polymerase activity was detected in infected cells treated with these compounds. In the in vitro cell-free polymerase assay (TONEW et al. 1974a), working concentrations of the drugs inhibited uridine ^{14}C triphosphate incorporation into acid-precipitable material by 50%. Furthermore, UV absorption maxima of these compounds at 360 nm were unaffected by addition of nucleic acids, but showed enhanced optical densities and slight shifts toward red in the presence of protein. TONEW et al. (1974a) felt that these results excluded the possibility that the compounds were inhibitory because they bound to nucleic acids, but rather that complexes of enzyme components and isothiosemicarbazones were involved in the inhibition of RNA polymerase.

VI. Thiazole Thiosemicarbazones

All mode of action studies have been carried out with 3-methyl-4-bromo-5-formy-lisothiazole-TSC, one of two thiosemicarbazones to reach clinical trials (Sect. H). Like IBT (Sect. F.III), it protected mice against lethal infection with vaccinia virus, even though fully infectious virus could be recovered from the brains of treated mice – the difference in titers between control and treated mice being over 2 log units (RAO et al. 1965). SQUIRES and McFADZEAN (1966) summarized evidence (without presenting experimental data) that led them to suggest the possible involvement of an interfering substance induced by the drug–virus combination. This hypothesis was based on four observations. (1) Mouse brain suspensions were prepared from three groups: one treated with drug alone, one infected with vaccinia alone, and one receiving both virus and drug. The suspensions were clarified by centrifugation sufficient to pellet virus, and the supernatants were injected intradermally into mice. Dermal vaccinia was then scarified over the injection site. The virus "took" over the sites injected with material from the first two preparations, but not over the site from the third (combination) preparation. (2, 3) SQUIRES and McFADZEAN (1966) assumed that the interfering substance in their brain homogenates might be interferon. Since it had been reported that either steroids or high oxygen tension were generally considered to reduce interferon synthesis SQUIRES and McFADZEAN determined what effect they would have on the efficacy of isothiazole-TSC. Both cortisone treatment and increased partial pressure of oxygen virtually eliminated the protective activity of the drug. Concurrent research by LIEBERMAN et al. (1966) showed that cortisone had no effect on the antipox activity of EIBT. (4) They had shown previously that the isothiazole-TSC was completely inactive in mice infected with the RNA-containing encephalomyocarditis (EMC) virus. Yet isothiazole-TSC-treated mice which survived an otherwise lethal vaccinia virus infection were more resistant to challenge with EMC virus than the controls. Critical experiments to prove or disprove the interferon hypothesis were not performed. Since the hallmark of interferon production in virus-infected animals is a marked reduction or elimination of virus, a 1 log unit reduction in brain virus (if the isothiazoles act like the IBTs, see Sect. H.II) does not support the hypothesis. Parenthetically, interferon could not be detected in the brains of vaccinia-infected mice treated with the N_1-ethyl derivative of IBT, but was present in the absence of drug (POLLIKOFF et al. 1965).

Using tissue culture APPLEYARD et al. (1965) investigated the mode of action of 3-methyl-4-bromo-5-formylisothiazole-TSC at the same time they investigated IBT. Using techniques described in detail in Sect. F.III, they showed its action to be similar to that of IBT in all respects that were tested. The compound prevented formation of the same viral antigens as did IBT; it did not interfere with viral DNA synthesis; and it inhibited virus growth to the same extent as IBT in several cell lines. Another indication that the mode of action of both types of compounds might be similar was the finding that IBT-resistant mutants of vaccinia virus were almost as refractory to the isothiazole-TSC (APPLEYARD and WAY 1966).

VII. Pyrrolidine and Pyrazolone Thiosemicarbazones

No mode of action studies have been reported for these compounds.

VIII. Noncyclic Thiosemicarbazones

LEVINSON et al. (1977a) found that kethoxal-bis-thiosemicarbazone (KTS, Fig. 20) inhibited the replication of vesicular stomatitis virus (VSV). VSV is a negative-stranded RNA virus, that is its genome has none of the hallmarks of an mRNA [3'-poly (A) sequences and a capped 5' end, see Sect. F.III]. Five capped, poly (A)-containing RNA species which anneal to virion RNA can be resolved in infected cells. In a cell-free system, these mRNAs can direct the synthesis of each of the five proteins (L, G, N, NS, and M) which make up the intact virus particle. The enzyme responsible for transcribing the mRNAs is contained within the virion. This transcriptase is easily demonstrated in vitro. Unlike the results with IBTs and Rous sarcoma virus (Sect. F.III), KTS had no effect on the VSV polymerase. However, using labeling and polyacrylamide gel electrophoretic conditions that would differentiate three of the VSV mRNAs, LEVINSON et al. (1977a) found that KTS would completely inhibit their synthesis. The synthesis of all classes of protein was also inhibited. Pretreatment with the drug had no inactivating effect on the virus itself but rather enhanced subsequent virus replication. Since the chelating agent EDTA would produce the same effect it was felt that KTS was removing a toxic heavy metal cation. KTS has also been shown to inhibit the transforming activity and reverse transcriptase activity of Rous sarcoma virus (Kaska et al. 1978). On the basis of studies with Rous sarcoma virus and other thiosemicarbazones (Sect. F.III), it may be that KTS inhibits template rather than enzyme function.

IX. Miscellaneous Thiosemicarbazones

γ-Thiochromanone-1-thiosemicarbazone (TCT, Fig. 21) was shown to inhibit vaccinia virus replication beyond the adsorption–penetration–uncoating stage because it could be effectively added to chick embryo cell cultures up to 8 h after infection (Tsunoda et al. 1971). Katz et al. (1975) using techniques developed in studies on the mode of action of IBT against vaccinia virus in HeLa cells (Sect. F.III) found that TCT did not inhibit the replication of vaccinia DNA. However, as shown by prolonged sensitivity to deoxyribonuclease, it was not incorporated into maturing virions. Although both early and late viral proteins were produced in cells treated with TCT, the cleavage of a later precursor peptide (P4a) into the structural peptide 4a (Sect. F.III) was largely inhibited. In biochemical terms, not only were the modes of action of TCT and IBT similar, but there was also good cross-resistance between mutants that had been isolated which were capable of growing in the presence of one drug or the other.

G. Animal Studies

The distribution and metabolism of thiosemicarbazones with antitumor activity have been extensively investigated (Agrawal and Sartorelli 1978). However, as they relate to antiviral studies, the thiosemicarbazones have received little or no attention with regard to metabolic transformations of the compounds, adsorption from various sites of administration, pharmokinetics, or pharmodynamics. The main emphasis here will be to review the evidence that indicates the potent immunosuppressive nature of thiosemicarbazones. This is stressed since it is now known that the intensive meningitis produced in mice after intracerebral inoculation of vaccinia or ectromelia virus is mediated by T-cells. Thus, the thiosemicarbazones may act (at least in mice) as a two-edged sword, inhibiting both target cells by suppressing virus synthesis and effector cells by blocking lymphocyte proliferation.

I. Aryl Thiosemicarbazones

In the early work on benzaldehyde thiosemicarbazones (Fig. 1), it was noted that the concentrations of this compound in the diet, necessary to spare mice from otherwise lethal intracerebral injection with vaccinia virus, would prevent their normal increase in weight (Thompson et al. 1953b). If we assume that toxic substances are especially effective against rapidly dividing cells (as is the case in cancer chemotherapy), then the thiosemicarbazone could have altered lymphocytes that were proliferating in response to stimulation by the virus. Since the virus titers in the brains of these spared mice were not consistently lower than those in untreated mice (MINTON et al. 1953), and since the inflammatory response in the meninges is T-cell-mediated (see Sect. G.III), it is conceivable that sparing was due to immunosuppressive and not antiviral activity of the compound.

II. Quinoline, Pyridine, and Thiophene Thiosemicarbazones

MINTON et al. (1953) found that, when 5-bromothiophene-2-formylthiosemicarbazone was introduced into their diet, mice could be spared from otherwise lethal intracerebral injection with vaccinia virus. Yet the virus titers in the brains of these mice were not consistently lower than in those of the untreated group. The same observations were also noted with 4-formylquinoline-TSC (Fig. 5). These workers (THOMPSON et al. 1953b) also noted that each compound in a series of 5- or 3-substituted thiophene-2-formylthiosemicarbazones was quite toxic when given parenterally. As discussed in Sect. G.I and in the next paragraph, these mice may have survived the virus infection, not so much by the antiviral properties of the compounds, but by their ability to compromise the immunologic reaction to the infection.

Using 5-cyanothiophene-2-formylthiosemicarbazone (Fig. 7) at twice the dose (76 mg/kg) necessary to protect 100% of mice receiving 10^3 LD_{50} vaccinia virus (BORYSIEWICZ and TADEUSIEWICZ 1976), ZGORNIAK-NOWOSIELSKA et al. (1978) investigated the compound's ability to suppress both humoral and cell-mediated responses. The humoral response was measured by injecting compound subcutaneously into three inbred strains of mice in a schedule identical to that used in antiviral studies: twice a day for 4 days beginning immediately after antigen injection – in this case sheep red blood cells (SRBC). On day 5, lymphoid cells were removed and the number producing IgM immunoglobulins against SRBCs was determined by the in vitro "direct" Jerne hemolytic plaque assay. Although minor differences were found, there was about a 50% reduction in plaque numbers in relation to the control groups in all three strains of mice receiving the compound. This decreased primary immune response was also reflected by the numbers of IgG-producing cells (most immunogens elicit detectable antibodies of the IgM class before those of the IgG class) as measured by the "indirect" Jerne SRBC–hemolytic plaque assay. The effect of the compound on the secondary immune response was determined by reinjecting SRBCs into previously drug-treated mice on day 9 and removing lymphocytes on day 13. Again the number of IgM-producing cells detected by the Jerne assay was about 55% below that of the control group. The cell-mediated immune response in mice was assessed by allergic contact dermatitis to 2-phenyl-4-ethoxymethyleneoxazolone (oxazolone). The schedule of administration of the thiosemicarbazone to mice was the same as that used in the humoral response studies. The thickness of the ear was measured before and 24 h after painting with oxazolone (on day 7). Up to a 70% decrease in swelling was noted in mice treated with the thiosemicarbazone. In earlier studies BORYSIEWICZ and TADEUSIEWICZ (1976) noted that the relative activity of 5-cyanothiophene-2-thiosemicarbazone, as measured by survival time of infected mice, decreased above 20 mg/kg body weight.

III. Isatin-β-Thiosemicarbazones

The initial quantitative studies on the ability of thiosemicarbazones to inhibit the immune response in mice were carried out by McNeill (1972, 1973) and McNeill et al. (1972). The humoral response to sheep red blood cells (see Sect. G.II for details of the assay procedure) was measured 5–7 days after a single injection of cells and daily injection of 1 mg/kg body weight of MIBT (Fig. 8). McNeill et al. (1972) found that the number of IgM-producing lymphocytes was reduced almost 5-fold compared with the number found in drug-free mice. There was almost a 20-fold difference when the number of IgG-producing cells was determined. In line with these observations, the amount of circulating antibody against SRBCs 5 days after beginning the drug treatment was 15-fold lower than in the control group of mice. Since antibody-secreting cells are derived from the bone marrow, McNeill et al. (1972) next determined that the total number of cells which could be flushed from femurs was the same whether or not mice had received six daily injections of MIBT. They also established the number of cells in these preparations capable of forming colonies in a semisolid suspension cell assay. Again, very little numerical difference was seen in these cells which are generally regarded as specific progenitors of granulocytes and macrophages. However, using colony forming cells from the spleen, a marked decrease was noted in the drug-treated group. NcNeill (1972) went on to show that MIBT added directly to the semisolid suspension cell assay would inhibit development of colony formation. Although MIBT reduced the number of colonies, it did not affect the size of the colonies that did develop. He felt that this indicated a selective mode of action of the drug, although there was no change in the relative frequency of granulocyte and macrophage colonies. McNeill (1973) extended these studies on colony inhibition, using 25 derivatives of IBT (see Sect. G.IV). He found that EIBT was as effective as MIBT but that azo and iodo substituents on the aromatic ring substantially reduced activity (a finding parallel to the compounds ability to spare mice after vaccinia infection, Sect. C.III).

NcNeill et al. (1972) questioned if the ability of MIBT to compromise the immune system might play a role in its antipoxvirus activity. The poxvirus chosen for study was ectromelia because the bone marrow (and later the spleen) can become heavily infected with virus; and MIBT does not spare mice from the infection (Bauer and Sadler 1961). They assumed that the latter result meant that the drug had no effect on virus replication and would make explanation of the results less complicated. However, interpretation of the experiment was not clear since low concentrations of drug (0.5 mg/kg) had no effect on the death rate in ectromelia-infected mice (33%) while a higher dose (2 mg/kg) increased mortality somewhat (50%). Using experimental protocols and obtaining results almost identical to those found when studying 5-cyanothiophene-2-formylthiosemicarbazone (Sect. G.II), it was established that MIBT inhibited both the B-cell and T-cell response (Borysiewicz et al. 1977; Zgorniak-Nowosielska et al. 1978). The B-cell, or humoral response, was measured in the same way as reported by McNeill et al. (1972) except that mice received 20 mg kg^{-1} day^{-1} MIBT after a single injection of SRBCs. The T-cell, or cell-mediated response was measured by the degree of allergic contact dermatitis provoked by oxazolone, using the same regimen of drug administration as previously described. Both ectromelia and vaccinia virus multiply in the meninges and ependyma of mice after intracerebral inoculation. Meningitis is characterized by perivascular cuffing and marked infiltration of mononuclear cells (the category of cells including the B- and T-lymphocytes, monocytes, and macrophages). HAPEL and GARDNER (1974) demonstrated that the severity of meningitis in mice infected with ectromelia coincided with the number of cells in the cerebrospinal fluid (CSF) capable of destroying ectromelia-infected tissue culture cells labeled with ^{51}Cr. These CSF cells with cytolytic activity were shown to be T-lymphocytes because they possessed a surface antigen (θ) not found on B-cells or macrophages. The critical role of these T-cells in disease was further substantiated by treatment of ectromelia-infected mice with antithymocyte serum (the thymus being the site of T-cell differentiation). There was a marked reduction of T-cells in the CSF after treatment, and the normal 35% mortality was reduced to zero. Essentially the same conclusions were reached by MORISHIMA and HAYASHI (1978) while studying vaccinia meningitis. Their study was even more persuasive than HAPEL and GARDNER'S since cytotoxic T-cells (measured in a ^{51}Cr release assay using vaccinia-infected tissue culture cells as targets) were obtained directly from the meninges.

HERRLICH et al. (1965) noted that, like benzaldehyde-TSC and 4-formylquinoline-TSC (THOMPSON et al. 1953 b), MIBT did not prevent lesion formation in rabbits after intradermal inoculation of vaccinia virus. Drug was given twice a day, by intubation, for 10 days at concentrations up to 300 mg kg^{-1} day^{-1} (the acute oral LD$_{50}$ of MIBT in rabbits is in excess of 2,000 mg/kg; BAUER 1977). They noted that above 100 mg/kg the weight of the rabbits after 10 days was 20%–30% lower than the control animals. Also, above 100 mg/kg the hemagglutination antibody titer against the virus was as much as 15-fold lower than in drug-free animals. KACKELL et al. (1966) confirmed the lack of activity of MIBT against intradermal vaccinia virus except if the drug was injected at the site of vaccination. Giving MIBT by intubation for 6 days at 100 mg kg^{-1} day^{-1}, they measured the antibody response to the virus at the end of the second week of infection (during an initial 5-day observation period the rabbits were viremic). They found that the vaccinia hemagglutination antibody titer was reduced 20-fold while the neutralizing antibody titer was lowered 8-fold.

There are other examples, beside the response to poxviruses, where MIBT may influence the disease process by altering the immune response to the infection. The natural history of the F1 hybrid of New Zealand Black and New Zealand White mice is characterized by the appearance of serum antinuclear antibodies, and the development of proteinurea and fatal glomerulonephritis. This renal disease is believed to be caused by the deposition of antibody–antigen–complement complexes in the glomeruli. GABRIEL (1971) found that such mice, if given MIBT (100 mg/kg by weekly injections, starting within 24 h after birth and continuing for the rest of their lives), would develop this autoimmune disease much more slowly than the control group. For example, at 10 months 75% of the control group had died while only 25% of the drug-treated mice had expired. While studying the ability of MIBT to inactivate on contact both the transforming ability and RNA-dependent DNA polymerase of murine leukemia virus (Sects. D.III, F.III), LEVY et al. (1976) found that MIBT enhanced rather than inhibited development of leukemia in the mouse.

They found that, 17 days after injection with Friend (leukemia) virus, the spleens of MIBT-treated mice weighed almost twice as much as those from mice receiving virus alone. Since the Friend virus preferentially replicates in B-cells, one wonders if the increased weight of the spleen was due to an increasing number of B-cells which might occur if the drug selectively destroyed T-cells (an overabundance of B-cells is seen in some children with thymic hypoplasia); or an increased susceptibility of B-cells to the infection.

Since Levinson and his collaegues had shown that MIBT (in the presence of diavalent copper) was able to change the physical configuration of nucleic acids (Sect. F.III), possibly accounting for the biologic activity of the drug, they decided to determine if adenyl cyclase which utilizes adenosine triphosphate to form cyclic adenosine monophosphate (cAMP) was also inhibited. Their initial approach was to establish the amount of cAMP in human peripheral blood lymphocytes after incubation in the presence of drug (Webb et al. 1974). Since the level of cAMP increased significantly after exposure to MIBT, they questioned if this was due to increased adenyl cyclase or a decrease in the specific phosphodiesterase which hydrolyzes cAMP to AMP. They found that MIBT blocked phosphodiesterase activity. Since changes in cAMP levels in lymphocytes had previously been shown to influence the immune response, Webb et al. (1974) felt that the possibility existed that MIBT might suppress the host's natural defenses.

Little has been published on the pharmacology and toxicology of MIBT. The acute oral LD_{50} of MIBT in mice and rats is in excess of 2,000 mg/kg (Bauer 1977). MIBT is poorly absorbed from the gastrointestinal tract. The extent of adsorption is greatly influenced by particle size. When given to rats in the form of a suspension in sucrose syrup of 3 μm diameter particles, between 40% and 50% of the dose can be recovered in the feces. With 100 μm particles the recovery is near 80% (Axon 1972). The highest nonlethal dose of MIBT when given subcutaneously or intraperitoneally in mice is 2,000 mg/kg body weight and 235 mg/kg, respectively. The highest nonlethal doses of the derivative, N,N'-bis-(β-thiosemicarbazone-methylisatin)-2-methylpiperazine, when given subcutaneously and intraperitoneally in mice are 2,000 mg/kg and 475 mg/kg, respectively (Borysiewicz and Witalinski 1979). In chronic toxicity studies in which rhesus monkeys were given 250 mg/kg daily by mouth for 1 month there was some evidence of liver damage, but the liver was unaffected at the end of similar treatment in rats and dogs (Bauer 1977).

Methisazone has an embryotoxic effect in very high doses. In mated rats given 2,000 mg/kg daily by mouth for 12 days, there were no implantations in the majority of cases, and animals treated later in pregnancy showed an increase in resorptions in comparison to untreated controls. Similar effects were found in rabbits and fetal malformations were occasionally produced (Bauer 1977).

The duration of sleep after administration of sodium pentobarbital is greatly prolonged in mice given 25 mg/kg MIBT, probably owing to competition for detoxifying systems in the liver. In rats with unrestricted access to food and water, the stomach emptying time is greatly prolonged by the oral administration of 500 mg/kg MIBT. The delay in emptying in fasted rats was much less, indicating that methisazone should be given on an empty stomach (Bauer 1977).

IV. Isatin-β-4′,4′-Dialkylthiosemicarbazones

When studying the ability of MIBT to inhibit the immunologic response of the mouse to sheep red blood cells MCNEILL also found that granulocyte-macrophage colony formation in vitro could be prevented (Sect. G.III). This drug and a series of 4′,4′-dialkylthiosemicarbazones would inhibit when added directly to cells flushed from bone marrow prior to use in a semisolid suspension cell assay. The dialkylthiosemicarbazones could be divided into three groups, depending on the concentration range necessary to prevent 50% of the colonies from forming. The concentration of MIBT required for this degree of inhibition was 3 μg/ml, whereas 4′,4′-morpholino or 4′,4′-tetramethylene substituents in the side chain when associated with N_1-ethyl or N_1-methyl substitutions on isatin were very active (less than 0.5 μg/ml required for 50% colony inhibition). Seven other dialkyl-TSC side chain substituents (dimethyl, diethyl, pentamethylene, hexamethylene, 3-oxopentamethylene, 2-methylpentamethylene, and diallyl) with the same isatin substitutions gave 50% inhibition of colony formation in the 0.7–1.0 μg/ml range. Methoxy substitutions at the 5 position of the aromatic ring (Fig. 8) resulted in compounds of intermediate activity (1.0–5.0 μg/ml), while azo or iodo substitutions at the 5 or 7 positions yielded compounds of very low activity (greater than 20 μg/ml being required). The immunologic implications of these findings are discussed in Sect. G.III.

V. Isatin-β-Isothiosemicarbazones

Using N_1-ethylisatin-S-n-butylisothiosemicarbazone (Fig. 13) at 150 mg/kg body weight (a concentration that would spare 50% of mice infected with 10^3 LD$_{50}$ vaccinia virus) ZGORNIAK-NOWOSIELSKA et al. (1978) investigated the compound's ability to suppress both humoral and cell-mediated responses in the mouse. The humoral, or B-cell response, was measured exactly as described in Sect. G.II. The primary response to sheep red blood cells was reduced by 30%–60% depending on the strain of mouse used in the experiment. The secondary response to the red blood cells, as measured in BALB/c mice was reduced by 60% (twice as much as after the initial injection of cells). The cell-mediated, or T-cell response was measured by the degree of allergic contact dermatitis provoked by oxazolone (Sect. G.II). There was no indication that the compound diminished the cellular response.

VI. Thiazole Thiosemicarbazones

3-Methyl-4-bromo-5-formylisothiazole-TSC (Fig. 14) has been the only compound in this series to receive attention concerning its effect on bodily functions. Chronic toxicity was evaluated in rats and monkeys which were given the drug by mouth in daily doses of 250–1,000 mg/kg (5–20 times the human dose) for 3 months. The lower dose schedule had no deleterious effect on the animals (RAO et al. 1965). In rats, there was no evidence of liver or kidney dysfunction at the higher dose schedule, but there was some toxic suppression of bone marrow (see Sects. G.III, IV) and testicular damage (BAUER 1972). In monkeys, there was no kidney dysfunction, but there was some fatty change in the liver and moderate testicular atrophy (RAO et al. 1965; BAUER 1972).

H. Clinical Studies

On the basis of studies with mice and rabbits infected with various poxviruses, two of the thiosemicarbazones, N_1-methylisatin-β-thiosemicarbazone and 3-methyl-4-bromo-5-formylisothiazole thiosemicarbazone reached clinical trials. I will not describe them in any great detail and the interested reader should consult the concise and comprehensive discussions of this subject by BAUER (1972, 1977). Even though these trials are an important part of the history of antiviral chemotherapy, the success of the World Health Organization's campaign for the eradication of smallpox has resulted in a virtual disappearance of indications for treating poxvirus infections of humans (ARITA and BREMAN 1979). However, the thiosemicarbazone's potential efficacy against poxvirus infections should not be forgotten, especially in the case of isolated laboratory outbreaks or germ warfare. In this vein, studies on thiosemicarbazone-resistant poxvirus mutants will be described. Six features of the virus have made the eradication of smallpox possible (FENNER 1979): (a) the disease was severe enough to warrant quarantine precautions; (b) there was a safe and effective vaccine; (c) the virus did not cause persistent disease or recurrent infection in humans; (d) there appeared to be no animal reservoirs; (e) subclinical but infectious cases did not occur, and cases were not infectious (or rarely so) before eruption occurred, thus making isolation of cases an important part of control; and (f) there were no major barriers of eradication, either social (as with venereal diseases) or financial (as with tuberculosis).

I. N_1-Methylisatin-β-Thiosemicarbazone

As in the laboratory animal studies (Sect. D.III), human infections, other than with poxviruses, have not been convincingly shown to respond to MIBT (HUTFIELD and CSONKA 1964; SANDEMAN 1966). If given in the proper dosage schedule, MIBT appears to have definite merit in the prophylaxis of smallpox and alastrim, and unquestionable value in the complications of vaccination.

Smallpox occurs in two clinical variants, variola major and variola minor or alastrim. Variola major is typically a very severe illness with a mortality around 30%, although its course may be greatly modified by previous vaccination. Alastrim used to occur in South America, mainly in Brazil, and was a much milder illness with a mortality of 0.5%. The initial site of multiplication of the virus after entry is not known, but is probably somewhere in the respiratory tract. After an incubation period of about 12 days the virus escapes into the bloodstream, and further cycles of multiplication take place in the dermis and also in the internal organs. The viremic phase is associated with severe prodromal illness with extreme backache, headache, and prostration. The severity of the clinical course is directly related to the amount of virus liberated into the bloodstream during viremia, and also to the degree of preexisting immunity (BAUER 1977). Because MIBT has been found to lower the attack rate 25-fold among household contacts (a contact being an individual exposed to a person with clinical smallpox and thus likely to become infected) during a smallpox epidemic, and 8-fold among contacts during an alastrim epidemic, it is assumed that the drug arrests virus multiplication during the

12-day incubation period (BAUER 1977). MIBT has not proven effective in the treatment of clinical smallpox (BAUER 1965, 1972, 1977). Since people admitted to the hospital with characteristic lesions of smallpox are in the late stage of disease (the lesions usually erupt simultaneously over the entire body, in distinction to chickenpox, which shows multiple crops of lesions), it is too late for the drug to prevent spread of the infection to target organs. The main side effect of MIBT administration is vomiting, usually occurring almost immediately or 4–6 h later (BAUER 1965). This disconcerting side effect has been repeatedly observed (LANDSMAN and GRIST 1964; HUTFIELD and CSONKA 1964; BAUER 1972, 1977). The percentage of patients in which this occurred varied from approximately 20% to as high as 100%. The effect of the drug on the prophylaxis of smallpox appears to be inversely related to the percentage of people vomiting and thus losing the drug. For adults, 6 g/day MIBT for 4 days has proven prophylactic activity, but it must not be administered in a single daily dose. The best schedule is every 3–4 h but twice a day will also be effective (BAUER 1972).

The efficacy of MIBT in the complications of vaccination have been repeatedly confirmed (BAUER 1965, 1977; MCLEAN 1977). The virus used for vaccination is always vaccinia. Its origin is uncertain: it may have derived from Jenner's original strain of cowpox virus or it may have evolved from recombination between cowpox and smallpox. Its importance lies in the fact that intradermal inoculation of it into humans produces a localized infection in the skin followed by the development of antibodies capable of neutralizing related poxviruses, including smallpox.

If persons suffering from eczema are vaccinated against smallpox, the infection may not remain confined to the site of inoculation, but may spread to involve the eczematous areas and other parts of the body, producing a generalized eruption resembling smallpox in many ways. This condition known as eczema vaccinatum may be fatal in the absence of treatment. It commonly occurs in infants with infantile eczema. Vaccination is usually witheld in such cases. The recommended course of treatment is an initial loading dose of 200 mg/kg, followed by 50 mg/kg at 6-h intervals to a total dose of 600 mg/kg.

In primary smallpox vaccination, the course of infection is brought to a halt by humoral and cell-mediated immunity. In certain cases these mechanisms may be impaired or absent, as in congenital agammaglobulinemia and hypogammaglobulinemia, and in patients undergoing immunosuppressive treatment. In such cases the lesion fails to heal and undergoes indefinite enlargement. Metastatic lesions arise as a result of viremia and can occur in almost any organ of the body. The condition is known as vaccinia gangrenosa, and is invariably fatal in the absence of treatment with antivaccinial gamma globulin or MIBT. The recommended drug dosage schedule is the same as for eczema vaccinatum. The course may be repeated as necessary after an interval of 7 days. It appears that patients who can be cured are those having a single immunologic defect. In patients with multiple defects treatment is ineffective.

APPLEYARD and WAY (1966) were the first to show that IBT-resistant poxviruses could arise in both IBT-treated tissue culture and mice. Mice (20 g body weight) were injected intranasally with 10^7 plaque forming units (pfu) rabbitpox virus. At the first pass the mice received 0.5 mg MIBT twice a day for 4 days; at the second pass 1 mg MIBT was injected daily for 4 days; and at the third pass treatment was 1 mg of MIBT for only two days. After each pass virus obtained from the lungs of one mouse was grown in HeLa cells to produce a suspension with sufficient titer to be used for the next passage. Plaque reduction tests were then carried out in HeLa cells using an IBT-containing agar overlay and virus obtained from mouse lungs at the various passage levels. A gradual resistance to IBT developed with each successive passage. Furthermore, the virus had lost its sensitivity to MIBT when tested in mice. The virus was also passed 16 times in HeLa cells in the presence of IBT. The concentration of drug in the medium for the first five passages was 0.05–0.1 µg/ml, but it was gradually raised to 20 µg/ml at the tenth and subsequent passages. Again, a plaque reduction test was used to assess resistance. About 100 pfu·were used to infect HeLa cells monolayers with the agar overlays containing up to 10 µg/ml IBT. The passaged virus become increasingly resistant to IBT, until about the tenth passage, after which there was no significant change (plaque numbers were almost identical with or without 10 µg/ml IBT in the overlay).

GHENDON and CHERNOS (1972) confirmed the tissue culture observations of APPLEYARD and WAY (1966) and extended them to include vaccinia virus. Chick embryo fibroblast cells were used, with the viruses being passed eight times in concentrations of MIBT increasing gradually from 0.2 to 1.0 µg/ml. Resistance to the drug was measured by a plaque reduction test or the yields of virus 24 h after infection in a liquid medium. Using virus passed in the presence of drug, no difference in virus yields were noted in either test using 1 µg/ml MIBT. The mutants appeared to be stable and retain resistance after a number of passages without the inhibitor. Furthermore, treatment with antiserum against vaccinia virus was shown to reduce the titer of both the original strains and the resulting inhibitor-resistant mutants to the same extent.

Further studies by KATZ et al. (1973 d) not only led to the isolation of IBT-resistant mutants, but also to mutants dependent on IBT for their replication. Vaccinia-infected chick embryo cells were treated with the mutagen, iododeoxyuridine (5 µg/ml) and IBT (14 µM). The culture was harvested 48 h later and used for infection of new cultures in the presence of IBT alone. Virus from one of these cultures was titrated using a plaque assay containing IBT. Well-separated plaques were excised and grown into stocks in the presence of IBT. One of these stocks formed plaques only in the presence of IBT (the IBT-dependent mutant) while another formed plaques both in the presence and absence of the drug (IBT-resistant mutant). The sedimentation rates of the three strains [wild-type (WT), IBT-dependent, and IBT-resistant] were the same, as was their neutralization by WT antiserum (KATZ et al. 1973c). The polypeptide analysis of all three strains showed a few minor differences in the relative amounts of several polypeptides. The IBT-resistant mutant appeared to lack one of the peptides, designated 6b (Sect. F.III). The IBT-dependent mutant was found to be able to grow in the absence of IBT during mixed infection with WT or IBT-resistant viruses (KATZ et al. 1973c). Mode of action studies (KATZ et al. 1973a) showed that the IBT-dependent mutant was blocked in its replication cycle in the absence of IBT at the same place the WT was blocked in its presence (Sect. F.III). KATZ (1979) has recently summarized his studies on these IBT-sensitive, IBT-resistant, and IBT-dependent strains of vaccinia virus.

II. 3-Methyl-4-Bromo-5-Formylisothiazole Thiosemicarbazone

This isothiazole was very effective in preventing death of smallpox-infected mice. Unlike MIBT, it would also spare rabbits infected with rabbitpox virus (RAO et al. 1965). It was then assessed in the treatment of smallpox in humans using a controlled double-blind trial in Madras, India (RAO et al. 1966a). The total number of patients admitted to the trial was 1293, 601 receiving a placebo and 692 being treated with the drug. The usual treatment was 6 g every 6 h for 10 days. The mortality rates in these two groups were 23.3% (140 deaths) and 22.4% (155 deaths), respectively. Marks of previous vaccination were seen on 478 patients; 218 of these received the placebo and eight died (3.7%) and the remaining 260 received the drug, of whom 5 died (1.9%). The mortality rates among the 815 patients who had not been previously vaccinated were 132 of 383 (34.5%) given placebo and 150 of 432 (34.7%) given the drug. The differences in the figures were not significant. Some slight differences in favor of the drug were seen in analysis of the mean number of febrile days, the time of scabbing, and the virus content of the scabs, but the differences were not significant. The isothiazole was also assessed in the prophylaxis of contacts – contacts being persons associated with a patient who develops smallpox and who thus run a risk of acquiring the infection and developing the disease. The persons treated were all family contacts of smallpox patients and the trial was restricted to those contacts who had not been previously vaccinated (RAO et al. 1966b). The drug was given to 196 contacts while 201 received the placebo. In the drug-treated group there were 40 cases of smallpox (20.4%) with 7 deaths (17.5% of the cases). In the placebo group there were 60 cases (29.9%) with 12 deaths (20% of the cases). The mortality rates were not significantly different. As with the MIBT trials the drug was not well tolerated. Vomiting, reported in 75% of the patients, was the major side effect. This loss of drug could have accounted for the lack of chemoprophylactic activity.

IBT-resistant mutants (Sect. H.I) were found to be almost as resistant in tissue culture to 3-methyl-4-bromo-5-formylisothiazole as to IBT itself (APPLEYARD and WAY 1966), thus suggesting a similar mode of action of the two compounds (Sect. F.VI).

J. Perspectives

Of all the antiviral agents discovered in the last two decades, the thiosemicarbazones are certainly one of the most interesting groups of compounds. The thiosemicarbazones have been shown to inhibit the replication of poxviruses in both tissue culture and animal studies. Furthermore, one of these compounds, N_1-methylisatin-β-thiosemicarbazone (MIBT) has been successfully used in the prophylaxis of smallpox in humans. Even though interest in the clinical application of MIBT has disappeared as the worldwide incidence of smallpox has decreased to an undetectable level, the potential value of thiosemicarbazones in medical virology remains high. The isatin-β-thiosemicarbazones in the presence of divalent cations of the first transition series metals (copper being the most effective) can inactivate on contact virtually any type of mature virus particle. With the exception of interferon, no selective, defined substance has such broad antiviral properties. The ability of thiosemicarbazones to inhibit only the poxviruses at an intracellular stage in their morphogenesis may be attributed to the claims that poxviruses contain copper. Divalent copper, as well as other first transition series metals, complexed with various thiosemicarbazones can change the physical configuration of nucleic acids and interfere with their template function. With the use of ionophores copper–thiosemicarbazone complexes within the cell might be able selectively to prevent virus synthesis resulting from infection with fully functional virus. Furthermore, if copper–thiosemicarbazone complexes selectively contact inactivate mature virions by interfering with genome function alone, the way may be open to the rapid production of potent inactivated vaccines.

Acknowledgments. The literature survey for this review was carried out while the author was on leave at the National Institute of Neurological and Communicative Disorders and Stroke. Special thanks go to PAUL DEPORTE of the Translating Service of The National Institutes of Health Library. I gratefully acknowledge Dr. EHUD KATZ for his comments after reading the manuscript. Drs. SYDNEY ARCHER, JAMES MOORE, and HARRY ROY also have helpfully reviewed specific sections. Studies conducted on the thiosemicarbazones in the author's laboratory were aided by a grant from The National Institute of Allergy and Infectious Diseases. I also thank JUDY MALONEY for typing and proofreading.

References

Agrawal KC, Sartorelli AC (1978) The chemistry and biological activity of α-(N)-heterocyclic carboxaldehyde thiosemicarbazones. Prog Med Chem 15:321–356

Andreani A, Cavrini V, Giovanninetti G, Mannini Palenzona A, Franchi L (1975) Ricerche su sostanze ad attività antivirale. Nota II-derivati di 2-chloro-3-formilindoli N-sostituiti. Farmaco [Sci] 30:440–448

Andreani A, Bonazzi D, Cavrini et al. (1978) Ricerche su sostanze ad attività antivirale. Nota IX-sintesi ed attivita antivirale di tiosemicarbazoni di 1-acil-2-alogeno-3-formilindoli. Farmaco [Sci] 33:754–760

Appleyard G, Way HJ (1966) Thiosemicarbazone-resistant rabbitpox virus. Br J Exp Pathol 4:144–151

Appleyard G, Westwood JCN, Zwartouw HT (1962) The toxic effect of rabbitpox virus in tissue culture. Virology 18:159–169

Appleyard G, Hume VBM, Westwood JCN (1965) The effect of thiosemicarbazone on the growth of rabbit pox virus in tissue culture. Ann NY Acad Sci 130:92–104

Arita I, Breman JG (1979) Evaluation of smallpox vaccination policy. Bull WHO 57:1–9

Axon A (1972) Presentation of methisazone (an antiviral chemical) as a medicine for oral administration. J Mond Pharm 15:221–232

Bablanian R (1968) The prevention of early vaccinia-virus induced cytopathic effects by inhibition of protein synthesis. J Gen Virol 3:51–61

Bach MK, Magee WE (1962) Biochemical effects of isatin β-thiosemicarbazone on development of vaccinia virus. Proc Soc Exp Biol Med 110:565–567

Bauer DJ (1955) The antiviral and synergic actions of isatin thiosemicarbazone and certain phenoxypyrimidines in vaccinia infection in mice. Br J Exp Pathol 36:105–114

Bauer DJ (1958) The chemotherapeutic activity of compounds of copper, rhodium, and certain other metals in mice infected with neurovaccinia and ectromelia viruses. Br J Exp Pathol 39:480–489

Bauer DJ (1961) The zero effect dose (E_o) as an absolute numerical index of antiviral chemotherapeutic activity in the pox virus group. Br J Exp Pathol 42:201–206

Bauer DJ (1963) The chemotherapy of ectromelia infection with isatin-β-dialkylthiosemicarbazones. Br J Exp Pathol 44:233–242

Bauer DJ (1965a) Monocyclic thiosemicarbazones as antiviral agents. Ann NY Acad Sci 130:105–109

Bauer DJ (1965b) Clinical experience with the antiviral drug marboran (1-methylisatin 3-thiosemicarbazone). Ann NY Acad Sci 130:110–117

Bauer DJ (1972) Thiosemicarbazones. In: Bauer DJ (ed) Chemotherapy of virus diseases. Pergamon, London (Int Encyclopedia Pharmacol Ther, vol 1, sect 61, pp 35–113)

Bauer DJ (1977) The specific treatment of virus diseases. MTP Press, Lancaster

Bauer DJ, Apostolov K (1966) Adenovirus multiplication: inhibition by methisazone. Science 154:796–797

Bauer DJ, Sadler PW (1960a) The structure-activity relationship of the antiviral chemotherapeutic activity of isatin β-thiosemicarbazone. Br J Pharmacol 15:101–110

Bauer DJ, Sadler PW (1960b) New antiviral chemotherapeutic agent active against smallpox infection. Lancet 1:1110–1111

Bauer DJ, Sadler PW (1961) Derivatives of isatin β-thiosemicarbazone with antiviral chemotherapeutic activity against ectromelia infection. Nature 190:1167–1169

Bauer DJ, Sheffield FW (1959) Antiviral chemotherapeutic activity of isatin-β-thiosemicarbazone in mice infected with rabbit-pox virus. Nature 184:1496–1497

Bauer DJ, Dumbell KR, Fox-Hulme P, Sadler PW (1962) The chemotherapy of variola major infection. Bull WHO 26:727–732

Bauer DJ, Apostolov K, Selway JWT (1970) Activity of methisazone against RNA viruses. Ann NY Acad Sci 173:314–319

Bishop DHL, Shope RE (1979) Bunyaviridae. In: Fraenkel-Contrat H, Wagner RR (eds) Comprehensive virology, vol 14. Plenum, New York, pp 1–156

Bock M (1957) Thiosemicarbazon-Wirkung bei experimentellen Pocken-Infektionen der Maus. Z Hyg Infektionskr 143:480–488

Bopp LH (1976) Contact inactivation of influenza virus by isatin β-thiosemicarbazones and CuSO$_4$. Masters thesis. Rensselaer Polytechnic Institute, Troy, N.Y.

Borysiewicz J, Lucka-Sobstel B (1978) The effect of certain Mannich N-bases, derivatives of isatin β-thiosemicarbazone, on the replication of vaccinia virus in in vitro studies. Acta Microbiol Pol Ser A Microbiol Gen 27:111–121

Borysiewicz J, Tadeusiewicz R (1976) Computer evaluation of antiviral activities of some thiosemicarbazones in experiments in vivo. Acta Virol 20:402–410

Borysiewicz J, Witalinski W (1979) Effect of N,N'-bis(methylisatin-β-thiosemicarbazone) on vaccinia virus replication in vitro and in vivo. Arch Virol 62:83–86

Borysiewicz J, Porebska A, Potec Z (1973) Activity of isatin-β-thiosemicarbazone derivatives against vaccinia virus studied in chick cells by the methyl-cellulose assay. Acta Microbiol Pol Ser A Microbiol Gen 22:205–207

Borysiewicz J, Mizerski J, Pryjma J (1977) Effect of methisazone on immune response in mice. Chemotherapy 23:276–281

Brockman RW, Sidwell RW, Arnett G, Shaddix S (1970) Heterocyclic thiosemicarbazones: correlation between structure, inhibition of ribonucleotide reductase, and inhibition of DNA viruses. Proc Soc Exp Biol Med 133:609–614

Brownlee KA, Hamre D (1951) Studies on chemotherapy of vaccinia virus. I. An experimental design for testing antiviral agents. J Bacteriol 61:127–134

Buu-Hoi NP, Saint-Ruf G, Perche JC, Bourgeade JC (1968) Nouvelles thiosemicarbazones, oxo-4Δ^2-thiazolinylhydrazones-2 et thiazolidinones-4 potentiellement antivirales. Chim Ther 3:110–115

Campaigne E, Thompson RL, Van Werth JE (1959) Some heterocyclic thiosemicarbazones possessing anti-viral activity. J Med Chem 1:577–599

Caton MPL, Jones DH, Slack R, Squires S, Wooldridge KRH (1965) Antiviral chemotherapy. II. Structure-activity relationships in a series of isothiazolealdehyde and ketone thiosemicarbazones. J Med Chem 8:680–683

Caunt AE (1967) The effect of marboran on the growth of varicella virus in tissue culture. In: Spitzy KH, Haschek H (eds) 5th international congress of chemotherapy. Verlag der Wiener medizinischen Akademie, Vienna, pp 313–317

Cho CT, Bolano CR, Kamitsuka PS, Wenner HA (1970) Methisazone and monkey pox virus: studies in cell cultures, chick embryos, mice, and monkeys. Am J Epidemiol 92:137–144

Cooper JA, Moss B, Katz E (1979) Inhibition of vaccinia virus late protein synthesis by isatin-β-thiosemicarbazone: characterization and in vitro translation of viral mRNA. Virology 96:381–392

Domagk G, Behnisch R, Mietzsch F, Schmidt H (1946) Über eine neue, gegen Tuberkelbazillen in vitro wirksame Verbindungsklasse. Naturwissenschaften 33:315

Easterbrook KB (1962) Interference with the maturation of vaccinia virus by isatin-β-thiosemicarbazone. Virology 17:245–251

Fenner F (1979) Portraits of viruses: the poxviruses. Intervirology 11:137–157

Fox MP, Bopp LH, Pfau CJ (1977) Contact inactivation of RNA and DNA viruses by N-methyl isatin β-thiosemicarbazone and $CuSO_4$. Ann NY Acad Sci 284:533–543

Francis RD, Bradford HB (1976) Some biological and physical properties of molluscum contagiosum virus propagated in cell culture. J Virol 19:382–388

Franke R, Labes D, Tonew M, Zschiesche W, Heinisch L (1975) Antivirale Thiosemikarbazone und verwandte Verbindungen. III. Quantitative Beziehungen zwischen Struktur und antiviraler Aktivität von Isatin-β-isothiosemikarbazonen gegen Mengovirus. Acta Biol Med Germ 34:491–499

Freund M, Schander A (1902) Thiosemicarbazid als Reagens auf Aldehyde und Ketone. Chem Ber 35:2602–2606

Gabriel R (1971) 1-Methylisatin 3-thiosemicarbazone treatment of NZBxNZW hybrid mice. Br J Exp Pathol 52:271–275

Gerzon K (1965) Discussion-thiosemicarbazones. Ann NY Sci 130:128–130

Ghendon YZ, Chernos VI (1972) Mutants of poxviruses resistant to acetone and N-methyl-isatin-beta-thiosemicarbazone. Acta Virol 16:308–312

Giannella M, Gualtieri F (1970) Ricerche nel campo della sostanze ad azione antivirale carbammati, tiosemicarbazoni e semicarbazoni di-α-ossimminochetoni ciclici. Farmaco [Sci] 25:509–518

Giannella M, Gualtieri F, Melchiorre C, Pigini M (1973) Ricerche nel campo sostanze ad attività antivirale. Farmaco [Sci] 28:597–610

Gladych JMZ, Hunt JH, Jack D, Haff RF, Boyle JJ, Stewart RC, Ferlauto RJ (1969) Inhibition of rhinovirus by isatin thiosemicarbazone analogues. Nature 221:286–287

Haase AT, Levinson W (1973) Inhibition of RNA slow viruses by thiosemicarbazones. Biochem Biophys Res Commun 51:875–880

Hamre D, Bernstein J, Donovick R (1950) Activity of p-aminobenzaldehyde, 3-thiosemicarbazone on vaccinia virus in the chick embryo and in the mouse. Proc Soc Exp Biol Med 73:275–278

Hamre D, Brownlee KA, Donovick R (1951) Studies on the chemotherapy of vaccinia virus. J Immunol 67:305–312

Hanson AG (1977) Contact inactivation of some RNA viruses by thiosemicarbazone derivatives and copper ions. Master's thesis. Rensselaer Polytechnic Institute, Troy, N.Y.

Hapel A, Gardner I (1974) Appearance of cytotoxic T cells in cerebrospinal fluid of mice with ectromelia virus-induced meningitis. Scand J Immunol 3:311–319

Harford CG, Rieders E, Osborn R (1972) Inhibition of arc-like fragments of immature forms of vaccinia virus by methisazone. Proc Soc Exp Biol Med 139:558–561

Heinisch L, Kramarczyk K (1972) Antivirale Thiosemicarbazone und verwandte Verbindungen. I. Synthese und Struktur substituierter Isatin-Thiosemicarbazone und -isothiosemicarbazone. J Prakt Chem 314:682–698

Herrlich A, Stickl H, Munz E (1965) Kann man den Ablauf der Pockenschutzimpfung medikamentös beeinflussen? Dtsch Wochensch 90:69–74

Herrman EC (1968) Sensitivity of herpes simplex virus, vaccinia virus, and adenoviruses to deoxyribonucleic acid inhibitors and thiosemicarbazones in a plaque suppression test. Appl Microbiol 16:1151–1155

Hoagland CL, Ward SM, Smadel JE, Rivers TM (1941) Constituents of elementary bodies of vaccinia. IV. Demonstration of copper in the purified virus. J Exp Med 74:69–80

Hutfield DC, Csonka GW (1964) Marboran in herpes genitalis. Lancet 1:329–330

Iwasaki K, Nishimura T, Igarashi Y, Nagaki D (1955) Studies on the chemotherapy of influenza virus I. Effect of thiosemicarbazones on influenza and Newcastle disease virus multiplication. Kitasato Arch Exp Med 28:31–44

Joklik WJ (1962) The purification of four strains of poxviruses. Virology 18:9–18

Kackell MY, Schneweis KE, Spiess H (1966) Untersuchungen über die Wirkung von Marboran, Activaccine-Hyperimmun-Serum und Vorimpfung mit Vaccineantigen auf die intracutane Pockenimpfung beim Kaninchen. Klin Wochenschr 44:1199–1204

Kaptsova TI, Marennikova SS (1967) On the prophylactic activity on N-methyl isatin β-thiosemicarbazone against smallpox infection. Acta Virol 11:554–556

Kaska WC, Carrano C, Michalowski J, Jackson J, Levinson W (1978) Inhibition of the RNA dependent DNA polymerase and malignant transforming ability of Rous sarcoma virus by thiosemicarbazone-transition metal complexes. Bioinorg Chem 8:225–236

Katz E (1979) Sensitivity, resistance, and dependence on the antiviral drug isatin-β-thiosemicarbazone (IBT) in the growth of vaccinia virus in tissue culture. In: Zuckerman A (ed) Dynamic aspects of host-parasite relationships, vol 3. Israel Universities Press, Jerusalem, pp 98–107

Katz E, Felix H (1977) Synthesis of vaccinia virus antigens in HeLa cells in the presence of isatin β-thiosemicarbazone. Antimicrob Agents Chemother 11:202–208

Katz E, Margalith E, Winer B (1973a) An isatin β-thiosemicarbazone (IBT)-dependent mutant of vaccinia virus: the nature of the IBT-dependent step. J Gen Virol 21:477–484

Katz E, Margalith E, Winer B, Goldblum N (1973b) Synthesis of vaccinia polypeptides in the presence of isatin β-thiosemicarbazone. Antimicrob Agents Chemother 4:44–48

Katz E, Margalith E, Winer B, Lazar A (1973c) Characterization and mixed infections of three strains of vaccinia virus: wild type, IBT-resistant and IBT-dependent mutants. J Gen Virol 21:469–475

Katz E, Winer B, Margalith E, Goldblum N (1973d) Isolation and characterization of an IBT-dependent mutant of vaccinia virus. J Gen Virol 19:161–164

Katz E, Margalith E, Winer B (1974) The effect of isatin β-thiosemicarbazone (IBT)-related compounds on IBT-resistant and on IBT-dependent mutants of vaccinia virus. J Gen Virol 25:239–244

Katz E, Margalith E, Winer B (1975) Isolation and characterization of a γ-thiochromanone-4-thiosemicarbazone-resistant mutant of vaccinia virus. Antimicrob Agents Chemother 7:85–90

Katz E, Margalith E, Winer B (1978a) Formation of vaccinia virus DNA-protein complex in the presence of isatin-β-thiosemicarbazone (IBT). J Gen Virol 40:695–699

Katz E, Margalith E, Felix H, Winer B (1978b) Synthesis of vaccinia viral RNA and proteins in the presence of isatin-β-thiosemicarbazone. In: Siegenthaler W, Luethy R (eds) Current chemotherapy. Proceedings of the 10th International Congress of Chemotherapy, vol 1. American Society for Microbiology, Washington CD, pp 330–332

Katz E, Margalith E, Winer B (1978c) Genetic recombination between a temperature sensitive mutant and an isatin β-thiosemicarbazone (IBT) resistant mutant of vaccinia virus. J Antimicrob Chemother 4:159–162

Kudriavtsev FS, Solov'ev IU V, Korovin RN, Shurchilov AF (1977) Effect of izatizon and OL-56 on the reproductive and transformational properties of Marek's disease virus (in Russian). Veterinariia 2:45–46

Landsman JB, Grist NR (1964) Controlled trial of marboran on group vaccinated against smallpox. Lancet 1:330

Levinson W (1973) Inhibition of viruses, tumors, and pathogenic microorganisms by isatin β-thiosemicarbazone and other thiosemicarbazones. In: Carter WA (ed) Selective inhibitors of viral function. CRC Press, Cleveland, Ohio, pp 213–226

Levinson W, Helling R (1976) Inactivation of λ phage infectivity and λ deoxyribonucleic acid transfection by N-methyl isatin β-thiosemicarbazone. Antimicrob Agents Chemother 9:160–163

Levinson W, Woodson B, Jackson J (1971) Inactivation of Rous sarcoma virus on contact with N-ethyl isatin β-thiosemicarbazone. Nature New Biol 232:116–118

Levinson W, Faras A, Morris R et al. (1973a) Effect of N-methyl isatin β-thiosemicarbazone on Rous sarcoma virus, several isolated enzymes and other viruses. In: Fox CF, Robinson WS (eds) Virus research-2nd ICN-UCLA symposium on molecular biology. Academic Press, New York, pp 403–414

Levinson W, Faras A, Woodson B, Jackson J, Bishop JM (1973b) Inhibition of RNA dependent DNA polymerase of Rous sarcoma virus by thiosemicarbazones and several cations. PNAS 70:164–168

Levinson W, Coleman V, Woodson B, Rabson A, Lanier J, Whitcher J, Dawson C (1974) Inactivation of herpes simplex virus by thiosemicarbazones and certain cations. Antimicrob Agents Chemother 5:398–402

Levinson W, Oppermann H, Jackson J (1977a) Inhibition of vesicular stomatitis virus by kethoxal bis (thiosemicarbazone). J Gen Virol 37:183–190

Levinson W, Rohde W, Mikelens P, Jackson J, Antony A, Ramakrishnan T (1977b) Inactivation and inhibition of Rous sarcoma virus by copper binding ligands: thiosemicarbazones, 8-hydroxyquinolines, and isonicotinic acid hydrazide. Ann NY Acad Sci 284:525–532

Levinson W, Mikelens P, Jackson J, Kaska W (1978a) Anti-tumor virus activity of copper-binding drugs. In: Schrauzer GN (ed) Inorganic and nutritional aspects of cancer, chap 12. Plenum, New York, pp 161–178

Levinson W, Oppermann H, Jackson J (1978b) Induction of four proteins in eukaryotic cells by kethoxal bis (thiosemicarbazone). Biochim Biophys Acta 518:401–412

Levinson W, Idriss J, Jackson J (1979) Metal binding drugs induce synthesis of four proteins in normal cells. Biol Trace Element Res 1:15–23

Levy JA, Levy SB, Levinson W (1976) Inactivation of murine RNA tumor viruses by isatin β-thiosemicarbazone, its derivatives and analogs. Virology 74:426–431

Lieberman M, Pollikoff R, Pascale AM (1966) Effect of concomitant treatment by cortisone and N-ethylisatin-β-thiosemicarbazone on neurovaccinia virus infected mice. Proc Soc Exp Biol Med 122:484–489

Logan JC, Fox MP, Morgan JH, Makohon AM, Pfau CJ (1975) Arenavirus inactivation on contact with N-substituted isatin β-thiosemicarbazones and certain cations. J Gen Virol 28:271–283

Lovas B, Hollos I (1969) Replication of vaccinia virus in the embryonated egg in the presence of methisazone. An electron microscope study. Acta Microb Acad Sci Hung 16:47–62

Lum GS, Smith PK (1957) Experimental chemotherapy of influenza virus with particular reference to thiosemicarbazones and diphenyl compounds. J Pharmacol Exp Ther 119:284–293

Lwoff A, Lwoff M (1964) Remarques sur l'isatine β-thiosemicarbazone et sur quelques inhibiteurs du développement viral. C R Acad Sci [D] (Paris) 258:1924–1927

Magee WE, Bach MK (1965) Biochemical studies on the antiviral activities of the isatin-β-thiosemicarbazones. Ann NY Acad Sci 130:80–91

McLean DM (1977) Methisazone therapy in pediatric vaccinia complications. Ann NY Acad Sci 284:118–121

McNeill TA (1972) Effect of methisazone and other drugs on mouse hemopoietic colony formation in vitro. Antimicrob Agents Chemother 1:6–11

McNeill TA (1973) Inhibition of granulocyte-macrophage colony formation in vitro by substituted isatin thiosemicarbazones. Antimicrob Agents Chemother 4:105–108

McNeill RA, Fleming W, McClure S, Killen M (1972) Suppression of immune and hematopoietic cellular response by methisazone. Antimicrob Agents Chemother 1:1–5

Mikelens PE, Woodson BA, Levinson WE (1976) Association of nucleic acids with complexes of N-methyl isation β-thiosemicarbazone and copper. Biochem Pharmacol 25:821–828

Minton SA, Officer JE, Thompson RL (1953) Effect of thiosemicarbazones and dichlorophenoxy thiouracil on multiplication of a recently isolated strain of variola-vaccinia virus in the brain of the mouse. J Immunol 70:222–228

Morishima T, Hayashi K (1978) Meningeal exudate cells in vaccinia meningitis of mice: role of local T cells. Infect Immun 20:752–759

Moss B (1974) Reproduction of poxviruses. In: Fraenkel-Conrat H, Wagner RR (eds) Comprehensive virology vol 3, chap 5. Plenum, New York, pp 405–474

Munro TW, Sabina LR (1970) Inhibition of infectious bovine rhinotracheitis virus multiplication by thiosemicarbazones. J Gen Virol 7:55–63

Ong SG (1958) The depressive effect of certain elements on influenza virus 1 (in Chinese). Sci J (K'o Hsueh T'ung Pao, Kexue Tunghao) 3:157–159

O'Sullivan DG, Sadler PW (1961) Agents with high activity against type 2 poliovirus. Nature 192:341–343

O'Sullivan DG, Sadler PW, Webley C (1963) A study of the chemotherapeutic activity of isatin-β-4',4'-dialkylthiosemicarbazones against ectromelia infection. Chemotherapia 7:17–26

O'Sullivan DG, Sadler PW, Russell V (1964) The influence of isatin β-thiosemicarbazone on the development of neurovaccinia virus in cells as shown by electron microscopy. Arch Gesamte Virusforsch 14:650–656

Pearson GD, Zimmerman EF (1969) Inhibition of poliovirus replication by N-methylisatin-β-4':4'-dibutylthiosemicarbazone. Virology 38:641–650

Pennington TH (1977) Isatin-β-thiosemicarbazone causes premature cessation of vaccinia virus-induced late post-replicative polypeptide synthesis. J Gen Virol 35:567–571

Petering DH (1980) Carcinostatic copper complexes. In: Sigel H, Sigel A (eds) Metal complexes as anticancer agents. Dekker, New York Basel (Metal ions in biologic systems, vol 11, pp 197–229)

Pfau CJ (1975) Arenavirus chemotherapy– retrospect and prospect. Bull WHO 52:737–744

Pfau CJ (1977) Current status on the chemotherapy of experimental arenavirus infections. Medicina (B Aires) 37:219–224

Pillai CKS, Nandi US, Levinson W (1977) Interaction of DNA with anti-cancer drugs: copper-thiosemicarbazide system. Bioinorg Chem 7:151–157

Polatnick J (1965) Effect of chemical agents on foot-and-mouth disease virus production in cell culture. Am J Vet Res 26:1051–1055

Pollikoff R, Lieberman M, Lem NE, Foley EJ (1965) Antiviral activity of N-ethylisatin-β-thiosemicarbazone in vaccinia-infected mice. J Immunol 94:794–804

Porterfield JS, Casals J, Chumakov MP et al. (1978) Togaviridae. Intervirology 9:129–148

Rao AR, McFadzean JA, Squires S (1965) The laboratory and clinical assessment of an isothiazole thiosemicarbazone (M & B 7714) against pox viruses. Ann NY Acad Sci 130:118–127

Rao AR, McFadzean JA, Kamalakshi K (1966a) An isothiazole thiosemicarbazone in the treatment of variola major in man. Lancet 1:1068–1072

Rao AR, McKendrick GDW, Velayudhan L, Kamalakshi K (1966b) Assessment of an isothiazole thiosemicarbazone in the prophylaxis of contacts of variola major. Lancet 1:1072–1074

Rapp F (1964) Inhibition by metabolic analogues of plaque formation by herpes zoster and herpes simplex viruses. J Immunol 93:643–648

Rigaudy J, Klesney SP (1979) Nomenclature of organic chemistry. Pergamon, New York, pp 305–322

Rohde W, Shafer R, Idriss J, Levinson W (1979) Binding of N-methyl isatin β-thiosemicarbazone-copper complexes to proteins and nucleic acids. J Inorg Biochem 10:183–194

Rolly H, Winkelmann E (1972) A new thiosemicarbazone active in vivo against vaccinia virus. Adv Antimicrob Antineoplast Chemother 1/1:305–307

Runti C, Collino F, Pescani G (1968) Potenziali antivirali nota II – tiosemicarbazoni di acetofenoni sostituti. Farmaco [Sci] 23:114–121

Sadler PW (1965) Antiviral chemotherapy with isatin-β-thiosemicarbazone and its derivatives. Ann NY Acad Sci 130:71–79

Sandeman TF (1966) Pilot trial of an antiviral agent in malignant disease. Br Med J 2:625–627

Sartorelli AC, Agrawal KC, Tsiftsoglou AS, Moore EC (1977) Characterization of the biochemical mechanism of action of α-(N)-heterocyclic carboxaldehyde thiosemicarbazones. Adv Enzyme Regul 11:117–139

Schmidt-Ruppin KH (1971) Chemotherapy of cytomegalovirus infections. Further results on intraperitoneal infection of Ehrlich ascites tumor mice with viruses of low virulence in vivo: MCMV/Smith, adenovirus 2, RSV/Long, and rhinoviruses. Chemotherapy 16:130–143

Sheffield FW (1962) Inhibition of rabbitpox virus replication by isatin β-thiosemicarbazone. Br J Exp Pathol 43:59–66

Sheffield FW, Bauer DJ, Stephenson S (1960) The protection of tissue cultures by isatin β-thiosemicarbazone from the cytopathic effects of certain pox viruses. Br J Exp Pathol 41:638–647

Singh M, Sudgen JK (1971) Some pyrrolidine thiosemicarbazones as potential antiviral agents. Pharm Acta Helv 46:627–631

Smejkal F, Budesinsky Z, Sulka J, Kuchar M (1972) Study of antiviral activity of some amantadine, pyrimidine, and isatine analogs. Adv Antimicrob Antineoplast Chemother 1/2:879–883

Squires SL, McFadzean JA (1966) The possible involvement of an interfering substance in the action of thiosemicarbazones against viruses. Trans R Soc Trop Med Hyg 60:419–421

Thompson RL, Price ML, Minton SA (1951) Protection of mice against vaccinia virus by administration of benzaldehyde thiosemicarbazone. Proc Soc Exp Biol Med 78:11–13

Thompson RL, Davis J, Russel PB, Hitchings GH (1953a) Effect of aliphatic oxime and isatin thiosemicarbazones on vaccinia infection in the mouse and in the rabbit. Proc Soc Exp Biol Med 84:496–499

Thompson RL, Minton SA, Officer JE, Hitchings GH (1953b) Effect of heterocyclic and other thiosemicarbazones on vaccinia infection in the mouse. J Immunol 70:229–234

Tonew M, Tonew E (1974) Effects of some antiviral isatinisothiosemicarbazones on cellular and viral ribonucleic acid synthesis in mengovirus-infected FL cells. Antimicrob Agents Chemother 5:393–397

Tonew E, Lober G, Tonew M (1974a) The influence of antiviral isatinisothiosemicarbazones on RNA dependent RNA polymerase in mengovirus-infected FL cells. Acta Virol 18:185–192

Tonew M, Tonew E, Heinisch L (1974b) Antiviral thiosemicarbazones and related compounds. II. Antiviral action of substituted isatinisothiosemicarbazones. Acta Virol 18:17–24

Tsunoda A, Miyazaki K, Aota T, Matsumoto S, Kumagai K, Ishida S (1971) Anti-vaccinia activity of γ-thiochromanone-1-thiosemicarbazone in vitro and in vivo. Jpn J Microbiol 16:61–66

Varma RS, Nobles WL (1967) Thiosemicarbazones derived from indanedione-1,3. J Pharm Sci 56:775–776

Veckenstedt A, Horn M (1974) Testing of antiviral compounds against mengo virus infection of mice. 1. Screening of compounds and statistical evaluation of their effects. Chemotherapy 20:235–244

Veckenstedt A, Zgorniak-Nowosielska I (1979) Antiviral activity of certain isatinisothiosemicarbazones against mengo and vaccinia virus infections in mice. Acta Virol 23:45–51

Wang L, Levinson W (1978) N-methyl isatin β-thiosemicarbazone copper complex inhibits RNA-dependent DNA polymerase but not ribonuclease H of Rous sarcoma virus. Bioinorg Chem 8:535–540

Webb DR, Bourne HR, Levinson W (1974) A new phosphodiesterase inhibitor in human lymphocytes: N-methyl-isatin-β-thiosemicarbazone. Biochem Pharmacol 23:1663–1667

Winkelmann E, Rolly H (1972) A new thiosemicarbazone with in vivo activity against smallpox. Adv Antimicrob Antineoplast Chemother 1/1:309–311

Woodson B, Joklik WK (1965) The inhibition of vaccinia virus by isatin β-thiosemicarbazone. PNAS 54:946–953

Zak MR (1959) Experience in the combined treatment of influenza. Probl Virol 4/3:84–86

Zgorniak-Nowosielska I, Marciszewska M, Pastuszak J, Lucka-Sobstel-Stobstel B (1973) The effect of isatin-β-thiosemicarbazone derivatives on vaccinia virus multiplication in L-132 cell line (human embryonic lung). Acta Microbiol Pol Ser A Microbiol Gen 22:199–204

Zgorniak-Nowosielska I, Gatkiewicz A, Potec Z (1976) The antiviral activity of isatin-β-thiosemicarbazone derivatives on vaccinia virus infection in mice. Arch Immunol Ther Exp 24:597–601

Zgorniak-Nowosielska I, Borysiewicz J, Cwik D, Drozd E (1978) The influence of some thiosemicarbazone derivatives with antiviral activity on immune response in mice. Arch Immunol Ther Exp 26:547–552

Zwartouw HT (1964) The chemical composition of vaccinia virus. J Gen Microbiol 34:115–123

CHAPTER 6

Interferon and Its Inducers

P. B. Sehgal, L. M. Pfeffer, and I. Tamm

A. Preface

Interferons are a group of inducible cellular proteins that interact with mammalian and other vertebrate cells and render them resistant to infection by a wide variety of RNA-containing or DNA-containing viruses. In addition to a marked antiviral effect, interferons cause numerous changes in the phenotype of target cells, including a reduction in the rate of cell proliferation and alterations in the structure and function of the cell surface, the distribution of cytoskeletal elements, and the expression of several differentiated cellular functions. The use of interferons and interferon inducers to treat human viral and neoplastic diseases is currently under intensive investigation. Considerable attention is thus focused on the structure and function of human interferons. Furthermore, investigations of the mechanisms which underlie the induction and the actions of interferons have led to novel insights into the regulation of gene expression in eukaryotic cells as well as into the pathophysiology of viral diseases. Thus, interferon research represents an important and rapidly advancing area of biomedical research today.

B. Introduction

The discovery of interferons (NAGANO and KOJIMA 1954; ISAACS and LINDENMANN 1957) came at the culmination of two decades of extensive research on viral interference (HOSKINS 1935; SCHLESINGER 1959). "Viral interference" refers to phenomena in which a live or inactivated virus interferes with the replication of related or unrelated viruses by a mechanism which does not involve virus-neutralizing immunoglobulins (FINDLAY and MACCALLUM 1937). NAGANO and KOJIMA (1954) observed that tissue extracts of vaccinia-inoculated rabbit skin contained a factor which inhibited the development of vaccinia lesions in rabbits challenged with the virus. This inhibitory factor was distinct from infectious virus since it could not be sedimented in the ultracentrifuge under conditions which removed virtually all infectious virus from the supernatant fluid. Independently, ISAACS and colleagues (ISAACS and LINDENMANN 1957; ISAACS et al. 1957) carried out elegant tissue culture experiments which demonstrated unequivocally that heat-inactivated influenza virus, when incubated with chick chorioallantoic membrane pieces in culture, induces a substance which renders the cells of a second culture unable to support the replication of related or unrelated viruses. These experiments convincingly demonstrated the existence of a virus-induced factor which was named "interferon" and which inhibited the replication of several RNA and DNA viruses. The clarity of the data obtained by Isaacs and his colleagues depended on the imaginative use of the then novel technique of maintaining fragments of chick chorioallantoic membrane in tissue culture (Fulton and Armitage 1951; Tyrrell and Tamm 1955).

The basic outline of the mechanisms involved in the induction and in the action of interferons emerged in the 1960s. Interferons could be induced in a wide variety of animal species in response to numerous viral and nonviral stimuli. Furthermore, interferons were effective against a wide range of viruses, both in cell culture and in animal experiments. The biochemical mechanisms underlying the induction and the antiviral effects of interferon have been extensively explored in the last 10 years. These investigations have uncovered novel cellular phenomena such as the post-transcriptional regulation of the stability of human fibroblast interferon mRNA (Sehgal et al. 1977; Cavalieri et al. 1977b), the role of $2',5'$-oligo(A) in degradation of mRNA species (Kerr et al. 1977) and the role of phosphorylation of initiation factor 2 (eIF-2) in regulating cellular protein synthesis (Farrell et al. 1978).

The potential use of interferon as an antiviral agent in humans was recognized from the very outset. However, since the protective effect of interferon is generally restricted to cells of homologous or related species (Tyrrell 1959), it was necessary to produce interferon destined for clinical use in human cells. Human interferon was first detected in cell culture by Ho and Enders (1959a, b) who induced HeLa cells and cells derived from various human organs using a chick embryo-adapted strain of poliovirus as inducer. Nevertheless, despite intensive efforts throughout the 1960s and the early 1970s, the goals of purification and characterization of human interferons on the one hand and their application in the clinic on the other, remained elusive. The lack of availability of sufficient amounts of interferon was the principal hurdle. This problem has been alleviated to some extent by the development of three procedures for large-scale production of human interferon: (a) human leukocytes induced with Newcastle disease virus or Sendai virus (Gresser 1961; Strander and Cantell 1966; Cantell and Hirvonen 1978); (b) human diploid fibroblast cultures induced with $poly(I) \cdot poly(C)$ together with the judicious use of cycloheximide and actinomycin D (Tan et al. 1970; Havell and Vilček 1972, Billiau et al. 1973a); and (c) human lymphoblastoid cell lines (e.g., Namalva) induced with Sendai or Newcastle disease virus (Strander et al. 1974; Finter and Bridgen 1978; Zoon et al. 1979b). These procedures for large-scale production have provided amounts of human interferon sufficient for the purification of these proteins as well as for preliminary clinical investigations. It appears that recombinant DNA technology may succeed in providing larger amounts of biologically active human interferons synthesized in *Escherichia coli* (Nagata et al. 1980).

The difficulties encountered in producing large amounts of human interferons and the observation that numerous natural and synthetic compounds induce interferon (reviewed in Ho and Armstrong 1975) stimulated extensive studies on the efficacy of interferon inducers per se in viral infections. $Poly(I) \cdot poly(C)$ has emerged as one of the more potent synthetic inducers of interferon (Field et al. 1967). A complex of $poly(I) \cdot poly(C)$ with carboxymethylcellulose and poly-L-lysine is receiving a great deal of attention as an antiviral and immunomodulatory agent (LEVY et al. 1975). At the same time, the search for more potent and less toxic inducers of interferon continues in several laboratories.

Whereas the initial interest in interferon centered on its antiviral effects, it is now recognized that interferons have numerous additional effects on cells. Interferons inhibit cell proliferation (PAUCKER et al. 1962) and exert antitumor effects in animal models (ATANASIU and CHANY 1960; GRESSER et al. 1967a; 1969a; CAME and MOORE 1971, 1972). Furthermore, interferons are not only produced in the course of several immune reactions (WHEELOCK 1965; GREEN et al. 1969), but also markedly modulate the immune system (BRAUN and LEVY 1972; for review see DE MAEYER and DE MAEYER-GUIGNARD 1979a; STEWART 1979). These observations have stimulated interest in the use of interferons as antineoplastic as well as immunomodulating agents. Human interferons are currently under clinical investigation for these purposes.

The actions of interferons as modulators of cell structure and function and the induction of interferons by stimuli such as specific antigens, contact with tumor cells, and various low molecular weight substances, raises the important question of the physiologic role of interferon in vivo. Does interferon represent mainly an antiviral defense mechanism or is it an important component of other regulatory processes that may function in vivo? Clearly, interferon production is involved in protection against some viral infections (GRESSER et al. 1976b; HALLER et al. 1979). However, it is unclear whether that is the most important role of interferon in vivo.

In the next several sections we shall focus attention on the production, characterization, pharmacokinetics, and actions of human interferons, as well as summarize some of the clinical investigations that have been conducted or are under way. We shall also discuss the current status of research on those interferon inducers which could be used as antiviral or antitumor agents per se.

C. Production and Characterization of Human Interferons

I. Classification

Historically, interferons have been classified into type I and type II interferons based upon the induction procedure used (type I: nonimmune induction, viral or nonviral; type II: immune induction) and the stability of the induced interferon (type I: pH stable; type II: pH labile). Human type I interferons have been further subdivided into leukocyte (Le) and fibroblast (F) interferons, depending on the phenotype of the induced cell and the host range of the induced interferon (Le interferon is more active on bovine cells than on human cells whereas F interferon is practically inactive on bovine cells). However, this classification is unable to deal adequately with the production of Le interferon by human fibroblasts, that of F interferon by human leukocytes and lymphoblastoid cells, as well as the production of type I interferon by lymphoid cells in response to stimuli such as exposure to extracts of *Corynebacterium parvum*, *Brucella abortus*, and *Nocardia rubea*. Furthermore, this classification cannot be readily generalized to interferons from other species such as the mouse.

Table 1. Classification of interferons

	Human	Murine	M_c (daltons)
α	Type I, Le	Type I, band C	20,000
β	Type I, F	Type I, band A	35,000–40,000
		and band B	26,000–33,000
γ	Type II, T, immune	Type II, immune	

  a Human fibroblast interferon

      H-Met-Ser-Tyr-Asn-Leu-Leu-Gly-Phe-Leu-Gln-Arg-Ser-Ser-

  b Mouse interferons A and B

      H-Ile -Asn-Tyr-Lys-Gln-Leu-Gln-Leu-Gln-Glu-Arg-Thr-Asn-

  c Human lymphoblastoid interferon

      H-Ser -Asp-Leu-Pro-Gln-Thr- His -Ser-Leu-Gly-Asn-Arg-Arg- Ala-Leu-Ile -Leu-Leu-Ala-Gln-

  d Mouse interferon C

      H-Ala-Asp-Leu-Pro-Gln-Thr- Tyr-Asn-Leu-Gly-Asn-Lys-Gly-Ala-Leu-Lys-Val-Leu-Ala-Gln-

Fig. 1 a–d. Comparison of the NH_2 terminal amino acid sequences of a human fibroblast interferon **a** with that of mouse interferons A and B **b**, and of a human lymphoblastoid interferon **c**, with that of mouse interferon C **d**. Identical amino acids in the same relative positions are italicized. (Taira et al. 1980)

Interferons are now classified as α, β, or γ depending upon their physical stability (pH lability), immunologic neutralization properties (Havell et al. 1975; Yamamoto and Kawade 1980), host range, and homology in amino acid sequence. Table 1 summarizes the relationship between the earlier nomenclature and the new terms. The α and β interferons are characteristically more stable to inactivation at low pH than γ interferons. Antiserum raised against α, β or γ human interferon neutralizes the biologic activity of only the homologous, i.e., α, β, or γ human interferon, respectively. In general, antisera raised against human interferons do not neutralize murine interferons and vice versa. Nevertheless, the NH_2 terminal amino acid sequence of one α human interferon species shows marked homology with the NH_2 terminal sequence of band C ($M_r = 20,000$ daltons) murine interferon (Zoon et al. 1980; Taira et al. 1980; Fig. 1). There is a lesser degree of homology between one of human β interferon species and murine band A and B interferons (Knight et al. 1980; Taira et al. 1980). Indeed some immunologic relatedness has been detected (STEWART and HAVELL 1980) between human α and a species of murine interferon of $M_r = 21,000$ daltons presumably identical with band C of TAIRA et al. (1980). At present, such amino acid sequence analyses of interferons are not yet complete and further insights may emerge in the near future. In addition, recent data from experiments which involved the characterization and cloning of interferon mRNA species indicate that there exist more than one distinct interferon protein in each of the α and β categories of human interferon (NAGATA et al. 1980; MANTEI et al. 1980; SEHGAL and SAGAR 1980; TANIGUCHI et al. 1980 a, b; WEISSENBACH et al. 1980).

II. Assay

Most current assays for interferon are based on its antiviral effects, though immunologic procedures such as radioimmunoassays may soon be developed. Several simple procedures are available for the quantitation of the antiviral effect of interferon (reviewed in STEWART 1979; SEHGAL and TAMM 1980a). These procedures generally involve the treatment of cell cultures for 16–24 h with an interferon preparation at varying dilutions, followed by the exposure of treated cultures to a suitable dose of an appropriate virus such as vesicular stomatitis virus. Virus replication can then be monitored by following the virus-induced cytopathic effect (visually or by dye-uptake techniques), virus-specific RNA synthesis, the development of viral plaques, or the yield of infectious virus (reviewed in STEWART 1979; SEHGAL and TAMM 1980a). The reciprocal of the highest dilution of an interferon preparation that exhibits an antiviral effect (usually a 50% protection of cell cultures or a 50% inhibition of viral replication) is taken as the interferon titer. For uniformity, interferon activity is expressed in terms of appropriate international reference standards. Several interferons which have been purified to homogeneity display a specific activity in the range of 10^8–10^9 U/mg protein (KNIGHT 1976a; DE MAEYER-GUIGNARD et al. 1978; CABRER et al. 1979; RUBINSTEIN et al. 1978; 1979; TAN et al. 1979; ZOON et al. 1979a, 1980; YONEHARA et al. 1980).

III. Production

Three distinct procedures are currently in use for large-scale production of human interferons and several alternative techniques are in various stages of development.

1. Human Leukocyte Interferon

Human buffy coat cells primed with interferon and induced with Sendai virus at a high multiplicity followed by incubation in medium supplemented with a human plasma protein fraction (e.g., fraction V according to the COHN classification) for 16–20 h provide approximately 1–4 × 10^6 U interferon per unit of buffy coat cells (CANTELL et al. 1974; CANTELL 1979). The virus induces interferon in B-lymphocytes present in these buffy coats (YAMAGUCHI et al. 1977). Several laboratories around the world are now involved in the large-scale production of human leukocyte interferon preparations. The Helsinki laboratories (CANTELL 1979) have a preeminent position in this regard. Close cooperation with the Finnish Blood

Transfusion Service allowed these laboratories to produce 2.5×10^{11} U of interferon from 90,000 buffy coats in 1978.

Crude human leukocyte interferon is concentrated and purified approximately 100-fold by precipitation with potassium thiocyanate at pH 3.5 followed by solubilization in 95% ethanol at pH 4.2 and -20 °C, with subsequent differential precipitation between pH 5.6 and 7.1 at 0°–4 °C. The ethanol precipitate at this stage contains almost all of the interferon activity and has a specific activity of $\sim 10^6$ U/ mg protein. This material, dissolved in phosphate-buffered saline, is called P-IF and has been used in many of the clinical trials carried out to date (Cantell et al. 1974). P-IF can be further fractionated into P-IF B and P-IF A by reprecipitation with potassium thiocyanate at pH 4.7 and 3.0, respectively (Cantell and Hirvonen 1977). P-IF B preparations are somewhat purer than P-IF A preparations. The main contaminant in P-IF A is albumin. This can be precipitated out of an ethanolic solution of interferon at pH 5.8 with minimal loss of interferon activity (Cantell and Hirvonen 1978). Thus crude human leukocyte interferon can be concentrated 5000-fold and purified over 100-fold on a large scale with over 50% recovery (Cantell and Hirvonen 1978).

2. Human Fibroblast Interferon

The observation that appropriate exposure of poly(I) · poly(C)-induced human, mouse, or rabbit cells to inhibitors of RNA or protein synthesis leads to a paradoxical enhancement of interferon yields (Youngner et al. 1965; Youngner and Hallum 1968; Vilček et al. 1969; Tan et al. 1970; Havell and Vilček 1972; Billiau et al. 1973a) is the basis for current large-scale production of human fibroblast interferon. This phenomenon, termed superinduction (Mcauslan 1963; Garren et al. 1964) was exploited for large-scale interferon production independently by two groups of investigators (Havell and Vilček 1972; Billiau et al. 1973a). Selected strains of diploid human fibroblasts are grown to confluence on a large scale in roller bottles, primed overnight with interferon (100 U/ml) and induced with poly(I) · poly(C) (20–50 µg/ml) in the presence of cycloheximide (50 µg/ ml) for 4 h. Actinomycin D (0.5–2 µg/ml) is then added to cultures for 0.5–2 h at the end of which period the inducer and all the inhibitors are removed, the cultures washed thoroughly with phosphate-buffered saline, and the cultures replenished with medium containing human plasma protein fraction (Cohn fraction V). The interferon produced during the next 24 h is collected, concentrated, and purified. Typically cells are grown in roller bottles (for example, disposable plastic bottles, 10 cm diameter, 490 cm² area) and the cells allowed to produce interferon in 20 ml medium containing human plasma protein (0.45 mg/ml). The average interferon yield is approximately 0.4×10^6 U for each 490 cm² bottle (750 U/cm²); (Billiau et al. 1979a). Human fibroblast interferon can be further concentrated and purified to a specific activity of 10^6–10^7 U/mg protein by fractional precipitation with ammonium sulfate, adsorption on controlled pore glass (Edy et al. 1977), affinity chromatography on zinc iminodiacetate–sepharose (Edy et al. 1977), or affinity chromatography on concanavalin A–agarose and other hydrophobic adsorbent columns (Davey et al. 1976; Sulkowski et al. 1976), or combinations of these procedures (Carter and Horoszewicz 1978; Billiau et al. 1979a).

The replacement of actinomycin D with a reversible inhibitor of hnRNA and mRNA synthesis such as 5,6-dichloro-1-β-D-ribofuranosylbenzimidazole (DRB) in the superinduction protocol has allowed the same culture of human diploid cells to be used for interferon production at least four times at weekly intervals with the same high yield of interferon in each cycle (SEHGAL et al. 1975 a, 1976 a; WIRANOWSKA-STEWART et al. 1977). Repeated superinduction of the same culture of diploid human cells which have a limited life span may help to economize human fibroblast interferon production.

3. Human Lymphoblastoid Interferon

STRANDER and his colleagues observed that several human Burkitt's lymphoma cell lines, when induced with Newcastle disease virus or Sendai virus, produced large amounts of interferon (STRANDER et al. 1974). The Namalva cell line produced the highest interferon yields. The continuous Namalva cell line grown in suspension cultures is now one of the major sources of human interferon (BRIDGEN et al. 1977; FINTER and BRIDGEN 1978; ZOON et al. 1978). These cells have been grown in suspension culture up to densities of 4×10^6 cells/ml in medium supplemented with 10% fetal bovine serum (ZOON et al. 1978) or 1% (w/v) bovine serum albumin (ZOON et al. 1979 b) and induced with Sendai or Newcastle disease virus at a high multiplicity (25 hemagglutinating units/10^6 cells) for 16–24 h at 35°–37 °C. Interferon yields reach a maximum approximately 12–16 h after induction. Approximateley 1–2×10^6 U interferon are produced for every 10^9 cells (ZOON et al. 1979 b). Interferon from lymphoblastoid cells can be markedly enhanced by treatment of cells with 5-bromodeoxyuridine (TOVEY et al. 1977), butyric acid (ADOLF and SWETLY 1979), and dimethylsulfoxide (ADOLF and SWETLY 1979). Since Namalva cells contain the Epstein–Barr virus genome, human lymphoblastoid interferon will need to be routinely purified to homogeneity (ZOON et al. 1979 b, 1980) before clinical application. In the meantime, it represents an excellent source of large quantities of human interferon for chemical purification and analysis.

4. Alternative Sources

Human buffy coat cells induced with phytohemagglutinin or staphylococcal enterotoxin A yield human γ (immune) interferon (WHEELOCK 1965; JOHNSON 1977; WIRANOWSKA-STEWART et al. 1980). Since human γ interferon may be particularly active as an immunomodulatory and antitumor agent (SONNENFELD et al. 1977; VIRELIZIER et al. 1977), several laboratories have now undertaken to produce this interferon on a large scale from human buffy coats for possible clinical use (WIRANOWSKA-STEWART et al. 1980).

Finally, the successful cloning of several α and β human interferon mRNA species in plasmids (TANIGUCHI et al. 1979, 1980 a, b; NAGATA et al. 1980; DERYNCK et al. 1980; MANTEI et al. 1980; WEISSENBACH et al. 1980) and the expression of at least some of these clones in *E. coli* to yield biologically active human α interferon (NAGATA et al. 1980; MANTEI et al. 1980) provide the basis for a novel procedure for the eventual large-scale production of human interferons. It is likely that several human interferon species will be produced using these techniques.

IV. Characterization

1. Protein Purification and Sequencing

Electrophoresis of native or heat- and urea-denatured interferon preparations in polyacrylamide gels containing sodium dodecylsulfate (SDS) under reducing or nonreducing conditions, followed by elution and assay of biologically active interferon activity from gel slices, has proven to be a powerful tool in the characterization and purification of interferons (Stewart 1974). Furthermore, novel techniques such as affinity chromatography using immobilized monospecific antibody (Sipe et al. 1973; Anfinsen et al. 1974; Tan et al. 1979), hydrophobic affinity chromatography (Huang et al. 1974; Davey et al. 1975), chromatography on lectin (Jankowski et al. 1975; Davey et al. 1976), or poly(U)–sepharose columns (De Maeyer-Guignard et al. 1978), as well as high performance liquid chromatography (Rubinstein et al. 1979) have contributed greatly to the purification of several interferon species.

It is generally considered that interferons are secretory glycoproteins. Evidence for the glycoprotein nature of interferons can be summarized as follows:

1. Interferon preparations exhibit marked charge heterogeneity in isoelectric focusing gels. This heterogeneity can be reduced by treatment of the preparations with various glycosidases or with periodate (Schonne et al. 1970; Dorner et al. 1973; Stewart et al. 1977, 1978; Morser et al. 1978). Furthermore, the heterogeneity returns when such treated interferon preparations are sialylated using sialyl transferases (Dorner et al. 1973). Treatment with glycosidases also reduced the apparent molecular weight of some interferons (Bose et al. 1976). 2. Interferons produced by cells treated with inhibitors of glycosylation such as tunicamycin, 2-deoxyglucose, and glucosamine have a reduced charge heterogeneity together with a lower apparent molecular weight in SDS–polyacrylamide gels (Havell et al. 1977; Fujisawa et al. 1978; Mizrahi et al. 1978; Stewart et al. 1978); 3. At least some pure homogeneous interferon preparations are stainable in acrylamide gels for protein by Coomassie blue and for carbohydrate by the periodic acid–Schiff (PAS) technique (Knight 1976a; De Maeyer-Guignard et al. 1978).

It appears possible that some interferon species are glycosylated to a greater extent than others (De Maeyer-Guignard et al. 1978; Morser et al. 1978; Cabrer et al. 1979). However, it is unclear whether all interferons are glycosylated (Jankowski et al. 1975; Rubinstein et al. 1979). It appears that little, if any, of the carbohydrate on interferon molecules is neccessary for biologic activity in conventional cell culture assays (Bose et al. 1976; Zoon et al. 1979a; Nagata et al. 1980). It is possible that the presence of sugar residues on interferon molecules may have some functional role in vivo.

a) Human Leukocyte (α) Interferons

Interferon preparations obtained from virus-induced human buffy coat cells can be clearly resolved in SDS–polylacrylamide gels into two species with apparent molecular weights of 21,000 and 15–16,000 daltons (Stewart and Desmyter 1975; Bose et al. 1976; Törma and Paucker 1976). The two species of α human interferon have equivalent antiviral activities when assayed on human, bovine, cat, and rabbit cells (GRESSER et al. 1974a; STEWART and DESMYTER 1975; DESMYTER and STEWART 1976; LIN et al. 1978). However, the leading edge of the faster-migrating species (approximately 13,500 daltons) contains interferon that is 100 times more active on bovine and cat cells than on human cells (DESMYTER and STEWART 1976; STEWART and DESMYTER 1975; LIN et al. 1978). This is consistent with the findings of RUBINSTEIN et al. (1979) who have resolved three species of interferon in leukocyte interferon preparations by high-performance liquid chromatography. One of these three components that has been purified to homogeneity has an apparent molecular weight of 17,500 daltons (RUBINSTEIN et al. 1979). Recent cDNA cloning experiments have also revealed the existence of at least three related mRNA sequences in virus-induced leukocytes which code for human α interferon (NAGATA et al. 1980; MANTEI et al. 1980). Human leukocyte interferon preparations also contain trace ($<1\%$) amounts of human β interferon (F or fibroblast type; HAVELL et al. 1975). This activity has not yet been characterized further.

There is suggestive evidence that at least some leukocyte interferons may lack or be poor in carbohydrate. Leukocyte interferons fail to bind to a variety of lectin columns (JANKOWSKI et al. 1975). Carbohydrate residues are undetectable in at least one species of α interferon that has been purified to homogeneity (RUBINSTEIN et al. 1979). Furthermore, the apparent molecular weight of α interferons from leukocytes is not decreased by periodate treatment (STEWART et al. 1977; RUBINSTEIN et al 1979) or when the interferons are produced in the presence of glycosylation inhibitors (STEWART et al. 1977). However, different conclusions have been reached by other investigators (BOSE et al. 1976; STEWART et al. 1977).

Two groups of investigators have purified some of the interferon species present in human leukocyte interferon preparations to homogeneity (LIN and STEWART 1978; RUBINSTEIN et al. 1978, 1979). The specific activities of these pure α interferons are approximately $2-4 \times 10^8$ (RUBINSTEIN et al. 1978, 1979) and 10^9 U/mg protein (LIN and STEWART 1978. RUBINSTEIN et al. (1979) have determined the amino acid composition of the 17,500 daltons human α interferon species purified by them and have found it to be similar to that of murine interferon (CABRER et al. 1979).

b) Human Fibroblast (β) Interferons

Interferon induced in human diploid fibroblast cultures by poly(I)·poly(C) using the superinduction protocol migrates in SDS–polyacrylamide gels as a single peak of activity with an apparent molecular weight in the range 20–25,000 daltons (REYNOLDS and PITHA 1975; KNIGHT 1976a; HAVELL et al. 1977). β Interferon produced in the presence of glycosylation inhibitors has an apparent mobility equivalent to approximately 16,000 daltons (HAVELL et al. 1977) which suggests that this interferon is glycosylated. Chromatographic behavior of β interferon on certain lectin columns supports this conclusion (JANKOWSKI et al. 1975). Furthermore, β interferon when purified to homogeneity reacts positively by the PAS procedure which is specific for glycoproteins (KNIGHT 1976a).

At least three groups of investigators have purified β interferon species to homogeneity; the pure material has a specific activity of $2-5 \times 10^8$ U/mg protein (KNIGHT 1976a; BILLIAU et al. 1979a; TAN et al. 1979). Homogeneous preparations

of human fibroblast (β) interferon have been radioiodinated using the Bolton–
Hunter reagent with the retention of 10%–30% of biologic activity (KNIGHT
1978; BERTHOLD et al. 1978; TAN et al. 1979). Such labeled preparations of interferon may be useful for investigations of the mechanism of interferon binding and
action and for drug disposition studies. KNIGHT et al. (1980) have recently reported
the sequence of the NH_2 terminal 13 amino acid residues of human β interferon
(Fig. 1). This sequence shows limited homology (3 of 13 residues identical) with the
37,000 daltons murine Ehrlich ascites cell interferon (TAIRA et al. 1980; Fig. 1).

Suggestive evidence of heterogeneity of human fibroblast (β) interferon proteins has been reported by DAVEY et al. (1976) and SENUSSI et al. (1979). Recent
mRNA characterization and cDNA cloning experiments provide some evidence to
support this posibility (see Sect. C. IV. 2).

Human fibroblast interferon preparations, produced using poly(I)·poly(C) as
inducer, are almost exclusively of the immunologic F-Type (β) interferon (HAVELL
et al. 1975). However, induction of fibroblast cultures with viral inducers leads to
the synthesis of significant amounts (up to 20%–30%) of the immunologic Le (α)
interferon (HAVELL et al. 1978 b). Thus, virus-induced interferon preparations are
likely to be more heterogeneous than poly(I)·poly(C)-induced fibroblast interferons.

c) Human Lymphoblastoid Interferons

Preparations of human lymphoblastoid interferon induced by Newcastle disease
virus in Namalva cells consist of both the α (leukocyte, 80%–85%) and β (fibroblast, 10%–15%) types of interferons (HAVELL et al. 1978 a). The α activities can
be resolved into two components on SDS–polyacrylamide gels: a major component
of apparent molecular weight 17,500–18,500 daltons and a minor component of
apparent molecular weight 21,500–23,500 daltons (HAVELL et al. 1978 a; ZOON et
al. 1979 a). The major 18,500 daltons component has been purified to homogeneity
and exhibits a specific activity of 2.5×10^8 U/mg protein (ZOON et al. 1979 a). The
NH_2 terminal sequence of the first 20 residues of this protein has been determined
recently (ZOON et al. 1980; Fig. 1). It is interesting to note that the faster-migrating
edge of the 18,500 daltons component contains a protein with a different sequence
(ZOON et al. 1979 a, 1980). It is therefore possible that there may exist at least three
α interferon proteins in virus-induced human lymphoblastoid interferon preparations.

There is a striking sequence homology between the 18,500 daltons component
of Namalva interferon and band C ($M_r = 18,000–22,000$ daltons) of murine Ehrlich
ascites tumor cell interferon (Fig. 1; ZOON et al. 1980; TAIRA et al. 1980). Certain
human lymphoblastoid cell lines spontaneously produce α interferon species. These
interferons do not comigrate on SDS–polyacrylamide gels with Sendai virus-induced α interferons produced by the same cell lines (PICKERING et al. 1980). Thus,
it is possible that there may exist even greater sequence heterogeneity among human α interferons than was originally appreciated.

d) Murine Interferons

Newcastle disease virus-induced murine (L cell) interferons can be usually resolved
into two components on SDS–polyacrylamide gels with apparent molecular

weights of 35,000–40,000 and 22,000–24,000 daltons (STEWART 1974; YAMAMOTO and KAWADE 1976, 1980). Murine interferons have been purified to homogeneity in several laboratories (DE MAEYER-GUIGNARD et al. 1978; KAWAKITA et al. 1978; IWAKURA et al. 1978). DE MAEYER-GUIGNARD et al. (1978) purified virus-induced C-243 cell interferon into two homogeneous species of apparent molecular weights of 35,000 and 22,000 daltons using sequential affinity chromatography on poly(U) and antibody–agarose columns. The 35,000 but not the 22,000 daltons component stained with PAS. The specific activity of each was of the order of 2.5×10^9 U/mg protein.

KAWAKITA et al. (1978) and CABRER et al. (1979) have purified Ehrlich ascites tumor cell interferon and obtained three homogeneous proteins of apparent molecular weights of 33,000 (band A), 26,000 (band B), and 20,000 daltons (band C). The specific activities range between 2 and 3×10^9 U/mg protein. The peptide maps of proteins in bands A and B are similar whereas that of protein in band C is different, at least in part. Figure 1 shows that the NH_2 terminal amino acid sequences of bands A and B are identical whereas that of band C is different (TAIRA et al. 1980). Figure 1 also shows that there is close homology between the NH_2 terminal sequences of band C and one of the human α species, and some homology between the NH_2 terminal sequence of bands A and B and one of the human β species. The difference in the molecular weights between bands A and B can at least in part be explained by unequal glycosylation (CABRER et al. 1979). It is of interest that a 22,000 daltons species of murine interferon (presumably band C) cross-reacts with antibody to human interferons (STEWART and HAVELL 1980).

IWAKURA et al. (1978) and YONEHARA et al. (1980) have described the purification to homogeneity of two components of mouse L cell interferon of apparent molecular weights of 40,000 and 24,000 daltons. These investigators have succeeded in labeling interferons with methionine ^3H and report that the tryptic peptide maps of the two interferons are partially similar.

2. Cloning of cDNA Corresponding to Interferon mRNA Species

Detailed information about the structure of some human interferon species has emerged recently as a result of the successful cloning of interferon mRNA molecules (TANIGUCHI et al. 1979; NAGATA et al. 1980; WEISSENBACH et al. 1980; HOUGHTON et al. 1980). Polyadenylated interferon mRNA species can be translated into biologically active interferons by microinjection into oocytes of *Xenopus laevis* (REYNOLDS et al. 1975; SEHGAL et al. 1977; CAVALIERI et al. 1977a). The oocyte assay is reliable and extremely sensitive. It is the cornerstone of virtually all attempts to characterize and clone interferon mRNA species.

The mRNAs for α and β human interferons are distinct (CAVALIERI et al. 1977a). Nevertheless, mRNA species for human interferons, both α and β, sediment at approximately 12 S in sucrose gradients (SEHGAL et al. 1978a; NAGATA et al. 1980). SEHGAL and SAGAR (1980) have recently resolved the mRNA for human β interferon into two translationally active species of lengths 1300 and 900 bases by electrophoresis in agarose gels (in 6 M urea or in 10 mM methylmercuryhydroxide). Similar electrophoretic analyses of other interferon mRNA species are now under way.

Recent cloning data are consistent with this heterogeneity. TANIGUCHI et al. (1979) have cloned the cDNA of a species of human β interferon mRNA. The cloned DNA of 770 base pairs (Fig. 2) contains a sequence which corresponds to the sequence of the NH$_2$ terminal 13 amino acids determined by KNIGHT et al. (1980). Upstream from this NH$_2$ terminus the nucleotide sequence corresponds to a fairly hydrophobic stretch of another 21 amino acids which would represent the "signal" sequence. The amino acid sequence can be deduced for 166 residues, starting with methionine which represents the first amino acid in the mature protein. Thus the mature polypeptide would correspond to a molecular weight of approximately 16–17,000 daltons, a value which is in agreement with that or deglycosylated human β interferon (HAVELL et al. 1977). Furthermore, the amino acid composition deduced from the nucleotide sequence (TANIGUCHI et al. 1980a) is in close agreement with that determined for the purified protein (KNIGHT et al. 1980).

There is a stretch of 203 residues equivalent to the 3' untranslated region of the mRNA. These data are consistent with recent experiments in which SOREQ et al. (1981) found that approximately 200 residues internal to the poly(A) junction are not necessary for the translational activity of human β interferon mRNA. The 3' untranslated region includes the AATAAA segment found in all eukaryotic mRNA species. HOUGHTON et al. (1980) indicate that this β interferon mRNA species has 72 untranslated residues at the 5' end. Consequently, this molecule has a length of approximately 900 residues. This value corresponds closely to the size of the shorter interferon mRNA observed by SEHGAL and SAGAR (1980). Finally, TANIGUCHI et al. (1980c) have recently also succeeded in synthesizing biologically active human β interferon in E. coli.

WEISSENBACH et al. (1980) have also cloned a species of human β interferon mRNA which has a nucleotide sequence distinct from that of the mRNA cloned by TANIGUCHI et al. (1979, 1980a). Moreover, WEISSENBACH et al. (1980) report that their ^{32}P-labeled cloned DNA hybridizes mainly to polyadenylated RNA of length 1,300 nucleotides (14 S) obtained from induced cells. Thus, the available data suggests that there exist at least two distinct human β interferons.

NAGATA et al. (1980) and MANTEI et al. (1980) have described the successful cloning of at least two distinct sequences corresponding to human α interferons. These investigators have succeeded in obtaining expression of the cloned sequences in E. coli with the production of biologically active human α interferon. Figure 2 illustrates the detailed sequence of one of the α interferon DNA clones (MANTEI et al. 1980) and compares this sequence with a β interferon DNA sequence (TANIGUCHI et al. 1980a, b). The α interferon sequence represents a 910 base pairs DNA insert. This cloned DNA contains a 567 (or 543) base pairs coding sequence which determines a putative pre-interferon polypeptide consisting of a signal peptide of 23 (or less likely 15) amino acids, followed by an interferon polypeptide of 166 amino acids. The coding sequence is followed by a 242 base pairs 3' trailer which contains the AATAAA sequence. A comparison between this α interferon sequence and that determined by ZOON et al. (1980) reveals that the two sequences are distinct. Thus there may exist three or more distinct human α interferons.

Figure 2 also illustrates that the coding sequences of the cDNAs of cloned human α and β interferons show homologies of 45% at the nucleotide level and 29%

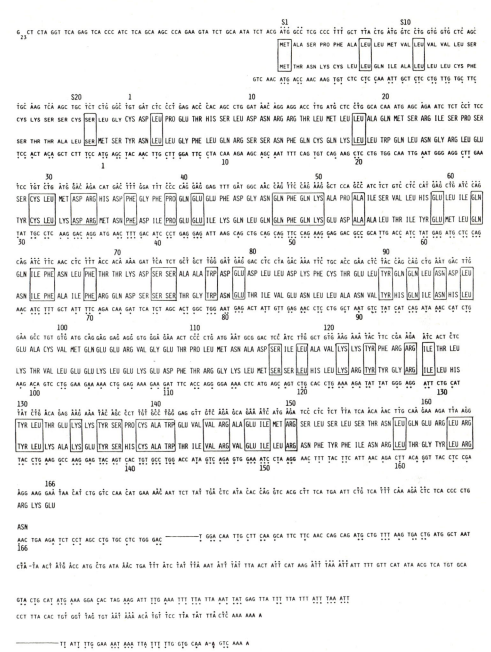

Fig. 2. Comparison of the nucleotide sequences of human leukocyte interferon I (Le-IF I) and human fibroblast interferon cDNA and of the derived amino acid sequences. The sequences are from MANTEI et al. (1980), TANIGUCHI et al. (1980a), and HOUGHTON et al. (1980). They were aligned to give maximal homology without introducing gaps in the coding sequence. Identical amino acids are *framed*, identical nucleotides are marked by *dots*. S1–S23 indicate the amino acids of the putative signal sequence and 1–166 the amino acids of the interferon polypeptides. (Adapted from TANIGUCHI et al. 1980b)

at the amino acid level (TANIGUCHI et al. 1980 b). The amino acid sequences show three domains of homology. The first one, with the least degree of homology, corresponds to the putative signal sequence, which is rich in hydrophobic residues and has 4 identical amino acid positions out of 21 (19%); the second domain, between amino acids 28 and 80 (counted on the α interferon sequence), has 21 identical residues out of 51 (41% homology) and the third, between positions 115 and 151 (α interferon sequence), has 19 out of 35 residues identical (54%). The longest stretches of contiguous conserved amino acids are Gln-Phe-Gln-Lys (positions 47–50 of α and 49–52 of β interferon) and Cys-Ala-Trp (positions 139–141 and 141–143, respectively); the latter sequence is notable because it contains Cys and Trp, which are preferentially conserved in related proteins. The sequence of β interferon cloned by WEISSENBACH et al. (1980) also possesses regions homologous to the stretches of contiguous conserved amino acids illustrated in Fig. 2 (M. REVEL, personal communication). It is quite likely that at least some of the conserved amino acids are essential for a function common to α and β interferons, perhaps the induction of the virus-resistant state in the target cell. These findings may provide guidelines for the tailoring of modified and possibly shorter polypeptides possessing specific activities of interferon.

The α interferon polypeptide synthesized in *E. coli* (NAGATA et al. 1980) is clearly unglycosylated and yet exhibits full biologic activity. Recent evidence suggests that this *E. coli* interferon comigrates in SDS–polyacrylamide gels with the leading edge of the faster-migrating peak of activity in human leukocyte interferon preparations (STEWART et al. 1980). Furthermore, in a manner analogous to authentic 13,500 daltons α interferon, the *E. coli* product is far more active on heterologous bovine and feline cells than on human cells.

The synthesis of biologically active interferons in *E. coli* clearly demonstrates that glycosylation is not required for the function of either α or β interferons in cell culture. Whether glycosylation is required for clinical efficacy of α or β interferons is an open question. Finally, the extensive heterogeneity of human interferons uncovered by recent investigations suggests that it may be necessary to evaluate each of these species for biologic functions and clinical efficacy.

V. Mechanisms of Interferon Induction

1. General Comments

Interferon production can be induced in vertebrate cells by a large variety of viral and nonviral stimuli. Despite the diversity of systems investigated, several general features of the induction mechanism have emerged (reviewed in STEWART 1979). Interferon production requires a cell capable of RNA and protein synthesis. This requirement reflects the synthesis of interferon mRNA in the cell nucleus and its translation in the cytoplasm in order to yield interferon. Following viral induction there is usually a lag of several hours before interferon appears in the cell culture medium and interferon production lasts approximately 24–28 h. Following induction with nonviral stimuli such as poly(I)·poly(C), interferon appears in the culture medium within 1–2 h of induction and its production terminates by 6–8 h. Thus, as a general rule the production of interferon takes place for a limited time. The levels of extractable cellular interferon mRNA usually correlate closely with the observed rate of interferon production. Interferon production is usually sensitive to inhibition by inhibitors of mRNA synthesis if the inhibitors are added at the same time as or shortly after the inducer. This reflects an inhibition of interferon mRNA transcription. Interferon production is usually resistant to inhibition by inhibitors of mRNA synthesis of these drugs are added once interferon production has begun. These observations lead to the important conclusion that, following induction, the interferon genes are transcribed only for a limited period of time. Subsequent to an initial triggering event, the continued presence of the inducer is not required nor does its presence affect the induction process. In this sense interferon induction is different from steroidal induction mechanisms.

The biochemical basis for interferon induction is unknown at the present time. Conceptually, interferon induction is thought of as a derepression of interferon genes. Various attempts have been made to elucidate some of the events leading to this derepression. While limited progress has been made in this direction, this area of research calls for much additional work. Clearly, an elucidation of the biochemical events underlying interferon induction would contribute greatly to our understanding of the regulation of gene expression in eukaryotic cells. In the next several sections we shall review information concerning interferon induction by viral and nonviral stimuli, evaluate data pertaining to the genetics of interferon induction, and discuss recent attempts to isolate and characterize interferon mRNA species. We shall also review phenomena such as priming, hyporesponsiveness, and superinduction that modify interferon production. Investigations of these phenomena have provided remarkable insights into the versatility with which interferon production is regulated.

2. Interferon Induction by Viral Inducers

A very large number of viruses have been reported to induce interferon under various experimental conditions. A recent review listed as many as 179 examples (STEWART 1979) and further observations continue at an unabated pace. An important motivation in many of these investigations is the view that collation of data from numerous virus–host systems, as well as investigations of interferon induction by selected viral mutants, may help pinpoint specific events in the induction mechanism.

Various viruses such as influenza, Sendai, Newcastle disease, bluetongue, and Semliki Forest viruses, and reoviruses, are usually considered good inducers of interferon. Others, such as adenoviruses, vesicular stomatitis virus, and picornaviruses, are conventionally considered poor inducers. Unfortunately, no generalizations have emerged because of great variation among strains of the same virus; as well as great differences in interferon induction by the same virus in cells of different species. For example, strains of Newcastle disease virus differ greatly in their inducing potential (HO et al. 1970; STEWART 1979). Some strains of rabies virus are poor inducers in human or rabbit cell cultures (WIKTOR et al. 1964; FERNANDES et al. 1964), but are good inducers in hamsters (Stewart and Sulkin 1966). Whereas vesicular stomatitis virus (VSV) is generally considered a poor inducer of interferon (Vilček et al. 1977), a particular defective interfering particle of VSV which contains ± snapback RNA (D1–011) is an efficient inducer in human and chick cells at a multiplicity of one particle for each cell(Marcus and Sekellick 1977). However, at higher multiplicities interferon yields are lower. Also, the presence of ± snapback RNA in VSV particles does not always correlate with the relative potency in interferon induction (Frey et al. 1979). Perhaps the only generalization to emerge so far is that a good viral inducer causes minimal inhibition of cellular RNA and protein synthesis. Inactivation of a live virus by ultraviolet (UV) irradiation, by heat, or by hydroxylamine generally enhances its ability to induce interferon in a cell system in which the virus would otherwise cause a rapid cytocidal infection (Gandhi and Burke 1970).

An important question in any discussion of interferon induction by viruses is the following: does the compound responsible for interferon induction already exist in the virions or is it synthesized during the course of viral transcription and replication? An evaluation of this is highly colored by the fact that synthetic or natural double-stranded RNA is a potent interferon inducer. At the present time it appears that in some instances the input virion contains the inducer (Marcus and Sekellick 1977; Henderson and Joklik 1978), whereas in other instances expression of viral functions is necessary to induce interferon (Stewart 1979; Kohase and Vilček 1979). Even in one and the same system, e.g., induction of interferon in human fibroblasts by Newcastle disease virus, "early" interferon production appears to be due to molecules preexisting in the virions whereas "late" interferon production requires the expression of viral functions (Kohase and Vilček 1979). Kohase and Vilček (1979) observed that the ability to induce early interferon production was far more resistant to inactivation by UV irradiation and to treatment with hydroxylamine than was viral infectivity, whereas late interferon production was approximately as sensitive to inactivation as was viral infectivity. The issue is complicated even further by a striking observation concerning the interferon-inducing ability of UV-irradiated reovirus (Lai and Joklik 1973). A group C mutant, ts447, which is essentially unable to synthesize progeny double-stranded (ds)RNA and which cannot induce interferon at the nonpermissive temperature (38 °C), is an excellent inducer of interferon at the nonpermissive temperature if irradiated with UV light (Lai and Joklik 1973). A similar phenomenon is also observed with wild-type (wt) reovirus (Henderson and Joklik 1978). UV irradiation increases the ability of wt virus to induce interferon approximately 200-fold, whereas that of ts 447 is increased by more than 10,000-fold. It appears that UV irradiation of the virus causes changes in the virion capsid structure such that parental dsRNA can then directly function as an interferon inducer.

An investigation of the ability of specific virus mutants to induce interferon is, in principle, an attractive method for pinpointing specific viral functions involved in interferon induction. Following the discovery of synthetic dsRNA (Field et al. 1967), it was thought that the intracellular formation of dsRNA as replicative forms or intermediates may correlate with the ability to induce interferon at least by RNA-containing viruses. However, numerous studies with ts mutants of various RNA-containing viruses (Semliki Forest virus, Sindbis virus, reovirus) have failed to correlate the ability to induce interferon with the ability to synthesize viral RNA (LOCKART et al. 1968; LOMNICZI and BURKE 1970; LAI and JOKLIK 1973; AT-KINS et al. 1974; ATKINS and LANCASHIRE 1976; TARODI et al. 1977). In fact, these investigations have failed to attribute interferon induction definitively to any specific viral function. Furthermore, mutants of measles virus have been isolated that are identical to the *wt* virus in all other respects except that they are unable to induce interferon (McKIMM and RAPP 1977a, b).

An additional level of complexity has recently been added to discussions of interferon induction by viruses. Different viruses induce different interferon species in different proportions in different cells. For example, after induction of lymphoblastoid cells (Namalva line) with Newcastle disease virus (NDV), the bulk of interferon produced is α interferon, with β interferon accounting for less than 20% of total activity (HAVELL et al. 1978a). In contrast, induction of any of several strains of human fibroblasts with NDV, results in the production of a large amount of β interferon and only a relatively small amount of α interferon (HAVELL et al. 1978b). The relative amount of α interferon produced depends on the cell strain used as well as the multiplicity of infection (HAYES et al. 1979). The highest yields of α interferon were produced when the GM-258 cell strain which is trisomic for chromosome 21 is induced with NDV. However, several other lines with trisomy 21 were not high producers of α interferon. The diploid cell strain, FS-4, also produced relatively small quantities of α interferon. Proportionately more α interferon was produced in cells inoculated with NDV at a low multiplicity of infection. Clearly, the mechanisms of interferon induction by viruses are rather complex.

3. Interferon Induction by Synthetic Polynucleotides

The discovery by FIELD and his co-workers that synthetic and natural dsRNA species (FIELD et al. 1967) are potent inducers of interferon led to expectations that a careful analysis of the structure–activity relationships with these synthetic inducers would go a long way to help pinpoint the biochemical bases for interferon induction. Although several generalizations about the structure–activity relationships have emerged (DECLERCQ 1977), these have not yet provided a clue as to the underlying mechanism of interferon induction. In brief summary, these generalizations are: a good inducer is a double-stranded RNA molecule (as opposed to single- and triple-stranded RNA and double-stranded DNA) of sufficiently high molecular weight ($>$ 100,000 daltons), that possesses relatively high thermal stability, is resistant to degradation by nucleases, has free 2′-OH groups in both strands of the dsRNA, and possesses an intact purine ring (with N-1, N-3, N-7, N-9; reviewed in DECLERCQ 1977). Despite considerable effort to develop more efficient interferon inducers, poly(I)·poly(C) remains the most potent inducer available when used either alone or complexed with DEAE-dextran (FIELD et al. 1967; STEWART 1979). The length of the poly(I) chain appears to be more critical than that of the poly(C) chain (DECLERCQ 1974). A T_m value $>$ 60 °C (in 0.15 M Na$^+$) appears necessary but not sufficient for maximal interferon-inducing activity. A greater degree of substitution is tolerated in the poly(C) strand than in the poly(I) strand. Substitution of bromine at C-5 and of sulfur at C-2 of cytosine does not markedly affect the interferon-inducing activity of poly(I) · poly(C) (reviewed in DECLERCQ 1977). Some exceptions to these rules have emerged. Some batches of single-stranded poly(I) are effective inducers of interferon, although their effectiveness varies considerably from one cell system to the next (DECLERCQ et al. 1978). Replacement of the 2′-OH of the poly(I) chain by azido groups does not alter the interferon-inducing ability of poly(I) · poly(C). It appears that this replacement does not alter the secondary structure of poly(I) · poly(C). Antiserum prepared against poly(I) · poly(br^{5}C), a potent interferon inducers, displays a spectrum of immunospecific cross-reactivity with other synthetic dsRNA species which parallels the ability of these dsRNA species to induce interferon (JOHNSTON and STOLLAR 1978). This correlation is not seen with antisera raised against poly(A) · poly(U); poly(A) · poly (m2′U); and poly(c^{7}A) · poly(rT). Antiserum to poly(I) · poly(br^{5}C) reacts equally well with poly(I) · poly(C) as with the 2′-azide-substitued molecules (DECLERCQ et al. 1978). Thus, this antiserum recognizes a structure in the latter synthetic dsRNA species which may be responsible for triggering the induction of interferon. A careful comparison of the ability of various synthetic dsRNA species to induce interferon and to inhibit protein synthesis in cell-free lysates indicates that the fine structural requirements for interferon induction and for inhibition of protein synthesis are not identical (CONTENT et al. 1978; TORRENCE and FRIEDMAN 1979).

Certain mismatched analogs of poly(I) · poly(C) such as poly(I) · poly(C$_{13}$,U) and poly(I) · poly(C$_{20}$,G) are hydrolyzed 5–8 times faster than poly(I) · poly(C), but are quite effective in inducing interferon production (CARTER et al. 1972). It has been suggested that the mismatched analogs may have lowered toxicity as a result of more rapid degradation (O'MALLEY et al. 1979). However, poly(I) · poly(C), which is degraded rapidly in primates, does not adequately induce interferon. For this reason LEVY et al. (1975) have developed a complex of poly(I) · poly(C) with poly-L-lysine and carboxymethylcellulose, poly(ICLC), which imparts a greater resistance to nucleolytic attack and thus renders poly(I) · poly(C) an efficient inducer of interferon in a wide range of animal species (OLSEN et al. 1976, 1978), including primates (LEVY et al. 1975, 1976; STEPHEN et al. 1977b; SAMMONS et al. 1977). Poly(ICLC) is currently under investigation in humans.

How does poly(I) · poly(C) trigger interferon induction? There are ample data from cell culture experiments that exposure of cells to poly(I) · poly(C) leads to the appearance of interferon in the culture medium, usually within 1–2 h from the beginning of induction, that the rate of interferon production peaks by 3–4 h, and that interferon production is rapidly shut off by 6–10 h (reviewed in STEWART 1979; Fig. 3). Despite a certain amount of temporal variation in different cell types, the induction of interferon by poly(I) · poly(C) is clearly a rapid event. An exposure of diploid human fibroblast (FS-4 strain) cell cultures to poly(I) · poly(C) for 1–5 min at 37 °C suffices to induce a normal yield of interferon (VENGRIS et al. 1975; SEHGAL and TAMM 1980b; and unpublished work; J. VILČEK, personal communication). It has been estimated that the transcription of interferon mRNA begins within 10–20 min after FS-4 cells have been exposed to poly(I) · poly(C) (SEHGAL and TAMM 1980b). Thus, the events which trigger interferon induction are likely to occur within the first 10–20 min of exposure to the inducer.

Various investigators have suggested that poly(I) · poly(C) triggers interferon induction by binding to sites on the cell membrane (VENGRIS et al. 1975; BACHNER et al. 1975). The main basis for this suggestion is the observation that sepharose-bound poly(I) · poly(C) functions as an efficient inducer of interferon (BACHNER et al. 1975). Furthermore, it appears that the initial binding reaction can be separated from the later step of interferon induction by incubating cells at 4 °C (BAUSEK and MERIGAN 1969) and exposing them to antiserum against poly(I) · poly(C) (VENGRIS et al. 1975) or to high concentrations of salt (JOHNSTON et al. 1976). Nevertheless, this issue is controversial because of: (a) the report by HUTCHINSON and MERIGAN (1975) of leakage of dsRNA from poly(I) · poly(C) bound to insoluble supports; (b) the inability to distinguish between nonspecific and specific cell membrane binding of the inducer (KOHNO et al. 1975; JOHNSTON et al. 1976); (c) the ability of poly(I) · poly(C) to induce interferon when dsRNA is delivered directly into the cellular cytoplasmic compartment using liposomes as vehicles for delivery (MAGEE et al. 1976; MAYHEW et al. 1977). Since viral dsRNA is generated intracellularly and, in at least some cases does function as the inducing molecule (HENDERSON and JOKLIK 1978), it appears that cell surface binding of dsRNA is not an obligatory step in the induction mechanism.

The events that intervene between the appearance of poly(I) · poly(C) in the cellular environment and the switching on of interferon mRNA transcription are obscure. It does appear that poly(I) · poly(C) induces not just interferon, but numerous other proteins as well (RAJ and PITHA 1979; WEISSENBACH et al. 1980).

4. Interferon Induction by Other Stimuli

Very little information is available about the mechanisms of interferon induction by immune stimuli, by exposure to various high molecular weight substances – preparations derived from *C. parvum*, *Nocardia*, carrageenan, or tumor cells, or preparations of staphylococcal enterotoxin A or phytohemagglutinin, or low molecular weight substances – tilorone, 2-amino-5-iodo-6-phenyl-4-pyrimidinol (AIPP) – or others. A generalization that does emerge is that inducers act on cells of specific phenotypes. Thus, several of these agents are able to induce interferon in vivo, but fail to do so in cell culture, perhaps because the cultured cells used no longer possess the phenotype and functional capabilities of the target cells that exist in vivo, or because the cells responding in vivo are not present in cultures in vitro.

The low molecular weight inducers such as AIPP represent a promising avenue of basic research. AIPP induces interferon in thymic explants from mice (HAMILTON et al. 1980). This compound rapidly enters the target cells, as demonstrated by following the fate of radioactively labeled AIPP (R. D. HAMILTON, personal communication). Radioactively labeled AIPP could be used as a tool in searching for selective ligand-binding protein which may be involved in interferon induction, much in the manner of steroid-binding proteins. This could go a long way in elucidating the mechanism for interferon induction. Finally, there exist several cell lines which produce low levels of interferon in the absence of any apparent stimulus (HENLE and HENLE 1965; reviewed in STEWART 1979). Investigation of cell lines which spontaneously produce interferon represents another area of interferon research that could be highly informative if pursued in depth.

5. Genetics of Interferon Induction

Investigations of the genetic basis of interferon induction have revealed that this phenomenon is complex. Furthermore, the interpretation of some of the key data is controversial. The earliest attempt to analyze interferon induction from a classical genetic standpoint was initiated by De Maeyer and De Maeyer-Guignard (1979 b). These investigators made use of two inbred mouse strains, the BALB/c and C57BL/6, together with the seven recombinant inbred and various congenic lines derived by Bailey (1971) from these two strains (reviewed in De Maeyer and De Maeyer-Guignard 1979 b). The ability to induce interferon in mouse strains by intravenous inoculation of Newcastle disease virus (NDV), Sendai virus, and murine mammary tumor virus (MMTV) was investigated. NDV induces a ten-fold higher level of serum interferon in C57BL/6 than in BALB/c mice. This phenotype defines the autosomal *If*-1 locus. Similarly, the *IF*-2 locus is responsible for a three-fold higher level of response by C57BL/6 mice to MMTV, while two loci (*If*-3 and *If*-4) are responsible for a ten-fold higher level of circulating interferon induced by Sendai virus in C57BL/6 mice. Thus, different genes appear to be involved in interferon induction by different inducers.

The *If*-1 phenotype can be reproduced in cultures of peritoneal macrophages derived from *If*-1^l (BALB/c) and *If*-1^h (C57BL/6) mouse strains and induced with NDV (De Maeyer et al. 1979). Unfortunately, the complexity of interferon induction is such that mouse embryo fibroblast cultures derived from these same strains induced with NDV do not exhibit the *If*-1 phenotype.

Virelizier and Gresser (1978) have determined that the resistance of C3H and A/J mice to mouse hepatitis virus 3 is due to interferon. Similarly, Haller et al. (1979, 1980) have determined that the genetically based resistance of certain mouse strains (A2G mice having an Mx/Mx locus) to influenza virus is related to interferon, but in this instance it appears that the genetic resistance resides in the greater sensitivity of macrophages derived from resistant mice to interferon. An unusual aspect of these results is that enhanced sensitivity to interferon action is observed only when cells are infected with influenza virus and not when vesicular stomatitis virus or encephalomyocarditis virus is used.

Somatic cell genetics has been used in attempts to map the chromosomal localization of genes coding for human α and β interferons. Tan et al. (1974 b) tested 40 human–mouse cell hybrids for interferon induction with NDV and poly(I)·poly(C), and concluded that both chromosomes 2 and 5 were necessary for induction of β interferon by either inducer. Slate and Ruddle (1979), using human–mouse and human–hamster hybrids, concluded that either chromosome 2 or 5 alone was sufficient for induction of β interferon. More recently Meager et al. (1979 a, b) have also investigated this issue and have concluded that genes on chromosome 5 are *not* required for interferon induction. While these investigators could not rule out contributions from chromosome 2, they concluded that one or more genes on chromosome 9 was involved in the production of human β interferon. Two additional problems cloud the issues even further. It is unclear whether a diploid cell possesses genes for interferon induction on each of chromosomes 2, 5, and 9 or whether there exists heterogeneity in this regard, with some cell strains possessing genes which reside only on one or the other chromosome. Furthermore, all cell hybrids derived from human leukocytes fail to produce α interferon in cell culture (SLATE and RUDDLE 1979). Thus, the localizations of the genes for human α interferon are unknown.

Against this backdrop some attempts have been made to use somatic cell genetics to investigate the regulation of interferon production and action (FRANKFORT et al. 1978; SLATE and RUDDLE 1979; GRAVES and MEAGER 1980). While several interesting observations have emerged, the data are contradictory and of limited value at the present time.

6. Characterization of Interferon mRNA Species and Their Transcription Units

Exposure of cells to interferon inducers results in the rapid appearance of interferon mRNA in induced cells. Several procedures are now available to assay translationally active interferon mRNA. Translation of interferon mRNA applied to cultures of intact heterologous cells using various procedures to enhance the uptake of RNA was the earliest technique used (DE MAEYER-GUIGNARD et al. 1972; ORLOVA et al. 1974; MONTAGNIER et al. 1974; REYNOLDS and PITHA 1974; KRONEN-BERG and FRIEDMANN 1975; GREENE et al. 1978). This procedure results in a low yield of biologically active interferon. Translation of interferon mRNA in a cell-free system into biologically active interferon was first described in 1975 (THANG et al. 1975; PESTKA et al. 1975; REYNOLDS et al. 1975). Although the yield of interferon activity in cell-free systems is variable and inconsistent (SEHGAL et al. 1977), this technique has found occasional use by some investigators (LEBLEU et al. 1978; WEISSENBACH et al. 1979). The discovery by REYNOLDS et al. (1975) that microinjection of polyadenylated mRNA preparations into oocytes of *Xenopus laevis* results in the synthesis of large amounts of interferon was a landmark contribution to this area of research. The *Xenopus* oocyte assay has proven to be a reliable and extremely sensitive assay for interferon mRNA (SEHGAL et al. 1977; CAVALIERI et al. 1977a).

Murine and human interferon mRNA species are polyadenylated RNA molecules (reviewed in STEWART 1979). Evidence for the existence of poly(A)-free interferon mRNA is unconvincing (MONTAGNIER et al. 1974). As would be expected, interferon mRNA is membrane associated in cells (ABREU and BANCROFT 1978). In sucrose gradients, most interferon mRNA species sediment between 10 and 14 S (REYNOLDS and PITHA 1974; SEHGAL et al. 1978a; LEBLEU et al. 1980; MORSER et al. 1979; BERGER et al. 1980; PANG et al. 1980) and have a poly(A) length of more than 100 residues (SEHGAL et al. 1978a). Two species of human β interferon mRNA of length 900 and 1300 bases can be resolved in agarose gels under fully denaturing conditions (SEHGAL and SAGAR 1980). The longer species is 2–10 fold more abundant than the shorter RNA. It appears that the longer RNA may correspond to clone A341 of WEISSENBACH et al. (1980) and that the shorter RNA corresponds to clone TpIF319 of TANIGUCHI et al. (1979, 1980a). The entire nucleotide sequence of a human β interferon mRNA molecule corresponding to clone TpIF319 is now known (Fig. 2; TANIGUCHI et al. 1980a, b; HOUGHTON et al. 1980). Thus the short β interferon mRNA consists of 836 residues excluding the 3′-terminal poly(A) (see Fig. 2 for full sequence). This sequence corresponds to the NH$_2$ terminal amino acid sequence of a species of β (fibroblast) interferon as determined by KNIGHT et al. (1980).

Two populations of human α interferon mRNA derived from lymphoblastoid cells can be resolved on sucrose gradients (Morser et al. 1979; Berger et al. 1980; Pickering et al. 1980). The predominant population sediments at 12–13 S, whereas a small but clearly detectable population of molecules sediments at approximately 18 S. These two populations can also be resolved by electrophoresis in methylmercury–agarose gels in addition to a third species of mRNA for a β interferon (Sagar et al. 1981). Furthermore, at least two distinct sets of clones differing in nucleotide sequences have been obtained from the 12 S RNA population derived from induced human leukocytes (Nagata et al. 1980; Mantei et al. 1980). Both α and β interferon mRNAs derived from the same cell type (GM-248 human fibroblasts; Namalva) appear to differ in length (Pang et al., 1980; Sagar et al. 1981). Murine interferon mRNA also sediments in sucrose gradients, predominantly in the 12–13 S region (Lebleu et al. 1978). In addition, a population of murine interferon mRNA of length corresponding to approximately 18 S has been resolved in methylmercury–agarose gels (Sagar et al. 1981). This is reminiscent of early results obtained by Montagnier et al. (1974) in this system.

The reasons for the heterogeneity in interferon mRNA species is obscure. These multiple mRNA molecules may represent the products of transcription of distinct interferon genes or they may arise from alternative pathways of processing long precursor RNA species. A target size analysis using UV irradiation indicates that the transcription unit for human β interferon mRNA species is of a size between 4,000 and 11,000 bases and 11 kb (Sehgal and Tamm 1980b). This observation constitute the first evidence that there exist long RNA molecules which represent precursors to interferon mRNA. Recent success in cloning interferon cDNA sequences suggests that there will be rapid progress in the near future in defining the structure and nucleotide sequences of interferon genes.

VI. The Regulation of Interferon Production

The regulation of interferon production is complex. Numerous experimental factors alter interferon yields in ways that are not yet clearly understood. Nevertheless, sufficient information is available to delineate certain fundamental aspects of transcriptional and posttranscriptional regulation of interferon production as a prelude towards the elucidation of the regulation of expression of interferon genes in mammalian cells.

So far, only limited attempts have been made to investigate the regulation of interferon production using mutant cell lines that display an altered interferon induction phenotype. Tan and Berthold (1977) have described interferon induction in a cell line (line 108) derived from SV40-transformed human WI-38 cells. Line 108 is an exceptionally good interferon producer and contains several copies of chromosome 5. Exposure of cell cultures of line 108 to inhibitors of macromolecular synthesis such as cycloheximide, 2-(4-methyl-2,6-dinitrovanilino)-N-methyl-propionamide (MDMP) and 5,6-dichloro-1-β-D-ribofuranosylbenzimidazole (DRB), in the absence of any interferon inducer, by itself results in the production of significant amounts of interferon. These findings lead to the suggestion that the induction of human interferon may be mediated by a reduction in the critical concentration of rapidly turning over repressor (or repressors) which normally re-

Table 2. Agents which affect interferon production

Agent	Reference
Enhancement	
Interferon	Isaacs and Burke (1958)
5-Bromodeoxyuridine	Tovey et al. (1977)
	Baker et al. (1979)
5-Iodo-2-deoxyuridine	Klein and Vilček (1980)
Polyene macrolides	Borden et al. (1978)
Amphotericin B and its methylester	
Nystatin	
Filipin	
Calcium salts	Booth and Borden (1978)
	Meager et al. (1978)
Insulin	Azuma et al. (1978)
Dibutyryl cGMP	Yoshida et al. (1978)
DEAE-dextran	Dianzani et al. (1968)
	Trapman (1979)
Short chain fatty acids	Adolf and Swetly (1979)
Acetic acid	
Propionic acid	
N-Butyric acid	
N-Valeric acid	
N-Caproic acid	
Isobutyric acid	
Hexamethylene bis-acetamide	Adolf and Swetly (1979)
Dimethylsulfoxide	Adolf and Swetly (1979)
Phorbolmyristate acetate	Klein and Vilček (1980)
Ascorbic acid	Siegel (1975)
Theophylline	Reizin et al. (1975)
Inhibition	
Interferon	Vilček (1962)
Vinblastine	Havell and Vilček (1975)
Adrenaline	Reizin et al. (1975)
Retinoic acid	Blalock and Gifford (1976)
Cytochalasin D	Ito et al. (1976)
Cycloleucine	P. B. Sehgal, unpublished work

presses the interferon gene in uninduced cells. The repressor or repressors in line 108 may turn over more rapidly than in other diploid cell strains. Burke et al. (1978) have observed that undifferentiated murine teratocarcinoma cells (lines 247-DEScl$_2$, 299-3; OC15S1) cannot be induced to produce interferon whereas differentiated cells (lines T-76-12 A and B; PYS-2; SV40-Cl$_2$; OC15S1 following differentiation in culture) can be so induced. This finding is of interest because undifferentiated murine teratocarcinoma cells are unable to splice certain mRNA precursor molecules in the nucleus and thus fail to allow expression of these mRNA species (Segal et al. 1979; Segal and Khoury 1979). Differentiated cells acquire this splicing function. These cells may represent an excellent system for the investigation of the role of RNA splicing in the expression of interferon genes. Finally,

Table 3. Agents known to cause superinduction of interferon production

Agent	Interferon superinduction[a]		Reference
	Cell cultures	Animals	
Inhibitors of RNA synthesis			
Actinomycin D	+		Ho and KONO (1965)
			VILČEK et al. (1969)
5,6-Dichloro-1-β-D-ribo-furanosylbenzimidazole (DRB)	+	ND	SEHGAL et al. (1975a)
5-(or 6-)Bromo-4,5(or 5,7)-dichloro-1-β-D-ribofuranosyl-benzimidazole (MBDRB)	+	ND	TAMM and SEHGAL (1977)
5,6-Dibromo-1-β-D-ribo-furanosylbenzimidazole	+	ND	TAMM and SEHGAL (1977)
Camptothecin	+	ND	ATHERTON and BURKE (1978)
α-Amanitin	+	ND	ATHERTON and BURKE (1978)
3-Deazaadenosine	+	ND	P. B. SEHGAL, unpublished work
Inhibitors of protein synthesis			
Cycloheximide	+	+	YOUNGNER et al. (1965)
			VILČEK (1960)
Puromycin	+	+	YOUNGNER et al. (1965)
			VILČEK (1960)
Acetoxycycloheximide	ND	+	YOUNGNER (1970)
Streptovitacin A	ND	+	YOUNGNER (1970)
Streptimidone	ND	+	YOUNGNER et al. (1970)
Tenuazonic acid	ND	+	YOUNGNER et al. (1970)
Pactamycin	+	ND	VILČEK and NG (1971)
Emetine	+	ND	TAN et al. (1971)
Trichodermin	+	ND	ATHERTON and BURKE (1978)
Oxytetracycline	+	ND	ATHERTON and BURKE (1978)
p-Fluorophenylalanine	+	ND	ATHERTON and BURKE (1978)
Other inhibitors			
UV irradiation	+	ND	MOZES and VILČEK (1974)
			LINDNER-FRIMMEL (1974)
Neutral red	+	ND	SEHGAL et al. (1975b)
Chloroquine	+	ND	SEHGAL et al. (1975b)

[a] Symbols indicate: + active; ND not done

an attempt has been made to characterize and investigate mutant murine 3T6 cells which are engaged in the semiconstitutive synthesis of interferon (JARVIS and COLBY 1978; JARVIS et al. 1978). Such mutants may prove valuable in delineating the genetic elements involved in the repression of interferon genes.

Various agents enhance or inhibit interferon yields (Tables 2, 3). The enhancing agents listed in Table 2 appear to act at the transcriptional level or posttranscriptional nuclear RNA processing level, while several of those listed in Table 3, in addition to affecting interferon mRNA transcription, markedly enhance the stability of interferon mRNA. The inhibitors of interferon production listed in Table 2 do not inhibit interferon yields by inhibiting RNA or protein synthesis, but rather by affecting production in a more subtle manner. Terms such as "priming", "blocking", "hyporesponsiveness", and "superinduction" are used widely in the interferon literature. "Priming" refers to a phenomenon in which cell cultures exposed to low concentrations of interferon produce higher interferon yields when subsequently exposed to an inducer (ISAACS and BURKE 1958; reviewed in STEWART 1979). "Blocking" refers to a phenomenon in which cell cultures exposed to high concentrations of interferon exhibit reduced interferon yields following subsequent induction (VILČEK 1962; VILČEK and RADA 1962). "Hyporesponsiveness" describes a decreased responsiveness with respect to interferon production when cell cultures (CANTELL and PAUCKER 1963; BURKE and BUCHAN 1965) or animals (HO et al. 1965; YOUNGNER and STINEBRING 1965) are reexposed to an interferon inducer. "Superinduction" refers to the paradoxical enhancement of interferon yields by the appropriate use of inhibitors of RNA or protein synthesis (YOUNGNER et al. 1965; YOUNGNER and STINEBRING 1965; VILČEK et al. 1969; TAN et al. 1970). While the biochemical bases for blocking and hyporesponsiveness (BILLIAU 1970; BORDEN and MURPHY 1971; BARMAK and VILČEK 1973; BREINIG et al. 1975; KOHASE and VILČEK 1977) are still quite obscure, some information about the biochemical correlates of priming and superinduction is now available.

1. Priming

Cell cultures respond to priming by interferon in two distinct ways. In some primed systems, e.g., induction of L cells by MM virus or by NDV (LEVY et al. 1966; STEWART et al. 1971) there may not only be an increase in interferon yields, but interferon is produced earlier than usual. Another kind of response is seen in rabbit kidney cultures (BARMAK and VILČEK 1973) and human cell strains (HAVELL and VILČEK 1972; BILLIAU et al. 1973a; KOHASE and VILČEK 1979; SEHGAL and GUPTA 1980) in which the usual response to the inducer is very rapid to begin with. In these instances, priming enhances interferon yields without any detectable alteration in the kinetics of interferon production.

The effects of priming mouse cells with interferon on the production of interferon and its mRNA were investigated by ABREU et al. (1979). Interferon-primed mouse L cells produced 3–10 times more interferon than did unprimed cells following induction with NDV. Interferon appeared 2–4 h sooner in primed cultures than in unprimed cultures. Similarly, interferon mRNA was detected in primed, induced cultures about 2 h earlier than in unprimed, induced cells. Interferon mRNA levels reached a peak 2–4 h earlier in primed cells, but also disappeared sooner in these cells. The peak levels of interferon mRNA isolated from primed, induced cells and unprimed, induced cells were similar. Thus, enhanced interferon production was interpreted as resulting from an enhanced efficiency of translation of interferon mRNA in the primed cells. These data are also open to an alternative interpretation. Since exposure of L cells to NDV results in a gradual inhibition of cellular protein synthesis (70% inhibition after 6 h, ABREU et al. 1979), the earlier appearance of interferon mRNA in primed cultures (2–8 h after induction) may allow its translation to occur under conditions of lessened virus-induced inhibition of cellular protein synthesis compared with unprimed cultures in which interferon mRNA appears 4–12 h after induction, when cellular protein synthesis is inhibited to a greater extent. These kinetic considerations would explain the higher yield of interferon from primed cultures, even though they contain the same level of interferon mRNA as unprimed cultures.

In a number of other systems, both murine and human priming has been shown to be correlated with an increase in the levels of extractable interferon mRNA (SAITO et al. 1976; FUJITA et al. 1979; SEHGAL and GUPTA 1980). These observations have been of use in the preparation of large amounts of human interferon mRNA (TANIGUCHI et al. 1979, 1980a; HOUGHTON et al. 1980).

2. Superinduction

The phenomenon of interferon superinduction is the key to large-scale production of human fibroblast interferon for clinical use. This phenomenon provides a novel insight into the regulation of gene expression in mammalian cells. It represents an outstanding example of the regulation of gene expression through an alteration in the stability of a specific mRNA. It also represents an experimental system which could lead to the eventual detection and isolation of a McAuslan–Tomkins post-transcriptional repressor (MCAUSLAN 1963; GARREN et al. 1964; TOMKINS et al. 1972).

The inhibitors of macromolecular synthesis listed in Table 3, when used appropriately, lead to a paradoxical enhancement of interferon yields in animal models as well as in cell cultures. Although this phenomenon has been observed with endotoxin, poly(I)·poly(C), or Newcastle disease virus as the inducer (YOUNGNER et al. 1965; YOUNGNER and HALLUM 1968; VILČEK et al. 1969; TAN et al. 1970; KOHASE and VILČEK 1979), in most investigations of this phenomenon poly(I)·poly(C) has been used as the inducer. Superinduction of poly(I)·poly(C)-induced interferon production has been observed in rabbit kidney cultures (VILČEK et al. 1969; TAN et al. 1970), in several strains of human diploid fibroblasts (HAVELL and VILČEK 1972; BILIAU et al. 1973a, 1977a; TAN and BERTHOLD 1977), and in several mouse fibroblast cultures (EDY et al. 1973; TOVEY et al. 1974). On the other hand, poly(I)·poly(C)-induced murine L cells do not exhibit this phenomenon (VILČEK 1970). Furthermore, superinduction is not observed in most cell systems in which viruses are used as inducers. Thus, although the phenomenon of superinduction is not unique to poly(I)·poly(C)-induced human diploid fibroblasts, it is not a general phenomenon observed in all systems of interferon induction. However, superinduction as a mechanism is operative in the expression of a wide variety of mammalian gene products (reviewed in TOMKINS et al. 1972; SEHGAL 1977; SEHGAL and GUPTA 1980). Thus, information about the mechanisms of interferon superinduction should help us understand a wide range of phenomena in mammalian cell biology.

Data relevant to the mechanism of interferon superinduction have been reviewed extensively (VILČEK et al. 1976; SEHGAL 1977; HAVELL 1977; SEHGAL and TAMM 1978; TAMM and SEHGAL 1978, 1979; STEWART 1979). Most of these investigations have been carried out in poly(I)·poly(C)-induced diploid human fibroblasts (FS-4 strain). DRB, a reversible inhibitor of hnRNA and mRNA synthesis has been an important tool in these investigations (SEHGAL and TAMM 1978; TAMM and SEHGAL 1978, 1979).

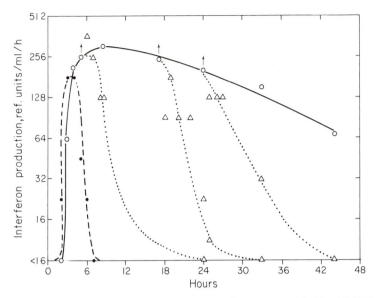

Fig. 3. Rate of interferon production during prolonged treatment with 30 μ*M* DRB and effect of termination of treatment. Four 11-day-old cultures (60-mm dishes) were induced with poly(I·C) in the presence *(open circles)*, and one in the absence *(full circles)*, of DRB and the rate of interferon production was followed by repeated medium replacement (2 ml, with or without DRB) and interferon titration. At 5, 17, and 24 h, one dish, which had contained DRB, was washed four times with warm PBS and the rate of interferon production was from then on monitored in the absence of DRB *(triangles)*. (SEHGAL et al. 1975 a)

Interferon production in FS-4 cells reaches detectable levels approximately 1 h after the beginning of induction, rises to a peak by 2.5–3 h, and is rapidly shut off by 6–8 h (Figs. 3, 4). Detailed analysis of the kinetics of interferon production by poly(I)·poly(C)-induced FS-4 cells have led to the suggestion that the rate of interferon production in response to poly(I)·poly(C) is determined by two processes (Figs. 3, 4). The inducer brings about the rapid synthesis of interferon mRNA, which is largely complete 3 h after the beginning of induction. Concurrently with the induction of the synthesis of interferon mRNA, poly(I)·poly(C) appears also to bring about the synthesis of an RNA and a corresponding protein species that are responsible for the posttranscriptional inactivation of interferon mRNA. This repressor mechanism is thought to cause the rapid shutoff of interferon production 6–8 h after induction, despite the intrinsic stability of interferon mRNA. It has been proposed that inhibitors of macromolecular synthesis, given at appropriate times, interfere with the synthesis of components of the shutoff mechanism and thereby are able to enhance interferon yields. At least one of the molecular species mediating the shutoff appears to be unstable and to have an overall lifetime of only 3–4 h (SEHGAL and TAMM 1976). It has been suggested that a translational repressor of the kind hypothesized by MCAUSLAN (1963) and by TOMKINS (GARREN et al. 1964; TOMKINS et al. 1972) is responsible for the shutoff of poly(I)·poly(C)-induced interferon production in human diploid fibroblasts (VILČEK et al. 1969; TAN et al. 1970).

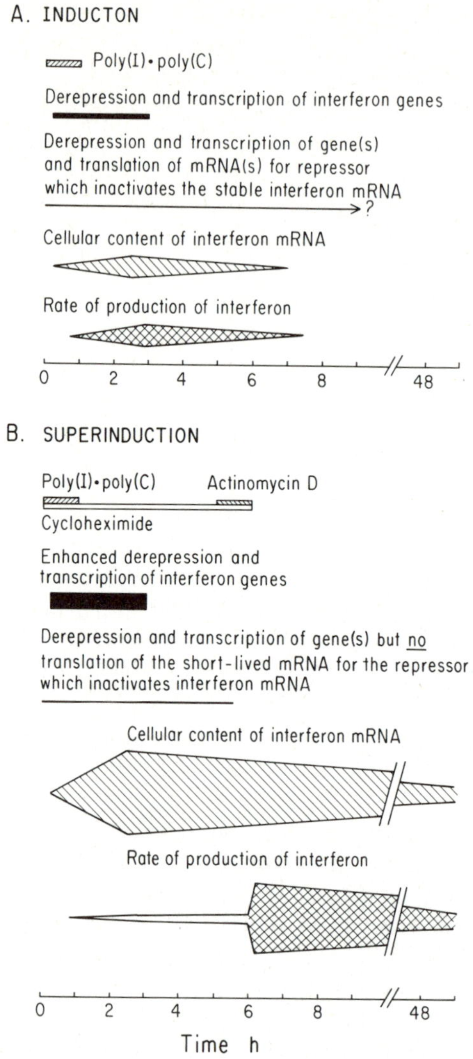

A. INDUCTON

B. SUPERINDUCTION

Fig. 4 a, b. Events thought to underlie the induction **a** of interferon production by poly(I) · - poly(C) in diploid human fibroblast cultures, and its superinduction **b** by cycloheximide and actinomycin D

With advent of the *Xenopus* oocyte assay for interferon mRNA, several investigators have measured the levels of interferon mRNA during the induction, shutoff, and superinduction of interferon production (Sᴇʜɢᴀʟ et al. 1977, 1978a; Sᴇʜɢᴀʟ and Tᴀᴍᴍ 1979; Cᴀᴠᴀʟɪᴇʀɪ et al. 1977b; Gʀᴇᴇɴᴇ et al. 1978). As a result of these experiments, two components have now been defined in the biochemical mechanisms of interferon superinduction (Sᴇʜɢᴀʟ et al. 1977, 1978a; Sᴇʜɢᴀʟ and Tᴀᴍᴍ 1979; Cᴀᴠᴀʟɪᴇʀɪ et al. 1977b). First, interferon mRNA is approximately 14-fold *more stable* in inhibitor-treated cultures than in inhibitor-free controls (Sᴇʜɢᴀʟ et al. 1978a). Second, estimates of the content of interferon mRNA during the first 3 h of induction in control cultures and in those exposed to DRB alone or cyclo-heximide alone are consistent with a 3–4-fold enhanced derepression of interferon mRNA synthesis in treated cultures (SEHGAL et al. 1976 b, c; SEHGAL and TAMM 1979). The experimental data are in good agreement with a mathematical model describing these events (SEHGAL et al. 1978 a; SEHGAL and TAMM 1979).

The biochemical basis for the increased functional stability of interferon mRNA is now under intensive investigation (SEHGAL et al. 1978 a, b; SEHGAL and GUPTA 1980; SEHGAL 1981). Alterations in the stability of interferon mRNA do not appear to involve alterations in the metabolism of the 3'-poly(A) tails of these molecules (SEHGAL et al. 1978 a, b; SOREQ et al. 1981). Furthermore, the mechanism which degrades or inactivates human fibroblast interferon mRNA does not affect the functional stability of bulk cellular mRNA. Finally, 2',5'-oligo(A)-mediated nuclease activation does not appear to be involved in the inactivation of interferon mRNA during the shutoff phase (SEHGAL and GUPTA 1980). The elucidation of the biochemistry underlying the regulation of the stability of specific mammalian mRNA species is an important task in modern molecular biology.

The understanding of the phenomenon of interferon superinduction that has been reached so far helps to clarify a long-standing confusion in the interferon field. Interferon synthesis in superinducible systems *appears* to be resistant to inhibition by inhibitors of RNA (Fig. 3) or protein synthesis. Does this imply that there exists "preformed" interferon waiting to be released (YOUNGNER et al. 1965; YOUNGNER and HALLUM 1968; FINKELSTEIN et al. 1968), or does it mean that the synthesis and subsequent translation of interferon mRNA are specifically resistant to the effects of the inhibitors used (ATHERTON and BURKE 1975; VENNSTRÖM et al. 1979)? The extensive analysis of the kinetic features and biochemical bases of interferon superinduction carried out in several laboratories indicate clearly that neither of these positions is correct (see SEHGAL et al. 1976 b, c; 1978 a; SEHGAL and TAMM 1979; TAMM and SEHGAL 1979; ATHERTON and BURKE 1978 for detailed discussions). Interferon production in the system treated with inhibitors of macromolecular synthesis is the net result of two mutually opposing effects: an inhibition of interferon mRNA and of interferon synthesis, and an enhancement of the depression of interferon genes and of the function of interferon mRNA. The specific enhancing effects outweigh and mask the inhibitory effects of superinducing agents on RNA and protein synthesis. Experimental protocols have been designed that remove superinduction as an experimental variable and allow a clear definition of the effects of various inhibitors on different aspects of interferon production (SEHGAL et al. 1976 c; ATHERTON and BURKE 1978; SEHGAL and TAMM 1979). With such procedures evidence has been obtained, for example, that interferon mRNA synthesis is intrinsically just as sensitive to inhibition by DRB as is bulk cellular mRNA synthesis (SEHGAL et al. 1976 b; SEHGAL and TAMM 1979; TAMM and SEHGAL 1979).

D. Spectrum of Antiviral Activity

Interferons inhibit the replication of a wide variety of RNA-containing and DNA-containing viruses (ISAACS and LINDENMANN 1957; reviewed in FINTER 1973; STEWART 1979). Despite extensive work in this area, very few generalizations are warranted about the relative efficacy of interferons against the replication of various viruses. Among the RNA-containing viruses, the togaviruses, such as Semliki Forest virus and Sindbis virus, are usually the most sensitive. The rhabdoviruses (e.g., vesicular stomatitis virus and rabies virus), orthomyxoviruses, paramyxoviruses (Sendai and Newcastle disease viruses), the reoviruses, and several strains of picornaviruses and oncornaviruses are also sensitive to inhibition by interferons. Among the DNA-containing viruses, the poxviruses and several strains of herpes simplex types 1 and 2 viruses, as well as the cytomegalovirus, are inhibited by interferon. The replication of tumor viruses such as SV40 and polyoma is also sensitive to inhibition. Although sensitive strains of adenovirus have been encountered, laboratory strains such as adenovirus type 2 are rather resistant.

The foregoing discussion is subject to several important qualifications. First, rather extreme variations in sensitivity to interferon are observed among different strains of the same virus. Newcastle disease virus is a notable example of this variability (reviewed in LOCKART 1966). Second, sensitivity to inhibition by interferon is dependent on the cell type in which the assay is carried out. For example, CAME et al. (1976) observed that, in HeLa cells, rhinovirus type 15 was resistant to interferons at high concentrations whereas rhinovirus type 10 was sensitive. In contrast, both types 10 and 15 were equally sensitive to inhibition by interferon in fibroblast cultures. Third, it is possible that various interferons may display different spectra of effectiveness against viruses. Although this has not yet been documented in a clear-cut fashion, the discovery of several human interferon species suggests that this may be an issue that deserves attention.

A rationale for the establishment of the antiviral spectrum of interferon in cell culture is that the use of interferon can then be targeted towards animal models and human diseases caused by interferon-sensitive viruses. A recent example indicates that this expectation needs to be qualified. SCHELLEKENS et al. (1979) have recently reported that human leukocyte interferon was effective in inhibiting vaccinia lesions in the skin of rhesus monkeys, but was completely inactive in inhibiting the replication of the same strain of vaccinia virus in cell cultures of human or rhesus fibroblasts. Thus, interferons may be effective in vivo against viruses which are insensitive to its action in cell cultures.

MOEHRING et al. (1971 b) have reported that the antiviral action of human fibroblast interferon against vesicular stomatitis virus is greater in human diploid cell strains than in aneuploid lines. It is important to note that a quantitatively graded response to interferon with the antiviral titers spread over a ten-fold range, was observed in both kinds of cells. Thus, human cell strains and lines display individual differences in responsiveness to interferon, but there is clustering of the values around the means.

E. Mechanisms of Antiviral Action of Interferon

Numerous modes of antiviral action have been proposed for interferons and supported by substantial evidence. Moreover, the role of interferons in the natural recovery process of the host from virus infections appears to be mediated, not only through the establishment of the antiviral state in host cells, but probably also through modulatory effects on immune systems.

We have elected in this section first to deal with interferon binding to cells and the induction of the antiviral state in cells. Next, we will discuss interferon-induced alterations at the cell surface and in three enzyme systems concerned with the regulation of translation. Not all of these alterations may be relevant to the antiviral state. Finally, we will summarize the diverse mechanisms that appear to be involved in the inhibition of replication of different viruses.

I. Interferon Binding

Although many of the details of the pathways leading to the induction of the antiviral state by interferon are poorly understood, an interaction of interferon with the external cell surface appears to be the first event in this process. Several lines of evidence indicate that newly produced interferon must be externalized and then interact with the outer cell surface to be effective in establishing the antiviral state. Incubation of induced cells with antibody directed against interferon prevents the establishment of the antiviral state in the induced cells (VENGRIS et al. 1975). Treatment of induced cells with ouabain, an inhibitor of membrane-bound ATPase, also prevents the development of the antiviral state without affecting interferon synthesis and release (LEBON et al. 1975). Several laboratories have reported that interferon bound covalently to sepharose beads is able to induce the antiviral state (ANKEL et al. 1973; KNIGHT 1974; BESANCON and ANKEL 1976; CHANY 1976). However, leakage of small quantities of soluble interferon from the beads cannot be completely ruled out as being instrumental in the induction of antiviral activity.

The binding of interferon to cells is fairly rapid at either 4° or 37 °C and is complete in several minutes, but the full expression of the antiviral state takes several hours and requires incubation at 37 °C, i.e., cell metabolism (FRIEDMAN 1967; BERMAN and VILČEK 1974; KOHNO et al. 1975; GARDNER and VILČEK 1969). For the induction of a high level of antiviral resistance, a longer exposure of human fibroblasts to human leukocyte interferon than to human fibroblasts interferon is required (GARDNER and VILČEK 1969). Exposure of cells to interferon at high concentration results in the induction of the antiviral state more rapidly than exposure to interferon at low concentration (DIANZANI et al. 1976). The higher concentrations of interferon may be near physiologic levels as local levels of induced interferon liberated from producing cells are probably much higher than the levels detected in circulating blood. A short exposure (e.g., 1 h) of cells to interferon also suffices to impair the proliferative capacity of the cells (PFEFFER et al. 1979; HOROSZEWICZ et al. 1979).

After incubation of cells with interferon at 37 °C, steps take place after which the response of cells to interferon is no longer blocked by protease digestion or by antibody directed against interferon (FRIEDMAN 1967; BERMAN and VILČEK 1974; DIANZANI and BARON 1977; REVEL 1979). There is no direct evidence that interferon is bound to a membrane receptor, but it is likely that discrete binding sites exist for interferons. The possibility has been raised that the binding site for interferon on the cell surface may be made up in part by a ganglioside-like structure (BESANCON and ANKEL, 1974a, b; VENGRIS et al. 1976) and in part by a glycoprotein component (GROLLMAN et al. 1978). If ganglioside and glycoprotein are components of the interferon receptor, then the interferon receptor would be structurally analogous to the receptors for glycoprotein hormones or cholera toxin. Pretreatment of cells with cholera toxin or thyrotropin diminishes the induction of antiviral activity by interferon by more than ten-fold (FRIEDMAN and KOHN 1976; KOHN et al. 1976), and conversely, interferon treatment alters the binding characteristics of cholera toxin and thyrotropin to the plasma membrane. However, interferon binding to a cell does not necessarily elicit the antiviral response. This observation has led to the proposal that interferon receptors may be composed of a high affinity binding component and a low affinity component (CHANY 1976; FRIEDMAN 1979). Binding of interferon to the high affinity component is thought to activate the series of events which results in the induction of the antiviral state.

II. Induction of the Antiviral State

It is well established that after treatment of cells with interferon, metabolic activity is a necessary prerequisite for the development of the antiviral state (LINDENMANN et al. 1957; LOCKART 1964; TAYLOR 1964; FRIEDMAN and SONNABEND 1965). It is generally accepted that interferon is not directly antiviral, but rather induces the intracellular production of one or more antiviral substances. Several inhibitors of protein and RNA synthesis have been shown to block the development of antiviral activity in interferon-treated cells (LOCKART 1964; TAYLOR 1964; FRIEDMAN and SONNABEND 1965). However, the established antiviral state is not diminished by inhibition of cellular RNA synthesis with actinomycin D (LOCKART 1964). Also, it has been demonstrated that enucleated cells cannot develop the antiviral state, but, once established, the antiviral state is not reversed by removal of the nucleus (RADKE et al. 1974; YOUNG et al. 1975). Study of the kinetics of the effect of actinomycin D treatment on the induction of the antiviral state has suggested that the messenger RNA for the "antiviral protein" is produced within 1 h after exposure of cells to interferon (DIANZANI et al. 1976). Recently, GORDON and STEVENSON (1980), using, DRB, a selective inhibitor of hnRNA and mRNA synthesis (TAMM et al. 1976; SEGHAL et al. 1976 d), have shown that the signal for development of the antiviral state activated in cells by interferon treatment, decays within 5–6 h.

Several investigators have suggested that the initial steps in the induction by interferon of complex changes in cells may be similar to the early steps in the action of peptide hormones (FRIEDMAN 1977; BLALOCK and STANTON 1980; PFEFFER et al. 1981 a, 1982). In the transmission of their messages to cells, peptide hormones require a series of cellular events which include binding to a specific membrane receptor, perturbation of the state of the membrane, and message transmission through the alteration in intracellular levels of cyclic nucleotides. As already discussed, interferon may bind to membrane receptors comprised of ganglioside and glycoprotein components. Treatment of human cells with interferon results in structural alterations in the cell surface, including increased rigidity of the plasma membrane (PFEFFER et al. 1981 a, b). It has been reported that interferon treatment of cells also results in a transient increase in the intracellular level of cAMP (FRIEDMAN and PASTAN 1969; MELDOLESI et al. 1977; WEBER and STEWART 1975). Furthermore, drugs which raise the intracellular level of cAMP have been shown in several cell systems to potentiate the antiviral state induced at a given interferon concen-

tration (FRIEDMAN and PASTAN 1969; WEBER and STEWART 1975; DAHL and DEGRE 1976). However, in interferon-treated mouse L1210 cells, maintained under steady state conditions, an increased intracellular level of cAMP is preceded by several hours by an increased level of cGMP, detectable within minutes following treatment (TOVEY et al. 1979). There have so far not been any definitive reports of the activation of membrane-associated cyclases by interferon treatment of cultured cells.

Recently, BLALOCK and STANTON (1980) have proposed that there may be a common cellular pathway of interferon and hormonal action and that the shared pathway may involve similar secondary messenger molecules. This hypothesis is based on the following evidence. Mouse interferon causes a species-specific hormonal response, i.e., noradrenaline-like stimulation of the beat frequency on cultured mouse myocardial cells (BLALOCK and STANTON 1980). Noradrenaline induces an antiviral state in mouse myocardial cells, but not in human amnion cells. Human interferon added to co-cultures of human amnion cells and mouse myocardial cells increases the beat frequency of the myocardial cells, but only when the myocardial cells are in contact with human cells. In the co-cultures, noradrenaline does induce an antiviral state in human cells. These results show that interferon can have hormonal activity and that hormonal stimulation can result in interferon-type antiviral activity. Although cAMP can account for some of the observed effects, it cannot account for all of them (BLALOCK and STANTON 1980).

Several reports have suggested a role for chromosome 21 in the induction of antiviral activity in human cells. Using human–mouse cell hybrids, synteny was demonstrated between chromosome 21 and sensitivity of cells to the antiviral action of human interferon (TAN et al. 1974; CHANY et al. 1975; CHANY 1976; REVEL et al. 1976; SLATE et al. 1978). The gene locus for interferon sensitivity is apparently localized on the distal portion of the long arm of chromosome 21, since translocation of this locus onto other chromosomes transfers interferon sensitivity (EPSTEIN and EPSTEIN 1976; TAN and GREENE 1976). In addition, it has been observed in several laboratories that interferon sensitivity may be related to gene dosage, i.e., with respect to interferon sensitivity, trisomic > diploid > monosomic (TAN et al. 1974a; CHANY et al. 1975; REVEL et al. 1976; TAN 1976; WIRANOWSKA-STEWART and STEWART 1977; SLATE et al. 1978). However, several exceptions have been noted in the literature (CHANY et al. 1975; DECLERCQ et al. 1975, 1976; PFEFFER et al. 1979a). It has been proposed that the chromosome 21 locus which determines interferon sensitivity may code for the membrane receptor for interferon (CHANY 1976; REVEL et al. 1976). REVEL et al. (1976) found that one particular antiserum directed against a cell surface component coded by human chromosome 21 inhibited the antiviral action of interferon in normal human diploid cells. However, DECLERCQ et al. (1975, 1976) have shown that monosomic 21, disomic 21, and trisomic 21 cells apparently bind interferon equally well and are equally sensitive to the nonantiviral activities induced by interferon.

There is evidence that the cell cytoskeleton may be involved in the induction of antiviral activity. Cytoskeleton-disrupting agents block the establishment of the antiviral state and induce a decay in the antiviral state (SOLOVIEV and MENTKEVICH 1965; BOURGEADE and CHANY 1976). Inhibition of proliferation of human fibroblasts by interferon is associated with increased abundance and organization of intracellular actin-containing microfilament bundles (Pfeffer et al. 1980a). Cytoskeletal structure is altered as part of the phenotypic expression of interferon action on transformed cells, making treated cells take on a "normal phenotype" (Chany et al. 1980).

III. Effects on the Cell Surface

Interferon treatment of cells results in alterations in the structural and functional properties of the plasma membrane and its associated proteins. These are summa-

Table 4. Interferon-induced changes involving the cell surface

Alteration	Reference
1. Increase in intramembranous particles	Chang et al. (1978)
2. Increased rigidity of plasma membrane lipid bilayer	Pfeffer et al. (1981a, b)
3. Increase in mean buoyant density of isolated plasma membrane preparation	Chang et al. (1978)
4. Higher electrophoretic mobility toward anode	Knight and Korant (1977)
5. Decreased surface exposure of gangliosides to galactose oxidase treatment	Grollman et al. (1978)
6. Altered binding characteristics of thyrotropin and cholera toxin	Kohn et al. (1976)
7. Protection from toxicity of diphtheria toxin	Yabrov (1966), Moehring et al. (1971a)
8. Enhanced sensitivity to toxicity of dsRNA and poly(I)·poly(C)	Stewart et al. (1973)
9. Enhanced expression of histocompatibility antigens	Lindahl et al. (1973, 1974, 1976a, b), Vignaux and Gresser (1977)
10. Enhanced expression of HLA and β_2 microglobulin	Heron et al. (1978)
11. Increased binding of concanavalin A	Huet et al. (1974)
12. Impaired capacity to redistribute lectin receptors	Matsuyama (1979), Pfeffer et al. (1980b)
13. Altered distribution of cell surface fibronectin	Pfeffer et al. (1980a, 1982)
14. Reduced rate of cell movement	Pfeffer et al. (1980a), Werenne et al. (1980), Brouty-Boyé and Zetter (1980)
15. Diminished thymidine transport	Tovey et al. (1975), Brouty-Boyé and Tovey (1977), Pfeffer et al. (1979)
16. Inhibition of plasminogen activator release	Schroeder et al. (1978)
17. Macrophage activation	Rabinovitch et al. (1977)
18. Enhanced phagocytic activity	Huang et al. (1971), Donahoe and Huang (1976)
19. Enhanced sensitivity of target cells to cytotoxic antibody	Skurkovitch et al. (1976)
20. Enhanced cytotoxicity of lymphocytes for target cells	Svet-Moldavsky and Chernyakovskaya (1967), Lindahl et al. (1973)

rized in Table 4. Some of the alterations of the cell surface may be phenotypic changes associated with the inhibition of cell proliferation by interferon. Further work is needed to identify which of these represent the primary effects of interferon.

IV. Effects on Translation-Inhibitory Enzymes

Cell-free systems have been utilized in an attempt to study the mechanisms by which the translation of virus-specific mRNA is inhibited in interferon-treated cells. Several laboratories have shown that preincubated (to depress endogenous synthesis) cell-free extracts from normal and interferon-treated cells translate poly(U) equally well. However, interferon-treated cell extracts show impaired translation of exogenously added virus-specified mRNAs, although extracts of control cells translate viral mRNA efficiently (FALCOFF et al. 1973; GUPTA et al. 1973; SAMUEL and JOKLIK 1974).

KERR et al. (1974) found that naturally occuring (the replicative intermediate formed by RNA viruses) and synthetic dsRNAs are potent inhibitors of protein synthesis in extracts of interferon-treated cells. The finding of enhanced sensitivity to inhibition by dsRNA has led to the demonstration of greatly elevated levels of certain dsRNA-dependent enzymes in extracts of interferon-treated human and mouse cells. These enzymes are: (a) $2',5'$-oligoadenylate synthetase which synthesizes $2',5'$-linked oligoadenylates with the structure pppA $(2'p5'A)n$ from ATP in the presence of double-stranded RNA (HOVANESSIAN et al. 1977; ZILBERSTEIN et al. 1978), and a phosphodiesterase, PPi which degrades $2',5'$-oligoadenylates (SCHMIDT et al. 1979; KIMCHI et al. 1979); and (b) a protein kinase which, in the presence of ATP and dsRNA, phosphorylates several specific protein species. It has also been reported that interferon induces the synthesis of several proteins that are not found in untreated control cell extracts (FARRELL et al. 1979; GUPTA et al. 1979; KNIGHT and KORANT 1979). However, the roles of these induced proteins have not yet been identified.

1. Oligo(A) Synthetase

Extracts of interferon treated cells incubated with dsRNA and ATP synthesize a low molecular weight, heat-stable inhibitor of protein synthesis (ROBERTS et al. 1976a, b). KERR et al. have isolated and chemically characterized this inhibitor as an oligonucleotide, pppA $(2'p5'A)n$, where $n = 1-16$ (KERR et al. 1977; KERR and BROWN, 1978). This class of inhibitors, collectively referred to as $2',5'$-A, is effective at subnanomolar concentrations and has been shown to activate an endonuclease that degrades mRNA (CLEMENS and WILLIAMS 1978; BAGLIONI et al. 1978b; SCHMIDT et al. 1978; RATNER et al. 1978). The $2',5'$-A oligonucleotides have been shown to inhibit protein synthesis when artificially introduced into intact cells (WILLIAMS and KERR 1978; HOVANESSIAN et al. 1979) and when added to cell-free systems derived from various animal species (KERR and BROWN 1978; BALL and WHITE 1978; ZILBERSTEIN et al. 1978).

Recent studies have led to the isolation, purification, and characterization of a synthetase in extracts of interferon-treated cells, which is responsible for the pro-

duction of 2′,5′-A (Ratner et al. 1978; Zilberstein et al. 1978; Hovanessian and Kerr 1979; Dougherty et al. 1980). Synthetase activity has been demonstrated in extracts of cells of various animal species not treated with interferon; however, the level of this enzyme is enhanced severalfold in extracts of interferon-treated cells (Ball, 1980). Synthetase activity is also found in normal differentiated tissues in widely varying amounts, suggesting a wider biologic role in the regulation of cell growth or development (Stark et al. 1979). Recently, the synthetase was shown to catalyze the addition of AMP residues in 2′,5′ linkage to a variety of nucleotide primers that contain adenosine as their 3′ residue, such as NAD, ADP ribose, and ApppppA (Ball, 1980). The induction of synthetase activity by interferon treatment has been correlated with the antiviral action of interferon (Baglioni et al. 1979; Kimchi et al. 1979).

Several studies have established the involvement of 2′,5′-A in the activation of an endonuclease and the subsequent inhibition of viral RNA accumulation and viral replication. This endonuclease, which degrades RNA, is activated in a two-stage process in interferon-treated cells (Brown et al. 1976; Sen et al. 1976b). In the first step, 2′,5′-A is produced by the oligo(A) synthetase in the presence of ATP and dsRNA. The second step requires activation of the endonuclease by the continued presence of endogenously or exogenously added 2′,5′-A (Clemens and Williams 1978; Eppstein and Samuel 1978; Baglioni et al. 1978a, b; Zilberstein et al. 1978). Partially purified endonuclease binds 2′,5′-A reversibly (Slattery et al. 1979). The activation of the endonuclease by added 2′,5′-A is transient in cell extracts as well as in intact cells (Hovanessian et al. 1979), presumably owing to degradation of 2′,5′-A, but readdition of 2′,5′-A can reactivate endonuclease avtivity (Schmidt et al. 1978; Slattery et al. 1979). The activated endonuclease cleaves both cellular and viral mRNA without preference (Baglioni et al. 1978b; Clemens and Williams 1978; Eppstein and Samuel 1978). Nilsen and Baglioni (1979), using synthetic substrates, have shown, that in extracts of interferon-treated cells, mRNA covalently bound to dsRNA is preferentially degraded compared with mRNA not bound to dsRNA. This result is consistent with the possibility that in infected cells endonuclease activation may be localized near the replicative intermediates of RNA viruses. However, this result does not readily explain the inhibition by interferon of the replication of DNA viruses.

There is evidence that the intracellular levels of 2′,5′-A are regulated, not only by the synthetase, but also by a phosphodiesterase which degrades $2′,5′-A_n$ into 5′AMP and ATP (Schmidt et al. 1978; Williams et al. 1978). Recently Schmidt et al. (1979) have purified the phosphodiesterase from interferon-treated cells and demonstrated a 4–5-fold enhanced enzyme level in interferon-treated cells. The enzyme, besides cleaving 2′,5′-dinucleotides, also degrades the CCA terminus of tRNA (see Sect. E. IV. 4).

2. dsRNA-Dependent Kinase

The phosphorylation of specific host cell proteins has been suggested as another pathway that mediates the impaired translation of viral mRNA in interferon-treated cell extracts. Samuel and Joklik (1974) showed that the inability of extracts of

interferon-treated cells to translate viral mRNA was due to an inhibitory activity, (probably of a protein) that was associated with ribosomes and could be removed from ribosomes by washing with 0.5 M KCl. Further experiments indicated that the translation-inhibitory activity in crude cell lysates from interferon-treated cells could be activated severalfold by preincubation with dsRNA and ATP (ROBERTS et al. 1976). In such cell lysates, dsRNA and ATP stimulate the phosphorylation of several proteins including the smallest subunit of initiation factor eIF-2 (M_r = 35.000 daltons) which binds initiator Met-tRNA, and of a 67.000 daltons protein (Pl) (LEBLEU et al. 1976; ROBERTS et al. 1976 a, b; ZILBERSTEIN et al. 1976). The phosphorylation of eIF-2 reduces its ability to function efficiently at the level of initiation of protein synthesis by possibly decreasing the binding of initiator tRNA to 40 S ribosomal subunits (FARRELL et al. 1977). The detailed mechanism of the impairment is still under active investigation. HUNT and EHRENFELD (1971) had previously shown that dsRNA stimulates the phosphorylation of these same polypeptides in reticulocyte lysates which are particularly sensitive to the impairment of protein synthesis by dsRNA addition. The phosphorylation of the Pl protein can serve as a marker for interferon action and has been shown to increase in proportion to the interferon dose. Treatment of human and mouse cells with homologous interferon also results in increased levels of a 67.000 daltons protein in cell extracts (GUPTA et al. 1979; KNIGHT and KORANT 1979).

The phosphorylation of these proteins is the result of activation of a protein kinase by dsRNA in extracts of interferon-treated cells (LEBLEU et al. 1976; ROBERTS et al. 1976a, b; ZILBERSTEIN et al. 1976). The protein kinase phosphorylates Pl (SHAILA et al. 1977; SLATE et al. 1978) and eIF-2 (FARRELL et al. 1978) with high efficiency, and also several cellular histones (ROBERTS et al. 1976a, b; ZILBERSTEIN et al. 1978). Assay of this kinase activity is complicated by the presence of a phosphatase activity in unfractionated cell extracts which dephosphorylates protein Pl and eIF-2 (REVEL 1977). However, this problem is circumvented by assaying the enzyme in isolated ribosomes. The kinase and its substrate cosediment with ribosomes while the phosphatase apparently remains in the postribosomal supernatant (BAGLIONI 1979). Incubation of ribosomes with ATP and dsRNA has been found to result in activation of the protein kinase. The level of the protein kinase is related to the dose of interferon. The time-dependent induction of the enzyme is correlated with the development of antiviral activity (BAGLIONI 1979; SAMUEL 1979). The kinase activity increases 5–10-fold in interferon-treated cells compared with basal levels observed in control cells (ZILBERSTEIN et al. 1978; REVEL 1979).

The kinase has been purified several hundred-fold (SEN et al. 1978; ZILBERSTEIN et al. 1978). It is present at low levels in untreated cells (JARVIS et al. 1978). The kinase binds to dsRNA–agarose and has been shown to be activated by dsRNA at low concentration (0.5–100 ng/ml; SEN et al. 1978). The relationship between dose and effect is linear in this range. The kinase activity is independent of cyclic nucleotide levels (REVEL 1977) and is highest in the absence of added KCl (SEN et al. 1978). Increasing the salt concentration reduces the level of inhibition of protein synthesis by protein kinase (BAGLIONI et al. 1978a). So far, no evidence has been obtained indicating that protein kinase activity in interferon-treated, virus-infected cells is increased compared with the level in uninfected, interferon-treated cells.

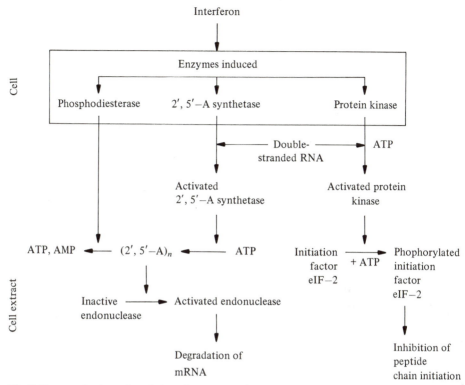

Fig. 5. Enzymatic alterations in interferon-treated cells and in cell extracts derived therefrom

To summarize, interferon treatment of cells induces at least two dsRNA-dependent enzymes, $2',5'$-A synthetase and a protein kinase. These enzymes constitute two distinct pathways (Fig. 5) for the inhibition of mRNA translation in cell extracts.

3. Cap Methylation of Viral mRNA

The methylation of nucleotides at the $5'$ end of mRNA, appears to be altered in extracts of some interferon-treated mouse and human cells (Sen et al. 1977 a, b). Desrosiers and Lengyel (1977) have reported that reovirus mRNA in interferon-treated cells contains 50% less cap II termini ($m^7 GpppN_1mpN_2mp$-capped chains in which both N-1 and N-2 are 2-O'-methylated) than control cells. In interferon-treated chicken cells, Kroath et al. (1978) have reported decreased cap methylation of both vaccinia and host mRNAs. In cell extracts, infected with vaccinia virus, viral mRNA with methylated caps has been found to bind ribosomes more efficiently than corresponding viral mRNA without methylated caps (Muthukrishnan et al. 1978). A study of interferon treatment late after lytic infection with SV40 indicates that there is an increase in the methylation of internal m^6A rather than a reduction in the methylation of SV40 mRNA cap (Revel 1979). It is important to note that the alterations of mRNA methylation have so far been found only in extracts of cells.

4. The tRNA Effect

The inhibition of translation of exogenously added mRNA in extracts of unin-fected, interferon-treated cells can be reversed by the addition of animal tRNA (GUPTA et al. 1974; CONTENT et al. 1975; SEN et al. 1977a). The inhibition is ap-parently a consequence of a block in the elongation of polypeptide chains (REVEL 1977), and the inhibition of polypeptide chain initiation seems to be secondary to the effect on elongation (CONTENT et al. 1975). LENGYEL and colleagues have re-ported that the basic defect could be traced to an impaired amino acid acceptor activity of specific tRNAs (SEN et al. 1976a, 1977a). This was ascribed to a faster tRNA inactivation in interferon-treated cell extracts compared with controls. Re-cently, the phosphodiesterase PPi, whose level is increased 2–3-fold after interferon treatment, has been shown to be a strong inhibitor of tRNA aminoacylation (SCHMIDT et al. 1979), and its action on the inhibition of translation could be re-versed to a great extent by tRNA addition (KIMCHI et al. 1979).

5. Postscript: The Problem of Selectivity

Several interferon-induced biochemical alterations have been identified in the pro-tein-synthesizing machinery through examination of extracts from interferon-treated cells. The changes observed in vitro after interferon treatment of cells may be artifacts of cell-free systems, or, as is more likely, they may be biologically sig-nificant. However, the problem is that in the cell-free translation systems (derived from interferon-treated cells) that have been utilized to demonstrate the impaired translation of viral mRNAs, the translation of cellular mRNAs is inhibited as well (FALCOFF et al. 1973; GUPTA 1974). Strong evidence has accumulated in several virus–host cell systems that interferon treatment of cells can result in selective in-hibition of viral protein synthesis in the living cells. The selectivity observed in these systems has not been convincingly reproduced, as yet, in a cell-free system.

V. Effects of Interferon in Various Virus–Host Cell Systems

Interferons have been shown to inhibit the replication of a wide spectrum of viruses at various steps in the viral replication cycle. At least four possible sites of inhibi-tory action have been identified. Although there have been numerous attempts to pinpoint a primary site of interferon action, it has become exceedingly clear that interferons act pleiotropically and block viral replication at several steps. The steps in the viral replication cycle inhibited by interferon are determined by the partic-ular virus–host cell system studied.

1. Viral Uncoating

Numerous studies with various viruses seemingly eliminated viral uncoating as a step at which interferon may inhibit viral replication. Infectious RNA from poliovirus and western equine encephalitis virus was found to be as sensitive to in-terferon inhibition as was infectious virus (HO 1961; DE SOMER et al. 1962; GROSS-BERG and HOLLAND 1962). In addition, reovirus was shown to be inhibited at a stage after viral uncoating (WIEBE and JOKLIK 1975). However, studies with simian virus 40 (SV40) have suggested that SV40 uncoating or an event soon after uncoating is a sensitive target for interferon action. Oxman and colleagues have shown that interferon-treated cells infected with SV40 exhibit a marked inhibition of SV40 early mRNA and T antigen production (Oxman and Levin 1971; Metz et al. 1976). When cells were transfected with infectious SV40 DNA, interferon treatment resulted in only a slight reduction of SV40 early mRNA and T antigen synthesis (Yamamoto et al. 1975). Furthermore, interferon does not inhibit T antigen formation in SV40-transformed mouse cells (Oxman et al. 1967). Finally, interferon apparently does not affect adsorption and penetration of SV40 (Yamamoto et al. 1975). These results are consistent with interferon inhibiting uncoating or an event soon afterwards in SV40 infection.

2. Viral Transcription

Interferon treatment decreases the accumulation of early virus-specific mRNA in cells infected with various RNA and DNA viruses. The reduction in virus-specific transcripts in VSV-infected cells treated with homologous interferon has been interpreted to reflect inhibition of primary transcription (Marcus et al. 1971; Manders et al. 1972). In these studies, cycloheximide was employed to block protein synthesis and thereby to restrict the the synthesis of virus-specific RNA products to primary transcripts of the parental viral genome. However, cycloheximide may increase the stability of viral mRNA in control cells, but not in interferon-treated cells. Other investigators have suggested that inhibition of the synthesis of the viral RNA species that are products of secondary transcription (which itself is dependent on viral protein synthesis) is responsible for the subsequent inhibition of VSV protein synthesis (Repik et al. 1974; Baxt et al. 1977) or reovirus protein synthesis (Wiebe and Joklik 1975). Interferon-induced inhibition of viral transcription has also been reported for vaccinia virus (Bialy and Colby 1972) and frog polyhedral cytoplasmic deoxyvirus (Gravell and Cromeans 1972). However, it was not established whether the effects observed were on primary rather than on secondary transcription.

Interferon treatment has been found in numerous studies to result in a marked reduction in the accumulation of SV40 early RNA during cytocidal infection (Oxman and Levin 1971; Yamamoto et al. 1975; Metz et al. 1977; Yakobson et al. 1977; Kingsman and Samuel 1980). However, in SV40-transformed mouse cells, T antigen production is insensitive to interferon treatment, although such treatment renders these cells resistant to VSV infection (Oxman et al. 1967).

Interferon treatment inhibits the expression of all early viral functions, including the synthesis of T antigen, stimulation of cell DNA synthesis, and cell transformation, after infection of either permissive (monkey) or nonpermissive (mouse) cells with SV40 (Metz 1975; Oxman 1977). In the permissive monkey cells, in the presence of an inhibitor of DNA synthesis that blocks SV40 DNA replication, interferon inhibits the accumulation of both SV40 T antigen and early SV40 RNA (Oxman and Levin 1971). When cells are transfected with SV40 DNA the interferon sensitivity of T antigen production appears to be somewhat reduced (Yamamoto et al. 1975). Although early SV40 RNA synthesis is markedly reduced in interferon-treated monkey cells, it has been reported that the number of available parental

DNA templates is not detectably altered in treated cells compared with controls (METZ et al. 1976). Fractionation of SV40-infected cells has demonstrated that interferon causes a comparable reduction in the cytoplasmic and nuclear content of early SV40 RNA (METZ et al. 1977; KINGSMAN and SAMUEL 1980). Furthermore, KINGSMAN and SAMUEL (1980) have found that the decay rate of early SV40 RNA in nuclear and cytoplasmic fractions is similar in interferon-treated and control cells. These results suggest that the effect of interferon was to decrease synthesis of early SV40 RNA rather than to enhance its degradation, however, it has not been established by what mechanism the synthesis is decreased.

3. Viral Protein Synthesis

Although viral protein synthesis has often been characterized as a site of interferon action, viral protein and RNA synthesis are so interdependent that it can be difficult to distinguish which of the two is the primary target for interferon action. To establish which of the two is the primary target of interferon action it is necessary to use conditions under which changes in viral RNA and protein synthesis are clearly separable. Viral protein synthesis has been analyzed either in intact virus-infected cells or in cell-free-systems. Pertinent experimental systems for the analysis of cell-free in vitro translation have been reviewed in detail in Sect. E. IV.

Vaccinia virus was the first virus to be intensively studied with respect to the action of interferon on viral multiplication. Several studies have demonstrated that, under conditions where interferon does not inhibit the transcription of early vaccinia-specific mRNA, there is inhibition of early viral protein synthesis, of secondary uncoating, and of viral DNA replication (JOKLIK and MERIGAN 1966; MAGEE et al. 1968; BODO et al. 1972; METZ and ESTEBAN 1972). These data suggest that translation of early virus-specific mRNAs is impaired in vaccinia-infected, interferon-treated cells.

Several studies have also been carried out of the effects of interferon treatment on the expression of reovirus-specified functions. Under conditions where interferon markedly inhibited reovirus replication and the synthesis of viral proteins, there was no impairment of reovirus adsorption, penetration, and uncoating into subviral particles (SVPs; GUPTA et al. 1974; WIEBE and JOKLIK 1975; GALSTER and LENGYEL 1976). Using a temperature-sensitive mutant of reovirus defective in the synthesis of progeny dsRNA at the nonpermissive temperature, WIEBE and JOKLIK (1975) found that early transcription of reovirus mRNA is much less sensitive to interferon than early translation of the several mRNA species. The most sensitive mRNA codes for polypeptide $\lambda 1$, which is a constituent of the structure within which double-stranded reovirus RNA is formed. The high interferon sensitivity of the translation of $\lambda 1$ mRNA may explain the high sensitivity of the late functions, including the secondary transcription of viral mRNA, the formation of progeny double-stranded RNA, and the formation of progeny virions.

In several other virus–host cell systems, it has been demonstrated that under conditions where there is slight inhibition of viral RNA synthesis, there is a greater inhibition of the synthesis of viral polypeptides. In VSV-infected cells, viral protein synthesis is inhibited by interferon in spite of the presence of near normal amounts of total virus-specified RNA. Only the synthesis of those viral RNA species dependent on viral protein synthesis is reduced (BAXT et al. 1977). THACORE (1978) reported that in interferon-treated monkey cells, VSV-specified mRNA transcripts were found in near normal amounts although viral protein synthesis was completely inhibited. However, in human cells a reduction in accumulation of VSV-specified mRNA transcripts was observed (THACORE 1978). SIMLI et al. (1980) have reported that, under conditions where near normal amounts of viral mRNA are found in interferon-treated, VSV-infected cells, there is a dose-dependent reduction in viral protein synthesis. In interferon-treated cells infected with Semliki Forest virus (SFV), the production of virus-specific proteins is largely inhibited under conditions where interferon treatment has no effect on viral RNA synthesis (FRIEDMAN 1968). Interferon treatment reduces the amount of viral RNA polymerase activity in cells infected with SFV (MARTIN and SONNABEND 1967) and in cells infected with Mengo virus (MINER et al. 1966). In addition, in cells treated with interferon and infected with Mengo virus, viral protein synthesis is completely inhibited although there is only a transient shutoff of host protein synthesis (FALCOFF et al. 1980).

In SV40 infection, interferon treatment has been demonstrated to inhibit virus-directed protein synthesis. When mRNA copied enzymatically from SV40 was microinjected into control and interferon-treated monkey cells, a marked inhibition of the translation of the mRNA was obtained after interferon pretreatment (GRAESSMANN et al. 1974). Addition of homologous interferon to monkey cells as late as 24 h after injection of SV40 led to the establishment of the antiviral state under conditions where more than 90% of cells were infected by SV40 (YAKOBSON et al. 1977). These experimental conditions were then utilized to show that "late" interferon addition caused a marked inhibition of early and late SV40-specific protein synthesis. However, viral mRNA synthesis continued, although viral DNA synthesis was somewhat reduced. Although late viral mRNA synthesis was unaffected, these mRNAs were no longer found associated with polyribosomes, thus suggesting post-transcriptional regulation of biosynthesis in these cells. It appears that interferon treatment of cells affects the replication cycle of SV40 at several levels, including viral uncoating and virus-directed transcription and translation.

4. Viral Assembly or Release

As has been described, most of the data support the concept that interferon treatment of cells affects viral RNA transcription or translation in the replication process of a wide range of viruses. However, interferon treatment has been found to inhibit a late step in the replication of murine leukemia viruses (MLV). Interferon can inhibit the release of MLV from chronically infected cells, even when the cells are infected with virus many generations before interferon treatment (HORVATH and FRIEDMAN 1971; BILLIAU et al. 1973b, 1975). Pretreatment of mouse cells with interferon also has been shown to inhibit virus production in cells newly infected with MLV (SARMA et al. 1969). The inhibition of MLV production mediated by interferon does not correlate with inhibition of viral RNA accumulation (PITHA et al. 1977), or the production of most virus-specific proteins (FRIEDMAN and RAMSEUR 1974). In fact, the number of virus particles associated with the cell membrane is increased (BILLIAU et al. 1975; CHANG et al. 1977) as is the intracellular content of several viral proteins and their precursor polypeptides (BILLIAU et al. 1975; FRIEDMAN et al. 1975).

Interferon does not seem to prevent the appearance of intracisternal type A particles in mouse cells induced by bromodeoxyuridine or dimethylsulfoxide treatment (BILLIAU et al. 1973b). However, interferon inhibits the induction of latent RNA tumor viruses by halogenated thymidine analogs (BLAINEAU et al. 1974). Such evidence also indicates that interferon affects a late event in virus formation, such as packaging of viral RNA, assembly of proteins, budding of the virus particle, or its release from the cell surface.

The effect on mouse leukemia virus production has been observed to last as long as interferon is present, and within 24 h after interferon removal full virus production resumes and reaches levels found in untreated cells (FRIEDMAN et al. 1975). It is important to note that interferon treatment of MLV-infected cells has been shown in some virus–host cell systems to result in a marked inhibition of particle release (FRIEDMAN et al. 1975; PITHA et al. 1977), while in others particle release is nearly normal but the infectivity of the particles is decreased (PITHA et al. 1976; WONG et al. 1977). STRAUCHEN et al. (1977) found that gluccocorticoid-stimulated mouse mammary tumor virus (MMTV) expression in a murine mammary tumor cell line was inhibited after interferon treatment, as measured by extracellular RNA-dependent DNA polymerase activity, incorporation of uridine ^{3}H into virus particles, and direct virus particle counts. Cell-associated RNA-dependent DNA polymerase activity was also depressed, but less so than the amount of extracellular virus. However, YAGI et al. (1980), using another chronically infected mouse mammary tumor line, found that the levels of extracellular virus particles (determined by incorporation of C^{14}-labeled amino acids and glucosamine-^{3}H into virus particles) was not significantly reduced, although electron microscopic examination of cells did indicate a decrease in the numbers of type A and budding type B virus particles. SDS–polyacrylamide gel electrophoresis of virus particles purified from interferon-treated cultures showed an increase in the relative level of the 60.000 daltons glycoprotein, gp 60. All of these results suggest that the morphogenesis and release of RNA tumor viruses are complex events that are sensitive to interferon action at various levels.

Recently, MAHESHWARI and FRIEDMAN (1980) have shown that the inhibition of virus maturation by interferon treatment is not limited to RNA tumor viruses. Interferon treatment of VSV-infected mouse cells resulted in the production of noninfectious particles which are deficient in two virus-specific proteins: G (glycoprotein) and M (matrix) proteins. The production of VSV deficient in glycoprotein may be due to decreased activity of UDP-N-acetylglucosaminedolichol phosphate transferase in interferon-treated cells (MAHESHWARI et al. 1980).

F. Diversity of Interferon Action: Effects on Normal and Transformed Cells

Although originally characterized as specific antiviral agents, interferons have been shown to have complex effects on cells. Many of the biologic effects on cells (other than antiviral) have often been attributed to some contaminating substance present in crude or partially purified interferon preparations. However, with the advent of preparations of interferons which have been purified to homogeneity, proof has been obtained that interferons themselves exert multiple biologic effects on cells. It is now clear that the interferon-treated cell is an altered cell and that antiviral activity is but one manifestation of interferon's action as a modulator of cell structure and function (GRESSER 1977).

I. Cell Proliferation

Historically, the first "nonantiviral" activity ascribed to interferon preparations was the inhibitory effect on cell multiplication. PAUCKER et al. (1962) showed that interferon inhibited the proliferation of L cells and that this effect was directly proportional to the antiviral activity. It is clear now that interferon is not a cytotoxic substance in the usual sense of the term, and that it inhibits the proliferation of both normal and tumor cells in cell culture and in animal models (for review see GRESSER 1977; STEWART 1979).

The effect of interferon on cell proliferation is not very rapidly reversible upon removal of interferon (PFEFFER et al. 1979, 1982). However, when cells are washed free of interferon, the cultures multiply at a rate similar to control cells after a varying lag period (GRESSER et al. 1970; KNIGHT 1976b). Human fibroblast (PFEFFER et al. 1979; 1982) and lymphoblastoid cultures (HOROSZEWICZ et al. 1979), exposed to interferon for a short period of time (1 h), show a decreased rate of cell proliferation, and the inhibition is similar to that observed with cultures continuously exposed to interferon. As viruses vary in sensitivity to interferon inhibition, so do cells. Several studies have shown that tumor cells vary in sensitivity to the antiproliferative effect of interferon (ADAMS et al. 1975; HILFENHAUS et al. 1977). Significant inhibition of cell proliferation has been found with certain tumor cell lines at low concentration (< 100 U/ml) of interferon (ADAMS et al. 1975; GRESSER 1977; HILFENHAUS et al. 1977). For example, mouse L1210 cells can be detectably inhibited by as little as 1 U/ml, and almost entirely inhibited by 100 U/ml (STEWART et al. 1976). Although the multiplication of certain human lymphoblastoid lines is inhibited by about 1 U or less, others are resistant to a concentration of several thousand U/ml (ADAMS et al. 1975; HILFENHAUS et al. 1977).

The dose–response relationship has been delineated in several human cell strains and lines (PFEFFER et al. 1979). An approximately exponential dose–response relationship was found for interferon doses in the range from 40–640 U/ml, but increasing the dose beyond 640 U/ml had little further effect on the degree of inhibition of cell proliferation. It has been observed in several laboratories that interferon-treated cells reach a plateau at a lower saturation density than do control cells (GRESSER et al. 1970; KNIGHT 1973; PFEFFER et al. 1979). Time-lapse cinematography of mouse EMT6 tumor cells (D'HOOGHE et al. 1977) and of human diploid fibroblasts (PFEFFER et al. 1979, 1982) has shown that interferon treatment causes a progressive increase in the intermitotic interval of cells. Furthermore, after several days of interferon treatment, an increasing proportion of the cell population ceases to divide.

Evidence is accumulating that interferon treatment affects a process in the G_1 phase of the cell cycle. However, interferon treatment alters cell cycle traverse in a complex manner as delays in progression through S and G_2 + M have also been observed. An extension of G_1 and G_2 has been observed in asynchronously growing interferon-treated cultures of L1210 and Friend leukemic cells and of cells (MCF-7) derived from pleural effusions of breast cancer patients (KILLANDER et al. 1976; MATARESE and ROSSI 1977; BALKWILL et al. 1979). In addition, an extension of S of lesser magnitude was observed in MCF-7 cells (BALKWILL et al. 1979). In actively growing human melanoma cells (H_s294T), interferon appeared to impede the progress of cells through all phases of the cell cycle (CREASEY et al. 1980).

In experiments in which cells were rendered quiescent in G_0/G_1 by culturing in serum-deficient medium and then stimulated to grow with serum in the presence or absence of interferon, a delayed passage through both G_1 and S + G_2 was observed with mouse cell lines (BALB/c 3T3 and Swiss 3T3K) and human fibroblasts (HEL 27; BALKWILL and TAYLOR-PAPADIMITRIOU 1978). However, SOKAWA et al. (1977) have reported that with the BALB/c 3T3 line used by them, the only parameter affected in similar experiments was the entry of cells into S phase. LUNDGREN et al. (1979), working with several strains of human fibroblasts, found that interferon prolonged the G_1 phase and diminished the rate of DNA synthesis during the S phase. In serum stimulation experiments with human melanoma cells, the transition rate of cells from G_0/G_1 into S and the rate of movement through S were both decreased in interferon-treated cultures (CREASEY et al. 1980). Evidence was reported that interferon-treated cells go slowly through one cell cycle, return to G_0/G_1, and fail to enter a new cycle.

The cell cycle phase distribution of several different lines of human melanoma cells at confluence revealed a remarkable heterogeneity in that certain lines of melanoma cells were blocked in G_0/G_1, whereas others were distributed in G_1, S, and G_2 + M as determined by flow cytometry of cells which had not been treated with interferon. Furthermore, those human melanoma lines that entered G_0/G_1 at high cell density were found to be more sensitive to the antiproliferative action of interferon than those that continued to cycle at high density (CREASEY et al. 1980).

Evidence obtained with Burkitt's lymphoma cells (Daudi) indicates that delaying the addition of interferon after seeding of cultures with cells in the plateau phase of growth results in a diminution of the inhibitory effect (HOROSZEWICZ et al. 1979). Thus, rapidly and exponentially multiplying Daudi cells were less sensitive to inhibition by interferon than cells in the process of resuming cycling after a quiescent period. Taken together, the evidence suggests that interferon treatment impedes the commitment of cells to DNA synthesis, but that it also results in other alterations in the cycling behavior of cells.

It has been suggested that a number of the biologic effects observed upon interferon treatment of human fibroblasts in culture may be representative of the phenotype of slowly dividing cell population (GRESSER 1977; PFEFFER et al. 1980a, 1982). A similar phenotype is observed in cellular senescence in vitro (GRESSER, 1977; PFEFFER et al. 1980a, 1982). Interferon has also been shown to affect the multiplication of normal and transformed cells in animal models. Interferon induces "runting" in the growth of suckling mice and rats (GRESSER et al. 1975a) and inhibits liver regeneration in partially hepatectomized adult mice (FRAYSSINET et al. 1973). Interferon and its inducers inhibit the multiplication of allogeneic and syngeneic bone marrow cells in irradiated mice (CEROTTINI et al. 1973). Interferon also inhibits the ability of transformed cells to induce tumors in mice or to form colonies in soft agar (GRESSER et al. 1971).

The precise mechanism of the inhibition of cell proliferation by interferon is not clear as yet. It is possible that, at least in some systems, interferon may render cells more sensitive to the normal control mechanisms that limit cell cycling as the population density increases, rather than acting as a cytostatic drug. Many investigators have searched for restraints imposed by interferon on cellular metabolism, but the results have often been contradictory and the effects seen may have been secondary to the slowing of cell cycle traverse. Treatment of L1210 cells sensitive to interferon decreased the rates of cellular RNA and protein synthesis and had no such effect in cells resistant to interferon (BROUTY-BOYÉ et al. 1973; GRESSER et al. 1974 b). DNA and RNA synthesis was found to be reduced in human RSa cells treated with interferon (FUSE and KUWATA 1976). In human fibroblasts, interferon treatment caused minor reductions in the rates of DNA, RNA, and protein synthesis (PFEFFER et al. 1979). The minor inhibitory effect on macromolecular synthesis probably has a trivial explanation, as it is known that a decreased rate of cell proliferation is accompanied by a step-down in macromolecular synthesis. Moreover, it has been shown that interferon-treated human fibroblasts increase in cell size, mass (protein and DNA), and volume (PFEFFER et al. 1979, 1980a, 1982). Treatment of human RSa cells with interferon is also accompanied by an increase in protein content (FUSE and KUWATA 1976). Thus, interferon does not appear to inhibit the growth of cells, but rather interferes with cell cycle traverse.

II. Cell Functions

In addition to inhibiting cell proliferation, interferon is also capable of modulating a variety of cell functions, as indicated in Table 5. The relationship between interferon-induced enhancement and inhibition of specific cell functions is poorly understood. It is clear, however, that interferon can modify cell structure and function at multiple levels.

Of great current interest are the findings which indicate that interferons modulate many humoral and cellular aspects of the immune system. As far as the humoral immune response is concerned, interferon treatment has varied effects on antibody-forming B-cells. Interferon treatment prior to exposure either to T-dependent or T-independent antigens results in the inhibition of antibody production (GISLER et al. 1974; JOHNSON et al. 1975). It should be noted that immune T-cell interferon (type II or γ) has been found to be about 100 times (on the basis of anti-VSV activity) more suppressive on antibody production than Le (α) or F (β) interferon (JOHNSON 1977). Interferons also inhibit the function of splenic memory lymphocytes when administered before antigen sensitization (BRODEUR and MERIGAN 1974). However, addition of interferon several days after antigen sensitization has been found to enhance the antibody response (BRAUN and LEVY 1972; GISLER et al. 1974). Interferons suppress the proliferative response of lymphocytes to mitogens and alloantigens (LINDAHL-MAGNUSSON et al. 1972).

Interferons have also been found to influence T-cell function by inhibiting a variety of cell-mediated immune reactions, including graft–host reaction, allograft rejection, and delayed hypersensitivity (DE MAEYER and DE MAEYER-GUIGNARD

Table 5. Interferon-induced changes in cell functions

A. Enhancement	
Phagocytosis of carbon particles	HUANG et al. (1971), IMANISHI et al. (1975), DONAHUE and HUANG (1976)
Phagocytosis of tumor cells	GRESSER and BOURALI (1970)
Macrophage activation	RABINOVITCH et al. (1977), SCHULTZ et al. (1977)
Cytotoxic activity of lymphocytes	SVET-MOLDAVSKY and CHERNYAKOVSKAYA (1967), LINDAHL et al. (1972)
Activation of natural killer cells	HERON et al. (1976), GIDLUND et al. (1978)
Number of antibody-producing cells	GISLER et al. (1974), JOHNSON (1977)
Specific proteins	
Interferon (priming)	ISAACS and BURKE (1958)
Aryl hydrocarbon hydroxylase	NEBERT and FRIEDMAN (1973)
Hemoglobin	LIEBERMAN et al. (1974)
Prostaglandin E	YARON et al. (1977)
tRNA methylase	ROZEE et al. (1969)
Lysozyme	LOTEM and SACHS (1978)
Protein kinase	LEBLEU et al. (1976), ROBERTS et al. (1976a, b), ZILBERSTEIN et al. (1976)
Phosphodiesterase PPi	SCHMIDT et al. (1979), KIMICHI et al. (1979)
Oligo(A) synthetase	HOVANESSIAN et al. (1977), ZILBERSTEIN et al. (1978)
Histamine release	IDA et al. (1977)
B. Inhibition	
Production of specific proteins	
Interferon (blocking)	VILČEK (1962), VILČEK and RADA (1962)
Tyrosine aminotransferase	VASSEFF et al. (1974)
Glycerol-3-phosphate dehydrogenase	ILLINGER et al. (1976)
Glutamine synthetase	MATSUNO et al. (1976)
Hemoglobin	ROSSI et al. (1977)
Cell proliferation	PAUCKER et al. (1962), GRESSER (1977)
Cell motility	PFEFFER et al. (1980a), BROUTY-BOYÉ and ZETTER (1980)

1977). Interferon treatment enhances the specific cytotoxicity of sensitized T-cells against allogeneic target cells (LINDAHL et al. 1972). Enhanced cytotoxicity may be related to interferon-mediated enhanced antigen expression on the surface of normal and tumor cells (LINDAHL et al. 1972, 1974). More recently, it has been established that interferon augments the cytotoxicity of natural killer cells for appropriate target cells (GIDLUND et al. 1978; DJEU et al. 1979).

In addition, interferon treatment stimulates several macrophage functions, including phagocytosis of carbon (HUANG et al. 1971; DONAHOE and HUANG 1976) and latex particles (IMANISHI et al. 1975), and ingestion of tumor cells (GRESSER and BOURALI 1970). Interferon-treated macrophages also exhibit morphological and cytochemical changes consistent with the activated state of macrophages (RABINOVITCH et al. 1977; SCHULTZ et al. 1977). In conclusion, interferons modulate several aspects of the immune system. Some of the effects may be related to the inhibitory action of interferon on cell proliferation, while others may represent the specific immunoregulatory role of interferons.

G. Pharmacokinetics of Interferons

Numerous investigators have studied the pharmacokinetics of interferon administration in animal models and in humans. Ho and ARMSTRONG (1975) have reviewed
the earlier work, whereas STEWART (1979) and PRIESTMAN (1979) have reviewed
more recent information. This information can be summarized as follows:

1. Following intravenous administration, interferons are cleared very rapidly
(half-life in the range 10–20 min). Following the early rapid clearance of most of
the intravenously administered interferon, there is a late phase during which interferon levels decay more slowly (half-life 1–2 h, CANTELL and PYHALA 1973).

2. Circulating interferon levels are sustained longer following intramuscular or
subcutaneous administration. For example, following intramuscular administration of leukocyte interferon preparations in humans, peak blood levels of interferon are attained in 2–4 h and are maintained for a further 4–6 h. Interferon levels
gradually decline thereafter. Nevertheless, detectable levels of circulating interferon are maintained even up to 24 h after administration. Thus, daily administration of human leukocyte interferon preparations by the intramuscular route in humans leads to the continuous presence of circulating interferon. A leukocyte interferon dose of 10^5 U/kg gives a mean blood level of approximately 50 U/ml over
a 12-h period.

3. Intramuscular administration of human fibroblast interferon preparations
results in 100–1,000-fold lower levels of circulating interferon compared with the
levels obtained with an equivalent amount of a leukocyte interferon preparation.

4. Interferons diffuse poorly from blood across tissue barriers. Thus, circulating interferons have little or no access to the respiratory tract, the cerebrospinal
fluid and the brain, the aqueous and vitreous humors of the eye, and the placenta.
Conversely, interferons produced in the brain or administered into the cerebrospinal fluid do not readily distribute in the whole body. Finally, oral administration
of interferon does not lead to the appearance of circulating interferon at detectable
levels.

5. Some interferon ($< 10\%$) is excreted through the kidney in the rabbit, but
no renal excretion has been detected in humans.

6. The role of carbohydrate in the clearance of circulating interferon is controversial (BOCCI et al. 1977; MOGENSEN et al. 1974). It is unclear whether deglycosylated interferons are cleared more or less rapidly than native interferons. Perhaps
the apparent variability is due to differences in the behavior of different interferons
in host animals of different species.

7. The recent observation (GUTTERMAN et al. 1980) that the levels of circulating
leukocyte interferon attained are 2–3-fold higher in patients with breast cancer
than following administration of equivalent amounts of interferon to patients with
multiple myeloma and malignant lymphoma suggests an even greater host-depen-
dent variability in the pharmacokinetic behavior of interferons than previously
suspected.

To summarize, an initial high loading dose of human leukocyte interferon (up
to 2×10^5 U/kg body weight, intramuscular route) followed by administration of
interferon (3×10^6–10^7 U/day) every 12 or 24 h, results in an average circulating

interferon level in the range 50–250 U/ml. Administration of similar doses of human fibroblast interferon (3×10^5 U/kg) leads to a much lower level of serum interferon (peak level 20 U/ml, BILLIAU et al. 1979 b). Whether the maintenance of high circulating levels of interferon is required or desirable for clinical efficacy is an open question.

H. Efficacy of Interferons in Animal Models

Numerous investigations have been conducted in the past two decades to test the efficacy of interferons in animal models of viral and neoplastic diseases. Several investigators have obtained encouraging inhibitory effects of exogenous interferon against a variety of localized and systemic viral infections (reviewed in STEWART 1979). Interferons have been observed to suppress tumor development in several animal tumor models induced by viruses, chemicals, or radiation, as well as against transplantable tumors (reviewed in GRESSER and TOVEY 1978; STEWART 1979). Because this information has been discussed in detail in numerous recent reviews (KRIM and SANDERS 1977; GRESSER and TOVEY 1978; STEWART 1979), we shall attempt here to summarize briefly the major conclusions derived from these investigations.

I. Antiviral Studies

The original observations of NAGANO and KOJIMA (1954, 1958) provided the first indication that interferons inhibit the development of viral lesions in animals. Preparations of the "inhibitory factor" administered intradermally prior to or at the same time as live vaccinia virus inhibited the development of viral lesions in rabbit skin. Administration of the inhibitory factor subsequent to vaccinia virus challenge failed to interfere with the appearance of viral lesions (reviewed in NAGANO 1975). Although in retrospect these observations do represent the first demonstration of the efficacy of interferons in an animal model of virus infection, the first deliberate experiment with exogenous interferons in virus-infected animals was carried out by LINDENMANN et al. (1957). These investigators also demonstrated that the appearance of vaccinia lesions in rabbit skin could be inhibited by a heterologous (chicken) interferon preparation. Subsequently, ISAACS and WESTWOOD (1959) reported that the homologous rabbit interferon was much more potent than the heterologous chicken interferon in inhibiting vaccinia lesions in rabbit skin. ISAACS and WESTWOOD (1958) also observed that complete protection was obtained when interferon was given the day before a large dose of vaccinia virus, but not when it was given along with or after the virus (10,000–100,000 infective doses, ID). With a smaller dose of vaccinia virus (10–10,000 ID) complete protection was obtained when interferon was given the day before or along with the challenge virus, but not when it was given the day after. These observations highlight a recurring theme in antiviral studies with interferons, that the best results are obtained when interferon is used as a prophylactic. However, GRESSER et al. (1975 b) have emphasized the important fact that, given an adequately high dose of interferon, mice exhibit an increased survival (52%) when treatment was initiated after the onset of multiplication of vesicular stomatitis virus (4 days after intranasal inoculation of virus) compared with 11%–18% in interferon-free controls. Thus, high doses of exogenous interferon can be used successfully for therapy.

Interferons have proven effective in several models of localized virus infections in animals. Vaccinia infections on the skin and the eye, and herpesvirus and paramyxovirus (Newcastle disease virus) infections of the eye in species such as rabbits, mice, and monkeys have been suppressed or prevented with the appropriate topical administration of interferons (reviewed in STEWART 1979). Systemically administered interferons have proven effective in generalized rhabdovirus (vesicular stomatitis virus and rabies virus), togavirus, picornavirus, herpesvirus and vaccinia virus infections (GLASGOW and HABEL 1962; FINTER 1964, 1967; HILFENHAUS et al. 1975; reviewed in STEWART 1979). An important general principle to emerge from these investigations is that repeated administration of interferon is more effective than a single injection (GRESSER et al. 1967 b, 1968 b).

Interferons have also proven effective in inhibiting tumor formation by oncogenic viruses in vivo. These include DNA tumor viruses such as polyomavirus and Shope fibroma virus (ATANASIU and CHANY 1960; KISHIDA et al. 1965) on the one hand and RNA tumor viruses such as Friend, Rauscher, Gross, Moloney, and radiation leukemia viruses, and Rous and Moloney sarcoma viruses on the other (LAMPSON et al. 1964; GRESSER et al. 1967 a, b, c, d, 1968 a, 1969 b; WHEELOCK and LARKE 1968; LIEBERMAN et al. 1971; BERMAN 1970; RHIM and HEUBNER 1971; DE-CLERCQ and DE SOMER 1971).

Interferons have been combined with other agents to obtain synergistic antiviral effects. Ammonium 5-tungsto-2-antimonate (HPA 23) partially protects mice against encephalomyocarditis virus or vesicular stomatitis virus (WERNER et al. 1976). Complete protection was observed when 75,000 U interferon was administered prior to HPA 23 and both agents were given prior to the virus. Similarly, interferon and isoprinosine act synergistically against encephalomyocarditis virus infection in mice (CHANY and CERUTTI 1977). However, although interferon inhibits herpesvirus synergistically with adenine arabinoside (ara-A) in cell cultures (LERNER and BAILEY 1974), no such synergism was observed in mice (LEFKOWITZ et al. 1976).

Numerous investigators have used interferon-inducing viruses rather than exogenous interferons per se in attempts to demonstrate the usefulness of interferon against viral diseases. For example, HITCHCOCK and ISAACS (1960) used an avirulent strain of influenza virus to induce circulating interferon in mice which then protected them against subsequent challenge with Bunyamwera virus. Similarly, BARON et al. (1966 a, b) used Newcastle disease virus to induce interferon in mice which protected them against encephalomyocarditis (EMC) virus when challenged 24 h later, and JAMESON et al. (1977) used an attenuated strain of bluetongue virus (a very good inducer of interferon) to protect mice from an otherwise lethal dose of EMC.

In summary, interferons have shown considerable prophylactic efficacy in a wide variety of viral infections in animals; however, interferons are usually less effective when administered after the onset of the viral disease. Nevertheless, high doses of interferon can be beneficial, even after the onset of a viral disease (FINTER 1967; GRESSER et al. 1976 b).

II. Antitumor Studies

Interferons have proven beneficial in animals against virus-induced, spontaneous, and transplantable tumors. A detailed summary of all of the investigations in this area has been presented by KRIM and SANDERS (1977), GRESSER and TOVEY (1978), and STEWART (1979).

1. Virus-Induced Tumors

Early investigators observed that when interferon was injected into animals prior to the inoculation of polyomavirus (ATANASIU and CHANY 1960), Rous sarcoma virus (LAMPSON et al. 1963), or Shope fibroma virus (KISHIDA et al. 1965), the appearance of tumors was delayed, the size of tumors was reduced, and the number of animals bearing tumors was decreased. Several investigators have shown that the development and progression of various virus-induced murine leukemias and sarcomas can be suppressed or delayed, provided that high doses of interferon are administered at frequent intervals (GRESSER et al. 1967a, b, c, d, 1968a; WHEELOCK and LARKE 1968; BERMAN 1970). Interferons may act in these cases by inhibiting viral multiplication, by directly inhibiting tumor cell proliferation, or by enhancing immune mechanisms. The complexity of the effects of interferon in these model systems is illustrated by the findings that interferon inducers, and interferon itself under certain experimental conditions, can enhance growth of murine leukemias and sarcomas caused by type C RNA viruses (LARSON et al. 1969; DECLERCQ and MERIGAN 1971; GAZDAR et al. 1972, 1973).

2. Virus- and Radiation-Related "Spontaneous" Tumors

The AKR strain of mice develops lymphomas between 6 and 8 months of age, owing to the vertically transmitted Gross leukemia virus. Administration of interferon to newborn AKR mice for 1 year (10^4 U/day, 5 days per week) reduced the incidence of disease from 95% to 65% (GRESSER et al. 1969b). Administration of high doses of interferon (6×10^6 U/day) *after* the diagnosis of lymphoma also resulted in a delayed evolution of the disease and a doubling in the survival time (untreated controls survived approximately 2–3 weeks) (GRESSER et al. 1976c). Furthermore, a combination of interferon (3×10^6 U/day) and a single injection of cyclophosphamide increased survival to approximately 7–8 weeks (GRESSER et al. 1978a). No tumor regression was observed.

Prophylactic interferon treatment of female mice (10^3–10^4 U once per week), begun at 6 weeks of age, inhibited and delayed the appearance of mammary tumors in the RIII mice (this strain carried the murine mammary tumor virus which is transmitted via milk; CAME and MOORE 1971, 1972). Futhermore, low doses of interferon (300 U 3 times per week) were sufficient to suppress the development of irradiation-induced lymphosarcoma or radiation leukemia virus-induced lymphosarcoma in the C57BL strain of mice (LIEBERMAN et al. 1971). Similarly, methylcholanthrene-induced tumors in mice can be suppressed or delayed by interferon (SALERNO et al. 1972; KISHIDA et al. 1971).

3. Transplantable Tumors

Gresser et al. (Gresser and Bourali 1969; Gresser and Bourali-Maury 1972; Gresser et al. 1969 a, 1978 b) have extensively explored the effects of interferon on the growth of a number of transplantable ascites as well as solid tumors in several strains of mice and have observed that daily intraperitoneal or intramuscular injections (on the order of 4×10^4 U/day) of interferon inhibited tumor growth and prolonged the survival of animals. Interferon treatment was effective only if continued over a long period and when the tumor burden was low. The best results were obtained when interferon was in close contact with the tumor cells (e.g., when both were given intraperitoneally). However, systemic administration of interferon did inhibit subcutaneously inoculated Lewis lung carcinoma cells (Gresser and Bourali-Maury 1972). Once a tumor was well established, lysis or regression of the tumor was not observed. Several other investigators have essentially confirmed these results using murine type I interferon (reviewed in Krim and Sanders 1977; Stewart 1979). Furthermore, Salvin et al. (1975) have reported that murine type II or γ interferon is also markedly effective in suppressing implants of MC-36 sarcoma cells in mice at a very low dose of interferon (300 antiviral U/day as assayed with vesicular stomatitis virus). A similar dose of type I interferon (also assayed with vesicular stomatitis virus) was ineffective. This is an interesting observation which deserves careful exploration.

III. Toxicity of Interferons in Animals

The administration of amounts of interferon that exhibit an antiviral or antitumor effect is well tolerated by animals. Adult mice for example tolerate well the administration of 10^6 U/day for prolonged periods of time (Gresser and Tovey 1978). Nevertheless the administration of 10^6 U/day to suckling Swiss mice is lethal. Most of the mice succumb between days 8 and 14 owing to diffuse liver degeneration (Gresser et al. 1975 a). If interferon is stopped at days 6–8, most of the mice survive longer, but eventually die of progressive glomerulonephritis and cardiac failure beginning at day 35 (Gresser et al. 1976 a). An impairment of cell-mediated immunity has been observed in AKR leukemic mice following administration of 5×10^5 U interferon daily (Bekesi et al. 1976). This was associated with runting and atrophy of the thymus and spleen.

J. Efficacy of Interferons in Humans

Table 6 illustrates the numerous efforts that have been made to test the clinical efficacy of interferons. These investigations have generally yielded mixed results. Interferons have proven beneficial only in a limited number of patients with various viral or neoplastic diseases. Table 6 contains a detailed account of these investigations.

I. Antiviral Studies

While interferons, both leukocyte and fibroblast, have proven beneficial in herpetic keratitis in combination with other agents such as trifluorothymidine, interferons

Table 6. Clinical trials with exogenous interferon. (After DUNNICK and GALASSO 1979)

Subject of study	Preparation, dose, method, schedule, and design (number of patients)	Results, side effects	Investigators
A. Antiviral studies			
Herpes keratitis	HLI, 6×10^6 U/ml, 9 drops/day either alone or with debridement, double-blind study (16 patients with HLI only; 22, HLI plus debridement; 17, mock-HLI plus debridement)	HLI plus debridement was not an improvement over debridement alone: HLI alone significantly worse than debridement alone	SUNDMACHER et al. (1976a, b, c)
Herpes keratitis	HLI, $1.1 – 3.1 \times 10^7$ U/ml, eyedrops, daily for 7 days, double-blind, stratified, randomyzed, and placebo-controlled trial (68 patients, all had minimal wiping debridement)	HLI reduced recurrences: 49% recurrence with placebo; 30% with 1.1×10^7 U/ml; 20% with 3.3×10^7 U/ml	JONES et al. (1976)
Herpes keratitis	HLI and HFI comparison, relation of dose to prevention of recurrences	Ongoing studies	COSTER et al. (1977)
Herpes keratitis	HFI, $1–2 \times 10^5$ U/day in 6–8 topical applications (5 patients, 2 resistant to idoxuridine)	All patients healed in 4–7 days	ROMANO, Sheba Medical Center, Ber Sheba, Israel[a] M. REVEL, Weizmann Institute, Rehovet, Israel[a]
Herpes keratitis prophylaxis in steroid-treated herpes patients	HLI, 3×10^6 U/ml, double-blind study (20 patients with HLI plus steroid; 20 with albumin plus steroid)	HLI had no effect (probably has low diffusion through intact epithelial surface layers)	SUNDMACHER et al. (1978a, b)
Herpes keratitis	HLI or HFI, 10^6 U/ml, drops, 2 days with debridement, double-blind trial (18 patients treated with HLI; 20 with HFI)	Both interferons equally effective	SUNDMACHER et al. (1978c)
Herpes keratitis	HLI, 3×10^6 U/ml, double-blind study (18 patients treated with HLI plus debridement; 24 with HLI plus minimal debridement)	Benefit of HLI shown but dependent upon efficiency of debridement	SUNDMACHER et al. (1978d)

P. B. Sehgal et al.

Table 6 (continued)

Subject of study	Preparation, dose, method, schedule, and design (number of patients)	Results, side effects	Investigators
Herpes keratitis	HLI, 1.4×10^6 U/ml, drops, twice a day, double-blind study (total of 46 patients)	6.45% recurrence in control group; 7.06% in treated group	Kaufman et al. (1976)
Herpes keratitis	HLI, 10^6 U/ml, several drops, for 8 days (1 patient)	Accelerated healing	Kobza et al. (1975)
Labial and genital herpes	HLI crude ointment, 4,000 U/g, 3–5 days treatment	Satisfactory clinical effect	Ikic et al. (1975a, b)
Varicella in childhood malignancy	HLI, 4.2×10^4–2.55×10^5 U/kg, every 12 h for average of 6.4 days, double-blind and placebo-controlled trial (9 patients treated with HLI; 9 with placebo)	6 of 9 placebo-treated vs 2 of 9 HLI-treated patients had serious complications; no effect on number of days of formation of new lesions; 2 placebo-treated patients died, 1 HLI-treated patient died; side effects included fever	Arvin et al. (1978)
Herpes zoster	HLI, 1–3×10^6 U/day, i.m. for 5–8 days, placebo-controlled trial (37 patients)	HLI accelerated healing, reduced new vesicular formation; disappearance of pain; side effects: local reaction	Emödi et al. (1975)
Localized herpes zoster in malignancy	HLI, 4.8×10^4–5.1×10^5 U kg^{-1} day^{-1} in 2 divided doses for 5–8 days, double-blind and placebo-controlled trial (45 patients treated with HLI; 45 with placebo)	Decreased spread within primary dermatome; prevention of cutaneous dissemination; decreased pain; highest dose decreased visceral complications; side effects include fever and transient granulocytopenia at highest dosage	Jordan et al. (1974) Merigan et al. (1978a, b)
HSV	HFI, 3×10^6 U total, i.m., in combination with ara-A	Ongoing studies	G. Emödi et al.[a]
HSV reactivation following trigeminal nerve root neurosurgery	HLI, 3.5×10^4 U/kg, i.m., twice a day, administered day before surgery, day of surgery, and 3 additional days (19 patients treated with HLI, 18 with placebo)	Reactivation in 15 of 18 placebo-treated patients vs 8 of 19 HLI-treated patients; lesions larger, earlier, and more frequent in placebo-treated group; oropharyngeal HSV secretion earlier, more frequent,	Pazin et al. (1979)

	Treatment	Results	Reference
CMV in infants	HLI, $1.7–3.5 \times 10^5$ U/kg, i.m., for 7–14 days (5 patients)	and prolonged in placebo-treated; side effects: 11 of 19 HLI-treated patients and 6 of 18 had malaise, vomiting; 5 HLI patients had fever	ARVIN et al. (1976)
CMV after bone marrow transplantation	HLI, 10^6 U/day, i.m., for 5–10 days	1 of 2 patients treated with highest dose had decrease in viruria; some side effects noted	O'REILLY et al. (1976)
CMV in newborns and adults	HLI, $1–3 \times 10^6$ U, i.m., for 10 days (12 patients)	4 patients had inhibition of viremia; 6 patients transient inhibition only; 2 patients no inhibition; side effects: fever	EMÖDI et al. (1974, 1976)
CMV	HFI plus ara-A	Clinical improvement; side effects; alteration of blood cell counts	EMÖDI et al. (1974, 1976)
Hepatitis virus B infections			
Chronic active hepatitis	HFI, 10^6 U/day for 3 months or more	Clearing of virologic markers of disease; no side effects	DOLEN et al. (1979)
Chronic active hepatitis	HFI, 10^7 U/day, 1 patient i.m., 1 patient s.c., for 14 days, parameters measured were HB_sAg^+, anti-HB_cAg^+, liver biopsy (2 patients)	HB_sAg initially decreased and then rebounded; anti-HB_cAg decreased; interferon in the serum was 10–100 U/ml sporadically for 14 days	SCOTT et al. (1977) KINGHAM et al. (1978)
Chronic active hepatitis	HFI, $2.1–8 \times 10^6$ U/day, i.m., for 2 weeks, parameters measured were HB_sAg^+, HB_cAg^+, SGOT, $DNAP^+$, liver biopsy$^+$ (3 patients; 3 controls)	In HFI-treated groups: 1 of 3 DNAP fluctuating; 1 of 3 loss of HB_cAg 7 weeks after study; 3 of 3 SGOT decreased; other parameters stable; side effects: decrease in white blood cells	W. WEIMAR et al. Erasmus Hospital, Rotterdam, The Netherlands[a]
Chronic active hepatitis	HLI, 3.1×10^6 U/day for 2 weeks (2 patients); 3.1×10^6 U per dose, 14 doses in 20 days (1 patient); controls were not inoculated; parameters measured were HB_sAg^+, HB_cAg^+, SGOT increase, liver biopsy$^+$, $DNAP^+$	In HLI-treated groups: 3 of 3 DNAP decrease (2 rebounded; 1 remained negative); 1 of 3 SGOT decrease; 3 of 3 HB_sAg and HB_cAg unchanged (serum interferon not assayed); side effects: 2 of 3 decrease in white blood cell count; 2 of 3 fever; controls unchanged for all markers	W. WEIMAR et al. (1977, 1978a, b)

Table 6 (continued)

Subject of study	Preparation, dose, method, schedule, and design (number of patients)	Results, side effects	Investigators
Chronic active hepatitis	HFI, 10^7 U every other day for 2 weeks (1 patient); 10^5 U/day for 1 week, 3×10^5 U/day for 1 week, 10^6 U/day for 1 week, 3×10^5 U/day for final week (1 patient); 3×10^6 U/day for 1 week (1 patient); 10^7 U/day for 1 week (1 patient); 3×10^6 U/day for 8 days (2 patients); parameters measured were HB_sAg^+ (5/5), $DNAP^+$ (4/5), HB_cAg^+ (4/5), liver HB_cAg^+ (5/5), SGOT increase (5/5)	Results during treatment: 1/5 HB_sAg decrease and 3/5 DNAP decrease; results during follow-up: 2/5 HB_sAg decrease, 1/5 DNAP decrease, 2/5 DNAP increase; no detectable interferon in blood; side effects: fever and malaise	DESMYTER et al. (1976), EDY et al. (1978), DE SOMER et al. (1977)
Chronic active hepatitis	HLI, 4.2×10^5–1.2×10^7 U/day, i.m., (dose and time course of treatment variable), or ara-A (varying treatment schedule); criteria for entrance into study: HB_sAg^+, $Dane^+$, SGOT increase, liver biopsy$^+$, $DNAP^+$, HB_cAg^+ in most cases 7 patients treated with HLI, 4 with ara-A)	3 of 7 patients and 2 of 4 ara-A patients showed permanent reduction in Dane particles, HB_sAg to below the level of detection, partial or complete disappearance of HB_sAg, disappearance of HB_cAg from liver biopsy; HLI side effects: leukopenia, fever, and malaise; ara-A side effects: reversible hematopoietic suppression, transient suppression, transient abdominal pain, and weight loss, possible neurologic effects	GREENBERG et al. (1976) POLLARD et al. (1978)
Chronic active hepatitis	HLI, 3×10^6 U/day, for 5–9 weeks, parameters measured were HB_sAg^+ (7/7), $Dane^+$ (5/7), HB_cAg^+ (3/7), SGOT increase (7/7), liver biopsy$^+$ (7/7) was read under code	5 of 5 DNAP decrease and then rebounded during treatment; 5 of 5 Dane decrease then rebounded during treatment; 2 of 3 loss of HB_sAg, 2 rebounded during treatment; 3 of 7 SGOT; coincided with DNAP; 7 of 7 unchanged biopsy; side effects: fever, malaise, joint pains after	SCULLARD et al., Kings College Hospital and London School of Hygiene and Tropical Medicine, London, England[a]

	Treatment	Result	Reference
Chronic active hepatitis	HLI, 12×10^6 U/day for 1 week, dose halved thereafter every week for 6–8 weeks; double-blind, total 16 patients, 8 given HLI	3–4 weeks treatment, 2 of 8 lowered neutrophil and platelet count (dose halved) Apart from a drop in DNA-polymerase activity in the first week, no effect was found on indices of hepatitis virus B infection; leukopenia was observed during the first 2 weeks in 6 interferon-treated patients	WEIMAR et al. (1980)
Fulminant hepatitis	HFI, 3×10^6 U/day for 5 days, then 3×10^6 U every other day, parameter measured was HB_sAg^+ (5 patients)	3 of 5 patients died	J. DESMYTER, Rega Institute, Leuven, Belgium[a] BILLIAU et al. (1978)[a]
Chronic persistent hepatitis	HLI, 3×10^6 U/day, 5–9 weeks, parameters measured were HB_sAg^+, SGOT increase, liver biopsy$^+$ (1 patient)	No long-term beneficial effect	SCULLARD et al.[a]
Hepatitis in hemodialysis patient	HFI, 10^5, 3×10^5, and 10^6 U/day for 1 week; parameters measured were HB_sAg^+, $DNAP^+$, HB_cAg^+, liver HB_sAg^+, SGOT increase	No change in markers; side effects: trial was stopped because of malaise	J. DESMYTER[a]
Non-B fulminant hepatitis	HFI, $2–4 \times 10^6$ U/day, for 8 days (2 patients)	1 patient died 4 days after treatment ended; side effects: fever	M. REVEL[a]
Respiratory virus infection			
Hong Kong influenza peophylaxis	HLI, contained 1,000 U/ml intranasal route, 3–7 days	Protection against influenza	SOLOV'EV (1969)
Influenza B	HLI, total of 8×10^5 U, in 16 doses, intranasal spray	No protection	MERIGAN et al. (1973)
Rhinovirus	HLI, total of 1.4×10^7 U, in 39 doses, intranasal spray, from −1 day to +3 day (16 controls, 16 in adult treatment group)	Inhibited symptoms of infection and virus shedding	MERIGAN et al. (1973)
Rhinovirus 4	HFI, 6×10^5–48×10^6 U intranasal drops	No protection	CARTWRIGHT et al. (1976) cited by DUNNICK and GALASSO (1979)

Table 6 (continued)

Subject of study	Preparation, dose, method, schedule, and design (number of patients)	Results, side effects	Investigators
Respiratory viral disease: prophylaxis and therapy	HLI, 160 U, 5 times a day, intranasal drops, for 3 days	Decreased severity of illness and complications	Arnaoudova (1976)
Respiratory viral disease: methods of administration to nasal mucosa	HLI, applied as drops or with cotton pledget, and with antihistamines	Ongoing studies	Harmon et al. (1977)
Other virus infections			
Vaccinia vaccination	Rhesus monkey interferon 1 day prior to vaccinia vaccination	Some reduction in vaccination takes	Scientific Committee on Interferon (1962)
Vaccinia vaccination	HFI, 10^5 U, single intradermal injection, 24 h prior to vaccination with Lister vaccinia vaccine	Some reduction in vaccination takes	Scott et al. (1978)
Congenital rubella in an infant	HLI, 3×10^6 U/day, i.m., for 2 weeks (1 infant, 14 months old, weight 7.0 kg)	Regression of disease, viremia disappeared	Larsson et al. (1976)
Rabies patients	HLI, i.m., started after symptoms of rabies appeared (2 patients)	Patients died	C. Chany, Institut National de la Santé at de la Recherche Médicale, Paris[a]
General virus infections			
Ebola (Marburg-like virus)	HLI, 3×10^6 U twice daily for 14 days, together with human convalescent serum (1 patient)	Course of illness after therapy was mild; protracted convalescence; bone marrow depression; complete recovery	Emond et al. (1977)
Viral infection after renal transplant	HLI, 3×10^6 U, i.m., twice a week for 6 weeks after transplant, double-blind trial (21 patients treated, 21 placebo controls)	Reduced incidence of CMV and herpes simplex virus infections; delayed shedding of CMV	Cheeseman et al. (1979)

Prevention of viral infections in recipients of kidney allograft	HFI, 3×10^4 U/mg protein, 3×10^6 U, i.m., twice weekly, for 3 months (8 patients treated, 3 controls)	No difference between treated and control groups, no effect on number of infections	WEIMAR et al. (1978[a,b])
Viral infections in children with acute lymphoblastic leukemia	HLI, 3×10^6 U/day, i.m., for 7 days, double-blind study	Ongoing study	L.J. GARDNER et al. Royal Victoria Infirmary, Newcastle-upon-Tyne, England[a]
B. Antitumor studies			
Metastatic diseases Osteogenic sarcoma	HLI, 3×10^6 U/day for 30 days followed by 3×10^6 U 3 times a week for 17 months; used in addition to local irradiation or amputation; if HLI-treated patients develop metastasis they are given methotrexate or adriamycin (33 HLI-treated and 36 control-treated patients – comparable contemporaries): 6 control patients given methotrexate or adriamycin and 30 of them received no drugs)	HLI-treated patients: 61% free of metastasis at 2 years; 69% alive at 3 years; control-treated patients: 37% free of metastasis at 2 years (67% of drug-treated group); 34% alive at 3 years (66% of drug-treated group); side effects in HLI-treated group: 59%, fever; 44%, pain at injection site; 38%, chills; 28% transient hair loss; 14%, itchy erythema; 14%, coughing	STRANDER et al. (1974, 1976) EINHORN and STRANDER (1978) STRANDER (1977)
Osteosarcoma	Lymphoblastoid interferon from Namalva[b] cells, 3×10^6 U, i.m., twice a week, matched pair randomized study with: therapy by surgery; prophylactic chemotherapy with high doses of methotrexate for 12 months; randomization in selection of matched pairs (4 patients, 2 interferon-treated and 2 control-treated to date; up to 15 matched pairs will be treated)	2 interferon-treated and 2 control-treated are well and without disease; side effects: fever seen in all patients (rise of 2–3 °C 4 h after injection)	G. BODO et al., Ernst Boehringer Institute, Vienna, Austria[a]
Multiple myeloma	HLI, 3×10^6 U/day for 3–19 months (4 patients)	Complete remission in 2 and partial remission in 2	MELLSTEDT et al. (1979)

Table 6 (continued)

Subject of study	Preparation, dose, method, schedule, and design (number of patients)	Results, side effects	Investigators
Multiple myeloma	HLI, 3×10^6 U/day for 4–12 weeks; maintenance: 3×10^6 U/day or 3 times a week (10 patients)	1 complete remission; 2 partial remission or improvement; rest no effect; side effects: fever, fatigue, anorexia, alopecia, myelosuppression	Gutterman et al. (1980)
Juvenile pharyngeal papilloma	HLI, 3×10^6 U, 3 times a week for 6–18 months	Regression on therapy; relapse after therapy stopped	Haglund et al. Karolinska Institute, Stockholm, Sweden[a]
Cervical cancer	Freeze-dried crude HLI, 1.25×10^6 U/day by pessary technique, for 50–80 days	Satisfactory clinical effect; side effects: fever	Ikic et al. (1979)[c]
Breast cancer	Crude HLI, 2×10^6 U, intrapleurally	Improvement shown in cytologic findings from pleural exudate; side effects; malaise, anorexia, local pain, fever	Jereb et al., Institute of Immunology, Zagreb, Yugoslavia[a]
Breast cancer	HLI, 3.9×10^6 U/day for 4 weeks or more (17 patients)	No complete remissions; 6 partial response; 1 slight improvement; 10 no effect; several side effects	Gutterman et al. (1980) Borden et al. (1980)
Mammary carcinoma	HLI, $1–3.25 \times 10^6$ U/day, intralesionally for 8–12 injections (5 patients)	Tumor regression (20%–60%) in 3 patients; carcinolytic effect in 2 patients; side effects: fever	Habif et al., Columbia University, New York[a]
Non-Hodgkin's lymphoma	HLI, 1×10^7 U, i.m., for 2–30 days (6 patients)	No change in established tumor in 3 patients with advanced diffuse, histocytic disease (previously heavily, treated); in 3 patients with nodular, lymphocytic lymphoma, there was 60% decrease in tumor mass as seen by abdominal lymphomyography 6 weeks after initiation of treatment; side effects: malaise, early febrile response, reversible leukopenia	Merigan et al. (1978b)

Disease	Treatment	Result	Reference
Non-Hodgkin's lymphoma	HLI, 3.9×10^6 U/day for 4 weeks or more (11 patients)	Patients with nodular lymphocytic or histiocytic lymphoma, 2 complete remissions, 2 partial remissions, 2 slight improvement, 5 no effect; various side effects	Gutterman et al. (1980)
Hodgkin's disease	HLI, 5×10^6 U/day for 1.5 months and raised to 7×10^6 U/day for 5.5 months; total dose was 1.4×10^8 U	Some remission	Blomgren et al. (1976)
Hodgkin's disease	HLI, $8-10 \times 10^6$ U/day, i.m., (1 patient)	Disappearance of bone infiltration	Emödi
Hodgkin's disease	HLI, $3-10 \times 10^6$ U/day, i.m., (3 patients)	1 patient complete remission, 2 patients, partial remission for 1–6 months	Emödi
Acute lymphatic leukemia	HLI, 10^6 U kg^{-1} day^{-1} for 2–3 weeks; 10^6 U/kg twice weekly for maintenance (2 patients)	Clearing of bone marrow of leukemic blasts in 2–3 weeks	Hill et al. (1978)
Melanoma	HFI, 5×10^5 U/day, intralesional injection, for several weeks	Melanoma cells disappeared and lymphocytes entered area formerly occupied by tumor cells	J. S. Horoszewicz et al., Roswell Park Memorial Institute[a]
Condylomata acuminata of uterine cervix and vagina	Crude HLI powder, 5×10^5 U/day for 2–3 weeks	Good clinical effect	Ikic et al. (1975b)

[a] Presented at the workshop held by the National Institute of Allergy and Infectious Diseases and the National Cancer Institute (National Institutes of Health, Bethesda, Md.) on March 22–23, 1978, for review of clinical trials of exogenous interferon

[b] Lymphoblastoid cell line

[c] D. Ikic, I. Padovan, J. Krusic, P. Nola, M. Knezevic, B. Rode, Z. Maricic, I. Brodarek, D. Jusic, and E. Soas, "Clinical Trials of the Effect of Human Leukocyte Interferon on Some Types of Tumors," manuscript in preparation

alone are not particularly effective (SUNDMACHER et al. 1978 a, b, c, d, 1979). Furthermore, long-term daily topical administration of interferon failed to affect the recurrence of herpetic keratitis (SUNDMACHER et al. 1977).

MERIGAN et al. (1973) observed in a human volunteer study that, although statistically significant therapeutic efficacy against respiratory rhinovirus infection could be achieved by intranasal instillation of interferon, the effects were not particularly impressive and were absent when influenza B virus was used as the infectious agent. Very high doses of interferon (5×10^5 U/kg^{-1}, day^{-1}) appear to have a beneficial effect in herpes zoster infections an immunocompromised patients (MERIGAN et al. 1978). Similarly, interferon appears to be helpful in reducing some of the serious complications of varicella infections in children receiving immunosuppressive therapy for malignancy (ARVIN et al. 1978). Interferons may also help reduce or delay viral complications (cytomegalovirus and herpes simplex infections; shedding of cytomegalovirus) in renal transplant patients (CHEESEMAN et al. 1979). The efficacy of interferon in chronic active hepatitis is controversial (GREENBERG et al. 1976; KINGHAM et al. 1978; WEIMAR et al. 1980). It is likely that interferons will prove helpful in the postexposure prophylaxis of rabies in humans (BAER et al. 1977; HILFENHAUS et al. 1977).

II. Antitumor Studies

STRANDER et al. have been instrumental in attracting attention to the possible use of interferons as antitumor agents in humans (STRANDER 1977). Patients with osteogenic sarcoma were treated with human leukocyte interferon (3×10^6/day for 30 days followed by 3×10^6 U three times weekly). Of 33 patients treated with interferon, 61% were free of metastasis at 2 years and 69% were alive at 3 years. In a concurrent control group collected from other Swedish hospitals (36 controls), 37% were free of metastasis at 2 years and 34% were alive at 3 years. It has not been demonstrated that these differences are statistically significant.

Interferons appear to have some therapeutic effect in some patients with multiple myeloma (MELLSTADT et al. 1979; GUTTERMAN et al. 1980), non-Hodgkin's lymphoma (MERIGAN et al. 1978 b; GUTTERMAN et al. 1980), and breast cancer (BORDEN et al. 1980; GUTTERMAN et al. 1980). Interferon therapy appears to be most effective in those patients who: (a) respond to chemotherapy, and (b) exhibit marked bone marrow depression following interferon administration (GUTTERMAN et al. 1980). Interferons have proven ineffective in the treatment of diffuse histiocytic lymphoma (MERIGAN et al. 1978 b) and lung cancer (KROWN et al. 1980).

It is too early to reach a conclusion as to whether interferons will play an important role in the management of human neoplasms either alone or in combination with other agents. While interferons exhibit some beneficial effects in a limited number of cases, direct comparisons between the efficacy of interferons and that of other existing therapeutic procedures have not yet been made. The findings that interferons do not cause regression of established tumors in any animal model and that the inhibitory effect of interferon on tumor growth even in optimal situations is reversed upon cessation of therapy suggest that long-term remissions in humans following interferon treatment may be the exception rather than the rule. Since interferons do not exhibit striking selectivity in inhibiting the multiplication of cells derived from tumor rather than normal tissues in cultures, their use in the management of neoplastic disease may be limited. Furthermore, interferons do not completely inhibit cell division in cell culture (PFEFFER et al. 1979a). Thus, neoplasms which initially may appear sensitive to inhibition by interferon could rapidly recur. The use of interferons against neoplastic diseases in humans is an interesting, albeit a highly preliminary development in interferon research.

III. Toxicity of Interferon in Humans

Both human leukocyte and fibroblast interferon preparations appear to exhibit similar side effects. Whether all of the side effects observed can be ascribed to interferon itself or are partly due to contaminating proteins in the preparations is an open issue. Bone marrow suppression is almost always apparent within a few weeks of the beginning of interferon administration (MERIGAN et al. 1978b; BILLIAU et al. 1979b; WEIMAR et al. 1980; GUTTERMAN et al. 1980). However, the degree of marrow toxicity is relatively small and is seen mainly as a reduction in circulating granulocyte, reticulocyte, and platelet levels. The blood picture stabilizes at these lower levels and returns to normal on reduction of interferon dose or on termination of the treatment. A majority (60%–80%) of patients also exhibit a transient (usually limited to the first week of treatment) pyrexial response to interferon administration (0.5 °–2.5 °C). The extent of fever is dependent on the dose of interferon administered. Chills, malaise, fatigue, anorexia, weight loss, and partial alopecia have also been observed frequently (MERIGAN et al. 1978b; PRIESTMAN 1979; BILLIAU et al. 1978, 1979b; INGIMARSSON et al. 1979; GUTTERMAN et al. 1980). However these symptoms are usually not so severe as to necessitate discontinuation of interferon treatment. Various other side effects such as local pain at site of injection, allergic skin rash, itching erythema, and headache have also been observed in several studies (INGIMARSSON et al. 1979; PRIESTMAN 1979).

Interferon administration leads to an elevation in the serum level of hepatic enzymes (KAJANDER et al. 1979; GUTTERMAN et al. 1980; KROWN et al. 1980) and a reduction in the serum levels of high density lipoprotein (HDL) cholesterol (CANTELL et al. 1980). The significance of these observations is unclear.

K. Interferon Inducers

Extensive studies have been carried out with interferon inducers in attempts to determine whether interferon inducers are useful in the prevention or treatment of virus infections and in the treatment of neoplastic diseases (reviewed in STEWART 1979). In early work, attention was focused on inducers of high molecular weight, such as poly(I)·poly(C). Subsequently, interferon inducers of low molecular weight were discovered, which could induce high levels of circulating interferon after oral administration. The first such compound, bis-diethylaminoethyl-fluorenone (tilorone; KRUEGER and MAYER 1970) was highly active in mice, but proved to be a poor inducer in humans (reviewed in STEWART 1979). Of particular interest was the finding that tilorone did not induce interferon in most of the cell culture systems investigated. Thus, it appears that a special class of cells, not com-

Table 7. Studies of antiviral and antineoplastic effects of interferon inducers since 1977

Substance	Route of administration of inducer	Infection or tumor	Route of virus inoculation	Animal species	Effect	Reference
Poly(I)·poly(C)	Intraperitoneal	Dengue virus	Intraperitoneal or intranasal	Mouse	Reduction in mortality	Liu (1978)
Poly(ICLC)	Topical	Vaccinia virus	Intracutaneous	Rabbit	Reduction in skin lesions	Levy and Lvovsky (1978)
Poly(I)·poly(C)	Intraperitoneal	Herpes simplex virus type 2	Intraperitoneal	Mouse	Increase in mean survival time and reduction in mortality	Olsen et al. (1978)
Poly(ICLC)	Intraperitoneal	Herpes simplex virus type 2	Intraperitoneal	Mouse	Increase in mean survival time and reduction in mortality	Olsen et al. (1978)
Poly(ICLC)	Intravenous	Venezuelan equine encephalomyelitis virus	Subcutaneous	Monkey	Reduction in viremia	Stephen et al. (1979)
Poly(I)·poly(C)	Intravenous	Ehrlich ascites and L1210 tumors	Intraperitoneal	Mouse	Increase in mean survival time	Gresser et al. (1978a, b)
P. aeruginosa liposaccharide	Intraperitoneal	Sarcoma 180	Intraperitoneal	Mouse	Decrease in volume of total packed cells from the peritoneal cavity	Tanamoto et al. (1979), Cho et al. (1979)
B. abortus preparation (BRU-PEL)	Intraperitoneal	Transplantable osteogenic sarcoma	Intraperitoneal	Mouse	Reduction in mortality	Glasgow et al. (1979)
B. abortus preparation (BRU-PEL)	Intraperitoneal	Madison lung carcinoma	Intravenous	Mouse	Reduction in number of lung lesions	Schultz et al. (1978)
ABPP	Oral or parenteral	Semliki Forest or encephalomyocarditis virus		Mouse	Reduction in mortality	Weed et al. (1980)

Table 7. (continued)

Substance	Route of administration of inducer	Infection or tumor	Route of virus inoculation	Animal species	Effect	Reference
ABPP	Nasal	Infectious bovine rhinotracheitis virus	Intranasal	Calf	Reduced duration of nasal and ocular discharges; reduced lung lesions	HAMDY and STRINGFELLOW (1980)
AIPP	Intraperitoneal	Herpes simplex virus type 1	Intraperitoneal	Mouse	Reduction in mortality	RENIS and EIDSON (1980)
Anthraquinone	Oral or parenteral	Encephalomyocarditis virus	Intranasal	Mouse	Reduction in mortality	STRINGFELLOW et al. (1979)
Acridanone	Parenteral	Japanese B encephalitis virus	Intraperitoneal	Mouse and hamster	Reduction in mortality	TAYLOR et al. (1980b)

monly used in culture, is responsible for interferon production after tilorone induction in experimental animals, such as mice. The interferon response to tilorone is highly sensitive to X-irradiation (Glasgow 1971), but not to treatment with antilymphocyte serum (Stringfellow and Glasgow 1972a, b). Recently, similar results have been obtained with new low molecular weight inducers such as 2-amino-5-bromo-6-phenyl-4-pyrimidinol (ABPP) and 2-amino-5-iodo-6-phenyl-4-pyrimidinol (AIPP) (Stringfellow et al. 1980).

Poly(I)·poly(C) has been complexed with poly-L-lysine and carboxymethyl cellulose (poly(ICLC)). The complex has high inducing activity in primates (Levy et al. 1975; Sammons et al. 1977). This has led to extensive studies of its several actions. *Brucella abortus* preparation (BRU-PEL) is under intensive study as an antitumor agent. It consists of ether-extracted organisms (Youngner et al. 1974).

It is important to emphasize that not all of the antiviral and antitumor effects that have been obtained with interferon inducers can be ascribed to the interferon produced in response to the action of the inducers. However, further work is required to elucidate the mechanism of action of a number of the high or low molecular weight inducers of interferon.

The search of more effective and less toxic interferon inducers for human use is continuing. Although the hyporeactivity that is commonly observed upon repeated administration of the same inducer limits the usefulness of interferon inducers, several factors are in favor of continued investigation of interferon inducers, notably: (1) a host rendered hyporeactive to one inducer may still be strongly reactive to a different inducer; (2) certain inducers are capable of inducing very high levels of interferon; (3) a number of inducers activate immunologic mechanisms that may be favorable to the host.

In this section, we will focus on results obtained since 1977, as earlier work has already been adequately summarized (see Stewart 1979; Declercq 1980). We shall first discuss the antiviral and antitumor effects of high molecular weight inducers and then deal with the antiviral effects of low molecular weight inducers. We will include information on the immunomodulating effects of the inducers where such information is available and relevant. To assess the activity of the inducers it is necessary to review some quantitative information about the experimental conditions. Table 7 presents a general overview of recent findings of note.

I. High Molecular Weight Substances

1. Antiviral Effects

a) Poly(I)·Poly(C) and Poly(ICLC).

α) Poly(I)·Poly(C) in Dengue Virus Infection in Mice
Poly(I)·poly(C), given in repeated intraperitoneal injections starting 4 h before intraperitoneal or intranasal inoculation of a small dose of dengue type 1 virus and continuing at 48-h intervals, afforded substantial protection against death (Liu 1978). In these experiments, the total dose of poly(I)·poly(C) was 130–190 µg per mouse. Poly(I)·poly(C) also showed some protective effect when treatment was begun 1 day, but not when it was begun 3 days after virus challenge.

β) Poly(ICLC) in Viral Infections in Rhesus Monkeys

In contrast to poly(I)·poly(C) which is not an effective inducer of interferon in monkeys (LEVY et al. 1976), poly(I)·poly(C) stabilized with poly-L-lysine and carboxymethylcellulose, poly(ICLC), induces high levels of circulating interferon in rhesus and cynomolgus monkeys and in chimpanzees (LEVY et al. 1975; SAMMONS et al. 1977). Poly(ICLC) has shown effectiveness in the prophylactic control of simian hemorrhagic fever (LEVY et al. 1976) and yellow fever (STEPHEN et al. 1977b). Of special interest are results which indicate that poly(ICLC), administered to rhesus monkeys who received a commercial rabies vaccine and were challenged with a high dose of rabies virus, markedly reduced the mortality rate in the experimental animals (BAER et al. 1977). Chronic hepatitis virus B infection has been modified in chimpanzees by the administration of poly(ICLC) (PURCELL et al. 1976). However, neither short-term therapy nor long-term (7 weeks) therapy terminated the infection and all indicators of hepatitis virus B infection returned to pretreatment levels shortly after discontinuation of treatment. Toxic effects of poly(I)·poly(C), including moderate anemia and evidence of hepatotoxicity, appeared to be completely reversible.

It has recently been shown that poly (ICLC) treatment of rhesus monkeys infected with Venezuelan equine encephalomyelitis virus reduces the incidence of viremia and prolongs the interval from infection to onset of viremia (STEPHEN et al. 1979). Poly(ICLC)-treated monkeys develop detectable serum-neutralizing antibody later than control animals. In these experiments poly(ICLC) was administered intravenously, 0.3 or 3.0 mg/kg body weight. Treatment was begun 8 h before inoculation with virus, with 9 subsequent injections given over a 17-day period. The virus (50, 1,000, or 1,800 pfu) was inoculated subcutaneously. Infection of rhesus monkeys with Venezuelan equine encephalomyelitis virus is generally benign and is characterized by a biphasic febrile response. Unexpectedly, some of the infected, treated monkeys died, although there were no deaths among monkeys that were either infected and left untreated or treated and infected. The possibility of a synergistic toxicity was suggested, resulting from the combination of infection, handling, and poly(ICLC) treatment (STEPHEN et al. 1979).

γ) Poly(ICLC) in Vaccinia Virus Infection in Rabbits

Infection of the rabbit skin with vaccinia virus can be controlled by poly(ICLC) (LEVY and LVOVSKY 1978). After intracutaneous injection of 10^3 skin lesion doses, there developed in about 3 days skin lesions which became severe by day 6. Three out of eight control animals died of vaccinia encephalitis. An ointment containing 1.7 mg/g poly(ICLC) was effective both prophylactically and therapeutically, and had a marked effect on the development of lesions when rubbed into the shaved area of the skin which had been injected with virus. Treatments were carried out daily for 4 or 5 days. Even when treatment was begun 3 days after infection, the viral titer in the skin sample 7 days after infection was only 4.5×10 pfu/g wet tissue compared with 5×10^4 pfu/g in controls. Interferon titers were 400–800 U/ml compared with 30–100 U/ml in treated and control skin samples, respectively. It was found that, 10 days after infection, the mean virus-neutralizing antibody titers were in the range of 600–1,700 (mean 1,500) in the treated compared with 80–300 (mean 160) in the control animals. These observations are consistent with previous findings indicating that poly(ICLC) is a potent immune adjuvant for mice, rats, and monkeys (Houston et al. 1976; Stephen et al. 1977a). Application of 1.5 g poly(ICLC)-containing ointment on the shaved skin of uninfected rabbits induced serum levels of interferon >100 U/ml 24 h after application.

δ) Poly(I)·Poly(C) and Poly(ICLC) in HSV-2 Infections in Mice

Inoculation of herpes simplex virus type 2 by the intraperitoneal route results in an infection that provides a highly sensitive model for evaluating the efficacy of antiviral compounds (Kern et al. 1978), although the intraperitoneal route is not a natural route of infection. In this model the virus initially replicates in visceral organs and subsequently infects the central nervous system by the hematogenous and the peripheral nerve routes. Olsen et al. (1978) have reported that poly(I)·- poly(C), poly(ICLC), and exogenous interferon can all significantly protect 7-week-old animals against death and increase the mean survival time when administered as late as 48 h after the inoculation of $\sim 3.0 \times 10^5$ pfu of virus. Mice were observed for 28 days after virus inoculation. The dosages used over a period of 7 days were as follows: poly(I)·poly(C), 100 µg per mouse daily for 2 days and then skipping a day; poly(ICLC), 100 µg per mouse every other day; or interferon 40×10^3 U twice a day. Poly(I)·poly(C) induced a peak of 5×10^3 U interferon 9 h after administration, and none was detectable at 24 h. In contrast, poly(ICLC) induced a peak of $\sim 25 \times 10^3$ U by 9 h and interferon was still detectable at 48 h. Upon repeated injections, hyporeactivity to interferon induction was more pronounced with poly(ICLC).

After intranasal infection by inhalation of virus ($\sim 4.5 \times 10^4$ pfu), the outcome was different in that these three therapeutic regimes did not reduce the final mortality or increase the mean survival time (Olsen et al. 1978). Given before intranasal infection, either poly(I)·poly(C) or poly(ICLC), but not interferon, increased the mean survival time, but the final mortality rate was not altered by any of the drugs.

When mice were inoculated intravaginally with $\sim 1.5 \times 10^5$ pfu, local treatment with poly(I)·poly(C), poly(ICLC), or interferon, started around the time of infection, appeared to reduce the mean titers of virus in genital secretions by reducing the number of infected animals and by earlier clearance of infection in some animals. With poly(I)·poly(C) and interferon, some prolongation of survival time was observed and some animals were protected against death (Olsen et al. 1978). After topical treatment with inducers, interferon was generally not detected in vaginal secretions or serum. Some of the intravaginally infected mice could be protected against death by poly(I)·poly(C), poly(ICLC), and interferon administered intraperitoneally.

These results suggest that treatment of herpesvirus type 2 infections with interferon inducers or interferon prior to involvement of the nervous system may modify the infection to the benefit of the host. Further studies are indicated to determine the anatomic site where interferon inhibits replication of this virus (Olsen et al. 1978).

ε) Immunomodulation by Poly(I)·Poly(C) and Poly(ICLC)

As would be expected, administration of interferon inducers results in a number of immunomodulating effects. For example, both interferon and poly(I)·poly(C) enhance natural killer cell activity (DJEU et al. 1979). However, as has been emphasized (LEVY et al. 1980), there are some clear differences between the effects of interferon and poly(I)·poly(C). Interferon blocks the action of a serum factor that stimulates the production in soft agar of granulocyte–macrophage colonies, whereas poly(I)·poly(C) enhances such activity (MCNEILL et al. 1972). It has been reported that, whereas interferon either inhibits or has no effect on graft–host reaction, poly(I)·poly(C) enhances such reaction (CANTOR et al. 1970; DE MAEYER and DE MAEYER-GUIGNARD 1977).

Interferon has been found to be mostly inhibitory to antibody production, however, poly(I)·poly(C) and its derivatives have been stimulatory (LEVY et al. 1980). Indeed, poly(ICLC) is an effective enhancer of the immune response when given with a number of weakly effective vaccines, including a monovalent influenza virus subunit vaccine designated A/swine X-53, prepared from a A/NJ/76 virus (STEPHEN et al. 1977a), an inactivated Venezuelan equine encephalomyelitis virus vaccine (HARRINGTON et al. 1979), a polysaccharide made from *Hemophilus influenzae* (H. B. LEVY, E. STEPHEN and D. HARRINGTON, unpublished work), a Rift Valley fever virus vaccine (D. HARRINGTON, E. STEPHEN, J. PETERS and H. B. LEVY, unpublished work), and a herpesvirus envelope protein [J. HILFENHAUS and H. B. LEVY, unpublished work; all these studies are cited in LEVY et al. (1980)].

Studies in rats, with Venezuelan equine encephalitis virus vaccine and poly(ICLC) have shown that injection of poly(ICLC) increases the size of lymph nodes draining the area where poly(ICLC) was injected and that this is associated with an increase in the number of small lymphocytes which are the cells capable of producing antibody (ANDERSON et al. to be published). The increased serum antibody is correlated with the increased number of such lymphocytes.

b) Double-Stranded RNA of Fungal Origin

Experimental rhinovirus infection can be induced in humans with virus strains, such as RU4, that have been passaged only a few times in humans and never in tissue culture since isolation from a subject who had a cold (AOKI et al. 1978). In a double-blind placebo-controlled trial, a double-stranded RNA obtained from a fungal virus had only a suggestive effect, rather than a statistically significant effect, on the experimental infection with ~ 50 tissue culture median infective doses ($TCID_{50}$) of virus given in 1 ml of nasal drops. The dose of dsRNA was limited to 5 mg/day in five doses for 3 days, because more intensive treatment regimes were associated with significant local irritating effects. The relatively low dose given locally had possibly only a small effect on the growth of virus, and delayed somewhat the onset of symptoms without affecting their maximal intensity. The interferon titers found in nasal washings from treated virus-challenged volunteers were low, and it appeared that the interferon was probably induced by the virus. Washings from those who received dsRNA and a saline challenge instead of virus contained no interferon.

2. Antitumor Effects

a) Poly(I)·Poly(C) and dsRNA from a Fungal Virus

Poly(I)·poly(C) and dsRNA from a fungal virus (statolon), given intravenously, prolong the survival time of mice with Ehrlich ascites or L1210 lymphoma cells, although ultimately all tumor-injected mice die with massive tumor ascites, despite repeated injections of interferon inducers (Gresser et al. 1978 b).

Administration of anti-interferon globulin intravenously eliminated the antitumor effects of poly(I)·poly(C) and statolon in mice inoculated intraperitoneally with varying numbers of Ehrlich ascites or L1210 leukemia cells (Gresser et al. 1978 b). Injection of normal sheep globulin or of anti-interferon globulin did not affect the survival time of mice inoculated with Ehrlich ascites or L1210 cells, but not treated with poly(I)·poly(C) or statolon. It has been established that these inducers induce in vivo an interferon which is neutralized by the anti-interferon globulin prepared in sheep against mouse interferon induced by Newcastle disease virus in mouse C-243 cells.

It was also shown that the anti-interferon globulin abolished the protective effect of poly(I)·poly(C) against infection with vesicular stomatitis or encephalomyocarditis virus (Gresser et al. 1978 b). No interferon was detected in the serum of poly(I)·poly(C)-treated mice which received antiserum globulin, but it was detected in mice which did not receive antiserum globulin.

These results provide strong evidence that the antitumor effects of poly(I)·-poly(C) and statolon in the systems investigated are mediated by interferon (Gresser et al. 1978 b). This does not rule out the possibility that endogenous interferon may render tumor cells sensitive to the cytotoxic effects of poly(I)·-poly(C).

In sharp contrast to these results, the antitumor effects of pyran copolymer and BCG were not modified by the administration of anti-interferon globulin (Gresser et al. 1978 b). Nevertheless, the small amounts of serum interferon induced by pyran copolymer were neutralized in vitro as well as in vivo by the anti-interferon globulin. The failure of the anti-interferon globulin to block the antitumor effects of pyran copolymer is consistent with previous evidence that its marked antitumor effects in mice may be due to stimulation of the reticuloendothelial system (Merigan 1967; Regelson 1967; reviewed in Pucetti and Giampietri 1978). Anti-interferon serum provides an important means of determining whether biologic effects attributed to viruses, dsRNA, and other agents are mediated through interferon (Gresser et al. 1978 b).

b) Pseudomonas aeruginosa Lipopolysaccharide

Recent studies have demonstrated that the lipopolysaccharide, isolated from the protein–lipopolysaccharide complex (endotoxin) obtained from *P. aeruginosa* autolysate, possesses antitumor, interferon-inducing, and adjuvant activities (Tanamoto et al. 1979; Cho et al. 1979). Lipid A, obtained from the lipopolysaccharide, still possesses interferon-inducing (Tanamoto et al. 1979) and adjuvant activities (Cho et al. 1979), but lacks antitumor activity. The degraded polysaccharide, obtained after extraction of lipid A, is completeley inactive.

In these studies, antitumor activity was estimated in mice inoculated intraperitoneally with ascites sarcoma 180. Test samples were injected intraperitoneally once a day for 5 days starting 24 h after tumor inoculation. The volume ratios of total packed cells from the peritoneal cavities of treated and control animals were determined on the day 7. The median effective dose (ED_{50}) for the protein–lipopolysaccharide complex from *P. aeruginosa* was 0.1 μg kg^{-1}day^{-1}, whereas that for the lipopolysaccharide was <0.1 μg kg^{-1}day^{-1}. Lipopolysaccharide from *E. coli* and *Salmonella typhimurium* was also active.

Both the antitumor and interferon-inducing activities remained after extensive treatment of the protein–lipopolysaccharide complex with protease (TANAMOTO et al. 1979). The lipopolysaccharide, isolated from the protein–lipopolysaccharide complex with aqueous phenol, showed qualitatively the same neutral sugar and fatty acid composition as that of the protein–lipopolysaccharide complex and lipopolysaccharide obtained from whole cells. Modification of the polysaccharide portion of the lipopolysaccharide by treatment with NaIO$_4$, succinic anhydride, or phthalic anhydride significantly reduced the antitumor activity, but did not affect the interferon-inducing activity. Deacylation of the lipopolysaccharide by treatment with hydroxylamine, which removes ester-linked fatty acids, also markedly decreased the antitumor activity without affecting the interferon-inducing activity. However, when all fatty acids were removed from the lipopolysaccharide by either hydrazinolysis or treatment with 4 *M* NaOH at 100 °C for 5 h, both activities were lost. Finally, when only about one-half of the fatty acids were removed with 0.1 *M* NaOH in ethanol at 37 °C for 0.5 h, both activities were retained by the preparation.

Thus, both lipid A and the polysaccharide portion, including 3-deoxy-D-mannooctulosonic acid, appear to be necessary for antitumor activity, whereas lipid A is sufficient for interferon induction. It is well known that the polysaccharide portion is not essential for endotoxicity of the lipopolysaccharide.

c) Brucella abortus Preparation (BRU-PEL)

Ether-extracted *B. abortus* cells (BRU-PEL) (YOUNGNER et al. 1974) possess interferon-inducing, antiviral, antitumor, and immunomodulating activities in mice (reviewed in YOUNGNER and FEINGOLD 1980). Extraction of BRU-PEL with chloroform–methanol (2:1 v/v) yields an insoluble residue (extracted cells) and a chloroform–methanol extract, neither of which alone induces interferon or affords protection against Semliki Forest virus infection in mice (FEINGOLD et al. 1976). Full activity is, however, restored by recombining the extracted cells and the chloroform–methanol extract. A chloroform–methanol extract from heat-killed *E. coli* is also effective in restoring the activity to extracted BRU-PEL. Although BRU-PEL contains a small residual amount of lipopolysaccharide, it has been shown that *B. abortus* lipopolysaccharide is relatively inactive as an interferon inducer in mice (KELETI et al. 1974), and lacks macrophage functional activity (SCHULTZ et al. 1978). Thus, it is unlikely that the effects of BRU-PEL are related to its residual lipopolysaccharide content.

Experiments on the antitumor activity of BRU-PEL in the sarcoma 180 ascites tumor system in mice showed that BRU-PEL, 2,000 μg per mouse, significantly inhibited ascites formation and delayed death when 10^4 cells were inoculated intraperitoneally per mouse and BRU-PEL was given within a time span of 7 days either before or after infection of the tumor cells (KELETI et al. 1977). BRU-PEL, 1,000 μg per mouse, reduced significantly the mortality of mice inoculated intraperitoneally with 10^5 cells of a plutonium-induced, transplantable osteogenic sarcoma (GLAS-

GOW et al. 1979). Mortality was reduced to 33%, 41%, or 50% when BRU-PEL was given 3 days after, at the time as, or 14 days befor tumor cells, respectively. *Corynebacterium parvum* (1,400 μg per mouse) was also effective; however, interferon induces Newcastle disease virus, and poly(ICLC) failed to protect against the development of lethal tumors (GLASGOW et al. 1979). BRU-PEL (100 mg/kg, given on day 5) also markedly reduced the number of lung lesions which developed following intravenous injection of Madison lung carcinoma cells into mice (SCHULTZ et al. 1978). *B. abortus* lipopolysaccharide (2 mg/kg) had no effect on the development of such metastatic lung nodules.

It is of considerable interest that BRU-PEL, at >1 ng/ml in culture medium, rendered macrophages nonspecifically tumoricidal for MBL-2 lymphoblastic leukemia target cells whereas *B. abortus* lipopolysaccharide failed to activate macrophages in vitro at all concentrations used (SCHULTZ et al. 1978). BRU-PEL appears to activate macrophages through a process not dependent on the thymus, as treatment of homozygous athymic mice with BRU-PEL induced cytotoxic macrophages. YOUNGNER and FEINGOLD (1980) have emphasized that BRU-PEL and a number of polyanions activate macrophages in vitro with similar kinetics, and that the basis of such activation may in fact be interferon induction (SCHULTZ and CHIRIGOS 1979; SCHULTZ et al. 1977).

BRU-PEL has been shown to potentiate an inactivated tumor cell vaccine (i.e., X-irradiated L1210 cells; CHIRIGOS et al. 1978 b). BRU-PEL also functions as an immunoadjuvant in conjunction with antitumor chemotherapy the nitrosourea derivative BCNU in the Moloney lymphoid leukemia in the mouse; CHIRIGOS et al. 1978 a). The adjuvant effect may be related to the ability of BRU-PEL to stimulate T- and B-cell production to the extent of partially reversing the depletion caused by the chemotherapeutic agent BCNU (STYLOS et al. 1978).

d) Bluetongue Virus

Bluetongue virus (BTV; attenuated vaccine strain) induces high titers of interferon in a number of animal species, in human leukocytes, and in certain cell lines and strains (JAMESON et al. 1978, 1980; JAMESON and GROSSBERG 1979). The infectivity of BTV can be destroyed by UV irradiation without seriously impairing the interferon-inducing ability of the virus. Plasma levels $>100,000$ U/ml can be obtained 8 h after intravenous injection of infective BTV, $10^{7.5}$–10^8 pfu per mouse. After 1 day, levels of 10% of the original are still detectable.

In C57BL mice, BTV suppressed the development of melanomas resulting from subcutaneous injection of B16 (F10) cells (high potential for metastasis) or B16 (F1) cells (low potential for metastasis; JAMESON et al. 1981). BTV was given one day after subcutaneous injection of cells, and repeated on day 14 after injection of B16 (F10) cells, and on day 23 after B16 (F1) cells. The development of tumors was delayed as indicated by tumor size and weight and prolongation of survival time.

Because mouse L cell interferon inhibits the proliferation of B16 (F10) cells in culture (BART et al. 1980; JAMESON et al. 1981), it is likely that the inhibition of tumor development in mice is at least in part due to the antiproliferative action of interferon. However, it is possible that other mechanisms are also involved, including a direct oncolytic effect of the virus as well as possible immunomodulating effects (JAMESON et al. 1981).

II. Low Molecular Weight Substances

1. Antiviral Effects
a) ABPP and AIPP

α) ABPP and AIPP in Encephalomyocarditis, Semliki Forest,
and HSV Infections in Mice

2-Amino-5-bromo-6-phenyl-4-pyrimidinol (ABPP) and 2-amino-5-iodo-6-phenyl-4-pyrimidinol (AIPP) protect mice against a number of RNA and DNA virus infections (WEED et al. 1980; RENIS and EIDSON 1980). AIPP is more effective than ABPP in protecting mice against encephalomyocarditis, Semliki Forest, and herpes simplex virus infections. However, ABPP is the more potent interferon inducer in the mouse. This suggests that induction of interferon is not the only possible mechanism responsible for the antiviral action of these pyrimidine derivatives in mice. However, as AIPP is approximately six times less soluble than ABPP in an aqueous medium (HAMILTON et al. 1980), differences in drug distribution may be a factor in determining the effectiveness of the drug with respect to different parameters. ABPP, but not AIPP, was effective by the oral route in protecting mice against Semliki Forest virus or encephalomyocarditis virus infection (WEED et al. 1980).

In studies with herpes simplex viruses, AIPP afforded maximum protection ($\sim 70\%$ of mice surviving) when a dose of 100 mg/kg was given intraperitoneally on 3 days consecutively, beginning 2 days prior to intraperitoneal inoculation of either herpesvirus 1 (1×10^5 pfu) or 2 (7×10^4 pfu) (RENIS and EIDSON 1980). Similar protection was obtained when 150 mg/kg was given at both 40 and 3 h prior to inoculation. Protection was diminished when AIPP was administered as a single dose of 300 mg/kg prior to inoculation, or as three daily treatments, 100 mg/kg, initiated 1 day before or on the day of virus inoculation. ABPP was less effective than AIPP on a weight basis and, even in the optimal dose range, afforded less protection than AIPP, particularly against herpesvirus 2.

Herpesvirus 1 could be isolated from kidney and liver homogenates, and after 72 h, also from spinal cord homogenates of control mice (RENIS and EIDSON 1980). Treatment with either AIPP or ABPP reduced the frequency of virus isolation from these organs. The effectiveness of AIPP and ABPP was greatly reduced when the drugs were given orally or subcutaneously, instead of intraperitoneally (RENIS and EIDSON 1980). Similarly, the protection afforded by AIPP was much less when mice were inoculated with herpesvirus 1 intravenously or intracerebrally, instead of intraperitoneally.

Cortisone, cyclophosphamide, silica, and anti-thymocyte serum exacerbate herpesvirus infections in mice. However, the protective effect of AIPP or ABPP was not altered by treatment of mice with cortisone, cyclophosphamide, or silica, but rabbit anti-mouse thymocyte serum greatly reduced the protection afforded by each drug (RENIS and EIDSON 1980). In contrast, such serum did not affect the protective effect of the drugs in encephalomyocarditis and Semliki Forest virus infections or the induction of interferon by the drugs.

ABPP, injected intraperitoneally at a dose level of 1,000 µg/kg, was a highly potent inducer of interferon and produced serum levels of interferon $>5,000$ U/ml (STRINGFELLOW et al. 1980). AIPP induced serum interferon levels of only ~ 30 U/

ml. As the level in serum rose after administration of ABPP, so did the levels in the spleen and thymus which suggested that the interferon in serum may have originated in the spleen and thymus. All levels peaked 6 h after infection of ABPP and decreased to less than one-third of the peak levels by 12 h. Although antilymphocyte serum treatment did not inhibit the interferon response, X-irradiation did, suggesting that, in vivo the interferon originated from or through the mediation of radiosensitive cell populations (STRINGFELLOW et al. 1980).

Structure–activity relationship studies with the 6-arylpyrimidines have yielded the following information (WIERENGA et al. 1980):

1. Antiviral activity against both Semliki Forest virus and herpesvirus 1 is maximized with the 6-phenyl analog when an iodo substituent is at position 5; alkyl substituents larger than propyl, at position 5, are associated with markedly diminished antiviral activity.

2. Antiviral activity is sometimes enhanced by monosubstitution (e.g., with fluoro or methoxy) on the phenyl ring.

3. Some relatively modest changes conformationally, and in some cases electronically or inductively, can completely eliminate activity.

4. There is an apparent lack of correlation between antiviral and interferon-inducing activities.

β) ABPP in Infectious Bovine Rhinotracheitis Virus Infection in Calves

The effects of nasal administration of ABPP have been determined on experimental infection of calves with infectious bovine rhinotracheitis virus (HAMDY and STRINGFELLOW 1980). Animals treated with ABPP before or after exposure to virus, or both before and after, showed lessened severity of infection as evidenced by indices such as the duration of nasal and ocular discharges and of malaise, nasal virus titers, and lung lesion scores. There was a positive correlation between early development of nasal interferon and reduction in symptoms and the severity of infection.

γ) Immunomodulation by ABPP and AIPP

Both ABPP and AIPP cause an increase in spleen natural killer (NK) cell activity in mice (LOUGHMAN et al. 1980). Because ABPP induces high levels of interferon, the possibility exists that NK cell activity is secondarily increased by the interferon produced in response to ABPP. It has been demonstrated that interferon is capable of increasing NK cell activity. However, because AIPP induces only very low levels of interferon, it would have to be assumed that very low levels of interferon are sufficient to cause increased NK cell activity. The precise mechanism by which ABPP and AIPP increase NK cell activity remains to be elucidated (LOUGHMAN et al. 1980).

ABPP and AIPP, when given 3 days prior to assay, stimulate antibody formation and increase the number of antibody forming cells detected by the Jerne plaque assay (FAST and STRINGFELLOW 1980). Antibody formation is stimulated both in immunized mice, as measured both by splenic plaque forming cells and by serum hemagglutinins, and in mice which have not been immunized. These compounds also inhibit the inflammatory phase of the graft–host reaction and the expression of delayed hypersensitivity to picrylchloride. These effects may in part be due to the interferon induced by the compounds; however, although ABPP and AIPP are similar in their immunomodulatory effects, ABPP is, as already mentioned, more effective than AIPP in interferon induction.

In another study on the immunomodulatory effects of pyrimidinols (TAGGART et al. 1980), evidence was obtained that pretreatment of mice with ABPP and AIPP significantly decreases the capacity of spleen cells to generate an in vitro humoral response to sheep red blood cells. Pretreatment of mice also abrogates the capacity of spleen cells to respond in vitro to alloantigens. Results of bone marrow cell transfer experiments have however indicated that ABPP or AIPP-pretreatment of bone marrow cells increases significantly their colony forming potential as determined in the recipient host. It has been proposed (TAGGART et al. 1980) that ABPP and AIPP may alter cell population dynamics and thereby increase the colony forming potential of bone marrow, together with effects on the humoral and cell-mediated immune responses. Drug treatment might cause an influx of immature precursor cells into the spleen with a compensatory proliferation of precursors in bone marrow.

ABPP and AIPP are not directly mitogenic for mouse splenocytes in vitro (TAGGART et al. 1980). Pretreatment of mice with ABPP significantly decreases the response of splenocytes to concanavalin A, *Salmonella typhosa* lipopolysaccharide, or phytohemagglutinin. This effect may be mediated through the interferon mechanism (TAGGART et al. 1980).

b) 1,5-Diamino Anthraquinones

Of the anthraquinones examined by STRINGFELLOW et al. (1979), 1,5-bis-[[2-(diethylamino)ethyl]amino]-anthraquinone was most active and partially protected mice against encephalomyocarditis virus infection at a dose of 8 mg/kg, which was 1/60 of its maximum tolerated dose. The virus was given intranasally. A single dose (1,000 mg/kg) given 6 days before infection had some protective activity. Protection was greatest when anthraquinone was given 1–2 days prior to infection. There was no protection when the compound was given 1 day after infection.

Anthraquinones induced the highest interferon levels when given orally (STRINGFELLOW et al. 1979). Maximal titers (1,000–10,000 U/ml serum) were reached 12–24 h after administration. X-irradiation of mice suppressed the response to the anthraquinones, but antilymphocyte serum had little effect (STRINGFELLOW et al. 1979). Examination of organ levels revealed high interferon levels in spleen and thymus tissue collected from animals injected with each of the anthraquinone derivatives used. Anthraquinones did not induce interferon production when added to murine tissues in vitro or to fibroblast cultures. It thus appears that nonlymphoid radiation-sensitive cells in the thymus and spleen, such as reticulocytes, may be involved in the interferon response (STRINGFELLOW et al. 1979).

If the same inducer was injected daily, mice rapidly developed hyporeactivity to interferon induction (STRINGFELLOW et al. 1979). However, by alternating between unrelated inducers (anthraquinone, 2-amino-5-bromo-6-methyl-4-pyrimidinol, tilorone hydrochloride) the loss of responsiveness could be avoided.

c) Propanediamine and Xylylenediamine Derivatives

N,N-Dioctadecyl-N',N'-bis (hydroxyethyl)-propanediamine and N,N-dihexade-cyl-m-xylylenediamine, administered by nasal spray, both stimulate interferon production detected by analysis of nasal washes (Gatmaitan et al. 1973; Douglas et al. 1979). The xylylenediamine derivative appears to be less potent than the propanediamine in inducing interferon production when administered intranasally (Douglas et al. 1979). Recent studies of the effectiveness of these compounds in the prevention or treatment of experimentally induced rhinovirus infections (type 21 in the study with the propanediamine derivative, and types 13 or 21 with the xylylenediamine derivative) have yielded limited evidence of effectiveness (Waldman and Ganguly 1978; Douglas et al. 1979).

The propanediamine was given at different times within 48 h of viral challenge. Given before challenge, this compound reduced by about one-half the average number and severity of symptoms, but it was without effect when given after the virus challenge. When given before infection, the propanediamine reduced virus shedding. These findings are consistent with the observation that there is a lag phase of 1–5 days before interferon is detected in humans treated with the propanediamine derivative (Gatmaitan 1973).

The xylylenediamine was administered at 24, 20, and 16 h before virus challenge, and 4 and 8 h after challenge (Douglas et al. 1979). No significant differences were seen between treated and placebo groups of volunteers with respect to the following parameters: (1) the number of subjects shedding virus in nasal washes; (2) the number developing four-fold or greater serum antibody responses; and (3) the number developing afebrile or febrile upper respiratory tract illnesses. Low levels of interferon were detected in nasal washes from 5 of 15 volunteers who received the xylylenediamine and in 2 of 15 in the placebo group. Interferon was most frequently detected on the day 5 after virus inoculation.

In view of the facts that, in mice, the xylylenediamine is a more potent interferon inducer than the propanediamine and offers a greater degree of protection against challenge with vaccinia or encephalomyocarditis virus, the results in humans emphasize the importance of species variation in response to interferon inducers (Douglas et al. 1979). Neither of the compounds stimulates interferon production in cell cultures or confers protection on cells in culture against vesicular stomatitis virus. Thus, these diamines may induce interferon only in particular cell types in vivo as has been shown for several other low molecular weight substances (see earlier in this section).

d) Carboxymethylacridanone

The acridine, 10-carboxymethyl-9-acridanone (Kramer et al., 1976) is a potent interferon inducer in mice and hamsters (Taylor et al. 1980a). Serum titers > 100,000 U/ml in young mice and titers of > 6,000 U/ml in baby hamsters have been reported (Taylor et al. 1980a, b). The acridanone gives partial protection against death from experimental Japanese B encephalitis infection in these rodents.

In the encephalitis models in weaned mice and suckling hamsters, Japanese B encephalitis virus was injected intraperitoneally (Taylor et al. 1980b). Carboxy-methylacridanone was given intraperitoneally, or by other less effective routes. The compound reduced the mortality from infection in a dose-dependent manner when given 24 h before, at the same time as, and 24 h after virus injection. Intraperitoneal administration of 224 mg/kg on this schedule reduced mortality by 60% compared with controls. A single dose of 670 mg/kg, given 24 h after virus, reduced mortality from 95% for controls to 40% for the treated group. Increasing the interval between virus and compound injection reduced therapeutic effectiveness.

In suckling hamsters, too, carboxymethylacridanone reduced mortality when given after the virus (TAYLOR et al. 1980b). In control animals, Japanese B encephalitis virus was detected in hamster plasma on day 1 following infection, and peak titer was reached on day 3. Deaths due to encephalitis began usually 5 days after infection. When the compound (920 mg/kg) was administered at the time of infection, the virus titers in the plasma were markedly reduced. Considerable reduction was also observed when the compound was given 2 days after infection.

The protection against Japanese B encephalitis afforded by carboxymethylacridanone is probably at least in part due to the interferon mechanism (TAYLOR et al. 1980b). The role of the immune system through enhanced B-lymphocyte function and phagocytosis cannot be excluded (TAYLOR et al. 1980b).

2. Antitumor Effects

It appears that so far no significant results have been obtained with low molecular weight interferon inducers in tumor systems.

L. Perspectives

The interferon field has entered a period of rapid development. Several molecular species of interferon have been sequenced and large-scale production of homogeneous preparations of different interferons may be achieved in the fairly near future. This will pave the way for a determination of the active site or sites on interferon polypeptides and of the activity of defined fragments of interferon molecules. It will be important to determine how many interferons there are in various animal species and what decides which interferon genes are turned on and for how long under the various circumstances which lead to interferon induction in living organisms and in cells in culture.

The possible organization of interferon genes into clusters of transcriptional units presents a challenging problem. A number of questions concerning the chromosomal localization of interferon genes also need to be resolved. The molecular mechanism involved in derepression of interferon genes needs to be established, and evidence obtained as to what other genes may be turned on by interferon inducers such as poly(I) · poly(C) and viruses. It is evident that interferon production is controlled not only at the transcriptional, but also at the posttranscriptional level. The translational repressor mechanism responsible for the rapid shutoff of interferon production in certain systems awaits elucidation.

The physiologic significance and the roles of interferons in health and disease should become clearer once the several different interferons have been characterized and their production and action linked to specific tissues and cell types. Strong evidence has recently been obtained in animal models of viral infections that endogenous interferons play a role in limiting infection and thus constitute an important component of the host defence against a number of different viruses. The antiviral effects of interferons may at least in part be mediated through modulation of the functions of the cellular and humoral immune systems. There is indeed evidence of a complex interplay between the interferon and the immune system. It remains to be established whether the interferon system plays a role in processes such as hormone action, cell differentiation, and cell senescence.

Interferons cause changes in the plasma membrane, alter the expression or distribution of membrane-associated proteins, and induce the synthesis of several proteins in cells. These findings focus attention on topics ranging from the precise nature of binding sites for interferons, to the mode of transmission of interferon-initiated signals to the cell nucleus, and the molecular mechanisms involved in the broad spectrum of cellular responses to interferon. It will be important to determine whether all types of interferon alter the structure and function of the plasma membrane, induce translation-regulatory proteins, and inhibit viral replication, cell proliferation, and cell locomotion. The present evidence suggests that there may indeed be significant differences in the actions of different interferons.

Cells whose proliferation has been inhibited by interferon treatment display a phenotype characteristic of a cell population in proliferative decline. Many of the structural and functional alterations in such cells appear to be secondary to the inhibition of cell proliferation by interferon and do not represent the primary effects of interferon. In future studies, it will be important to distinguish clearly between the early changes that may serve a role in initiating the proliferative decline and the coordinated alterations that are associated with the slowing of proliferation of interferon-treated cells. It will be important to determine the several mechanisms that may be involved in the inhibition of progression of normal or transformed cells through the phases of the cell cycle.

An important field for further research concerns, on the one hand, the inheritance of the capacity of cells to respond to inducers with the production of interferons and, on the other, the inheritance of the capacity of cells to respond to interferons. A number of chromosomal loci have been implicated as necessary for interferon production and at least one locus, different from these, has been implicated as necessary for responsiveness to interferon. Further work is needed to relate these loci to specific gene products.

There is strong evidence that the ability of comparable cell cultures, derived from different individuals, to produce a particular interferon upon induction with a given substance is a quantitatively graded character (MOEHRING et al. 1971 b; HAVELL and VILČEK 1972). This suggests that interferon production is a polygenic, multifactorial trait. In addition, some of the genes involved may have several alleles, which could give rise to genetic polymorphism; however, multiple allelism alone probably cannot explain the wide range of variation that has been observed. Quantitative differences have also been found in the responsiveness to interferon of cells from different strains of mice (GALLIEN-LARTIGUE et al. 1980) or from different persons (MOEHRING et al. 1971 a; BRADLEY and RUSCETTI 1981). Polygenic inheritance and genetic polymorphism may also underlie the quantitatively graded trait of responsiveness of cells to interferon. That polygenic inheritance appears to be involved in interferon production as well as in responsiveness to interferon is not surprising because of the complex cellular events involved in either trait. Work should be carried out to explore these questions systematically.

It is apparent that the duration and severity of a viral infection in an individual may at least in part be determined by his or her ability to produce interferons upon induction by the infecting virus, and in part by his or her ability to respond to the interferons produced. Furthermore, the effectiveness of an exogenously administered interferon appears to depend significantly on the responsiveness of individual recipients to interferon.

There have recently been conducted numerous, relatively small-scale trials of interferons as therapeutic agents in a variety of neoplastic diseases. Considerable variation has been encountered in the responsiveness of individual patients with the same type of tumor to interferon treatment. Of special interest are findings indicating that patients in whom an antitumor effect was obtained with interferon commonly also showed evidence of bone marrow depression, whereas patients whose tumors did not respond to interferon also failed to show such depression (GUTTERMAN et al. 1980). These observations are consistent with polygenic inheritance of the capacity to respond to interferon. As is well known (STERN 1960), the frequency distribution in polygenic inheritance is represented by the so-called normal curve; the largest number of individuals lies close to the mean measure of the range, and the greater the deviation from the mean, the smaller the groups become.

In future clinical trials of interferon in neoplastic diseases, it will be important to determine the sensitivity to the antiproliferative effect of interferon of the cells (both normal and tumor cells) from candidates for treatment. Such studies should contribute in a major way to our understanding of the inheritance of the capacity to respond to interferons and may be expected to aid in the selection of patients for treatment.

Acknowledgments. We thank Drs. K. CANTELL, S. E. GROSSBERG, H. B. LEVY, M. REVEL, T. TANIGUCHI, J. VILČEK, and J. S. YOUNGNER for providing us preprints of their forthcoming publications. We also thank Mrs. KATHLEEN E. PICKERING and Mr. HENRY BEDARD for their excellent secretarial assistance. Investigations in the authors' laboratory are supported by Grant AI-16262 from the National Institute of Allergy and Infectious Diseases, and by Grants CA-18608 and CA-18213 from the National Cancer Institute. P.B.S. is the recipient of a Junior Faculty Research Award from the American Cancer Society while L. P. was a Postdoctoral Fellow under the Institutional National Research Service Award CA-09256 from the National Cancer Institute.

References

Abreu SL, Bancroft FC (1978) Intracellular location of human fibroblast interferon messenger RNA. Biochem Biophys Res Commun 82:1300–1305

Abreu SL, Bancroft FC, Stewart WE II (1979) Interferon priming: effects on interferon messenger RNA. J Biol Chem 254:4114–4118

Adams A, Strander H, Cantell K (1975) The sensitivity of Epstein Barr virus transformed human lymphoid cells to interferon. J Gen Virol 28:207–214

Adolf GR, Swetly P (1979) Interferon production by human lymphoblastoid cells is stimulated by inducers of Friend cell differentiation. Virology 99:158–166

Anderson AO, Reynolds JA, Harrington DG Immunomodulating effect of polynucleotides on lymphocyte traffic and antiviral immunity. Proceedings of Symposium on Potentiation of Immune Response to Vaccines. J. Infect. Dis. to be published

Anfinsen CB, Bose S, Corley L, Gurari-Rotman D (1974) Partial purification of human interferon by affinity chromatography. Proc Natl Acad Sci USA 71:3139–3142

Ankel HC, Chany B, Galliot B, Chevalier MJ, Robert M (1973) Antiviral effect on interferon covalently bound to sepharose. Proc Natl Acad Sci USA 70:2360–2363

Aoki FY, Reed SE, Craig JW, Tyrrell DAJ, Lees LJ (1978) Effect of polynucleotide interferon inducer of fungal origin on experimental rhinovirus infection in humans. J. Infect. Dis. 137:82–86

Arnaoudova V (1976) Treatment and prevention of acute respiratory virus infections in children with leukocytic interferon (Abstr.). Virologie (Bucuresti) 27:83–88

Arvin AM, Yeager AS, Merigan TC (1976) Effect of leukocyte interferon on urinary excretion of cytomegalovirus by infants. J Infect Dis 133(Suppl):A205–A210

Arvin AM, Feldman S, Merigan TC (1978) Human leukocyte interferon in the treatment of varicella in children with cancer: a preliminary controlled trial. Antimicrob Agents Chemother 13:605–607

Atanasiu P, Chany C (1960) Action d'un interféron provenant de cellules malignes sur l'infection expérimentale du hamster nouveau-né par le virus du polyome. C R Acad Sci (Paris) 251:1687–1689

Atherton KT, Burke DC (1975) Interferon induction by viruses and polynucleotides: a differential effect of camptothecin. J. Gen. Virol. 29:297–304

Atherton KT, Burke DC (1978) The effects of some different metabolic inhibitors on interferon superinduction. J Gen Virol 41:229–237

Atkins GJ, Lancashire CL (1976) The induction of interferon by temperature-sensitive mutants of Sindbis virus: its relationship to double-stranded RNA synthesis and cytopathic effect. J Gen Virol 30:157–161

Atkins GJ, Johnston MD, Westmacott LM, Burke DC (1974) Induction of interferon in chick cells by temperature-sensitive mutants of Sindbis virus. J Gen Virol 25:381–384

Azuma M, Svenaga T, Yoshida I, Mizuno F (1978) Interferon synthesis in human diploid cells pretreated with insulin. Antimicrob Agents and Chemother 13:566–569

Bachner L, Declercq E, Thang MN (1975) Sepharose-bound poly(I)·poly(C): interaction with cells and interferon production. Biochem Biophys Res Commun 63:476–479

Baer GM, Shaddock JH, Moore SA, Yager PA, Baron SS, Levy HB (1977) Successful prophylaxis against rabies in mice and rhesus monkeys: the interferon system and vaccine. J Infect Dis 136:286–291

Baglioni C (1979) Interferon-induced enzymatic activities and their role in the antiviral state. Cell 17:255–264

Baglioni C, Lenz JR, Maroney PA (1978 a) The effect of salt concentration on the inhibition of protein synthesis by double-stranded RNA. Eur J Biochem 92:157–163

Baglioni C, Minks MA, Maroney PA (1978 b) Interferon action may be mediated by activation of a nuclease by pppA2′p5′A2′A. Nature 273:684–687

Baglioni C, Maroney PA, West DK (1979) 2′5′oligo(A) polymerase activity and inhibition of viral RNA synthesis in interferon treated HeLA cells. Biochemistry 18:1765–1770

Bailey DW (1971) Recombinant-inbred strains. An aid to finding identity, linkage, and function of histocompatibility and other genes. Transplantation 11:325–327

Baker PN, Bradshaw TK, Morser J, Burke DC (1979) The effect of 5-bromodeoxyuridine on interferon production in human cells. J Gen Virol 45:177–184

Balkwill F, Taylor-Papadimitriou J (1978) Interferon affects both G_1 and $S+G_2$ in cells stimulated from quiescence to growth. Nature 274:798–800

Balkwill FR, Watling D, Taylor-Papadimitriou J (1979) The effect of interferon on cell growth and the cell cycle. In: Chandra P (ed) Antiviral mechanisms in the control of neoplasia. Plenum Press, NY, pp 712–728

Ball LA Induction, purification and properties of 2′5′ oligoadenylate synthetase. In: Koch G & Richter D (eds) Regulation of macromolecular synthesis by low molecular weight mediators. Academic Press

Ball LA, White CN (1978) Oligonucleotide inhibitor of protein synthesis made in extracts of interferon treated chick embryo cells: comparison with the mouse low molecular weight inhibitor. Proc Natl Acad Sci USA 75:1167–1171

Barmak SL, Vilček J (1973) Altered cellular responses to interferon induction by poly(I)· poly(C): priming and hyporesponsiveness in cells treated with interferon preparations. Arch Virology 43:273–283

Baron S, Buckler CE, McCloskey RV, Kirschstein RL (1966a) Role of interferon during viremia. I. Production of circulating interferon. J Immunol 96:12–17

Baron S, Buckler CE, Friedman RM, McCloskey RV (1966b) Role of interferon during viremia. II. Protective action of circulating interferon. J Immunol 96:17–24

Bart RS, Porzio NR, Kopf AW, Vilček JT, Cheng EH, Farcet Y (1980) Inhibition of growth of B16 murine malignant melanoma by exogenous interferon. Cancer Research 40:614–619

Bausek GH, Merigan TC (1969) Cell interaction with a synthetic polynucleotide and interferon production in vitro. Virology 39:491–498

Baxt B, Sonnabend JA, Bablanian R (1977) Effects of interferon on vesicular stomatitis virus transcription and translation. J Gen Virol 35:325–334

Bekesi JG, Roboz JP, Zimmerman E, Holland JF (1976) Treatment of spontaneous leukemia in AKR mice with chemotherapy, immunotherapy or interferon. Cancer Res 36:631–636

Berger SL, Hitchcock MJM, Zoon KC, Birkenmeier CS, Friedman RM, Chang EH (1980) Characterization of interferon messenger RNA synthesis in Namalva cells. J Biol Chem 255:2955–2961

Berman B, Vilček J (1974) Cellular binding characteristics of human interferon. Virology 57:378–386

Berman LD (1970) Inhibition of oncogenicity of murine sarcoma virus (Harvey) in mice by interferon. Nature 227:1349–1350

Berthold W, Tan C, Tan YH (1978) Purification and in vitro labeling of interferon from a human fibroblastoid cell line. J Biol Chem 253:5206–5212

Besancon F, Ankel H (1974a) Inhibition of interferon action by plant lectins. Nature 250:784–786

Besancon F, Ankel H (1974b) Binding of interferon to gangliosides. Nature 252:478–480

Besancon F, Ankel H (1976) Inhibition de l'action de l'interféron par des hormones glycoprotéiques. CR Acad Sci (Paris) 283:1807–1810

Bialy HS, Colby S (1972) Inhibition of early vaccinia virus ribonucleic acid synthesis in interferon-treated chicken embryo fibroblasts. J Virol 9:286–289

Billiau A (1970) The refractory state after induction of interferon with double-stranded RNA. J Gen Virol 7:225–232

Billiau A, Joniau M, De Somer P (1973a) Mass production of human interferon in diploid cells stimulated by poly(I)·poly(C). J Gen Virol 19:1–8

Billiau A, Sobis M, De Somer P (1973b) Influence of interferon on virus particle formation in different oncornavirus carrier cell lines. Int J Cancer 12:646–653

Billiau A, Edy VG, De Clercq E, Heremans H, De Somer P (1975) Influence of interferon on the synthesis of virus particle in oncornavirus carrier cell lines. III. Survey of effects on A-, B-, and C-type oncornaviruses. Int J Cancer 15:947–950

Billiau A, Edy VG, Heremans H, Van Damme J, Desmyter J, Georgiades J, De Somer P (1977) Human interferon: mass production in a newly established cell line, MG-63. Antimicrob Agents Chemother 12:11–15

Billiau A, Edy V, De Somer P (1978) The clinical use of fibroblast interferon. In: Chandra P (ed) Antiviral Mechanisms in the Control of Neoplasia. Plenum Press, NY pp 675–696

Billiau A, Van Damme J, Van Leuven F, Edy VG, De Ley M, Cassiman J-J, Van Den Berghe H, De Somer P (1979a) Human fibroblast interferon for clinical trials: production, partial-purification, and characterization. Antimicrob Agents Chemother 16:49–55

Billiau A, De Somer P, Edy VG, De Clercq E, Heremans H (1979b) Human fibroblast interferon for clinical trials: pharmacokinetics and tolerability in experimental animals and humans. Antimicrob Agents Chemother 16:56–63

Blaineau C, Kishida T, Salle M, Peries J (1975) Inhibitory effect of interferon preparation on the induction of endogenous mouse type C virus by iododeoxyuridine. IRGS Med Sci 3:258–263

Blalock JE, Gifford GE (1976) Suppression of interferon production by vitamin A. J Gen Virol 32:143–146

Blalock J, Stanton JD (1980) Common pathways of interferon and hormonal action. Nature 283:406–408

Blomgren H, Cantell K, Johansson B, Lagergren C, Ringborg U, Strander H (1976) Interferon therapy in Hodgkin's disease. Acta Med Scand 199:527–532

Bocci V, Pacini A, Pessina GP, Bargigli V, Russi M (1977) Metabolism of interferon: hepatic clearance of natural and desialylated interferon. J Gen Virol 35:525–526

Bodo G, Scheirer W, Suh M, Schultze B, Morak I, Jangwirth C (1972) Protein synthesis in pox-virus infected cells treated with interferon. Virology 50:140–147

Booth BW, Borden EC (1978) Increase by calcium in production of poly rI · poly rC induced interferon by L_{929} cells. J Gen Virol 40:485–488

Borden EC, Murphy FA (1971) The interferon refractory state: in vivo and in vitro studies of its mechanism. J Immunol 106:134–138

Borden EC, Booth BW, Leonhardt PH (1978) Mechanistic studies of polyene enhancement of interferon production by poly(I) · poly(C). Antimicrob Agents Chemother 13:159–164

Borden E, Dao T, Holland J, Gutterman J, Merigan T (1980) Interferon in recurrent breast carcinoma: preliminary report of the American Cancer Society Clinical Trials Program. Interferon Sci Memoranda I-A896, p 10

Bose S, Gurari-Rotman D, Ruegg U.Th, Corley L, Anfinsen CB (1976) Apparent dispensability of the carbohydrate moiety of human interferon for antiviral activity. J Biol Chem 251:1659–1662

Bourgeade MF, Chany C (1976) Inhibition of interferon action by cytochalasin B, colchicine and vinblastine. Proc Soc Exp Biol Med 153:486–488

Bradley EC, Ruscetti FW (1981) Effect of fibroblast, lymphoid, and myeloid interferons on human tumor colony formation in vitro. Cancer Res 41:244–249

Braun W, Levy HB (1972) Interferon preparations as modifiers of immune responses. Proc Soc Exp Biol Med 141:769–773

Breinig MC, Armstrong JA, Ho M (1975) Rapid onset of hyporesponsiveness to interferon induction on reexposure to polyribonucleotide. J Gen Virol 26:149–158

Bridgen PJ, Anfinsen CB, Corley L, Bose S, Zoon KC, Ruegg VT, Buckler CE (1977) Human lymphoblastoid interferon: large scale production and partial purification. J Biol Chem 252:6585–6587

Brodeur BR, Merigan TC (1974) Suppressive effect of interferon on the humoral immune response to sheep red blood cells in mice. J Immunol 113:1319–1325

Brouty-Boyé D, Tovey MG (1977) Inhibition by interferon of thymidine uptake in chemostat cultures of L1210 cells. Intervirology 9:243–252

Brouty-Boyé D, Zetter BR (1980) Inhibition of cell motility by interferon. Science 208:516–518

Brouty-Boyé D, Macieira-Coehlo A, Fiszman M, Gresser I (1973) Effect of interferon on macromolecular synthesis in L1210 cells in vitro. Int J Cancer 12:250–258

Brown GE, Lebleu B, Kawakita M, Shaila S, Sen GC, Lengyel P (1976) Increased endonuclease activity in an extract from mouse Ehrlich ascites tumor cells which had been treated with a partially purified interferon preparation: dependence on double-stranded RNA. Biochem Biophys Res Commun 69:114–122

Burke DC, Buchan A (1965) Interferon production in chick embryo cells. I. Production by ultraviolet-inactivated virus. Virology 26:28–35

Burke DC, Graham CF, Lehman JM (1978) Appearance of interferon inducibility and sensitivity during differentiation of murine teratocarcinoma cells in vitro. Cell 13:243–248

Cabrer B, Taira H, Broeze RJ, Kempe TD, Williams K, Slattery E, Konigsberg WH, Lengyel P (1979) Structural characteristics of interferons from mouse Ehrlich ascites tumor cells. J Biol Chem 254:3681–3684

Came PE, Moore DH (1971) Inhibition of spontaneous mammary carcinoma of mice by treatment with interferon and poly I · C. Proc Soc Exp Biol Med 137:304–305

Came PE, Moore DH (1972) Effect of exogenous interferon treatment on mouse mammary tumors. J Natl Cancer Inst 48:1151–1154

Came PE, Schafer TW, Silver GH (1976) Sensitivity of rhinoviruses to human leucocyte and fibroblast interferons. J Infect Dis [Suppl] 133:A136–A138

Cantell K (1979) Why is interferon not in clinical use today? Interferon 1:1–28

Cantell K, Hirvonen S (1977) Preparation of human leukocyte interferon for clinical use. In: Baron S, Dianzani F (eds) The interferon system: a current review. Tex Rep Biol Med 35:138–141

Cantell K, Hirvonen S (1978) Large-scale production of human leukocyte interferon containing 10^8 units per ml. J Gen Virol 39:541–543

Cantell K, Paucker K (1963) Quantitative studies on viral interference in suspended L cells. IV. Production and assay of interferon. Virology 21:11–21

Cantell K, Pyhala L (1973) Circulating interferon in rabbits after administration of human interferon by different routes. J Gen Virol 20:97–104

Cantell K, Hirvonen S, Mogensen KE, Pyhala L (1974) Human leukocyte interferons: production, purification, stability and animal experiments. The production and use of interferon for the treatment of human virus infections. In: Waymouth C (ed) In Vitro Monograph 3:35–38

Cantell K, Ehnholm G, Mattila K, Kostiainen E (1980) Interferon and high-density lipoproteins. New Engl J Med 302:1032–1033

Cantor H, Asofsky R, Levy HB (1970) The effect of polyinosinic polyadenylic acid upon graft vs host activity in BALB/C mice. J Immunol 104:1035

Carter WA, Horoszewicz JS (1978) Human interferon and its inducers: clinical program overview at Roswell Park Memorial Institute. Cancer Treat Rep 62:1897–1898

Carter WA, Pitha PM, Marshall LW, Tazawa I, Tazawa S, Ts'o POP (1972) Structural requirements of then I·rC complex for induction of human interferon. J Mol Biol 70:567–575

Cavalieri RL, Havell EA, Pestka S, Vilček J (1977a) Synthesis of human interferon by *Xenopus laevis* oocytes: two structural genes for interferons in human cells. Proc Natl Acad Sci USA 74:3287–3291

Cavalieri RL, Havell EA, Vilček J, Pestka S (1977b) Induction and decay of human fibroblast interferon messenger RNA. Proc Natl Acad Sci USA 74:4415–4419

Cerrotini JC, Brunner KT, Lindahl P, Gresser I (1973) Inhibitory effect of interferon preparations and inducers on the multiplication of transplanted allogenic spleen cells and syngenic bone marrow cells. Nature 242:152–153

Chang EH, Mims SJ, Triche TJ, Friedman RM (1977) Interferon inhibits mouse leukemia virus release: an electron microscopic study. J gen Virol 34:363–371

Chang EH, Jay FT, Friedman RM (1978) Physical morphological, and biochemical alterations in the membrane of AKR mouse cells after interferon treatment. Proc Natl Acad Sci USA 75:1859–1863

Chany C (1976) Membrane-bound interferon specific cell receptor system: role in the establishment and amplification of the antiviral state. Biomedicine 24:148–160

Chany C, Cerutti I (1977) Enhancement of antiviral protection against encephalomyocarditis virus by a combination of isoprinosine and interferon. Arch Virol 55:225–232

Chany C, Ankel H, Bourgeade MF (1975) Interferon cell receptor interactions. In: Pollard M (ed) Perspectices in virology, Vol 9. Academic Press, NY, p 269

Chany C, Rousset S, Bourgeade MF, Mathieu D, Grégoire A (1980) Role of receptors and cytoskeleton in reverse transformation and steroidogenesis induced by interferon. In: Ann NY Acad Sci 350:254–265

Cheeseman SH, Rubin RH, Stewart JA, Tolkoff-Rubin NE, Cosimi AD, Cantell K, Gilbert J, Winkle S, Herrin JT, Black PH, Russell PS, Hirsch MS (1979) Controlled clinical trial of prophylactic human-leukocyte interferon in renal transplantation. Effects on cytomegalovirus and herpes simplex virus infections. N Engl J Med 300:1345–1349

Chirigos MA, Schultz RM, Pavlidis N, Feingold DS, Youngner JS (1978a) Comparative adjuvant effects of levamisole and *Brucella abortus* in murine leukemia. Cancer Treatment Reports 62:1943–1947

Chirigos MA, Stylos WA, Schultz RM, Fullen JR (1978b) Chemical and biological adjuvants capable of potentiating tumor cell vaccine. Cancer Res 38:1085–1091

Cho Y, Tanamoto K-I, Oh Y, Homma JY (1979) Differences of chemical structures of *Pseudomonas aeruginosa* lipopolysaccharide essential for adjuvanticity and antitumor and interferon-inducing activities. FEBS Letters 105:120–122

Clemens MJ, Williams BRG (1978) Inhibition of cell free protein synthesis by pppA$^{2'}$p$^{5'}$A$^{2'}$-p$^{5'}$A: a novel oligonucleotide synthesized by interferon treated L cell extracts. Cell 13:565–572

Content J, Lebleu B, Nudel U, Zilberstein A, Berissi H, Revel M (1975) Blocks on elongation and initiation of protein synthesis induced by interferon treatment in mouse L cells. Eur J Biochem 54:1–10

Content J, Lebleu B, De Clercq E (1978) Differential effects of various double-stranded RNAs on protein synthesis in rabbit reticulocyte lysates. Biochemistry 17:88–94

Coster DJ, Falcon MG, Cantell K, Jones BR (1977) Clinical experience of human leucocyte interferon in the management of herpetic keratitis. Trans Ophthalmol Soc UK 97:327–329

Creasey AA, Bartholomew JC, Merigan TC (1980) Role of G_0–G_1 arrest in the inhibition of tumor cell growth by interferon. Proc Natl Acad Sci USA 77:1471–1475

Dahl H, Degre M (1976) The effect of ascorbic acid on production of human interferon and antiviral activity in vitro. Acta Pathol Microbiol Scand B84:280–285

Davey MW, Huang JW, Sulkowski E, Carter WA (1975) Hydrophobic binding sites on human interferon. J Biol Chem 250:348–356

Davey MW, Sulkowski E, Carter WA (1976) Binding of human fibroblast interferon to concanavalin A-agarose. Involvement of carbohydrate recognition and hydrophobic interaction. Biochem 15:704–710

DeClercq E (1974) Synthetic interferon inducers. In: Topics in current chemistry 52. Springer, Berlin Heidelberg New York, p 173

DeClercq E (1977) Polynucleotides as inducers of interferon. In: Walton AG (ed) Proceedings of the first Cleveland symposium on macromolecules. Elsevier, Amsterdam, Oxford, NY, pp 217–243

DeClercq E (1980) Interferon inducers. Antibiotics Chemother 27:251–287

DeClercq E, De Somer P (1971) Role of interferon in the protective effect of the double-stranded polyribonucleotide against murine tumors induced by moloney sarcoma virus. J Natl Cancer Inst 47:1345–1355

DeClercq E, Merigan TC (1971) Moloney sarcoma virus-induced tumors in mice: inhibition or stimulation by (poly-I)·(poly-C). Proc Soc Exp Biol Med 137:590–594

DeClercq E, Edy VG, Cassiman JJ (1975) Nonantiviral activities of interferon are not controlled by chromosome 21. Nature 256:132–134

DeClercq E, Edy VG, Cassiman JJ (1976) Chromosome 21 does not code for an interferon receptor. Nature 264:249–251

DeClercq E, Stollar BD, Thang MN (1978) Interferon inducing activity of polyinosinic acid. J Gen Virol 40:203–212

De Maeyer E, De Maeyer-Guignard J (1977) Effect of interferon on cell-mediated immunity. Tex Rep Biol Med 35:370–374

De Maeyer E, De Maeyer-Guignard J (1979a) Interferons. Comprehensive Virology 15:205–284

De Maeyer E, De Maeyer-Guignard J (1979b) Considerations on mouse genes influencing interferon production and action. Interferon 1:75–100

De Maeyer E, Hoyez MC, De Maeyer-Guignard J, Bailey DW (1979) Effect of mouse genotype on interferon production. III. Expression of If-1 by peritoneal macrophages in vitro. Immunogenetics 8:257–263

De Maeyer-Guignard J, De Maeyer E, Montagnier L (1972) Interferon messenger RNA: Translation in heterologous cells. Proc Natl Acad Sci USA 69:1203–1207

De Maeyer-Guignard J, Tovey MA, Gresser I, De Maeyer E (1978) Purification of mouse interferon by sequential affinity chromatography on poly(U)- and antibody-agarose columns. Nature 271:622–625

Derynck R, Content J, DeClercq E, Volckaest G, Tavernier J, Devos R, Fiers W (1980) Isolation and structure of a human fibroblast interferon gene. Nature 285:542–547

Desmyter J, Stewart WE II (1976) Molecular modification of interferon: attainment of human interferon in a conformation active on cat cells but inactive on human cells. Virology 70:451–458

Desmyter J, Ray MB, De Groote J, Bradburne AF, Desmet VJ, Edy VG, Billiau A, De Somer P, Mortelmans J (1976) Administration of human fibroblast interferon in chronic hepatitis B infection. Lancet 2:645–647

De Somer PA, Prinzie P, Denys P Jr, Schonne E (1962) Mechanism of action of interferon. I. Relationship with viral ribonucleic acid. Virology 16:63–70

De Somer P, Edy VG, Billiau A (1977) Interferon induced skin reactivity in man. Lancet 1:47–48

Desrosiers RC, Lengyel P (1977) Impairment of reovirus mRNA cap methylation in interferon treated L cells. Fed Proc 36:812

D'Hooghe CM, Brouty-Boyé D, Malaise EF, Gresser I (1977) Interferon and cell division. XII. Prolongation by interferon of the intermitotic time of mouse mammary tumor cells in vitro. Microcinematographic analysis. Exptl Cell Res 105:73–76

Dianzani F, Baron S (1977) The continued presence of interferon is not required for activation of cells by interferon. Proc Soc Exp Biol Med 155:562–566

Dianzani F, Cantagalli P, Gagnoni S, Rita G (1968) Effects of DEAE-dextran on production of interferon induced by synthetic double-stranded RNA in L cell cultures. Proc Soc Exp Biol Med 128:708–710

Dianzani F, Levy HB, Berg S, Baron S (1976) Kinetics of the rapid action of interferon. Proc Soc Exp Biol Med 152:593–596

Djeu JY, Heinbaugh JA, Holden HT, Herberman RB (1979) Augmentation of mouse natural killer cell activity by interferon and interferon inducers. J Immunol 122:175–181

Dolen JG, Carter WA, Horoszewics JS, Vladutiu AP, Leibowitz A, Nolan JP (1979) Fibroblast interferon treatment of a patient with chronic active hepatitis. Am J Med 67:127–131

Donahoe RM, Huang KY (1976) Interferon preparations enhance phagocytosis in vivo. Infect Immun 13:1250–1253

Dorner F, Scriba M, Weil R (1973) Interferon: evidence for its glycoprotein nature. Proc Natl Accad Sci USA 70:1981–1985

Douglas RG Jr, Waldman RH, Betts RF, Ganguly R (1979) Lack of effect of an interferon inducer, N,N-dihexadecyl-m-xylyenediamine, on rhinovirus challenge in humans. Antimicrob Agent Chemother 15:269–272

Dunnick JK, Galasso GJ (1979) Clinical trials with exogenous interferon: summary of a meeting. J Infect Dis 139:109–123

Edy VG, Billiau A Desomer P (1973) Enhancement of interferon production in mouse cell line: a high-yielding source of mouse interferon. Appld Microbiol 26:434–436

Edy VG, Braude IA, DeClercq E, Billiau A, Desomer P (1976) Purification of human fibroblast interferon by glass. J Gen Virol 33:517–521

Edy VG, Billiau A, Desomer P (1977) Purification of human fibroblast interferon by zinc chelate affinity chromatography. J Biol Chem 252:5934–5936

Edy VG, Billiau A, De Somer P (1978) Non-appearance of injected fibroblast interferon in circulation. Lancet 1:451–452

Einhorn S, Strander H Interferon therapy for neoplastic diseases in man: in vitro and in vivo studies. In: Stinebring W (ed) Production of human interferon and investigation of its clinical use. Proceedings of a workshop, Tissue Culture Association. Plenum Press, NY, to be published

Emödi G, Just M (1974) Impaired interferon responses of children with congenital cytomegalovirus disease. Acta Paediatr Scand 63:183–187

Emödi G, Rufli T, Just M, Hernandez R (1975) Human interferon therapy for herpes zoster in adults. Scand J Infect Dis 7:1–5

Emödi G, O'Reilly R, Muller A, Everson LK, Binswanger U, Just M (1976) Effect of human exogenous leukocyte interferon in cytomegalovirus infections. J Infect Dis [Suppl] 133:A199–A204

Emond RTD, Evans B, Bowen ETW, Lloyd G (1977) A case of Ebola virus infections. Brit Med J 2:541–544

Eppstein DA, Samuel CE (1978) Mechanism of interferon action. Properties of an interferon mediated ribonucleic activity from mouse L929 cells. Virology 89:240–251

Epstein LB, Epstein CJ (1976) Localization of the gene AVG for the antiviral expression of immune and classical interferon to the distal portion of the long arm of chromosome 21. J Infect Dis 133:A56–A62

Falcoff E, Falcoff R, Lebleu B, Revel M (1973) Correlation between the antiviral effect of interferon treatment and the inhibition of in vitro mRNA translation in noninfected L cells. J Virol 12:421–430

Falcoff R, Sanceau J, Aujean O, Vaquero C (1980) Recovery by interferon of mengovirus induced shutoff of host protein synthesis. In: Vilček J (ed) Conference on regulatory functions of interferons. NY Acad Sci, pp 522–532

Farrell PJ, Balkow K, Hunt T, Jackson R (1977) Phosphorylation of initiation factor eIF-2 and the control of reticulocyte protein synthesis. Cell 11:187–200

Farrell PJ, Sen GC, Dubois MF, Ratner L, Slattery E, Lengyel P (1978) Interferon action: two distinct pathways for the inhibition of protein synthesis by double stranded RNA. Proc Natl Acad Sci 75:5893–5897

Farrell PJ, Broeze RJ, Lengyel P (1979) Accumulation of mRNA and protein in interferon-treated Ehrlich ascites tumor cells. Nature 279:523–525

Fast PE, Stringfellow DA (1980) Immune modulation by two antiviral isocytosines with different abilities to induce interferon. In: Nelson JD, Grassi C (eds) Current chemotherapy and infections diseases. Proceedings of the 11th International Congress of Chemotherapy and the 19th Interscience Conference on Antimicrobial Agents and Chemotherapy, vol II. The American Society for Microbiology, Washington DC, pp 1396–1398

Feingold DS, Keleti G, Youngner JS (1976) Antiviral activity of Brucella abortus preparations: separation of active components. Infection and Immunity 13:763–767

Fernandes MY, Wiktor TJ, Koprowski H (1964) Endosymbiotic relationship between animal viruses and host cells. J Exp Med 120:1099–1116

Field AK, Tytell AA, Lampson GP, Hilleman MR (1967) Inducers of interferon and host resistance. II. Multistranded synthetic polynucleotide complexes. Proc Natl Acad Sci USA 58:1004–1009

Findlay GM, MacCallum FO (1937) An interference phenomenon in relation to yellow fever and other viruses. J Path Bact 44:405–424

Finkelstein MS, Bausek GM, Merigan TC (1968) Interferon inducers in vitro: difference in sensitivity to inhibitors of RNA and protein synthesis. Science 161:465–468

Finter NB (1964) Protection of mice by interferon against systemic virus infections. Brit Med J 2:981–985

Finter NB (1967) Interferon in mice: protection against small doses of virus. J Gen Virol 1:395–397

Finter NB (1973) Interferons. North Holland Publ Co, Amsterdam

Finter NB, Bridgen D (1978) The large scale production of human interferons and their possible uses in medicine. Trends in Bioch Sc 3:76–80

Frankfort HM, Havell EA, Croce CM, Vilcek JV (1978) The synthesis and actions of mouse and human interferons in mouse-human hybrid cells. Virology 89:45–52

Frayssinet C, Gresser I, Tovey M, Lindahl P (1973) Inhibitory effect of potent interferon preparations on the regenerations of mouse liver after partial hepatectomy. Nature 245:146–147

Frey TK, Jones EV, Cardamone JJ Jr, Youngner JS (1979) Induction of interferon in L cells by defective-interfering (DI) particles of vesicular stomatitis virus: lack of correlation with content of [±] snapback RNA. Virology 99:95–102

Friedman RM (1967) Interferon binding: the first step in establishment of antiviral activity. Science 156:1760–1761

Friedman RM (1968) Interferon inhibition of arbovirus protein synthesis. J Virol 2:1081–1085

Friedman RM (1977) Antiviral activity of interferon. Bacter Rev 41:543–567

Friedman RM (1979) Interferons: interactions with cell surfaces. Interferon 1:53–74

Friedman RM, Kohn L (1976) Cholera toxin inhibits interferon action. Biochem Biophys Res Commun 70:1078–1081

Friedman RM, Pastan I (1969) Interferon and cyclic 3'5' adenosine monophosphate potentiation of antiviral activity. Biochem Biophys Res Commun 36:735–739

Friedman RM, Ramseur JM (1974) Inhibition of murine leukemia virus production in chronically infected AKR cells: a novel effect of interferon. Proc Natl Acad Sci USA 71:3542–3544

Friedman RM, Sonnabend JA (1965) Inhibition of interferon action by puromycin. J Immunology 95:696–703

Friedman RM, Chang EH, Ramseur JM, Myer MW (1975) Interferon-directed inhibition of chronic murine leukemia virus production in cell cultures: lack of effect on intracellular viral markers. J Virol 16:569–574

Fujisawa J, Iwakura Y, Kawade Y (1978) Nonglycosylated mouse L cell interferon produced by the action of tunicamycin. J Biol Chem 253:8677–8679

Fujita T, Saito S, Kohno S (1979) Priming increases the amount of interferon mRNA in poly(rI)·poly(rC)-treated L cells. J Gen Virol 45:301–308

Fulton F, Armitage P (1951) Surviving tissue suspensions for influenza virus titration. J Hyg Camb 49:247–262

Fuse A, Kuwata T (1976) Effects of interferon on the human clonal cell line, RSa. J Gen Virol 33:17–22

Gallien-Lartigue O, Carrez D, De Maeyer E, De Maeyer-Guignard J (1980) Strain dependence of the antiproliferative action of interferon on murine erhthroid precursors. Science 209:292–293

Galster RL, Lengyel P (1976) Formation and characteristics of reovirus subvirus particles in interferon-treated mouse L cells. Nucl Acids Res 3:581–598

Gandhi SS, Burke DC (1970) Interferon production by myxoviruses in chick embryo cells. J Gen Virol 6:95–104

Gardner LJ, Vilček J (1979) Initial interaction of human fibroblast and leukocyte interferon with FS-4 fibroblasts. J Gen Virol 44:161–168

Garren LD, Howell RR, Tomkins GM, Crocco RM (1964) A paradoxical effect of actinomycin D: the mechanism of regulation of enzyme synthesis by hydrocortisone. Proc Natl Acad Sci USA 52:1121–1129

Gatmaitan BG, Stanley ED, Jackson GG (1973) The limited effect of nasal interferon induced by rhinovirus and a topical chemical inducer on the course of infection. J Infect Dis 127:401–407

Gazdar AF, Steinberg AD, Spahn GF, Baron S (1972) Interferon inducers: enhancement of viral oncogenesis in mice and rats. Proc Soc Exp Biol Med 139(4):1132–1137

Gazdar AF, Sims M, Spahn GJ, Baron S (1973) Interferon mediates enhancement of tumor growth and virus-induced sarcomas in mice. Nature New Biol 245(142):77–78

Gidlund M, Orn A, Wigzell H, Senik A, Gresser I (1978) Enhanced NK cell activity in mice injected with interferon and interferon inducers. Nature 273:759–764

Gisler RH, Lindahl P, Gresser I (1974) Effects of interferon on antibody synthesis in vitro. J Immunol 113:438–444

Glasgow LA (1971) Immunosuppression, interferon, and viral infections. Fed Prod 30:1846–1851

Glasgow LA, Habel K (1962) Interferon production by mouse leukocytes in vitro and in vivo. J Exp Med 117:149–160

Glasgow LA, Crane JL Jr, Schleupner CJ, Kern ER, Youngner JS, Feingold DS (1979) Enhancement of resistance to murine osteogenic sarcoma in vivo by an extract of *Brucella abortus* (Bru-Pel): association with activation of reticuloendothelial system macrophages. Infection and Immunity 23:19–26

Gordon I, Stevenson D (1980) Kinetics of decay in the expression of interferon-dependent mRNAs responsible for resistance to virus. Proc Natl Acad Sci USA 77:452–456

Graessmann A, Graessmann M, Hoffmann H, Niebel J, Brandner G, Mueller N (1974) Inhibition by interferon of SV40 tumor antigen formation in cells injected with SV40 cRNA transcribed in vivo. FEBS Letters 39:249–251

Gravell M, Cromeans TL (1972) Inhibition of early viral ribonucleic acid synthesis in interferon treated cells infected with frog polyhedral cytoplasmic deoxyribovirus. Virology 50:916–919

Graves HE, Meager A (1980) Interferon production by human-mouse hybrid cells: dominant mouse control of superinduction and priming. J Gen Virol 47:489–495

Green JA, Cooperband SR, Kibrick S (1969) Immune-specific induction of interferon production in cultures of human blood lymphocytes. Science 164:1415–1417

Greenberg HB, Pollard RB, Lutwick LI, Gregory PB, Robinson WS, Merigan TC (1976) Effect of human leukocyte interferon on hepatitis B virus infection in patients with chronic active hepatitis. New Engl J Med 295:517–522

Greene JJ, Dieffenbach CW, Ts'o POP (1978) Inactivation of interferon mRNA in the shutoff of human interferon synthesis. Nature 271:81–83

Gresser I (1961) Production of interferon by suspensions of human leukocytes. Proc Soc Exp Biol Med 108:799–803

Gresser I (1977) On the varied biologic effect of interferon. Cellular Immunol 34:406–415

Gresser I, Bourali C (1969) Exogenous interferon and inducers of interferon in the treatment of Balb/c mice inoculated with RC19 tumor cells. Nature 223:844–846

Gresser I, Bourali C (1970) Antitumor effects of interferon preparation in mice. J Natl Cancer Inst 45:365–375

Gresser I, Bourali-Maury C (1972) Inhibition by interferon preparations of a solid malignant tumor and pulmonary metastasis in mice. Nature New Biol 236:78–79

Gresser I, Tovey MG (1978) Antitumor effects of interferon. Biochim Biophys Acta 516:231–247

Gresser I, Coppey Y, Falcoff E, Fontaine D (1967a) Interferon and murine leukemia. I. Inhibitory effect of interferon preparations on development of Friend leukemia in mice. Proc Soc Exp Biol Med 124:84–91

Gresser I, Fontaine D, Coppey Y, Falcoff R, Falcoff E (1967b) Interferon and murine leukemia. II. Factors related to the inhibitory effect of interferon preparations on development of Friend leukemia in mice. Proc Soc Exp Biol Med 124:91–94

Gresser I, Coppey J, Brouty-Boyé DF, Falcoff R (1967c) Interferon and murine leukemia. III. Efficacy of interferon preparations administered after inoculation of Friend virus. Nature 215:174–175

Gresser I, Falcoff R, Brouty-Boyé DF, Zaydela F, Coppey Y, Falcoff E (1967d) Interferon and murine leukemia. IV. Further studies on the efficacy of interferon preparations administered after inoculation of Friend virus. Proc Soc Exp Biol Med 126:791–797

Gresser I, Berman L, DeThe G, Brouty-Boyé D, Coppey Y, Falcoff E (1968a): Interferon and murine leukemia. V. Effect of interferon preparations on the evolution of Rauscher disease in mice. J Nat Cancer Inst 41:505–509

Gresser I, Bourali C, Thomas MT, Falcoff E (1968b) Effect of repeated inoculation of interferon preparations on infection of mice with encephalomyocarditis virus. Proc Soc Exp Biol Med 127:491–496

Gresser I, Bourali C, Levy JP (1969a) Increased survival in mice inoculated with tumor cells and treated with interferon preparations. Proc Natl Acad Sci USA 63:51–56

Gresser I, Coppey J, Bourali C (1969b) Interferon and murine leukemia. VI. Effect of interferon preparations on the lymphoid leukemia of AKR mice. J Natl Cancer Institut 43:1083–1089

Gresser I, Brouty-Boyé D, Thomas MT, Macieira-Coehlo A (1970) Interferon and cell division. I. Inhibiton of the multiplication of mouse leukemia L1210 cells in vitro by interferon. Proc Nat Acad Sci USA 66:1052–1058

Gresser I, Thomas MT, Brouty-Boyé D (1971) Effect of interferon on L1210 cells in vitro on tumor and colony formation. Nature 231:20–21

Gresser I, Bandu MT, Brouty-Boyé D, Tovey M (1974a) Pronounced antiviral activity of human interferon on bovine and porcine cells. Nature 251:543–545

Gresser I, Bandu MT, Brouty-Boyé D (1974b) Interferon and cell division. IX. Interferon-resistant L1210 cells: characteristics and origin. J Natl Cancer Inst 52:553–559

Gresser I, Tovey MG, Maury C, Chouroulinkov I (1975a) Lethality of interferon preparations for newborn mice. Nature 258:76–78

Gresser I, Tovey MG, Bourali-Maury C (1975b) Efficacy of exogenous infection. Treatment initiated after onset of multiplication of vesicular stomatitis virus in the brains of mice. J Gen Virol 27:395–398

Gresser I, Maury C, Tovey M, Morel-Maroger L, Pontillon F (1976a) Progressive glomerulonephritis in mice treated with interferon preparations at birth. Nature 263:420–422

Gresser I, Tovey MG, Bandu MT, Maury C, Brouty-Boyé D (1976b) Role of interferon in the pathogenesis of virus disease in mice as demonstrated by the use of anti-interferon serum. I. Rapid evolution of EMC virus infection. J Exp Med 144:1305–1315

Gresser I, Maury C, Tovey M (1976c) Interferon and murine leukemia. VII. Therapeutic effect of interferon preparations after diagnosis of lymphoma in AKR mice. Int J Cancer 17:647–653

Gresser I, Maury C, Tovey MG (1978a) Efficacy of combined interferon cyclophosphamide therapy after diagnosis of lymphoma in AKR mice. Europ J Cancer 14:97–102

Gresser I, Maury C, Bandu MT, Tovey M, Maunoury MT (1978b) Role of endogenous interferon in the antitumor effect of Poly I-C and statolon as demonstrated by the use of anti-mouse interferon serum. J Natl Cancer Inst 21:72–77

Grollmann EF, Lee G, Ramos S, Lazo PS, Kaback HR, Friedman R, Kohn LD (1978) Relationships of the structure and function of the interferon receptor to hormone receptors and the establishment of the antiviral state. Cancer Res 38:4172–4185

Grossberg SE, Holland JJ (1962) Interferon and viral ribonucleic acid. Effect on virus-susceptible and insusceptible cells. J Immunol 88:708–714

Gupta SL, Sopori ML, Lengyel P (1973) Inhibition of protein synthesis directed by added viral and cellular messenger RNAs in extracts of interferon-treated Ehrlich ascites tumor cells. Biochem Biphys Res Commun 54:777–783

Gupta SL, Graziadei WD III, Weideli H, Sopori ML, Lengyel P (1974) Selective inhibition of viral protein accumulation in interferon treated cells; nondiscriminate inhibition of the translation of added viral and cellular messenger RNAs in their extracts. Virology 57:49–63

Gupta SL, Rubin BY, Holmes SL (1979) Interferon action: induction of specific proteins in mouse and human cells by homologous interferons. Proc Natl Acad Sci USA 76:4817–4821

Gutterman JU, Blumenchein GR, Alexanian R, Yap H-Y, Buzdar AU, Cabanillas F, Hortobagyi GN, Hersh EM, Rasmussen SL, Harmon M, Kramer M, Pestka S (1980) Leukocyte interferon induced tumor regression in human metastatic breast cancer, multiple myeloma, and malignant lymphoma. Ann Int Med, 93:399–406

Haller O, Arnheiter H, Gresser I, Lindenmann J (1979) Genetically determined, interferon-dependent resistancce to influenza virus in mice. J Exp Med 149:601–612

Haller O, Arnheiter H, Lindenmann J, Gresser I (1980) Host gene influences sensitivity to interferon action selectively for influenza virus. Nature 283:660–662

Hamdy AH, Stringfellow DA (1980) Effect of 2-amino-5-bromo-6-phenyl-4-pyrimidinol in calves infected with infectious bovine rhinotracheitis virus. In: Nelson JD, Grassi C (eds) Current chemotherapy and infectious diseases, Proceedings of the 11th International Congress of Chemotherapy and the 19th Interscience Conference on Antimicrobial Agents and Chemotherapy, vol II. The American Society for Microbiology, Washington DC, pp 1404–1406

Hamilton RD, Buthala DA, Eidson EE, Tomilo A, Andrews JC (1980) Interferon induction in vitro with 6-methyl- and 6-arylpyrimidines. In: Nelson JD, Grassi C (eds) Current chemotherapy and infectious diseases, Proceedings of the 11th International Congress of Chemotherapy and the 19th Interscience Conference on Antimicrobial Agents and Chemotherapy, vol II. The American Society for Microbiology, Washington DC, pp 1409–1411

Harmon MW, Greenberg SB, Johnson PE, Couch RB (1977) Human nasal epithelial cell culture system: evaluation of response to human interferons. Infec Immun 16:480–485

Harrington DL, Crabbs CL, Hilmas DE, Brown JR, Higbee CA, Cole EF Jr, Levy HB (1979) Adjuvant effects of low doses of a nuclease resistant derivative of polyinosinic polycytidylic acid on antibody responses of monkeys to inactivated Venezuelan Equine Encephalomyelitis virus vaccine. Infect Immun 24:60–66

Havell EA (1977) Cellular regulation mechanisms controlling synthesis of interferons. In: Stewart WE II (ed) Interferons and their actions. CRC Press, Inc, Cleveland, Ohio, pp 37–48

Havell EA, Vilček J (1972) Production of high-titered interferon in cultures of human diploid cells. Antimicrob Agents Chemother 2:476–484

Havell EA, Vilček J (1975) Inhibition of interferon secretion by vinblastine. J Cell Biol 64:716–721

Havell EA, Berman B, Ogburn CA, Berg K, Paucker K, Vilček J (1975) Two antigenically distinct species of human interferon. Proc Natl Acad Sci USA 72:2185–2190

Havell EA, Yamazaki S, Vilček J (1977) Altered molecular species of human interferon produced in the presence of inhibitors of glycosylation. J Biol Chem 252:4425–4433

Havell EA, Yip YK, Vilček J (1978a) Characteristics of human lymphoblastoid (Namalva) interferon. J Gen Vriol 38:51–60

Havell EA, Hayes TG, Vilček J (1978b) Synthesis of two distinct interferons by human fibroblasts. Virology 89:330–334

Hayes TG, Yip YK, Vilček J (1979) Le interferon production by human fibroblasts. Virology 98:351–363

Henderson DR, Joklik WK (1978) The mechanism of interferon induction by UV-irradiated reovirus. Virology 91:389–406

Henle G, Henle W (1965) Evidence for a persistent viral infection in a cell line derived from Burkitt's lymphoma. J Bacteriol 89:252–260

Heron I, Berg K, Cantell K (1976) Regulation effect of interferon on T cell in vitro. J Immunol 117:1370–1377

Heron I, Hokland M, Berg K (1978) Enhanced expression of β_2-microglobulin and HLA antigen on human lymphoid cells by interferon. Proc Natl Acad Sci USA 75:6215–6219

Hilfenhaus J, Karges HE, Weinmann E, Barth R (1975) Effect of administered human leukocyte interferon on experimental rabies in monkeys. Infect Immun 11:1156–1162

Hilfenhaus J, Damm H, Johannsen R (1977) Sensitivities of various human lymphoblastoid cells to the antiviral and anticellular activity of human leukocyte interferon. Arch Virol 54:271–277

Hill NO, Loeb E, Pardue A, Khan A, Dorn GL, Comparini S, Hill JM (1978) Leukocyte interferon production and its effectiveness in acute lymphatic leukemia. J Clin Hemat Onc 8:66

Hitchcock G, Isaacs A (1960) Protection of mice against the lethal action of an encephalitis virus. Brit Med J II:1268–1270

Ho M (1961) Inhibition of the infectivity of poliovirus RNA by interferon. Proc Soc Exp Biol Med 107:639–644

Ho M, Armstrong JA (1975) Interferon. Ann Rev Microbiol 29:131–161

Ho M, Enders JF (1959a) An inhibitor of viral activity appearing in infected cell cultures. Proc Natl Acad Sci USA 45:385–389

Ho M, Enders JF (1959b) Further studies on an inhibitor of viral activity appearing in infected cell cultures and its role in chronic viral infection. Virology 9:446–477

Ho M, Kono Y (1965) Effect of actinomycin D on virus and endotoxin-induced interferon-like inhibitors in rabbits. Proc Natl Acad Sci USA 53:220–224

Ho M, Kono Y, Breinig MK (1965) Tolerance to the induction of interferons by endotoxin and virus: role of a humoral factor. Proc Soc Exp Biol Med 119:1227–1232

Ho M, Breinig MK, Postic B, Armstrong JA (1970) The effect of preinjections on the stimulation of interferon by a complexed polynucleotide, endotoxin, and virus. Ann NY Acad Sci 173:680–688

Horoszewicz JS, Leong SS, Carter WA (1979) Noncycling tumor cells are sensitive targets for the antiproliferative activity of human interferon. Science 206:1091–1093

Horvath SE, Friedman RM (1971) Nucleic acid and proteins isolated from a strain of murine sarcoma virus (MSV-O). Proc Soc Exp Biol Med 137:1075–1081

Hoskins M (1935) A protective action of neurotropic against viscerotropic yellow fever virus in Macacus rhesus. Amer J Trop Med Hyg 15:675–680

Houghton M, Stewart AG, Doel SM, Emtage JS, Eaton MAW, Smith JC, Patel TP, Lewis HM, Poster AG, Birch JR, Cartwright T, Carey NH (1980) The amino-terminal sequence of human fibroblast interferon as deduced from reverse transcripts obtained using synthetic oligonucleotide primers. Nuc Acids Res 8:1913–1931

Houston WE, Crabbs CL, Stephen SL, Levy HB (1976) Modified polyriboinosinic-polyribocytidylic acid, an immunologic adjuvant. Infec Immun 14:318–319

Hovanessian AR, Kerr IM (1979) The (2′5′)Oligoadenylate (pppA2′-5′A2′5′A) synthetase and protein kinase(s) from interferon-treated cells. Eur J Biochem 93:515–526

Hovanessian AG, Brown RE, Kerr IM (1977) Synthesis of low molecular weight inhibitor of protein synthesis with enzyme from interferon-treated cells. Nature 268:537–540

Hovanessian AG, Wood J, Meurs E, Montagnier L (1979) Increased nuclear activity in cells treated with pppA2′p5′A2′p5′A. Proc Natl Acad Sci USA 76:3261–3265

Huang JW, Davey MW, Hejna CJ, Von Muenchhausen W, Sulkowski E, Carter WA (1974) Selective binding of human interferon to albumin immobilized on agarose. J Biol Chem 249:4665–4667

Huang KY, Donahoe RM, Gordon FB, Dressler HR (1971) Enhancement of phagocytosis by interferon-containing preparations. Infect Immunity 4:581–588

Huet C, Gresser I, Bandu MT, Lindahl P (1974) Increased binding of concanavalin A to interferon-treated murine leukemia L1210 cells. Proc Soc Exp Biol Med 147:52–57

Hunt T, Ehrenfeld F (1971) Cytoplasm from poliovirus infected HeLa cells inhibits cell-free haemoglobin synthesis. Nature 230:91–94

Hutchinson DW, Merigan TC (1975) The lack of antiviral effect of poly I · poly C when attached to insoluble supports. J Gen Virol 27:403–410

Ida S, Hooks JJ, Siraganian RP, Notkins AL (1977) Enhancement of IgE mediated histamine release from human basophils by viruses: role of interferon. J Exp Med 145:892–906

Ikic D, Smerdel S, Rajninger-Miholic M, Soos E, Jusic D (1975a): Treatment of labial and genital herpes with human leukocytic interferon. In: Proceedings of the symposium on clinical use of interferon. Yugoslav Academy of Sciences and Arts, Zagreb, pp 195–202

Ikic D, Bosnic N, Smerdel S, Jusic D, Soos E, Delimar N (1975b) Double blind clinical study with human leukocyte interferon in the therapy of condylomata acuminata. In: Proceedings of the symposium on clinical use of interferon. Yugoslav Academy of Sciences and Arts, Zagreb, pp 229–233

Illinger D, Coupin G, Richards M, Poindron P (1976) Rat interferon inhibits steroid-inducible glycerol 3-phosphate dehydrogenase synthesis in a rat glial cell line. FEBS Letters 64:391–395

Imanishi J, Yokota Y, Kishida T, Mukainaka T, Matsuo A (1975): Phagocytosis-enhancing effect of human leukocyte interferon preparation on human peripheral monocytes in vitro. Acta Virology 19:52–55

Ingimarsson S, Cantell K, Strander H (1979) Side effects of long-term treatment with human leukocyte interferon. J Infect Dis 140:560–563

Isaacs A, Burke DC (1958) Mode of action of interferon. Nature 182:1073–1074

Isaacs A, Lindenmann J (1957) Virus interference I. The interferon. Proc Roy Soc Serie B 147:258–267

Isaacs A, Westwood MA (1959) Inhibition by interferon of the growth of vaccinia virus in the rabbit skin. Lancet II:324–325

Isaacs A, Lindenmann J, Valentine RC (1957) Virus interference II. Some properties of interferon. Proc Roy Soc Series B 147:268–273

Ito Y, Nishiyama Y, Shimokata K, Kimura Y, Nagata I, Kunii A (1976) The effects of cytochalasin and colchicine on interferon production. J Gen Virol 33:1–9

Iwakura Y, Yonehara S, Kawade Y (1978) Presence of a common structure in the two molecular species of mouse L cell interferon. Biochem Biophys Res Commun 84:557–563

Jameson P, Grossberg SE (1979) Production of interferon by human tumor cell lines. Arch Virol 62:209–219

Jameson P, Schoenherr CK, Grossberg SE (1977) Bluetongue virus induction of interferon and resistance to viral infection. Interferon Workshop, Lake Placid, NY

Jameson P, Schoenherr CK, Grossberg SE (1978) Bluetongue virus, an exceptionally potent interferon inducer in mice. Infection and Immunity 20:321–323

Jameson P, Taylor JL, Dixon M, Sedmak J, Grossberg SE (1980) Bluetongue virus, a potent inducer of leukocyte and fibroblastoic interferons. In: Khan A, Hill NO, Dorn GL (eds) Interferon: properties and clinical uses. Proceedings of the International Symposium on Interferons, Wadley Institutes of Molecular Medicine. Leland Fikes Foundation Press, Dallas, pp 11–20

Jameson P, Taylor JL, Grossberg SE (1981) Bluetongue virus induction of interferon: Potential for cancer therapy. In: Hersh EM, Chirigos M, Mastrangelo M (eds) Augmenting agents in cancer therapy. Current status and future prospects, Vol 16. Raven Press, New York, pp 193–203

Jankowski WJ, Davey MW, O'Malley J, Sulkowski E, Carter WA (1975) Molecular structure of human fibroblast and leukocyte interferons: probe by lectin and hydrophobic chromatography. J Virol 16:1124–1130

Jarvis AP, Colby C (1978) Regulation of the murine interferon system: isolation and characterization of a mutant 3T6 cell engaged in the semiconstitutive synthesis of interferon. Cell 14:355–364

Jarvis AP, White C, Ball A, Gupta SL, Ratner L, Sen GC, Colby C (1978) Interferon associated, dsRNA-dependent enzyme activities in a mutant 3T6 cell engaged in the semiconstitutive synthesis of interferon. Cell 14:879–887

Johnson HM (1977) Effect of interferon on antibody formation. Tex Rep Biol Med 35:357–365

Johnson HM, Smith BG, Baron S (1975) Inhibition of primary in vitro antibody response by interferon preparations. J Immunol 114:403–409

Johnston MD, Atherton KT, Hutchinson DW, Burke DC (1976) The binding of poly I · poly C to human fibroblasts and the induction of interferon. Biochim Biophys Acta 435:69–73

Johnston MI, Stollar BD (1978) Antigenic structure of double-stranded RNA analogues having varying activity in interferon inducers. Biochem 17:1959–1964

Joklik WK, Merigan TC (1966) Concerning the mechanism of action of interferon. Proc Natl Acad Sci USA 56:558–565

Jones BR, Coster DJ, Falcon MG, Cantell K (1976) Topical therapy of ulcerative herpetic keratitis with human interferon. Lancet 2:128

Jordan GW, Fried RP, Merigan TC (1974) Administration of human leukocyte interferon in herpes zoster. I. Safety, circulating antiviral activity, and host responses to infection. J Infect Dis 130:56–62

Kajander A, Von Essen R, Isomäki H, Cantell K (1979) Interferon treatment of rheumatoid arthritis. Lancet 1:984–985

Kaufman HE, Meyer RF, Laibson PR, Waltman SR, Nesburn AB, Shuster JJ (1976) Human leukocyte interferon for the prevention of recurrences of herpetic keratitis. J Infect Dis 133:A165–A168

Kawakita M, Cabrer B, Taira H, Rebello M, Slattery E, Weideli H, Lengyel P (1978) Purification of interferon from mouse Ehrlich ascites tumor cells. J Biol Chem 253:598–602

Keleti G, Feingold DS, Youngner JS (1974) Interferon induction in mice by lipopolysaccharide from *Brucella abortus*. Infection and Immunity 10:282–283

Keleti G, Feingold DS, Youngner JS (1977) Antitumor activity of a *Brucella abortus* preparation. Infection and Immunity 15:846–849

Kern ER, Richards JT, Overall JC Jr, Glasgow LA (1978) Alteration of mortality and pathogenesis of three experimental *Herpesvirus hominis* infections of mice with adenine or arabinoside 5'monophosphate, adenine arabinoside, and phosphonoacetic acid. Antimicrob Agents Chemother 13:53–60

Kerr IM, Brown RE (1978) pppA2'p5'p2'p5'A: An inhibitor of protein synthesis synthesized with an enzyme fraction from interferon treated cells. Proc Natl Acad Sci USA 75:256–260

Kerr IM, Brown RE, Ball LA (1974) Increased sensitivity of cell free protein synthesis to double stranded RNA after interferon treatment. Nature 250:57–59

Kerr IM, Brown RE, Hovanessian AG (1977) Nature of inhibitor of cell free protein synthesis found in response to interferon and double stranded RNA. Nature 268:540–542

Killander D, Lindahl P, Lundin L, Leary P, Gresser I (1976) Relationship between the enhanced expression of histocompatibility antigens of interferon-treated L1210 cells and their position in the cell cycle. Eur J Immunol 6:56–59

Kimchi A, Shulman L, Schmidt A, Chernajovsky Y, Fradin A, Revel M (1979) Kinetics of the induction of three translation-regulatory enzymes by interferon. Proc Natl Acad Sci USA 76:3208–3212

Kingham JGC, Ganguly NK, Shaari ZD, Holgate ST, McGuire MJ, Mendelson R, Cartwright T, Scott GM, Richards BM, Wright R (1978) Treatment of HBsAG-positive chronic active hepatitis with human fibroblast interferon. Gut 19:91–94

Kingsman SM, Samuel CE (1980) Mechanism of interferon action. Interferon-mediated inhibition of simian virus 40 early RNA accumulation. Virology 101:458–465

Kishida T, Kato S, Nagano Y (1965) Effet du facteur inhibiteur du virus sur le fibrome de Shope. C.R. Soc Biol 159:782–784

Kishida T, Toda S, Toida T, Hattori T (1971) Effect of interferon on malignant mouse cells. C.R. Soc Biol (Paris) 165:1489–1492

Klein G, Vilček J (1980) Attempts to induce interferon production by IdUrd induction and EBV superinfection in human lymphoma lines and their hybrids. J Gen Virol 46:111–117

Knight E Jr (1973) Interferon: effect on the saturation density to which mouse cells will grow on vitro. J Cell Biol 56:846–849

Knight E Jr (1974) Interferon sepharose: induction of the antiviral state. Biochem Biophys Res Commun 56:860–864

Knight E Jr (1976 a) Interferon purification and initial characterization from human diploid cells. Proc Natl Acad Sci USA 73:520–523

Knight E Jr (1976 b) Antiviral and cell growth inhibitory activities reside in the same glycoprotein of human fibroblast interferon. Nature 262:302–303

Knight E Jr (1978) Preparation of ^{125}Iodine-labeled human fibroblast interferon. J Gen Virol 40:681–684

Knight E Jr, Korant BD (1977) A cell surface alteration in mouse L cells induced by interferon. Biochim Biophys Res Commun 74:707–713

Knight E Jr, Korant BD (1979) Fibroblast interferon induces synthesis of four proteins in human fibroblast cells. Proc Natl Acad Sci 76:1824–1827

Knight E Jr, Hunkapiller MW, Korant BD, Hardy RWF, Hood LE (1980) Human fibroblast interferon: amino acid analysis and amino terminal amino acid sequence. Science 207:525–526

Kobza K, Emödi G, Just M, Hilti E, Leuenberger A, Binswanger U, Thiel G, Brunner FP (1975) Treatment of herpes infection with human exogenous interferon. Lancet 1:1343–1344

Kohase M, Vilček J (1977) Regulation of human interferon production stimulated with poly I·poly C: correlation between shutoff and hyporesponsiveness to reinduction. Virology 76:47–54

Kohase M, Vilček J (1979) Interferon induction with Newcastle disease virus in FS-4 cells: effect of 5,6-dichloro-1-β-D-ribofuranosylbenzimidazole (DRB). Arch Virol 62:263–271

Kohn LD, Friedman RM, Holmes JM, Lee G (1976) Use of thyrotropin and cholera toxin to probe the mechanism by which interferon initiates its antiviral activity. Proc Natl Acad Sci USA 73:3695–3699

Kohno S, Shirasawa N, Umino Y, Matsuno T, Kohase M (1975) Binding of polyribosinosinic-polyribocytidylic acid with cultured cells. Arch Virol 49:229–237

Kramer MJ, Cleeland R, Grunberg S (1976) Antiviral activity of 10-carboxymethyl-9-acridanone. Antimicrob Agents Chemother 9:233–238

Krim M, Sanders FK (1977) Prophylaxis and therapy with interferons. In: Stewart WE II (ed) Interferons and their actions. CRC Press, Cleveland, Ohio, pp 153–201

Kroath H, Gross HJ, Jungwirth C, Bodo G (1978) RNA methylation in vaccinia virus-infected chick embryo fibroblasts treated with homologous interferon. Nuc Acids Res 5:2441–2454

Kronenberg L, Friedmann T (1975) Relative quantitative assay of the biological activity of interferon messenger RNA. J Gen Virol 27:225–232

Krown SE, Stoopler MB, Cunningham-Rundles S, Oettgen HF (1980) Phase II trial of human leukocyte interferon (IF) in non-small cell lung cancer (NSCLC). Proc Amer Assoc Can Res 21:179

Krueger RF, Mayer GD (1970) Tilorone hydrochloride: an orally active antiviral agent. Science 169:1213–1214

Lai MH, Joklik WK (1973) The induction of interferon by temperature-sensitive mutants of reovirus, UV-irradiated and subviral reovirus particles. Virology 51:191–212

Lampson GP, Tytell AA, Nemes MM, Hillemann MR (1963) Purification and characterization of chick embryo interferon. Proc Soc Exp Biol Med 112:468–481

Larson VM, Clark WR, Dagle GE, Hilleman MR (1969) Influence of synthetic double-stranded ribonucleic acid, poly I:C on Friend leukemia in mice. Proc Soc Exp Biol Med 132:602–607

Larsson A, Forsgren M, Hard af Segerstad S, Strander H, Cantell H (1976) Administration of interferon to an infant with congenital rubella syndrome involving persistent viremina and cutaneous vasculitis. Acta Paediatr Scand 65:105–110

Lebleu B, Sen GC, Shaila S, Cabrer B, Lengyel P (1976) Interferon, double stranded RNA and protein phosphorylation. Proc Natl Acad Sci USA 73:3107–3111

Lebleu B, Hubert E, Content J, De Wit L, Braude IA, De Clercq E (1978) Translation of mouse interferon mRNA in *Xenopus laevis* oocytes and in rabbit reticulocyte lysates. Biochem Biophys Res Comm 82:665–673

Lebon P, Moreau MC, Cohen L, Chany C (1975) Different effect of ouabain on interferon production and action. Proc Soc Exp Biol Med 149:108–112

Lefkowitz E, Worthington M, Confiffe MA, Baron S (1976) Comparative effectiveness of six antiviral agents in herpes simplex TYPE 1 infection of mice. Proc Soc Exp Biol Med 152:337–352

Lerner AM, Bailey EJ (1974) Synergy of a 9-Beta-D-Arabinofuranosyladenine and human interferon against herpes simplex virus type 1. J Infect Dis 130:549–552

Levine DW, Wong JS, Wang DIC, Thilly WG (1977) Microcarrier cell culture: new methods for research scale application. Somatic Cell Genet 3:149–155

Levy HB, Lvovsky E (1978) Topical treatment of vaccinia virus infection with an interferon inducer in rabbits. J Infect Dis 137:78–81

Levy HB, Buckler CE, Baron S (1966) Effect of interferon on early interferon production. Science 152:1274–1276

Levy HB, Baer G, Baron S, Buckler CE, Gibbs CJ, Iadorola MJ, London WT, Rice J (1975) A modified polyriboinosinic-polyribocytidylic acid complex that induces interferon in primates. J Infect Dis 132:434–439

Levy HB, London W, Fuccillo DA, Baron S, Rice J (1976) Prophylactic control of simian hemorrhagic fever in monkeys by an interferon inducer, polyriboinosinic · polyribocytidylic acid-poly-L-lysine. J Infect Dis [Suppl] 133:A256–A259

Levy HB, Lvovsky E, Riley F, Harrington D, Anderson A, Moe J, Hilfenhaus J, Stephen E (1980) Immune modulating effects of poly ICLC. Ann NY Acad Sci 350:33–41

Lieberman M, Merigan TC, Kaplan HS (1971) Inhibition of radiogenic lymphoma development in mice by interferon. Proc Soc Exp Biol Med 138:575–578

Lieberman D, Voloch Z, Aviv H, Nudel U, Revel M (1974) Effect of interferon on hemoglobin synthesis and leukemia virus production in Friend cells. Mol Biol Rep 1:447–451

Lin LS, Stewart WE II (1978) Two dimensional gel electrophoresis of human leukocyte interferon. Abstr Ann Meeting Amer Soc Biol Chem

Lin LS, Wiranowska-Stewart M, Chudzio T, Stewart WE II (1978) Characterization of the heterogenous molecules of human interferons: differences in the cross-species antiviral activities of various molecular populations in human leukocyte interferons. J Gen Virol 39:125–130

Lindahl P, Leary P, Gresser I (1972) Enhancement by interferon of the specific cytotoxicity of sensitized lymphocytes. Proc Natl Acad Sci USA 69:721–725

Lindahl P, Leary P, Gresser I (1973) Enhancement by interferon of the expression of surface antigens on murine leukemia L1210 cells. Proc Natl Acad Sci USA 70:2785–2788

Lindahl P, Leary P, Gresser I (1974) Enhancement of the expression of histocompatibility antigen of mouse lymphoid cells by interferon in vitro. Eur J Immunol 4:779–794

Lindahl P, Gresser I, Leary P, Tovey M (1976a) Enhanced expression of histocompatibility antigens of lymphoid cells in mice treated with interferon. J Infect Dis 133:A66–A72

Lindahl P, Gresser I, Leary P, Tovey M (1976b) Interferon treatment of mice-enhanced expression of histocompatibility antigens on lymphoid cells. Proc Natl Acad Sci 73:1284–1299

Lindahl-Magnusson P, Leary P, Gresser I (1972) Interferon inhibits DNA synthesis in mouse lymphocyte suspensions by phytohaemagglutinin or by allogeneic cells. Nature New Biol 273:120–121

Lindenmann J, Burke D, Isaacs A (1957) Studies on the production, mode of action and properties of interferon. Brit J Exp Path 38:551–562

Lindner-Frimmel SJ (1974) Enhanced production of human interferon by UV-irradiated cells. J Gen Virol 25:147–150

Liu J-L (1978) Effects of mouse serum interferon and interferon inducers on dengue and Japanese encephalitis virus infections in weanling mice. Kobe J Med Sci 24:153–163

Lockart RZ Jr (1964) The necessity for cellular RNA and protein synthesis for viral inhibition from interferon. Biochem Biophys Res Commun 15:513–518

Lockart RZ Jr (1966) Biological properties of interferons: criteria for acceptance of a viral inhibitor as an interferon. In: Finter NB (ed) Interferons, North-Holland Publ Co, Amsterdam, pp 1–20

Lockart RZ Jr, Bayliss NL, Toy ST, Yin FH (1968) Viral events necessary for the induction of interferon in chick embryo cells. J Virol 2:962–965

Lomniczi B, Burke DC (1970) Interferon production by temperature-sensitive mutants of Semliki Forest virus. J Gen Virol 8:55–68

Lotem J, Sachs L (1978) Genetic dissociation of different cellular effects of interferon on myeloid leukemic cells. Int J Cancer 22:214–220

Loughman BE, Gibbons AJ, Taggart MT, Renis HE (1980) Modulation of mouse natural killer cell activity by interferon and two antiviral isocytosines. In: Nelson JD, Grassi C (eds) Current chemotherapy and infectious diseases, Proceedings of the 11th International Congress of Chemotherapy and the 19th Interscience Conference on Antimicrobial Agents and Chemotherapy, vol II. The American Society for Microbiology, Washington DC, pp 1398–1400

Lundgren E, Larsson I, Moirner H, Strannegard O (1979) Effects of leukocyte and fibroblast interferon on events in the fibroblast cell cycle. J Gen Virol 42:589–597

Magee WE, Levine S, Miller OV, Hamilton RD (1968) Inhibition by interferon of the uncoating of vaccinia virus. Virology 35:505–511

Magee WE, Talcott MJ, Strau SX, Vriend CY (1976) A comparison of negatively and positively charged lysosomes containing entrapped pIC for interferon induction in mice. Biochim Biophys Acta 451:610–621

Maheshwari RK, Friedman RM (1980) Effect of interferon treatment on vesicular stomatitis virus (VSV): release of unusual particles with low infectivity. Virology 101:399–407

Maheshwari RK, Banerjee DK, Waechter CJ, Olden K, Friedman RM (1980) Interferon treatment inhibits glycosylation of a viral protein. Nature 287:454–456

Manders EK, Tilles JG, Huang AS (1972) Interferon-mediated inhibition of virion-directed transcription. Virology 49:573–581

Mantei N, Schwarzstein M, Streuli M, Panem S, Nagata S, Weissmann C (1980) The nucleotide sequence of a cloned human leukocyte interferon cDNA. Gene 10:1–10

Marcus PI, Sekellick MJ (1977) Defective interfering particles with covalently linked ($\pm$) RNA induced interferon. Nature 226:815–818

Marcus PI, Engelhardt DL, Hunt JM, Sekellick MJ (1971) Interferon action: inhibition of vesicular stomatitis virus RNA synthesis induced by virion-bound polymerase. Science 174:593–598

Martin EM, Sonnabend JA (1967) Ribonucleic acid synthesis of double-stranded arbovirus ribonucleic acid. J Virol 1:97–109

Matarese GP, Rossi GB (1977) Effect of interferon on growth and division cycle of Friend erythroleukemic murine cells in vitro. J Cell Biol 75:344–354

Matsuno T, Shirasawa N, Kohno S (1976) Interferon suppresses glutamine synthetase induction in chick embryonic neural retina. Biochem Biophys Res Commun 70:310–314

Matsuyama M (1979) Action of interferon on cell membrane of mouse lymphocytes. Exp Cell Res 124:253–259

Mayhew E, Papahadjopoulos D, O'Malley JA, Carter WA, Vail WJ (1977) Cellular uptake and protection against virus infection by poly IC entrapped within phospholipid vesicles. Mol Pharmacol 13:488–495

McAuslan BR (1963) The induction and repression of thymidine kinase in the poxvirus-infected HeLa cell. Virology 21:383–389

McKimm J, Rapp F (1977a) Variation in ability of measles virus plaque progeny to induce interferon. Proc Natl Acad Sci USA 74:3056–3061

McKimm J, Rapp F (1977b) Inability of measles virus temperature sensitive mutants to induce interferon. Virology 76:409–421

McNeill TA, Fleming ZWA, McCance DJ (1972) Interferon and hemopoietic colony inhibitor responses to poly I · poly C in rabbits and hamsters. Immunology 22:711–721

Meager A, Graves HE, Bradshaw TK (1978) Stimulation of interferon yields from cultured human cells by calcium salts. FEBS Letter 87:303–307

Meager A, Graves H, Burke DC, Swallow DM (1979a) Involvement of a gene on chromosome 9 in human fibroblast interferon production. Nature 280:493–495

Meager A, Graves HE, Walker JR, Burke DC, Swallow DM, Westerveld A (1979b) Somatic cell genetics of human interferon production in human-rodent cell hybrids. J Gen Virol 45:309–321

Meldolesi MF, Friedman RM, Kohn LD (1977) An interferon-induced increase in cyclic AMP levels precedes the establishment of the antiviral state. Biochim Biophys Res Commun 70:239–246

Mellstedt H, Ahre A, Bjorkholm M, Holm G, Johansson B, Strander H (1979) Interferon therapy in myelomatosis. Lancet 1:245–247

Merigan TC (1967) Induction of circulating interferon by synthetic anionic polymers of known composition. Nature (Lond) 214:416–417

Merigan TC, Reed SE, Hall TS, Tyrrell DAJ (1973) Inhibition of respiratory virus infection by locally applied interferon. Lancet 1(803):563–567

Merigan TC, Rand KH, Pollard RB, Abdallah PS, Jordan GW, Fried RP (1978a) Human leukocyte interferon for the treatment of herpes zoster in patients with cancer. N Engl J Med 298:981–987

Merigan TC, Sikora K, Breeden JH, Levy R, Rosenberg S (1978b) Preliminary observations on the effect of human leukocyte interferon in non-Hodgkin's lymphoma. New Engl J Med 299:1449–1453

Metz DH (1975) Interferon and interferon inducers. Adv in Drug Res 10:101–156

Metz DH, Esteban RM (1972) Interferon inhibits viral protein synthesis in L cells infected with vaccinia virus. Nature 238:385–388

Metz DH, Levin MJ, Oxman MN (1976) Mechanism of interferon action: further evidence for transcription as a primary site of action in simian virus 40 infection. J Gen Virol 32:227–240

Metz DH, Oxman MN, Levin MJ (1977) Interferon inhibits the in vitro accumulation of virus specific RNA in nuclei isolated from SV40 infected cells. Biochem Biophys Res Commun 75:172–178

Miner N, Ray WJ Jr, Simon EM (1966) Effect of interferon on the production and action of viral RNA polymerase. Biochem Biophys Res Commun 24:261–268

Mizrahi A, O'Malley JA, Carter WA, Takatsuki A, Tamura G, Sulkowski E (1978) Glycosylation of interferons. Effects of tunicamycin on human immune interferon. J Biol Chem 253:7612–7615

Moehring TJ, Moehring JM, Stinebring WR (1971a) Response of interferon treated cells to diphtheria toxin. Infect Immun 4:747–752

Moehring JM, Stinebring WR, Merchant DJ (1971b) Survey of interferon production and sensitivity of human cell lines. Appl Microbiol 22:102–105

Mogensen KE, Pyhala L, Torma E, Cantell K (1974) No evidence for carbohydrate moiety affecting the clearance of circulating human leukocyte interferon in rabbits. Acta Pathol Microbiol Scand B82:305–310

Montagnier L, Collandre M, De Maeyer-Guignard J, De Maeyer E (1974) Two forms of mouse interferon messenger RNA. Biochem Biophys Res Commun 59:1031–1038

Morser J, Kabayo JP, Hutchinson DW (1978) Differences in sialic acid content of human interferons. J Gen Virol 41:175–178

Morser J, Flint J, Meager A, Graves H, Baker PN, Colman A, Burke DC (1979) Characterization of interferon messenger RNA from human lymphoblastoid cells. J Gen Virol 44:231–234

Mozes LW, Vilček J (1974) Interferon induction in rabbit cells irradiated with U.V. light. J Virology 13:646–651

Muthrukrishnan S, Moss B, Cooper JA, Maxell ES (1978) Influence of 5′ terminal structure on the initiation of translation of vaccinia virus mRNA. J Biol Chem 253:1710–1715

Nagano Y (1975) Virus-inhibiting factor. University of Tokyo Press, Tokyo, pp 1–260

Nagano Y Kojima Y (1954) Pouvoir immunisant de virus vaccinal inactive par des rayo ultraviolets. C.R. Soc Biol (Paris) 148:1700–1702

Nagano Y, Kojima Y (1958) Inhibition de l'infection vaccinale par le virus homologue. C.R. Seances Soc Biol Filiales 154:1627–1630

Nagata S, Taira H, Hall A, Johnsrud L, Streuli M, Escödi J, Boll W, Cantell K, Weissmann C (1980) Synthesis in E. Coli of a polypeptide with human leukocyte interferon activity. Nature 284:316–320

Nebert DW, Friedman RM (1973) Stimulation of aryl hydrocarbon hydroxylase induction in cell cultures by interferon. J Virol 11:193–197

Nilson TW, Baglioni C (1979) Mechanism for discrimination between viral and host mRNA in interferon treated cells. Proc Natl Acad Sci USA 76:2600–2604

Olsen GA, Kern ER, Glasgow LA, Overall JC Jr (1976) Effect of treatment with exogenous interferon Poly I · Poly C, or poly I · poly C – poly-lysine complex on EMC virus infections in mice. Antimicrob Agents Chemother 10:668–679

Olsen GA, Kern ER, Overall JC, Glasgow LA (1978) Effect of treatment with exogenous interferon, polyriboinosinic-polyribocytidylic acid, or polyriboinosinic-polyribocytidylic acid-poly-L-lysine complex on Herpesvirus hominis infections in mice. J Infect Dis 137:428–436

O'Malley JA, Leong SS, Horoszewicz JS, Carter WA (1979) Polyinosinic acid-polycytidylic acid and its mismatchend analogues: differential effects on human cell fusion. Molec Pharmacol 15:165–173

O'Reilly RJ, Everson LK, Emodi G, Hansen J, Smithwick EM, Grimes E, Pahwa S, Pahwa R, Schwartz S, Armstrong D, Siegel FP, Gupta S, Dupont B, Good RA (1976) Effect of exogenous interferon in cytomegalovirus infections complicating bone marrow transplantation. Clin Immunol Immunopathol 6:51–61

Orlova TG, Georgadze II, Kognovitskaya AL, Soloviev VD (1974) Formation of messenger RNA for interferon in cells treated with various viruses and poly I · poly C. Vopr Virusol (4):431–435

Oxman MN (1977) Interferon, tumors and tumor viruses. In: Finter NB (ed) Interferons and interferon inducers, North-Holland Publ Co, Amsterdam, pp 391–480

Oxman MN, Levin MJ (1971) Interferon and transcription of early virus-specific RNA in cells infected with simian virus 40. Proc Natl Acad Sci USA 68:299–302

Oxman MN, Baron S, Black PH, Takemoto KK, Habel K, Rowe WP (1967) The effect of interferon on SV40 T-antigen production in SV40-transformed cells. Virology 32:122–127

Pang RHL, Hayes TG, Vilček J Isolation of Le interferon mRNA from human fibroblasts. Proc Natl Acad Sci USA, to be published

Paucker K, Cantell K, Henle W (1962) Quantitative studies on viral interference in suspended L cells. V. Persistence of protection on growing cultures. Virology 21:22–29

Pazin GJ, Armstrong JA, Lam MT, Tarr GC, Jannetta PJ, Ho M (1979) Prevention of reactivated herpes simplex infection by human leukocyte interferon after operation on the trigeminal root. New Engl J med 301:225–230

Pestka S, McInnes J, Havell EA, Vilček J (1975) Cell-free synthesis of human interferon. Proc Natl Acad Sci USA 72:3898–3906

Pfeffer LM, Landsberger FR, Tamm I (1981a) β-interferon-induced time dependant changes in the plasma membrane lipid bilayer of cultured cells. J Ifn Res 1:615–620

Pfeffer LM, Murphy JS, Tamm I (1979) Interferon effects on the growth and division of human fibroblasts. Exp Cell Res 121:111–120

Pfeffer LM, Wang E, Landsberger FL, Tamm I (1981b) Assays to measure plasma membrane and cytoskeletal changes in interferon-treated cells. Methods in enzymology 79:461–413

Pfeffer LM, Wang E, Tamm I (1980a) Interferon effects on microfilament organization, cellular fibronectin distribution, and cell motility in human fibroblasts. J Cell Biol 85:9–17

Pfeffer LM, Wang E, Tamm I (1980 b) Interferon inhibits redistribution of cell surface components. J Exp Med 152:469–474

Pfeffer LM, Wang E, Fried J, Murphy JS, Tamm I (1982) Interferon as a modulator of fibroblast poliferation and growth. In: Padilla GS, McCarthy KS Jr. (eds) Genetic Expression in the Cell Cycle. Vol II. Academic Press NY, pp 289–314

Pickering LA, Sarkar FH, Stewart WE II (1980) Spontaneous production of human interferons. Abst Ann Meeting Am Soc Microbiol T11, p 237

Pitha PA, Rowe WP, Oxman MN (1976) Effect of interferon on exogenous, endogenous, and chronic murine leukemia virus infection. Virology 70:324–337

Pitha PA, Staal SP, Bolognesi DP, Denny TP, Rowe WP (1977) Effect of interferon murine leukemia virus infection. II. Synthesis of viral components in exogenous infection. Virology 79:1–16

Pollard RB, Smith JL, Neal EA, Gregory PB, Merigan TC, Robinson WS (1978) Effect of vidarabine on chronic hepatitis B virus infection. J.A.M.A. 239:1648–1650

Priestman TJ (1979) Interferon: an anti-cancer agent? Cancer Treat Rev 6:223–237

Puccetti P, Giampietri A (1978) Immunopharmacology of pyran copolymer. Pharmacological Res Commun 10:489–501

Purcell RH, Loncon WT, McAuliffe VJ, Palmer AE, Kaplan PM, Gerin JL, Wagner J, Popper H, Lvovsky E, Wong DC, Levy HB (1976) Modification of chronic hepatitis B virus infection in chimpanzees by administration of an interferon inducer. Lancet 2:757–761

Rabinovitch M, Manejias RE, Russo M, Abbey EF (1977) Increased spreading of macrophages from mice treated with interferon inducers. Cell Immunol 29:86–93

Radke KL, Colby C, Kates JR, Krider HM, Prescott DM (1974) Establishment and maintenance of the interferon-induced antiviral state: studies in enucleated cells. J Virol 13:623–645

Raj NBK, Pitha PM (1979) The messenger RNA sequences in superinduced and uninduced human fibroblast cells. Abst Ann Meeting Am Soc Microbiol S80, p 253

Ratner L, Wiegand RG, Farrell PJ, Sen GC, Cabrer B, Lengyel P (1978) Interferon, double stranded RNA and RNA degradation. Fractionation of the endonuclease int system into two macromolecular components, role of a small molecule in nuclease activation. Biochem Biophys Res Commun 81:947–953

Regelson W (1967) Prevention and treatment of Friend leukemia virus (FLV) infection by interferon-inducing synthetic polyanions. Advanc exp Med Biol 1:315–332

Reizin FN, Roikhel VM, Chumakov MP (1975) The influence of substances changing the intracellular concentration of cyclic adenosine 3′,5′-monophosphate on interferon synthesis in chick embryo cell culture. Arch Virol. 49:307–315

Renis HE, Eidson EE (1980) Protection of mice from herpes simplex virus infection by 5-halo, 6-aryl-isocytosines. In: Nelson JD, Grassi C (eds) Current chemotherapy and infectious diseases, Proceedings of the 11th International Congress of Chemotherapy and the 19th Interscience Conference on Antimicrobial Agents and Chemotherapy, vol II. The American Society for Microbiology, Washington DC, pp 1411–1413

Repik P, Flamand A, Bishop DH (1974) Effect of interferon upon the primary and secondary transcription of vesicular stomatitis and influenza viruses. J Virol 14:1169–1178

Revel M (1977) Interferon-induced translation regulation. Tex Rep Biol Med 35:212–220

Revel M (1979) Molecular mechanisms involved in the antiviral effects of interferon. Interferon 1:102–157

Revel M, Bash D, Ruddle FH (1976) Antibodies to a cell-surface component coded by human chromosome 21 inhibit action of interferon. Nature 260:139

Reynolds FH, Pitha PM (1974) The induction of interferon and its messenger RNA in human fibroblasts. Biochem Biophys Res Commun 59:1023–1030

Reynolds FH Jr, Pitha PM (1975) Molecular weight study of human fibroblast interferon. Biochem Biophys Res Commun 65:107–114

Reynolds FH Jr, Premkumar E, Pitha PM (1975) Interferon activity produced by translation of human interferon messenger RNA in cell-free ribosomal systems and in *Xenopus* oocytes. Proc Natl Acad Sci USA 72:4881–4887

Rhim JS, Heubner RJ (1971) Comparison of the antitumor effect of interferon and interferon inducers. Proc Soc Exp Biol Med 136:524–529

Roberts WK, Clemens MJ, Kerr IM (1976a) Interferon-induced inhibition of protein synthesis in L-cell extracts: an ATP-dependent step in the activation of an inhibitor by double stranded RNA. Proc Natl Acad Sci USA 70:3136–3140

Roberts WK, Hovanessian A, Brown RE, Clemens MJ, Kerr I (1976b) Interferon-mediated protein kinase and low molecular weight inhibitor of protein synthesis. Nature 264:477–480

Rossi GB, Matarese GP, Grapelli C, Belardelli F, Beneditto A (1977) Interferon inhibits dimethyl sulfoxide induced erythroid differentiation of Friend leukemia cells. Nature 267:50–52

Rozee KR, Katz W, McFarlane ES (1969) Interferon stimulation of methylase activity in L-cells. Can J Microbiol 15:969–971

Rubinstein M, Rubinstein S, Familletti PC, Gross MS, Miller RS, Waldman AA, Pestka S (1978) Human leukocyte interferon purified to homogeneity. Science 202:1289–1290

Rubinstein M, Rubinstein S, Familletti PC, Miller RS, Waldman AA, Pestka S (1979) Human leukocyte interferon: production, purification to homogeneity, and initial characterization. Proc Natl Acad Sci USA 76:640–644

Sagar AD, Pickering LA, Sussman-Berger P, Stewart WE II, Sehgal PB (1981) Heterogeneity of interferon-mRNA species from Sendai virus-induced human lymphoblastoid (Namalva) cells and Newcastle disease virus-induced murine fibroblastoid (L) cells. Nucleic Acids Res 9:149–160

Saito S, Matsuno T, Sudo T, Furuya E, Kohno S (1976) Priming activity of mouse interferon effect on interferon messenger RNA synthesis. Arch Virol 52:159–163

Salerno RA, Whitmire CE, Garcia IM, Huebner RJ (1972) Chemical carcinogenesis in mice inhibited by interferon. Nature New Biol 239:31–32

Salvin SB, Youngner JS, Nishio J, Neta R (1975) Tumor suppression by a lymphokine released into the circulation of mice with delayed hypersensitivity. J Natl. Cancer Inst 55:1233–1235

Sammons ML, Stephen EL, Levy HB, Baron S, Hilmas DE (1977) Interferon induction in cynomolgus and rhesus monkeys after repeated doses of a modified polyriboinosinic-polyribocytidylic acid complex. Antimicrob Agents Chemother 11:80–83

Samuel CE (1979) Mechanism of interferon action. Kinetics of interferon action in mouse L929 cells: phosphorylation of protein synthesis initiator factor eIF-2 and ribosome associated protein P1. Virology 93:281–285

Samuel CE, Joklik WK (1974) A protein synthesizing system from interferon-treated cells that discriminates between cellular and viral messenger RNAs. Virology 58:476–491

Sarma PS, Shiu G, Baron S, Huebner RJ (1969) Inhibitory effect of interferon in murine sarcoma and leukemia virus infection in vitro. Nature 223:845–846

Schellekens H, Weimar W, Cantell K, Stilz L (1979) Antiviral effect of interferon in vivo may be mediated by the host. Nature 278:742

Schlesinger RW (1959) Interference between animal viruses. The viruses, vol III. Academic Press, NY, pp 157–194

Schmidt A, Zilberstein A, Shulman L, Federman P, Berissi H, Revel M (1978) Interferon action: isolation of nuclease a translation inhibitor activated by interferon-induced (2′–5′) oligoisoadenylate. FEBS Letter 95:257–264

Schmidt A, Chernajovsky V, Shulman L, Federman P, Berissi H, Revel M (1979) An interferon-induced phosphodiesterase degrading (2′–5′)oligoadenylate and the C-C-A terminus of tRNA. Proc Natl Acad Sci USA 76:4788–4792

Schonne E, Billiau A, Desomer P (1970) The properties of interferon. IV. Isoelectric focusing of rabbit interferon (NDV-RK13). In: Symp Series Immunbiol 14. Karger, Basel, p 61

Schroeder EW, Chou IN, Jaken S, Black P (1978) Interferon inhibits the release of plasminogen activator from SV 3T3 cells. Nature 276:828–829

Schultz RM, Chirigos MA (1979) Selective neutralization by antiinterferon globulin of macrophage activation by L-cell interferon, *Burcella abortus* ether extract, *Salmonella typhimurium* lipopolysaccharide, and polyanions. Cellular Immunology 48:52–58

Schultz RM, Papamatheakis JD, Chirigos MA (1977) Interferon: an inducer of macrophage activation by polyanions. Science 197:674–676

Schultz RM, Chirigos MA, Pavlidis NA, Youngner JS (1978) Macrophage activation and antitumor activity of a *Brucella abortus* ether extract, Bru-Pel. Cancer Treatment Reports 62:1937–1941

Scientific Committee on Interferon (1962) Effect of interferon on vaccination in volunteers. Lancet 1:873–875

Scott GM, Butler JK, Cartwright T, Richards BM, Kingham JG, Wright R, Tyrrell DAJ (1977) Interferon skin reactivity and pyrexial reactions. Lancet 2:402–403

Scott GM, Cartwright T, Ledu G, Dicker D (1978) Effect of human fibroblast interferon on vaccination in volunteers. J Biol Stand 6:73–76

Segal S, Khoury G (1979) Differentiation as a requirement for simian virus 40 gene expression in F-9 embryonal carcinoma cells. Proc Natl Acad Sci USA 76:5611–5615

Segal S, Levine AJ, Khoury G (1979) Evidence for non-spliced SV40 RNA in undifferentiated murine teratocarcinoma stem cells. Nature 280:335–338

Sehgal PB (1977) Regulation of gene expression in human cells: RNA synthesis and interferon production. PhD dissertation, The Rockefeller University

Sehgal PB (1981) Regulation of the stability of human β interferon mRNA: anchorage independence of the shutoff mechanism. Virology 112:738–745

Sehgal PB, Gupta SL (1980) Regulation of the stability of poly(I)·poly(C)-induced human fibroblast interferon mRNA: selective inactivation of interferon mRNA and lack of involvement of 2′,5′-oligo(A) synthetase activation during the shutoff of interferon production. Proc Natl Acad Sci USA 77:3489–3493

Sehgal PB, Sagar ADS (1980) Heterogeneity of poly(I)·poly(C)-induced human fibroblast interferon mRNA species. Nature, to be published 287:95–97

Sehgal PB, Tamm I (1976) Evaluation of messenger RNA competition in shutoff of human interferon production. Proc Natl Acad Sci USA 73:1621–1625

Sehgal PB, Tamm I (1978) Halogenated benzimidazole ribosides. Novel inhibitors of RNA synthesis. Biochem Pharmacol 27:2475–2485

Sehgal PB, Tamm I (1979) Two mechanisms contribute to the superinduction of poly(I)·poly(C)-induced human fibroblast interferon production. Virology 92:240–244

Sehgal PB, Tamm I (1980a) Antiviral agents: determination of activity. In: Lorian V (ed) Antibiotics in laboratory medicine. Williams & Wilkins, Baltimore, pp 573–591

Sehgal PB, Tamm I (1980b) The transcription unit for poly(I)·poly(C)-induced human fibroblast interferon messenger RNA. Virology 102:245–249

Sehgal PB, Tamm I, Vilček J (1975a) Human interferon production: superinduction by 5,6-dichloro-l-β-D-ribofuranosylbenzimidazole. Science 190:282–285

Sehgal PB, Tamm I, Vilček J (1975b) Enhancement of human interferon production by neutral red and chloroquine: analysis of inhibition of protein degradation and macromolecular synthesis. J Exp Med 142:1283–1290

Sehgal PB, Tamm I, Vilček J (1976a) On the mechanism of enhancement of human interferon production by actinomycin D and cycloheximide. Virology 70:256–265

Sehgal PB, Tamm I, Vilček J (1976b) Regulation of human interferon production: I. Superinduction by 5,6-dichloro-l-D-ribofuranosylbenzimidazole. Virology 70:532–540

Sehgal PB, Tamm I, Vilček J (1976c) Regulation of human interferon production. II. Inhibition of interferon messenger RNA synthesis by 5,6-dichloro-1-β-D-ribofuranosylbenzimidazole. Virology 70:542–544

Sehgal PB, Darnell JE Jr, Tamm I (1976d) The inhibition by DRB (5,6-dichloro-1-β-D-ribofuranosylbenzimidazole) of hnRNA and mRNA production in HeLa cells. Cell 9:473–480

Sehgal PB, Dobberstein B, Tamm I (1977) Interferon messenger RNA content of human fibroblasts during induction, shutoff, and superinduction of interferon production. Proc Natl Acad Sci USA 74:3409–3413

Sehgal PB, Lyles DS, Tamm I (1978a) Superinduction of human fibroblast interferon production: further evidence for increased stability of interferon mRNA. Virology 89:186–198

Sehgal PB, Soreq H, Tamm I (1978b) Does 3′-terminal poly(A) stabilize human fibroblast interferon mRNA in oocytes of *Xenopus laevis?* Proc Natl Acad Sci USA 75:5030–5033

Sen GC, Gupta SL, Brown GE, Lebleu B, Rebello MA, Lengyel P (1976a) Interferon treatment of Ehrlich ascites tumor cells: effects on exogenous mRNA translation of tRNA inactivation in the cell extract. J Virol 17:191–203

Sen GC, Lebleu B, Brown GE, Kawakita M, Slattery E, Lengyel P (1976b) Interferon, double-stranded RNA and mRNA degradation. Nature 264:370–373

Sen GC, Desrosiers R, Ratner L, Shaila S, Brown GE, Lebleu B, Slattery E, Kawaita M, Cabrer B, Taira H, Lengyel P (1977a): Messenger RNA methylation, translation and degradation on extracts of interferon-treated cells. Tex Rep Biol Med 35:221–229

Sen GC, Shaila S, Lebleu B, Brown GE, Desrosier RC, Lengyel P (1977b) Impairment of reovirus mRNA methylation in extracts of interferon-treated Ehrlich ascites tumor cells: further characteristics of the phenomenon. J Virol 21:69–83

Sen GC, Taira H, Lengyel P (1978) Characteristics of a double-stranded RNA-activated protein kinase system partially purified from interferon-treated Ehrlich ascites tumor cells. J Biol Chem 253:5915–5921

Senussi OA, Cartwright T, Thompson P (1979) Resolution of human fibroblast interferon into two distinct classes by thiol exchange chromatography. Arch Virol 62:323–331

Shaila S, Lebleu B, Brown GE, Sen GC, Lengyel P (1977) Characteristics of extracts from interferon-treated HeLa cells, presence of a protein kinase and endoribonuclease activated by double-stranded RNA and of an inhibitor of mRNA methylation. J Gen Virol 37:535–546

Siegel BV (1975) Enhancement of interferon production by poly(rI) · poly(rC) in mouse cell cultures by ascorbic acid. Nature 254:531–532

Simli M, Deferra F, Baglioni C (1980) Inhibition of RNA and protein synthesis in interferon treated HeLa cells infected with vesicular stomatitis virus. J Gen Virol 47:373–384

Sipe JD, Demaeyer-Guignard J, Fauconnier B Demaeyer E (1973) Purification of mouse interferon by affinity chromatography on a solid-phase immunoadsorbent. Proc Natl Acad Sci USA 70:1037–1040

Skurkovich SV, Kalinina IA, Eremkina EI, Bulycheva TA (1976) Increased sensitivity of leukemia cells incubated in interferon to the action of immune serum. Byull eksp Biol Med 12:1459–1461

Slate DL, Ruddle FH (1979) Fibroblast interferon in man is coded by two loci on separate chromosomes. Cell 16:171–180

Slate DL, Shulman L, Lawrence JB, Revel M, Ruddle FH (1978) Presence of human chromosome 21 alone is sufficient for hybrid cell sensitivity of human interferon. J Virol 25:319–325

Slattery E, Ghosh N, Samanta H, Lengyel P (1979) Interferon, double-stranded RNA, and RNA degradation activation of an endonuclease by $(2'-5')A_n$. Proc Natl Acad Sci USA 76:4778–4782

Sokawa Y, Watanabe Y, Kawade Y (1977) Suppressive effect of interferon on the transition from quiescent to a growing state in 3T3 cells. Nature 268:236–238

Solov'ev VD (1969) The results of controlled observation on the prophylaxis of influenza with interferon. Bull W.H.O. 41:683–688

Soloviev VD, Mentkevich LM (1965) The effect of colchicine on viral interference and interferon formation. Acta Virol 9:308–312

Sonnenfeld G, Mandel AD, Merrigan TC (1977) The immunosuppressive effect of type II mouse interferon preparations on antibody production. Cell Immunol 34:193–206

Soreq H, Sagar AD, Sehgal PB (1981) Translational activity and functional stability of human fibroblast β_1 and β_2 interferon mRNA species lacking 3'-terminal RNA sequences. Proc Natl Acad Sci USA 78:1741–1745

Stark GR, Dower WJ, Schimke RT, Brown RE, Kerr IM (1979) pppA2',5'-A2'p5'A synthetase: convenient assay, species and tissue distribution and variation upon withdrawal of oestrogen from chick oviducts. Nature 278:471–473

Stephen EL, Hilmas DE, Mangiafico JA, Levy HB (1977a) Swine influenza virus vaccine: potentiation of antibody responses in rhesus monkeys. Science 197:1289–1290

Stephen EL, Sammons ML, Pannier WL, Baron S, Spertzel RO, Levy HB (1977b) Effect of a nuclease-resistant derivative of polyriboinosinic-polyribocytidylic acid complex on yellow fever in rhesus monkeys (Macaca mulatta). J Infect Dis 136:122–126

Stephen EL, Hilmas DE, Levy HB, Spertzel RO (1979) Protective and toxic effects of a nuclease-resistant derivative of polyriboinosinic-polyribocytidylic acid on Venezuelan equine encephalomyelitis virus in rhesus monkeys. J Infect Dis 139:267–272

Stern C (1960) Principles of human genetics. 2nd Edition. WH Freeman and Co, San Francisco, London

Stewart WE II (1974) Distinct molecular species of interferons. Virology 61:80–86

Stewart WE II (1979) The interferon system. Springer-Verlag, Wien New York, 421 pages

Stewart WE II, Desmyter J (1975) Molecular heterogeneity of human leukocyte interferon: two populations differing in molecular weights, requirements for renaturation and cross-species antiviral activity. Virology 67:68–78

Stewart WE II, Havell EA (1980) Characterization of a subspecies of mouse interferon cross-reactive on human cells and antigenically related to human leukocyte interferon. Virology 101:315–318

Stewart WE II, Sulkin SE (1966) Interferon production in hamsters experimentally infected with rabies virus. Proc Soc Exp Biol Med 123:650–653

Stewart WE II, Gosser LB, Lockard RZ Jr (1971) Priming: a non-antiviral function of interferon. J Virol 7:792–801

Stewart WE II, Declercq E, Desomer P (1973) Specificity of interferon-induced enhancement of toxicity for double-stranded ribonucleic acids. J Gen Virol 18:237–246

Stewart WE II, Gresser I, Tovey MG, Bandu MT, Legoff S (1976) Identification of the cell-multiplication inhibitory factors in interferon preparations as interferon. Nature 262:300–303

Stewart WE II, Lin LS, Wiranowska-Stewart M, Cantell K (1977) Elimination of size and charge heterogeneities of human leukocyte interferons by chemical cleavage. Proc Natl Acad Sci USA 74:4200–4204

Stewart WE II, Chudzio T, Lin LS, Wiranowska-Stewart M (1978) Interferoids: In vitro and in vivo conversion of native interferons to lower molecular weight forms. Proc Natl Acad Sci USA 75:4814–4818

Stewart WE II, Sarkar FH, Taira H, Hall A, Nagata S, Weissmann C (1980) Comparisons of several biological and physicochemical properties of human leukocyte interferons produced by human leukocytes and by E. coli. Gene 11:181–186

Strander H (1977) Interferons: anti-neoplastic drugs? Blut 35:277–288

Strander H, Cantell K (1966) Production of interferon by human leukocytes in vitro. Ann Med Exp Biol Fenn 44:265–273

Strander H, Cantell K (1974) Studies on antiviral and antitumor effects of human leukocyte interferon in vitro and in vivo. In: Waymouth C (ed) The production and use of interferon for the treatment and prevention of human virus infection. The Tissue Culture Association, Rockville, Md, pp 49–56

Strander H, Cantell K, Carlstrom G, Jakobsson PA (1973) Clinical and laboratory investigations on man; systemic administration of potent interferon to man. J Natl Cancer Inst 51:733–739

Strander H, Mogensen KE, Cantell K (1974) Production of human lymphoblastoid interferon. J Clin Microbiol 1:116–117

Strander H, Cantell K, Carlstrom G, Ingimarsson S, Jakobsson P, Nilsonnne U (1976) Acute infections in interferon-treated patients with osteosarcoma: preliminary report of a comparison study. J Infect Dis [Suppl] 133:A245–A248

Strauchen JA, Young NA, Friedman RM (1977) Interferon-mediated inhibition of mouse mammary tumor virus expression in cultured cells. Virology 82:232–236

Stringfellow DA, Glasgow LA (1972a) Hyporeactivity of interferon: potential limitation to therapeutic use of interferon-inducing agents. Infect Immun 6:743–751

Stringfellow DA, Glasgow LA (1972b) Tilorone hydrochloride: an oral interferon-inducing agent. Antimicrob Agents Chemother 2:73–85

Stringfellow DA, Weed SD, Underwood GE (1979) Antiviral and interferon-inducing properties of 1,5-diamio anthraquinones. Antimicrob Agents Chemother 15:111–118

Stringfellow DA, Vanderberg HC, Weed SD (1980) Interferon induction by 5-halo-6-phenyl pyrimidines. In: Nelson JD, Grassi C (eds) Current chemotherapy and infectious diseases, Proceedings of the 11th International Congress of Chemotherapy and the 19th Interscience Conference on Antimicrobial Agents and Chemotherapy, vol II. The American Society for Microbiology, Washington DC, pp 1406–1408

Stylos WA, Chirigos MA, Lengel CR (1978) Lymphocyte stimulatory effect of an ether-extracted preparation of *Brucella abortus*. Cancer Treatment Reports 62:1949–1954

Sulkowski E, Davey MW, Carter WA (1976) Interaction of human interferons with immobilized hydrophobic amino acids and dipeptides. J Biol Chem 251:5381–5390

Sundmacher R, Neumann-Haefelin D, Manthey KF, Muller O (1976a) Interferon in treatment of dendritic keratitis in humans: a preliminary report. J Infect Dis [Suppl] 133:A160–A164

Sundmacher R, Neumann-Haefelin D, Cantell K (1976b) Interferon treatment of dendritic keratitis. Lancet 1:1406–1407

Sundmacher R, Neumann-Haefelin D, Cantell K (1976c) Successful treatment of dendritic keratitis with human leukocyte interferon: a controlled clinical study. Albrecht von Graefes Arch Klin Exp Ophthalmol 201:39–45

Sundmacher R, Neumann-Haefelin D, Cantell K (1977) Quoted in Cantell K (1979)

Sundmacher R, Cantell K, Haug P, Neumann-Haefelin D (1978a) Role of debridement and interferon in the treatment of dendritic keratitis. Albrecht von Graefes Arch Ophthalmol 207:77–82

Sundmacher R, Neumann-Haefelin D, Cantell K (1978b) Prophylaxis of dendritic keratitis with topical human leukocyte interferon in monkeys and patients treated with steroids. Quoted in Dunnick and Galasso (1979)

Sundmacher R, Cantell K, Haug P, Neumann-Haefelin D (1978c) Interferon Prophylaxe von dendritica rezidivien bei lokaler steroid-therapie. Quoted in Dunnick and Galasso (1979)

Sundmacher R, Cantell K, Neumann-Haefelin D (1978d) Combination therapy of dendritic keratitis with trifluorothymidine and interferon. Lancet 2:687

Sundmacher R, Cantell K, Skoda R, Hallermann C, Neumann-Haefelin D (1979) Human leukocyte and fibroblast interferon in a combination therapy of dendritic keratitis. Quoted in Cantell (1979)

Svet-Moldavsky GJ, Chernyakovskaya IY (1967) Interferon and the interaction of allogeneic normal and immune lymphocytes with L cells. Nature 215:1299–1300

Taggart MT, Loughman BE, Gibbons AJ, Stringfellow DA (1980) Immunomodulatory effects of 2-amino-5-bromo-6-methyl-4-pyrimidinol and its isocytosine analogs. In: Nelson JD, Grassi C (eds) Current chemotherapy and infectious diseases, Proceedings of the 11th International Congress of Chemotherapy and the 19th Interscience Conference on Antimicrobial Agents and Chemotherapy, vol 11. The American Society for Microbiology, Washington DC, pp 1400–1401

Taira H, Broeze RJ, Jayaram BM, Lengyel P, Hunkapiller MW, Hood LE (1980) Mouse interferons: amino terminal amino acid sequences of various species. Science 207:528–530

Tamm I, Sehgal PB (1977) A comparative study of the effects of certain halogenated benzimidazole ribosides on RNA synthesis, cell proliferation, and interferon production. J Exp Med 145:344–356

Tamm I, Sehgal PB (1978) Halobenzimidazole ribosides and RNA synthesis of cells and viruses. Adv Virus Res 22:187–258

Tamm I, Sehgal PB (1979) New evidence for regulated transcription of mRNA and for regulated translation of interferon mRNA in human cells. In: Engberg J, Klenow H, Leick V (eds) Specific eukaryotic genes, Alfred Benzon Symposium 13, Munksgaard, Copenhagen, pp 424–439

Tamm I, Hand R, Caliguiri LA (1976) Action of dichlorobenzimidazole riboside on RNA synthesis in L-929 and HeLa cells. J Cell Biol 69:229–240

Tan YH (1976) Chromosome 21 and the growth inhibitory effect of human interferon preparations. Nature 260:141–142

Tan YH, Berthold W (1977) A mechanism for the induction and regulation of human interferon genetic expression. J Gen Virol 34:401–412

Tan YH, Greene AE (1976) Subregional localization of the genes governing the human interferon-induced antiviral state in man. J Gen Virol 32:153–157

Tan YH, Armstrong JA, Ke YM, Ho M (1970) Regulation of cellular interferon production: enhancement by antimetabolites. Proc Natl Acad Sci USA 67:464–471

Tan YH, Armstrong JA, Ho M (1971) Accentuation of interferon production by metabolic inhibitors and its dependence on protein synthesis. Virology 41:503–509

Tan YH, Schneider EL, Tishfield J, Epstein CJ, Ruddle FM (1974a) Human chromosome 21 dosage: effect on the expression of the interferon induced antiviral state. Science 186:61–63

Tan YH, Creagan RP, Ruddle FM (1974b) The somatic cell genetics of human interferon: assignment of human interferon loci to chromosomes 2 and 5. Proc Natl Acad Sci USA 71:2251–2255

Tan YH, Barakat F, Berthold W, Smith-Johannsen H, Tan C (1979) The isolation and amino acid/sugar composition of human fibroblastoid interferon. J Biol Chem 254:8067–8073

Tanamoto K-I, Abe C, Homma JY, Kojima Y (1979) Regions of the lipopolysaccharide of *Pseudomonas aeruginosa* essential for antitumor and interferon-inducing activities. Eur J Biochem 97:623–629

Taniguchi T, Sakai M, Fuji-Kuriyama Y, Muramatsu M, Kobayashi S, Sudo T (1979) Construction and identification of bacterial plasmid containing the human fibroblast interferon gene sequence. Proc Japan Acad, Ser B 55:464–489

Taniguchi T, Ohno S, Fuji-Kuriyama Y, Muramatsu Y (1980a) The nucleotide sequence of human fibroblast interferon DNA. Gene 10:11–15

Taniguchi T, Mantei N, Schwarzstein M, Nagata S, Muramatsu M, Weissmann C (1980b) Human leukocyte and fibroblast interferons are structurally related. Nature 285:547–549

Taniguchi T, Guarente L, Roberts TM, Kimelman D, Douhan J III, Ptashne M (1980c) Expression of the human fibroblast interferon gene in *Escherichia coli*. Proc Natl Acad Sci USA 77:5230–5233

Tarodi B, Metz DH, Douglas A, Russell WK (1977) A study of events in chick cells infected with human adenovirus type 5 and their relationship to the induction of interferon. J Gen Virol 36:425–436

Taylor J (1964) Inhibition of interferon action by actinomycin. Biochem Biophys Res Commun 14:447–453

Taylor JL, Schoenherr CK, Grossberg SE (1980a) High-yield interferon induction by 10-carboxymethyl-9-acridanone in mice and hamsters. Antimicrob Agents and Chemo 18:20–26

Taylor JL, Schoenherr C, Grossberg SE (1980b) Protection against Japanese encephalitis in mice and hamsters by treatment with carboxymethyl-acridanone, a potent interferon inducer. J Infect Dis 142:394–399

Thacore HR (1978) Effect of interferon on transcription and translation of vesicular stomatis virus in human and simian cell cultures. J Gen Virol 41:421–426

Thang MN, Thang DC, DeMaeyer E, Montagnier L (1975) Biosynthesis of mouse interferon by translation of its messenger RNA in a cell-free system. Proc Natl Acad Sci USA 72:3975–3979

Tomkins GM, Levinson BB, Baxter JD, Dethlefsen L (1972) Further evidence for post-transcriptional control of inducible tyrosine aminotransferase synthesis in cultured hepatoma cells. Nature New Biol 239:9–14

Törma ET, Paucker K (1976) Purification and characterization of human leukocyte interferon components. J Biol Chem 251:4810–4820

Torrence PF, Friedman RM (1979) Are double-stranded RNA-directed inhibition of protein synthesis in interferon-treated cells and interferon induction related phenomena? J Biol Chem 256:1259–1267

Tovey MG, Begon-Lours J, Gresser I (1974) A method for large-scale production of potent interferon preparations. Proc Soc Exp Biol Med 146:809–815

Tovey MG, Brouty-Boyé D, Gresser I (1975) Interferon and cell division X. Early effect of interferon on mouse leukemia cells cultured in a chemostat. Proc Natl Acad Sci USA 72:2265–2269

Tovey MG, Begon-Lours J, Gresser I, Morris AG (1977) Marked enhancement of interferon production in 5-bromodeoxyuridine treated human lymphoblastoid cells. Nature 267:455–456

Tovey MG, Egly CR, Castagna M (1979) Effect of interferon on concentration of cyclic nucleotides in cultured cells. Proc Natl Acad Sci 76:3890–3893

Trapman J (1979) A systematic study of interferon production by mouse L-929 cells induced with poly(I)·poly(C) and DEAE-dextran. FEBS Lett 98:107–110

Tyrrell DAJ (1959) Interferon produced by culures of calf kidney cells. Nature 184:452–453

Tyrrell DAJ, Tamm I (1955) Prevention of virus interference by 2,5-dimethylbenzimidazole. J Immunol 75:43–49

Vasseff A, Spencer C, Gelehrter TD, Lengyel P (1974) Selectivity of interferon action: hormonal induction of tyrosine aminotransferase in rat hepatoma cells is much less sensitive to interferon than the replication of vesicular stomatitis virus or reovirus. Biochem Biophys Acta 353:115–120

Vengris VE, Stollar BD, Pitha PM (1975) Interferon externalization by producing cell before induction of antiviral state. Virology 65:410–417

Vengris VE, Reynolds FH Jr, Hollenberg MD, Pitha PM (1976) Interferon action: role of membrane gangliosides. Virology 72:486–493

Vennström B, Persson H, Pettersson U, Philipson L (1979) A DRB (5,6-dichloro-β-D-ribofuranosylbenzimidazole)-resistant adenovirus mRNA. Nuc Acids Res 7:1405–1418

Vignaux F, Gresser I (1977) Differential effects of interferon on the expression of H-2K,H-2D and 1 α antigens on mouse lymphocytes. J Immunol 118:721–723

Vilček J (1962) Studies on an interferon from tick-borne encephalitis virus infected cells. IV. Comparison of IF with interferon from influenza virus-infected cells. Acta Virol 6:144–160

Vilček J (1970) Metabolic determinants of the induction of interferon by a double-stranded polynucleotide in rabbit cells. Ann NY Acad Sci 173:390–403

Vilček J, Ng MH (1971) Post-transcriptional control of interferon synthesis. J Virol 7:588–594

Vilček J, Rada B (1962) Studies on an interferon from tick-borne encephalitis virus infected cells. III. Antiviral action of IF. Acta Virol 6:9–15

Vilček J, Rossman TC, Varacalli F (1969) Differential effects of Actinomycin D and puromycin on the release of interferon induced by double-stranded RNA. Nature 222:682–683

Vilcek J, Havell EA, Kohase A (1976) Superinduction of interferon with metabolic inhibitors: possible mechanisms and practical applications. J Infect Disease 133:A22–A29

Vilček J, Yamazaki S, Havell EA (1977) Interferon induction by vesicular stomatitis virus and its role in virus replication. Infect Immun 18:836–867

Virelizier J-L, Gresser I (1978) Role of interferon in the pathogenesis of mice as demonstrated by the use of anti-interferon serum. IV. Protective role in mouse hepatitis virus Type 3 infection of susceptible and resistant strains of mice. J Immunol 120:1616–1619

Virelizier JL, Allison AC, DeMaeyer E (1977) Production by mixed lymphocyte cultures of a Type II interferon able to protect macrophages against virus infections. Infect Immun 17:282–296

Waldman RH, Ganguly R (1978) Effect of CP-20,961, an interferon inducer, on upper respiratory tract infections due to rhinovirus Type 21 in volunteers. J Infect Dis 138:531–535

Weber JM, Stewart RB (1975) Cyclic AMP potentiation of interferon antiviral activity and effect of interferon on cellular cyclic AMP levels. J Gen Virol 28:363–372

Weed SD, Kramer GD, Stringfellow DA (1980) Antiviral properties of 6-arylpyrimidines. In: Nelson JD, Grassi C (eds) Current chemotherapy and infectious diseases, Proceedings of the 11th International Congress of Chemotherapy and the 19th Interscience Conference on Antimicrobial Agents and Chemotherapy, vol II. Society for Microbiology, Washington DC, pp 1408–1409

Weimar W, Heijtink RA, Schalm SW, Van Blankenstein M, Schellekens H, Masurel N, Edy VG, Billiau A, De Somer P (1977) Fibroblast interferon in HBsAg-positive chronic active hepatitis. Lancet 2:1282

Weimar W, Schellekens H, Lameijer LDF, Masurel N, Edy VG, Billiau A, De Somer P (1978 a) Double-blind study of interferon administration in renal transplant recipients. Eur J Clin Invest, Quoted in Dunnick and Galasso (1979)

Weimar W, Heijtink RA, Schalm SW, Schellekens H (1978 b) Differential effects of exogenous fibroblast and leukocyte interferon in HBsAg chronic hepatitis [abstract]. Gastroenterology, Quoted in Dunnick and Galasso (1979)

Weimar W, Heijtink RA, Ten Kate FJP, Schalm SW, Masurel N, Schellekens H, Cantell K (1980) Double-blind study of leukocyte interferon administeration in chronic HBsAg-positive hepatitis. Lancet 1:336–338

Weissenbach J, Zeevi M, Landau T, Revel M (1979) Identification of the translation products of human fibroblast interferon mRNA in reticulocyte lysates. Eur J Biochem 98:1–8

Weissenbach J, Chernajovsky Y, Zeevi M, Shulman L, Soreq H, Nir U, Wallach D, Perricaudet M, Tiollais P, Revel M (1980) Two interferon mRNAs in human fibroblasts: in vitro translation and *Escherichia coli* cloning studies. Proc Natl Acad Sci USA 77:7152–7156

Werenne J, Edmonts-Alt X, Bartholeyns J (1980) Interferon regulates cell motility. Ann NY Acad Sci 350:623–624

Werner GH, Jasmin C, Chermann JC (1976) Effect of ammonium-S-tungsts-2-antimoniate on EMC and VSV infections in mice. J Gen Virol 31:59–64

Wheelock EF (1965) Interferon-like virus-inhibitor induced in human leukocytes by phytohemagglutinin. Science 149:310–311

Wheelock EF, Larke RPB (1968) Efficacy of interferon in the treatment of mice with established Friend virus leukemia. Proc Soc Exp Biol Med 127:230–236

Wiebe ME, Joklik WK (1975) The mechanism of inhibition of reovirus replication by interferon. Virology 66:229–240

Wierenga W, Skulnick HI, Weed SD, Stringfellow DA (1980) Antiviral and interferon induction structure-activity relationship profile of 6-aryl pyrimidenes. In: Nelson JD, Grassi C (eds) Current chemotherapy and infectious diseases, Proceedings of the 11th International Congress of Chemotherapy and the 19th Interscience Conference on Antimicrobial Agents and Chemotherapy, vol II. Society for Microbiology, Washington DC, pp 1402–1404

Wiktor TJ, Fernandes MV, Koprowski H (1964) Cultivation of rabies viruses in human diploid cell strain WI-38. J Immunol 93:353–360

Williams BRG, Kerr IM (1978) Inhibition of protein synthesis by 2′ 5′ linked adenine oligonucleotides in intact cells. Nature 276:88–90

Williams BRG, Kerr IM, Gilbert CS, White CN, Ball LA (1978) Synthesis and breakdown of ppp A2′p 5′A 2′p 5′A and transient inhibition of protein synthesis in extracts from interferon-treated and control cell. Eur J Biochem 92:455–462

Wiranowska-Stewart M, Stewart WE II (1977) The role of human chromosome 21 in sensitivity to interferons. J Gen Virol 37:629–634

Wiranowska-Stewart M, Chudzio T, Stewart WE II (1977) Repeated superinduction of interferon in human diploid fibroblast cultures. J Gen Virol 37:351–374

Wiranowska-Stewart M, Lin LS, Braude IA, Stewart WE II (1980) Production, partial purification and characterization of human and murine interferon-type II. Molecular Immunol, 14:625–633

Wong PKY, Yuen PM, MacLeod R, Chang EH, Myers MW, Friedman RM (1977) The effect of interferon on de novo infection of Moloney murine leukemia virus. Cell 10:245–252

Yabrov AA (1966) The enhancement of the stability of cells to diptheria toxin under the influence of a latent viral infection. Cytol 8:767–769

Yagi MJ, King NW Jr, Bekesi JG (1980) Alteration of a mouse mammary tumor virus glycoprotein with interferon treatment. J Virol 34:225–233

Yakobson E, Prives C, Hartman JR, Winocour E, Revel M (1977) Inhibition of viral protein synthesis in monkey cells treated with interferon late in simian virus 40 lytic cycle. Cell 12:73–81

Yamaguchi T, Handa K, Shimizu Y, Abo T, Kumagai K (1977) Target cell for interferon production in human leukocytes stimulated by Sendai virus. J Immunol 118:1931–1946

Yamamoto Y, Kawade Y (1976) Purification of two components of mouse L-cell interferon: electrophoretic demonstration of interferon proteins. J Gen Virol 33:225–234

Yamamoto Y, Kawade Y (1980) Antigenicity of mouse interferons: distinct antigenicity of the two L-cell interferon species. Virology 103:80–88

Yamamoto K, Yamaguchi N, Oda K (1975) Mechanism of interferon induced inhibition of early simian virus 40 functions. Virology 68:58–70

Yaron M, Yaron I, Gurari-Rotman D, Revel M, Lindner HR, Zor U (1977) Stimulation of prostaglandin E production in cultured human fibroblasts by poly I:C and and human interferon. Nature 267:457–459

Yonehara S, Iwakuna Y, Kawade Y (1980) Rapid purification of mouse L-cell interferon labeled with radioactive amino acid by immune precipitation. Virology 100:125–129

Yoshida M, Azuma M, Suenaga T, Mizuno F (1978) Regulation of interferon production by dibutyryl cyclic AMP in serum-free human diploid cell cultures. J Gen Virol 39:303–310

Young CHS, Pringle CR, Follett EAC (1975) Effect of interferon in enucleated cells. J Virol 15:428–441

Youngner JS (1970) Influence of inhibitors of protein synthesis on interferon formation in mice. II. Comparison of effects of glutarimide antibotics and tenuazonic acid. Virology 40:335–343

Youngner JS, Feingold DS (1980) Potential for cancer therapy with a *Brucella Abortus* preparation (BRU-PEL). In: Hersh EM, Chirigos M, Mastrangelo M (eds) Augmenting agents in cancer therapy. Current status and future prospects, vol 16. Raven Press, New York, pp 205–213

Youngner JS, Hallum JV (1968) Interferon production in mice by double-stranded synthetic polynucleotides: induction or release. Virology 35:177–185

Youngner JS, Stinebring WR (1965) Interferon appearance stimulated by endotoxin, bacteria, or viruses in mice pretreated with E. coli, endotoxin, or infected with *Mycobacterium tuberculosis*. Nature 208:456–458

Youngner JS, Stinebring WR, Taube SG (1965) Influence of inhibitors of protein synthesis on interferon formation in mice. Virology 27:541–564

Youngner JS, Keleti G, Feingold DS (1974) Antiviral activity of an ether-extracted nonviable preparation of *Burcella abortus*. Infection and Immunity 10:1202–1206

Zilberstein A, Federman P, Shulman L, Revel M (1976) Specific phosphorylation in vitro of a protein associated with ribosomes of interferon-treated mouse L-cells. FEBS Lett 68:119–124

Zilberstein A, Kimchi A, Schmidt A, Revel M (1978) Isolation of two interferon induced translational inhibitors: a protein kinase and an oligoisoadenylate sythetase. Proc Natl Acad Sci 75:4734–4738

Zoon KC, Buckler CE, Bridgen PJ, Gurari-Rotman D (1978) Production of human lymphoblastoid interferon by Namalwa cells. J Clin Microbiol 7:44–51

Zoon KC, Bridgen PJ, Smith ME (1979 a) Production of human lymphoblastoid interferon by Namalwa cells cultures in serum-free media. J Gen Virol 44:227–229

Zoon KC, Smith ME, Bridgen PJ, Zur Nedden D, Anfinsen CB (1979 b) Purification and partial characterization of human lymphoblastoid interferon. Proc Natl Acad Sci USA 76:5601–5605

Zoon KC, Smith ME, Bridgen PJ, Anfinsen CB, Hunkapiller MW, Hood LE (1980) Amino terminal sequence of the major component of human lymphoblastoid interferon. Science 207:527–528

CHAPTER 7

Immunotherapy and Immunoregulation

H. Friedman and S. Specter

A. Introduction

The importance of an individual's host defense mechanism (or mechanisms) in controlling virus multiplication and the resultant spread of disease has been recognized for centuries. In eighteenth century Europe, variolation was practiced as a crude form of immunization to protect against smallpox. This eventually led to Jenner's acclaimed experiments in which he successfully used vaccine for the first time, employing a "live, attentuated virus" for humans. Approximately 80 years later, Pasteur prepared the first "artificial" vaccine for rabies virus. Thus began the active assault on viruses employing the host immune system. In the century following Pasteur's vaccine development numerous successes have been achieved using specific immunotherapy (vaccines). The development of live attentuated vaccines has led to routine administration for mumps, poliomyelitis, rubella (German measles), rubeola (measles), and smallpox, drastically reducing the morbidity and mortality of these diseases. Smallpox has recently been declared by the World Health Organization to be eradicated by such immune intervention. Inactivated vaccines are in common use for influenza, poliomyelitis, and rabies. Vaccines are also available for several other viruses (adenoviruses, encephalitis viruses, yellow fever) but are used only under specialized circumstances. Additionally, vaccines are in various stages of development for cytomegalovirus (CMV), herpes simplex virus (HSV), respiratory syncytial virus (RSV), and hepatitis virus B. However, vaccines represent only a single approach to immune intervention in virus infections. An extensive array of agents which modulate the immune response and affect host resistance to microbial agents and tumors are currently being examined for antiviral activity. Many of these activities have been recently summarized in a review by WERNER (1979). Unlike vaccines, these immunomodulators act nonspecifically and thus have broad spectrum application in combating viruses. Furthermore, their application may be prophylactic or therapeutic.

Two important factors favor the use of immunotherapeutic approaches to antiviral activity. First is the lack of success in developing chemotherapeutic antiviral agents. With the exception of nucleic acid analogs (ara-A, ara-C, IUDR), which are used to treat herpes simplex encephalitis or conjunctivitis, no other effective therapeutic agents are available. However recent experimental studies indicate that acycloguanosine is an effective antiherpes agent. Only a handful of agents are in use which have prophylactic antiviral activity, these include: methisazone (smallpox), amantadine (influenza), and ribavirin (broad spectrum). The second factor is the ability of the host defense system to limit virus infections under normal circumstances and the presence of a natural broad spectrum antiviral substance within the host. Isaacs and Lindenmann (1957) first reported the presence of a host factor which was induced by virus infection and interfered with further virus replication – this factor was termed interferon. Interferon has broad spectrum antiviral activity and is believed to be an important factor in recovery from virus infection. This subject is discussed elsewhere in the volume and will be given only brief consideration. Another factor concerning host responsiveness to viral infections is the ability of many viruses actively to suppress various aspects of the immune system. Suppression may be selective for only certain components of the immune system or may be generalized. This subject was recently reviewed by Specter and Friedman (1978). The mechanisms by which immunostimulants boost responsiveness are central to understanding the antiviral activity they exert. Thus, this chapter will attempt to outline: the role of immune response in controlling virus infections, the mechanism (or mechanisms) by which various agents enhance immunity, and the success of experimental and clinical studies of immunotherapy and immunoregulation as related to virus infections.

B. Immunity and Virus Infections

Host defenses against virus infections may be approached from several aspects; natural resistance, nonspecific responses, specific immunity (either cellular or humoral), and primary versus secondary immune responses. Regardless of the approach to dissecting this complex interaction of responses which is activated to combat spread of the virus within the host, two basic cell types must be examined, macrophages, and lymphocytes.

Macrophages represent the first line of defense against microbial infections and thus present a formidable force in host natural resistance. Although many activities associated with these cells are nonspecific, their participation in specific responses as antigen processors and presenters has been delineated. In a review on macrophage functions in natural resistance in virus infections, Mims (1964) has provided a classic review illustrating the role of macrophages in natural resistance, and Mogensen (1979) recently extensively examined the many interactions which occur between viruses and these large phagocytic cells. Regulation of the macrophages' ability to resist viruses is at several levels, including genetic disposition, state of activation, and age.

Genetically determined resistance/susceptibility has been described in several animal systems. This host–virus interaction has been examined extensively in mice and reported to be under the control of a single dominant gene (Bang and Warwick 1960; Chang and Hildemann 1964; Goodman and Koprowski 1962a, b; Lindenmann et al. 1978; Mogensen 1977; Sabin 1952; Schell 1960; Oldstone et al. 1973) or due to a multigenic complex (Chesebro et al. 1974; Lilly and Pincus 1973; Lopez 1975; Lopez and Dudas 1979; Stevens and Cook 1971; Yoon and Notkins 1976). In humans, HLA (human leukocyte antigens) have been implicated in natural susceptibility to herpes simplex virus infection (England and Tait 1977; Russell and Schlaut 1977). Mogensen (1979) has a comprehensive discussion of genetic control of natural resistance in his review on the role of macrophages in resistance to virus infections.

The state of activation of macrophages may be defined by phagocytic capability (STIFFEL et al. 1970), enhanced spreading on glass or plastic surfaces (BLANDEN 1968), increased metabolic activity including lysosomal enzyme activity (COHN and BENSON 1965; KARNOVSKY et al. 1975; REIKVAM et al. 1975), antitumor activity (EVANS and ALEXANDER 1972; HIBBS et al. 1972; TAGLIABUE et al. 1979), and most importantly microbicidal activity (BENNEDSEN 1977; BLANDEN 1969, 1974). Generally any stimulation which enhances the activity of macrophages by any of these criteria will lead to enhancement of antiviral activity (MOGENSEN and ANDERSEN 1978; MORAHAN and KAPLAN 1977). However, stimulation of macrophages with diethylstilbestrol, which enhances phagocytosis, may also decrease resistance to endomyocarditis virus (FRIEDMAN et al. 1972) and influenza (S. SPECTER, unpublished work). In the converse situation where factors which depress macrophage function are used, virus pathogenicity may be enhanced (DU BUY 1975; HALLER et al. 1976; LARSON et al. 1972; MOGENSEN and ANDERSEN 1977; RAGER-ZISMAN and ALLISON 1973; SELGRADE and OSBORN 1974; TURNER and BALLARD 1976; WIRTH et al. 1976; ZISMAN et al. 1970, 1971).

Macrophages are strongly implicated in age-related resistance to virus infection. In vitro studies with peritoneal macrophages and herpesvirus indicated that adult and newborn cells were equally susceptible to infection; however, the adult macrophages limited spread of infection to neighboring cells more effectively (JOHNSON 1964). In vivo studies with suckling and adult mice are further suggestive of age-related susceptibility and macrophage function (ANDERVONT 1929; HENSON et al. 1966; KILBOURNE and HORSFALL 1961; LENNETTE and KOPROWSKI 1944; MANNINI and MEDEARIS 1961; MOGENSEN 1976, 1978; MOGENSEN et al. 1974). In humans, herpes susceptibility is enhanced in the neonate and has been attributed to macrophage function (NAHMIAS et al. 1975). Recent studies by CHING and LOPEZ (1979), however, suggest that absence of another cell type may also be relevant to this decreased natural resistance.

Natural resistance by cells designated as natural killer (NK) has been recognized in recent years for antiviral (CHING and LOPEZ 1979; LOPEZ and BENNETT 1978) as well as antitumor immunity (HERBERMAN and HOLDEN 1979; KUMAR et al. 1979; RODER 1979). NK cells have been described in mouse, rat, and human systems; these cells have Fc receptors and recent reports indicate they are pre-T-cells (HERBERMAN and HOLDEN 1979). Recent studies have further investigated the nature of these cells and their relationship to K cells which are involved in antibody-dependent cellular cytotoxicity (ADCC; ORTALDO et al. 1979). NK cells are bone-marrow dependent for their generation and their antiviral activity is directed toward antigens on virus-infected cells (CHING and LOPEZ 1979; LOPEZ and BENNETT 1978). CHING and LOPEZ (1979) have reported an association between the lack of anti-HSV immunity and low or absent NK cell activity. Cellular resistance to infection also resides in two other cell types. Thymus-derived T-lymphocytes react highly specifically against virus-infected cells. Classical cell-mediated immunity to virus infections involve T-cells, however, this occurs in sensitized individuals and is not natural resistance. The ability of cytotoxic T-lymphocytes to kill virus-infected cells is under genetic control, as is recognition of virus antigen during in vitro tests (DOHERTY et al. 1974; ZINKERNAGEL and ALTHAGE 1977; ZINKERNAGEL and WELSH 1976). Recovery from virus infection has been demonstrated to be enhanced by either stimulation of T-cells or transfer of sensitized T-lymphocytes to susceptible donors (BLANDEN and GARDNER 1976; HAMADA and UETAKE 1975; YAP et al. 1978). The fourth cell type involved in cytotoxicity of virus-infected cells is the K cell, so designated for its effector role as a killer cell (BARON et al. 1979). This cytotoxicity is effected via antibody and K cells and is referred to as ADCC. ADCC has been demonstrated experimentally in mice immunized with vaccinia virus (MOLLER-LARSON and HAAHR 1978; PERRIN et al. 1977).

Antibody is also extremely important in antiviral immunity, usually acting in concert with complement. The role of antibody, however, is probably more important in protection from reinfection (ALMEIDA and LAWRENCE 1969; RAWLS and TOMPKINS 1975). Antibodies are also used prophylactically in passive immunity and may be administered as specific sera as with varicella zoster immunoglobulin (VZIG), which is given to immunosuppressed individuals exposed to herpes zoster (chickenpox–shingles) or as pooled serum gamma globulin which is administered to individuals exposed to hepatitis virus B (BARON et al. 1979).

Interferon also has a significant role in recovery from virus infection. This substance may result from either nonspecific stimulation of macrophages and fibroblasts or from specific stimulation of lymphocytes by viruses or other antigens (BARON et al. 1979). Interferons may contribute further to antiviral effects via their ability to stimulate NK cells (DJEU et al. 1979; GIDLUND et al. 1978).

While this has been a very brief summary of the interactions of the immune response in resistance to virus infections, the foundation has been established for examining the effects of host stimuli on various aspects of immunity in antiviral responses. Comprehensive discussions of antiviral immunity have been presented in several recent reviews (BARON et al. 1979; MOGENSEN 1979; WERNER 1979; WHITE 1977).

C. Antiviral Agents

I. Microbial Products

1. Protozoa

Activation of macrophages by chronic infection with the protozoa *Besnoitia jellisoni* and *Toxoplasma gondii* has been reported by REMINGTON and his colleagues (HIBBS et al. 1971; REMINGTON and MERIGAN 1969). Most of these studies examined antitumor immunity. However, in an early paper REMINGTON and MERIGAN (1969) reported an increased resistance to Mengo virus which was maintained for a year or longer in chronically infected mice. The mechanism of this activity is not known; however, the authors seemed to demonstrate that interferon was not involved in this effect. In one recent report, a protozoan parasite, *Trypanosoma brucei*, suppressed resistance to louping ill virus in mice chronically infected with the organism (REID et al. 1979). In contrast to stimulation of antiviral responses by some protozoan parasites, experimental helminthic infections apparently consistently depressed resistance to viruses such as poliovirus, Japanese B encephalitis, swine influenza, encephalomyocarditis, and eastern swine encephalitis viruses (CYPRESS et al. 1973; WOODRUFF 1968). This decreased resistance was associated by the authors with helminth-induced trauma, not with a change in immune function. Thus, antiviral resistance may be affected in varying manners by parasitic infections, some protozoa boosting resistance, with helminths and other protozoa generally reducing host activity.

2. Gram-Negative Bacteria

a) *Lipopolysaccharides (Endotoxins)*

Immunomodulatory activity associated with Gram-negative bacteria has been recognized for many years. Much of this activity, as well as numerous other biologic activities, can be attributed to the lipopolysaccharide (LPS) moiety of the bacterial cell wall (BERRY 1977; MORRISON and ULEVITCH 1978). Enhancement of macrophage functions with regard to resistance to virus infections has been documented by several authors (CLUFF 1970; GLEDHILL 1959; ROLLY et al. 1974). Viruses to which increased resistance due to LPS treatment was demonstrated included: ectromelia, endomyocarditis, herpes simplex, influenza, and vaccinia. These effects were dependent on dose (BLIZNAKOV and ADLER 1972), temporal relationship between LPS and virus inoculation, and route of administration. For example, optimal resistance to influenza was established when 0.3–1.0 µg LPS was inoculated intranasally to mice 24 h prior to inoculation of influenza virus by the same route (ROLLY et al. 1974). BUTLER and FRIEDMAN (1979) reported decreased immune suppression in mouse spleen cell cultures infected with Friend (leukemia) virus and treated with LPS. These authors further indicated that LPS-free supernatant from LPS-treated spleen cells was also capable of enhancing antibody responses in these virus-infected cultures. It thus appears that LPS induces a soluble factor which has activity for reversing some effects of the virus. The mechanism of action of LPS in these responses is not delineated, although effectiveness as an antiviral agent may be related to the pyrogenicity and interferon-inducing capacity of LPS. Yet antiviral activity of LPS can not be directly related to interferon levels (WERNER 1979). The toxicity of LPS has precluded consideration of its use as a therapeutic agent in humans. This toxicity, along with many other biologic functions, is associated with the lipid A moiety of LPS (GALANOS et al. 1977). However, some activities have also been associated with the lipid-free, polysaccharide-rich portion of this molecule (NOWOTNY et al. 1975). FRANK et al. (1977) reported that the detoxified polysaccharide-rich fraction was capable of acting as a polyclonal stimulator of B-lymphocytes. However, the antiviral activity of this moiety of the LPS molecule has not been examined.

b) *Bordetella pertussis*

The vaccine of *Bordetella pertussis* has been demonstrated to induce a leukocytosis, induce splenic hypertrophy, enhance antibody responses to heterologous antigens both in vivo and in vitro, and stimulate activity of peritoneal macrophages (BENJAMIN and KLEIN 1979; FLOERSHEIM 1965; MORSE 1965; MURGO and ATHANASSIADES 1975). Furthermore, pertussis vaccine has been reported to depress cell-mediated immune function (FINGER et al. 1967), exert a mitogenic effect in vitro on splenic T-cells (HO et al. 1980) and induce interferon (BORECKY and LACKOVIC 1967). At least two active components are active in altering immunity by pertussis vaccine: heat-stable endotoxin and pertussis toxin, which is labile to heating at

80 °C for 30 min. The mechanism of action of endotoxins has been discussed, while the mechanisms by which pertussis antigen affects immunity is not clearly understood. It appears that most immunostimulatory activities of pertussis vaccine are attributed in part to both factors. Antiviral activity of pertussis vaccine has been examined in several animal models. ANDERLIK and co-workers have reported that pertussis vaccine enhances the pathogenicity of lymphocytic choriomeningitis (LCM) virus in newborn mice, while reducing pathogenesis of the virus in adults (ANDERLIK et al. 1972; BANOS et al. 1978). This may be related to the ability of the vaccine to decrease cellular immunity, thus reducing pathology in the adult mice, but also abrogating tolerance to the virus in the newborn. *Bordetella* has also been reported to enhance protection against herpes simplex virus infection in mice (KIRCHNER et al. 1978) and against mouse adenovirus (W. R. BENJAMIN, personal communication). Resistance to adenovirus after administration of pertussis vaccine was achieved in conventional and athymic hairless mice, indicating that T-lymphocytes were probably not involved in this response. Furthermore, heating to destroy pertussis toxin did not abrogate the protective effect, suggesting that endotoxin may have been responsible for this protection.

c) *Brucella* spp.

Like the other Gram-negative organisms discussed, *Brucella* spp. contain LPS and are capable of inducing interferon (STINEBURG and YOUNGNER 1964; YOUNGNER et al. 1974). However, protection against viral infection could be induced well after the interferon response abated (BILLIAU et al. 1970). Studies with Mengo virus and Semliki Forest virus, HSV-2, and vaccinia virus suggest that the mechanism of enhanced resistance induced with *Brucella* spp. could be attributed to stimulation of macrophages with some early effects associated with interferon activity (DE CLERCQ 1974; FEINGOLD et al. 1976; KERN et al. 1976; MUYEMBE et al. 1972). An extract of *Brucella abortus* designated BRU-PEL has been demonstrated to induce interferon and assist in protection against HSV-2 or infection with encephalomyocarditis virus (KERN et al. 1976). When this material is extracted with chloroform–methanol, neither the soluble nor insoluble fractions are active. However, recombination of the fractions yielded active fractions for both antiviral activity and interferon production (YOUNGNER et al. 1974). In contrasting studies, STARR et al. (1976) were not able to demonstrate any antiviral effect for *Brucella abortus* against HSV-2 when the immunostimulant was used 2, 4, or 6 days before viral challenge. No explanation for this lack of effect was offered.

3. Gram-Positive Bacteria

a) *Corynebacterium* spp.

Both *C. parvum* and *C. acnes* have been used as immunopotentiating agents to stimulate macrophages and/or NK cells in antitumor (BAUM and BREESE 1976; MACFARLAN et al. 1979; WOODRUFF and WARNER 1977) and antiviral resistance (BUDZKO et al. 1978; CERUTTI 1974; GLASGOW et al. 1977; MORAHAN and KAPLAN 1977). Heat- or formaldehyde-killed *C. parvum* was reported to enhance mouse survival when administered i.p. approximately 1 week before challenge with encephalomyocarditis virus (CERUTTI 1974), herpes simples virus (KIRCHNER et al. 1978), mouse cytomegalovirus and Semliki Forest virus (GLASGOW et al. 1977), and Junin virus (BUDZKO et al. 1978). The enhancement of antiviral activity by *Corynebacterium* spp. has not been clearly delineated, however, studies suggest that interferon and enhanced NK activity are important (GIDLUND et al. 1978; HIRT et al. 1978; MACFARLAN et al. 1979; OJO et al. 1978). Interferon has been demonstrated to enhance NK activity, thus possibly explaining the relationship between the increase in these two activities. MACFARLAN et al. (1979) have indicated that antitumor NK cells induced by *C. parvum* differ from unstimulated NK cells; thus their role in antiviral activity may be different from unstimulated cells.

These antiviral effects of *C. parvum* are tempered by observations in tumor systems whereby administration of the killed bacteria led to immune suppression and enhanced tumor growth (KIRCHNER et al. 1975; SCOTT 1972). The use of *Corynebacterium* spp. in clinical trials has been limited by the lack of understanding of which direction, i.e., enhanced resistance vs susceptibility, in which treatment might lead the virus infection. In the only reported clinical studies, *C. parvum* enhanced antibody responses to hepatitis B surface antigens (HB$_s$Ag) in individuals with previous antibody titers. However, chronic HB$_s$Ag carriers were not induced to form anti-HB$_s$Ag antibodies and carriers remained antigen positive (PAPAEVANGELOU et al. 1977).

Subcellular fractions of *C. parvum* cell walls have also been tested for antiviral activity. A low molecular weight (6,000 daltons) peptidoglycan fraction was effective in enhancing resistance to encephalomyocarditis virus and to a variant of Moloney (sarcoma) virus (MIGLIORE-SAMOUR et al. 1974). Although there are numerous Gram-positive organisms from which peptidoglycans have been extracted (DZIARSKI 1980; HEYMER and RIETSCHEL 1977), this appears to be the only report of an antiviral effect associated with this molecule. The peptidoglycans are capable of inducing many endotoxin-like effects, including the induction of interferon by *Nocardia* peptidoglycans (BAROT-CIORBARU et al. 1978); thus this cell wall fraction could be responsible, at least in part, for the antiviral resistance-stimulating effects of *C. parvum*.

b) Muramyl Dipeptide

A low molecular weight (400 daltons) muramyl dipeptide, *N*-acetylmuramyl-L-alanyl-D-isoglutamine (MDP), which is a constituent of the Gram-positive bacterial cell wall or mycobacterial cell wall, has been shown to be the minimal structure necessary to induce adjuvant activity associated with peptidoglycan derivatives (ELLOUZ et al. 1974). This molecule has widespread application as an immunostimulant and is easily synthesized (CHEDID et al. 1978). In addition to the adjuvant effect of MDP, this molecule has been reported to enhance tumor immunity (JOHNSON et al. 1978), increase resistance to bacterial infection (CHEDID et al. 1977), and enhance resistance to parasitic infection (KIERSZENBAUM and FERRARESI 1979). These activities indicate favorably that MDP might enhance resistance to viruses, but antiviral activity has not been reported. MDP has been reported to enhance immunity to influenza virus vaccines in mice and hamsters (AUDIBERT et al. 1977; WEBSTER et al. 1977). The advantage of this adjuvant material is that it does not require suspension in oil, as do many other adjuvants. Additionally, it may be administered by any route, including oral and is still effective when administered by a different route than antigen (Chedid et al. 1978). Many other MDP analogs have been tested but the L-analyl-D-isoglutamine appears to be the most effective structure. Two groups have sought to enhance the activity of MDP by different methods. Kotani et al. (1977) have produced 6-O-acyl derivatives in linear and branched forms, which enhance MDP activity. Chedid et al. (1979) have attempted to increase adjuvanticity by polymerization. These studies suggest that MDP or other synthetic cell wall analogs may be effective in enhancing the immunogenic potential of viral vaccines which are only weakly immunogenic. The mechanisms of immunopotentiation by MDP and other cell wall components are varied, but most likely involve B- and T-lymphocytes and macrophages, and have been reviewed on several occasions (Chedid et al. 1978; Kotani et al. 1975).

4. Mycobacteria

The most significant bacterial immunostimulants for experimental and clinical application are associated with the mycobacteria. These agents are used to prepare complete Freund's adjuvant. The bacille Calmette–Guérin (BCG) strain of *Mycobacterium bovis*, used to vaccinate humans against tuberculosis, is utilized extensively as a nonspecific immunostimulant in cancer therapy (Bast et al. 1973; Mastrangelo et al. 1976). Antiviral activity of BCG has been clearly demonstrated as well. In early experiments, Larson et al. (1971) demonstrated that BCG induced resistance in mice to leukemia caused by Friend virus. BCG was demonstrated effective in other tumor virus systems, inhibiting tumors in AKR mice (Lemonde 1973) and in mice infected with Moloney sarcoma virus (Schwartz et al. 1971). In humans with Burkitt's lymphoma, antibody titers to Epstein–Barr virus-associated membrane antigens were increased although there was no significant effect on tumor remission (Magrath and Ziegler 1976). Resistance to acute virus infections has also been reported after treatment with BCG. The earliest observation of enhanced resistance to virus infection was recorded by Old et al. (1963) who saw a reduction in virus titer using the Mengo strain of encephalomyocarditis virus. Although BCG is believed to express its effects via activation of macrophages, peritoneal exudate macrophages from BCG-treated mice replicated virus as well as control macrophages when cultured in vitro. This might suggest that other cells or host factors act with the macrophages in conferring resistance. Increased resistance was a long-term phenomenon, lasting from 1 week after BCG treatment to 3.5 months.

Several studies have been performed using BCG in HSV infection in mice. Barker et al. (1979) reported unsuccessful studies in which BCG appeared to enhance death following intravaginal HSV-2 infection. Similar reports of BCG having tumor-enhancing effects in human and experimental cancers have also been observed (Mastrangelo et al. 1976). Starr et al. (1976) used infection of newborn mice in their studies with HSV-2. Lethal infection was significantly reduced in these mice when BCG was given 2–6 days before challenge with virus. In these same studies, other immunostimulants (levamisole, staphage lysate, typhoid vaccine, and *Brucella* vaccine) failed to provide protection. This protection was attributed to activation of peritoneal macrophages by BCG. In addition to the mouse studies, clinical human trials also have been performed. Anderson et al. (1974) demonstrated a decrease in recurrence of herpes genitalis in men and women. BIERMAN (1976) showed similar effects after intradermal BCG infection. However COREY et al. (1976) showed no beneficial effects of BCG therapy for recurrent herpes. A marmoset model with *Herpesvirus saimiri* revealed no protection with regard to lymphoma development (SCHAUF et al. 1975). Thus BCG treatment of herpesvirus infections has met with varying success, although antiviral activity of BCG with this system seems apparent. This activity can be associated directly with macrophage activation. Influenza virus infection has also been used to examine BCG as an antiviral agent. In studies with A2 and A0 influenza strains, protective effects of BCG were also associated with enhanced clearance of virus by macrophages (FLOC'H and WERNER 1976; SPENCER et al. 1977).

Studies with other mycobacteria, living or heat killed, have also demonstrated antiviral effects. ALLEN and MUDD (1973) reported that H37Ra, an avirulent strain of *Mycobacterium tuberculosis*, enhanced resistance of mice to vaccinia virus challenge. This protection was maintained by elicitation of immunity in H37Ra-treated mice with tuberculin. In addition, mice immune to *Staphylococcus aureus* were protected against vaccinia when stimulated with staphage lysate. Complete Freund's adjuvant (CFA) containing heat-killed mycobacteria as well as a Wax D preparation from *M. tuberculosis* showed antiviral activity in adult mice (GORKE 1967; GORKE et al. 1968; WERNER 1979). GORKE and co-workers reported that these preparations limited virus multiplication of foot-and-mouth Disease virus and increased the number of virus particles required for a median lethal dose (LD_{50}). This effect was associated with an early high level of interferon. The effects were seen when the mycobacterial products were administered in two injections 1 week apart preceeding virus infection. WERNER was not able to establish any antiviral effect when delipidated mycobacteria in aqueous solution was administered in a single dose before infection of mice with either encephalomyocarditis, herpes simplex, swine influenza, or mouse hepatitis viruses. WEISS and YASPHE (1973) performed extensive antitumor studies with another mycobacterial fraction, a methanol-extracted residue (MER). These authors reported that animals treated with MER resisted an outbreak of pneumonitis in their animal colony. Although the cause of this disease was unknown, it was believed to be due to a virus.

These extensive studies with mycobacteria and their products are evidence of the possible role of stimulated specific (T-cell) and nonspecific (macrophages) immunity, yielding antiviral activity. A major beneficial side effect of using BCG in antitumor immunotherapy may therefore be related to increased natural resistance of otherwise debilitated individuals against virus infections. From most reports, it appears that 7–10 days is required to achieve significant levels of antiviral activity; however, this effect lasts for extended periods of time. Subsequent administrations of immunopotentiators may prolong or boost this effect.

II. Products of the Immune System

Immune therapy has been practiced in antiviral immunity for decades using products of the immune system. The most proven technique is administration of serum antibodies. However, more recent studies have utilized subcellular factors secreted or extracted from lymphocytes.

1. Immune Globulins

The most conventional method for antiviral immunotherapy involves passive immunization using immune serum globulins (ISG). This therapy mimics one of nature's earliest host defense mechanism, i.e., naturally acquired antibodies which are passed transplacentally from mother to fetus. These antibodies generally persist in the newborn for approximately 6 months and are vital in preventing virus infections of the infant. While preparations of ISG are very useful as prophylactic agents, they are seldom of any beneficial effect in abrogating the course of an established infection. In many instances, pooled human serum is used as a source of ISG; however, in some cases special globulin preparations are utilized. For preparation of ISG, the globulin is extracted from plasma and concentrated to levels 25 times greater than those found in whole plasma. As in the case of transplacentally transferred antibody, the major antibody constituent of ISG is IgG. Details of preparation and administration are reviewed by BARON et al. (1979). At present, ISG is used most frequently in prophylaxis against hepatitis virus A. Protection is only of short duration, and larger doses or repeated administration are preferred for protection over an extended period of time (KOFF 1978; KRUGMAN 1963). Specific immune globulins obtained from plasma of patients in convalencence from virus infections (1–4 weeks postinfection) has been used against five viruses; hepatitis B, mumps, rabies, vaccinia, and varicella zoster.

a) Mumps Immune Globulin

Mumps immune globulin has been utilized to help reduce severity of orchitis and parotitis associated with mumps infection. Globulin has been administered at the time of exposure to the virus but did not decrease incidence of disease or severity of infection, and has thus been discontinued (REED et al. 1967).

b) Hepatitis B Immune Globulin

Passive hemagglutination tests indicate that anti-hepatitis B antibodies in hepatitis B immune globulin (HBIG) are extremely high, sometimes reaching a titer in excess of 1:1,000,000. When used prophylactically in individuals exposed to hepatitis B by a needle prick or ingestion of contaminated materials, the risk of infection appears to be reduced (GRADY and LEE 1975; KOFF 1978). Administration of HBIG should be as soon after exposure as possible and involves intramuscular inoculation of 5 ml globulin, a booster should be given 1 month later. HBIG is also being used prophylactically for medical personnel exposed to the virus while working in dialysis units where hepatitis B is relatively common (KOFF 1978). Under most conditions tested, HBIG has been reported to be effective, with no severe side effects, and is now licensed for general use by the U.S. Food and Drug Administration.

c) Rabies Immune Globulin

Rabies immune globulin is administered to bite victims as soon as possible after a bite by a rabid animal is suspected. The bite site should be cleansed thoroughly with soap and water and 20 IU/kg body weight globulin administered. Passive immunity with globulin is used as an adjunct to vaccination with rabies vaccine. Thus, the recommended dose of globulin must not be exceeded as this may interfere with active immunization (HATTWICK et al. 1974). Globulin is used when it is ascertained that rapid antibody levels are desired, as in areas where rabies is known to be present, depending upon the site of the animal bite, and whether it was provoked or not. Attempts to develop more potent and effective rabies vaccines used alone or with interferon may, however, limit or eliminate the use of rabies immune globulin.

d) Vaccinia Immune Globulin

Although smallpox is no longer considered a significant human pathogen, owing to the extensive eradication program of the World Health Organization, vaccinia immune globuline (VIG) still has application. VIG has been used mainly to control complications associated with smallpox vaccination, usually seen in immunocompromised individuals (KEMPE 1960). In addition, this report indicated that in epidemics in India, VIG was effective in reducing disease frequency and severity. KEMPE (1960) also indicated that VIG was effective in treatment of vaccination-induced eczema vaccinatum, but not for vaccinia necrosum.

e) Varicella Zoster Immune Globulin

Varicella zoster immune globulin(VZIG) has been reported to prevent varicella in normal individuals when administered within 72 h of exposure to the virus (BRUNELL et al. 1969). In immunocompromised individuals, who are at high risk of systemic disease, VZIG has been reported to modify the course of varicella (BRUNELL et al. 1972; GERSHON et al. 1974). VZIG is in limited supply and is available from the Sidney Farber Cancer Institute, Boston, Massachusetts from individuals who meet criteria established by the Center for Disease Control (MORBIDITY and MORTALITY WEEKLY REPORT 1979). These criteria generally relate to immunosuppressed/immunodeficient individuals or newborns of mothers who have contracted varicella within 4 days of delivery.

2. Thymic Hormones

The thymus has been documented repeatedly as the site of maturation of lymphocytes involved in cell-mediated immunity; these are designated T-cells. Investigations in several laboratories have revealed that factors (hormones) from the epithelium in the thymus are involved in T-cell maturation. Each laboratory has described their factor differently so that the hormone or hormones are referred to as thymosin (LOW et al. 1979) which was first described 14 years earlier (KLEIN et al. 1965), thymopoetin (GOLDSTEIN 1975), thymic factor (BACH and CHARRIERE 1979), thymic hormone factor (TRAININ et al. 1979), and lymphocyte stimulating hormone (PIERSCHBACHER et al. 1979).

Zaizov et al. (1979) treated children with immunosuppression, lymphoproliferative malignancy, and generalized varicella with their thymic hormone factor. Of 13 children, 12 had a return of cellular immune function and recovered from varicella infection. Thymic hormone factor was administered daily for 12 days by intramuscular injection.

Experimental models using Moloney sarcoma virus (ZISBLATT et al. 1970) and virus-associated leukemia in AKR mice (BARKER et al. 1979) demonstrated antiviral effects of thymosin. Unlike the previous studies which implicated nonspecific immune functions, thymic hormone activity is directly related to enhancement of T-lymphocyte function. In this regard, the use of transfer factor (see Sect. C.II.3) appears to be mediated via T-cells.

3. Transfer Factor

Transfer factor is a product of specifically immune peripheral blood lymphocytes which can be collected by leukophoresis. This substance is extracted from disrupted cells and collected from dialysates of this material. LAWRENCE (1955) originally demonstrated this factor in humans, and numerous studies have been performed to examine its antitumor effects. Although the structure of transfer factor has not been established, a model has been proposed (BURGER et al. 1979). MAZAHERI et al. (1977) reviewed therapeutic effects of transfer factor as an antiviral agent in progressive vaccinia, herpes zoster, measles, subacute sclerosing panencephalitis, chronic active hepatitis, and cytomegalovirus, all of which involved persistent virus infections. Only one of these studies was controlled, so results are questionable. However, in a study of chronic active hepatitis, four patients treated with transfer factor showed some clinical improvement but remained positive for persistence of viremia as measured by HB_sAg (SCHULMAN et al. 1976). In a study of recurrent herpes simplex, transfer factor from individuals with nonrecurrent herpes infection was not effective in reducing recurrent disease (OLESKE et al. 1978). A problem with many of these transfer factor preparations is the concentration used. Since many of these preparations vary in their content of transfer factor, it is difficult to assess the efficacy of various preparations used in such studies. In subacute sclerosing panencephalitis and multiple sclerosis, transfer factor has been obtained from measles-immune individuals or "household contacts." Since the etiology of these diseases is poorly understood, although there appears to be some association with measles virus, the presence of a transfer factor relevant to the disease is in doubt. Nevertheless, anecdotal cases of successful therapy have been reported. STEELE and co-workers have reported successful use of transfer factor in prophylaxis against herpesviruses. Human transfer factor protected marmosets against challenge with a lethal dose of HSV-1 (STEELE et al. 1976). A more recent report utilized transfer factor to varicella zoster virus in children with acute lymphocytic leukemia. Since varicella zoster has a high mortality rate in this population, prophylaxis is indicated. Of 12 children, 10 showed a conversion of vigorous anti-varicella zoster cellular immunity (STEELE 1980). This immunity has persisted for 17 months with no reported cases of varicella zoster. While several studies have suggested careful immunotherapy or prophylaxis with transfer factor, the absence of controlled studies and standardized preparations has prevented any firm conclusions concerning the usefulness of these preparations as broad spectrum antiviral agents.

4. Immune RNA

Antitumor immunotherapy using specific immunostimulants has also included studies using RNA from sensitized lymphocytes, which is designated "immune

RNA" (FINK 1976; FRIEDMAN 1973, 1979). Although the nature of transfer of immunity is not well understood with such immune RNA, its effectiveness has been demonstrated in humans and animal models by several investigators. An advantage of immune RNA is the ability to get satisfactory stimulation with xenogenic lymphocytes. PILCH and associates have used sheep immune RNA against human tumor cells to treat patients with malignant melanoma (KERN and PILCH 1979). To date no reports of immune RNA as an antiviral agent are available; however, successes with other immunostimulants in antiviral therapy suggest this substance might also be effective.

5. Interferon

Interferon has been demonstrated to have antiviral activity for many years; however, only recently has it gained attention as an effective antiviral agent by modulating immune functions. Interferon has been reported to enhance lymphocyte activity (LINDAHL et al. 1972, 1976; BARON et al. 1979), macrophage function (HUANG et al. 1971), and most recently NK cell activity (GIDLUND et al. 1978; HERBERMAN and HOLDEN 1979). This relationship between interferon and immune responses in antiviral and antitumor activity has received a great deal of interest lately. Because of interferon's extensive activities as an antiviral substance, the topic has been treated as a separate review in this volume (see Chap. 6).

III. Synthesized Immunostimulants

1. Levamisole

Levamisole has been utilized as an antihelmintic agent for the past decade, and has been successfully used in humans in treating nematode infections. RENOUX and RENOUX (1971) first demonstrated the immunomodulatory effects of levamisole and its isomer, tetramisole. Mice given *Brucella* vaccine and levamisole showed greater protection against live *Brucella abortus* challenge than those given bacilli only. The interest stimulated by this study led to the use of levamisole as an immunoadjuvant in therapy for neoplasia (AMERY 1976; RENOUX and RENOUX 1972). These studies indicated that levamisole stimulates cellular immune responses: however, this effect was only seen when T-cell response are depressed. Normal T-cell immunity was not further augmented by this agent (RENOUX 1978; SYMOENS 1978).

In experimental studies employing levamisole as an antiviral agent in animal models, two reports concerning HSV indicate the effectiveness of this treatment. SADOWSKI and RAPP (1975) reported that HSV-1-transformed cells were inhibited by levamisole from causing lung metastases in weanling hamsters. This effect was observed whether 2 mg levamisole was given at the time of tumor challenge, 24 h later, or when tumors became palpable. In suckling rats, 3 mg/kg levamisole was also effective in inhibiting HSV-2 acute infection, increasing survival from 4% to 30%. When levamisole was used in combination with adenine arabinoside, however, survival was only 11%, indicating that these two antiviral agents have antagonistic effects (FISCHER et al. 1975, 1976). Two additional studies with large animals have also yielded positive results. Levamisole improved the health of minks chronically infected with Aleutian disease of mink when it was incorporated into their food (Kenvon 1978). Cattle and goats with foot-and-mouth disease also showed a decrease in symptoms within 48 h when injected intramuscularly with a single dose of levamisole (Rojas and Olivari 1974). Several studies with mice have yielded consistently negative results with levamisole as an antiviral agent against mouse hepatitis virus, HSV-2, and influenza virus (Morahan et al. 1977; Starr et al. 1976; Werner 1979).

Clinical studies using levamisole as an antiviral agent have been concentrated on herpes simplex virus, although other viruses have been examined. Clinical improvement of herpes skin lesions, facial, labial, and genital, as well as corneal lesions, have been recorded, as was a decreased frequency of recurrences (Kint and Verlinden 1974; Kint et al. 1974; Lods 1976). In contradictory results, Spitler et al. (1975) reported decreased immune responses to herpes antigen associated with clinical improvement, while O'Reilly et al. (1977) showed enhanced in vitro lymphocyte responsiveness to herpes antigen. However, none of these studies were properly controlled. When a double-blind, controlled study was performed over a 6-month period, no difference between placebo-treated and levamisole-treated groups was seen when evaluated clinically, subjectively, or in immunologic studies (Russell et al. 1978). If those data were adjusted to account for a higher number of recurrences in the levamisole-treated group before treatment, then there was a significant difference recorded.

Reports of successful treatment with levamisole in clinical trials against other viruses have been reported for: molluscum contagiosum which causes warts (Helin and Bergh 1974), hepatitis B (Par et al. 1977), and respiratory disease of undetermined etiology in children (Van Eygen et al. 1976). In addition, levamisole was reported to cause clinical improvement in Crohn's disease which is suspected of having a viral etiology (Bertrand et al. 1974).

In view of the numerous reports of immunosuppressive activities of viruses (Specter and Friedman 1978), reported therapeutic effects of levamisole as an antiviral agent are not surprising. Unsuccessful prophylactic experiments in animals might be explained by failure of levamisole to alter a normal state of responsiveness. In clinical studies however, individuals with existing infections and possibly reduced immune competence, but intact immune compartments, were stimulated by the levamisole to combat the virus. Although studies to date employing levamisole are not conclusive, they suggest clinical efficacy for this drug as an antiviral agent.

2. Vitamins

Synthetic vitamins or their analogs are now reported to have antiviral activity. The most publicized vitamin to have antiviral activity has been vitamin C (ascorbic acid); however vitamin A (retinoic acid) has also been demonstrated to be effective against tumor viruses.

a) Vitamin A and Retinoids

Antitumor effects of retinoic acid and analogs have been reported to be highly effective in treatment of chemically induced tumors (Sporn 1978). In recent studies, virally induced tumors have been reported to be diminished by treatment with retinoids (FRANKEL et al. 1980; TODARO et al. 1978). TODARO et al. (1978) reported that Moloney sarcoma virus was blocked from phenotypic cell transformation by retinyl acetate associated with sarcoma growth factor. Rous sarcoma virus was inhibited from causing tumors when Syrian hamsters were treated prophylactically with an aromatic retinoid (FRANKEL et al. 1980). Therapeutic treatment of tumors was also effective in this study. Therapy of acute virus infections is not reported for vitamin A or other retinoids.

b) Vitamin C

Vitamin C has been demonstrated by SIEGEL and MORTON (1977 a, b) to stimulate T-cell activity, macrophage activity, and interferon, but not antibody responses. Thus this vitamin is immunostimulatory and has been reported to have antiviral activity by many investigators (CAMERON et al. 1979; JUNGEBLUT 1939; MANZELLA and ROBERTS 1979). However, most of these effects have not substantiated in well-controlled studies. Several in vitro studies indicate that vitamin C directly reduces infectivity of virus particles per se, indicating that effects on the host may be minimal, and that the antiviral effects of ascorbate may not be attained by administration to humans (JUNGEBLUT 1935; SCHWERDT and SCHWERDT 1975). Although the claims for vitamin C as an antiviral therapeutic agent remain to be substantiated, its immune enhancing activity suggests it is an effective means of reducing severity of viral infections.

3. Tilorone

Tilorone has been reported to enhance antibody responses, stimulate interferon activity and decrease cellular immunity (BARON et al. 1979). REGELSON (1975) has demonstrated that this agent is effective against established Friend virus. In acute virus infections in mice, tilorone was shown to be effective against nine viruses when administered before the virus (KRUEGER and MAYER 1970). The authors suggest that activity was due to interferon stimulation. However, REGELSON has indicated that the antiviral effects of this agent extend beyond the interferon effects. The mechanism or mechanisms responsible for these antiviral effects which are not due to interferon have not been delineated.

4. Pyran

Pyran is another example of an antitumor agent that has also been investigated as an antiviral agent. Pyran is a copolymer of divinyl ether and maleic anhydride, and is an inducer of interferon. In addition, it is capable of modulating immune responsiveness (REGELSON et al. 1978). Intravaginal infection with HSV-2 could be abrogated in pyran-treated mice (BREINIG et al. 1978). These studies indicated that viral replication was limited locally, thus preventing spread of the virus to the central nervous system, which is fatal. This activity was associated with macrophages. In earlier studies, pyran was reported also to protect against herpesvirus infection whether the virus was inoculated intravaginally or intravenously into mice (McCORD et al. 1976; MORAHAN and McCORD 1975). Pyran could be administered intraperitoneally or intravenously, but was effective only when administered 24 h prior to virus challenge. A protective effect could also be demonstrated in these studies against herpesvirus in adult thymectomized, lethally irradiated, bone marrow reconstituted animals. Thus, pyran effects are not apparently related to T-lymphocyte activity.

5. Inosiplex (Isoprinosine)

Unlike most of the products listed in this chapter, inosiplex has been utilized from its earliest studies as an antiviral agent (GINSBERG and GLASKY 1977). Inosiplex was also reported to stimulate both humoral and cellular immune functions (GINSBERG and GLASKY 1977; HADDEN et al. 1976, 1977). HADDEN (1978) has also indicated that this compound is capable of stimulating macrophage proliferation.

Numerous initial experiments with inosiplex failed to demonstrate a consistent antiviral effect, as reported by GLASGOW and GALASSO (1972). MULDOON et al. (1972) first indicated that anti-influenza effects might be associated with potentiation of immunity when they demonstrated that cortisone abrogated the protective effects of inosiplex. Recently, SIMON et al. (1978) reported that inosiplex in dose ranges 0.005–1.0 µg/ml and 10–150 µg/ml inhibited, to a moderate degree, infection of tissue culture cells by influenza virus. These doses were also effective in enhancing concanavalin A stimulation of lymphocytes from mouse spleen. In vivo studies revealed that immune responses to influenza antigens were increased in inosiplex-treated mice as measured by hemagglutination antibodies. Thus, protective effects of the drug could be directly related to immunostimulatory doses.

Inosiplex was effective in protecting mice against encephalomyocarditis virus when used in conjunction with interferon. This occurred only when inosiplex was given 24 h before infection and interferon was given 1 h postinfection (CHANY and CERUTTI 1977). This enhancing effect on interferon protection was due to a membrane interaction. Inosiplex was not effective therapeutically in this system when given 7 h postinfection.

Clinical trials with inosiplex have been reported for several viruses. Again reports have been both negative and positive. FELDMAN et al. (1978) found that children with neoplasms who developed herpes zoster infection did not show improvement with inosiplex. The authors attribute this lack of effect to the depressed state of the immune system of these individuals.

The majority of clinical studies with inosiplex have concentrated on treatment of respiratory virus infections. Three separate studies investigated the efficacy of this drug in rhinovirus infection (PACHUTA et al. 1974; SOTO et al. 1973; WALDMAN andGANGULY 1977). When inosiplex was given prophylactically before and after intranasal rhinovirus no beneficial effects were seen in two studies (PACHUTA et al. 1974; SOTO et al. 1973). However, in a double-blind study in which the drug was administered either at the time of infection or 48 h later, treated patients showed reduced cold symptoms and a decreased incidence of virus isolation (WALDMAN and GANGULY 1977). Inosiplex-treated individuals also showed increased responsiveness to phytohemagglutinin, indicating that increased cellular immunity correlates well with enhanced antiviral activity. Two studies concerning the efficacy of inosiplex in influenza infection also showed mixed results, although beneficial effects were seen in both studies. LONGELY et al. (1973) reported that volunteers inoculated intranasally with influenza A/Hong Kong did not show clinical improvement when given inosiplex twice daily for 10 days, beginning 2 days before infection. However, virus shedding measured by virus isolation determinations was statistically lower in the drug-treated group. A study using prophylactic–therapeutic and therapeutic administration of inosiplex showed clinical reduction of influenza A symptoms in both groups compared with placebo controls (WALDMAN et al. 1978). The drug was administered daily for 9 days, beginning either 2 days before (prophylactic) or after (therapeutic) virus inoculation. In these studies, inosiplex treatment was also associated with enhanced responsiveness of phytohemagglutinin.

The overall clinical efficacy of inosiplex was evaluated by GLASKY et al. (1978), who reviewed 165 studies with the drug. Viruses studies included hepatitis, dengue, mumps, acute measles, and subacute sclerosing panencephalitis, influenza, herpes simplex, and varicella zoster. In general, results were favorable and inosiplex treatment was judged to be significant in reducing symptoms in intensity and duration.

D. Potential of Immunostimulants as Antiviral Agents

We have seen in this chapter that numerous studies have indicated that various immunostimulatory substances may exhibit antiviral activity. In both experimental models and clinical trials, immunoenhancing agents resulted in moderate to impressive results as antiviral agents against a broad spectrum of viruses. However, it must be noted that during studies with most of these substances, several failures were also recorded. Before one can expect general acceptance of any of these agents as antiviral substances a consistent effect must be recorded. To attain this goal it seems apparent that the mechanism or mechanisms by which these substances exert their influence on virus infections must be delineated.

The immune mechanisms involved in antiviral activity of the host was discussed in Sect. A and has been reviewed by WERNER (1979). Clearly there are at least four cell types involved in these responses: T-lymphocytes, NK cells, K cells which are involved in ADCC, and macrophages. Elements of the humoral immune system, i.e., antibodies and interferon, are most definitely involved in antiviral host defenses as well. Unfortunately, understanding the interactions among these cells and their products in optimizing antiviral immunity will require many more years of study. Fortunately, however, the immune mechanisms involved in combating viruses and tumors appear to be very similar, if not identical, and antiviral studies should benefit from the extensive studies that are performed in the area of immunotherapy of neoplastic disease. In addition, understanding of cells (expecially NK and K cells) and their functions which have only been recognized in the past decade should lead to further success in understanding these mechanisms.

It must be recognized that production and marketing of immunostimulants as antiviral agents must await their acceptance as a commercially profitable venture. At present, products such as interferon, transfer factor, thymic hormones, etc., all of which appear to have excellent potential as antiviral agents, are prohibitively expensive for general use. Further advances in some of these areas, such as genetic engineering to induce bacteria to produce interferon, as recently reported, may alleviate these problems. However, commercial interests will undoubtedly be served in such ventures.

Finally, one should advocate approaches to immunostimulants for antiviral therapy which uses multiple modalities. With a few exceptions, the therapeutic approaches reviewed here examined only a single agent to enhance antiviral activity. Studies using two or more agents which modulate various aspects of immunity may be considerably more effective in combating viral diseases. Various combinations of stimulants must be evaluated if a highly effective therapy is to be developed. While it is understood that such investigation is costly, involves several control groups and large numbers of subjects, it seems apparent that the relative lack of success to date using conventional antiviral drugs warrants such a multifaceted approach.

References

Allen EC, Mudd S (1973) Protection of mice against vaccinia virus by bacterial infection and sustained stimulation with specific bacterial antigens. Infect Immun 7:62–67

Almedia JD, Lawrence GD (1969) Heated and unheated antiserum on rubella virus. Am J Dis Child 118:101–106

Amery WK (1976) Double blind levamisole trial in resectable lung cancer. Ann NY Acad Sci 277:260–268

Anderlik P, Szeri I, Banos Z, Foldes I, Radnai B (1972) Interaction of *Bordetella pertussis* vaccine treatment and lymphocytic choriomeningitis virus infection in mice. Experentia 28:985–986

Anderson FD, Ushyima RN, Larson CL (1974) Recurrent herpes genitalis: treatment with attentuated *Mycobacterium bovis* (BCG). Obst Gynec NY 43:797–805

Andervont HB (1929) Activity of herpetic virus in mice. J Inf Dis 44:383–393

Audibert F, Chedid L, Hannoun C (1977) Augmentation de la response immunitaire au vaccin grippal par un glycopeptide synthetique adjuvant (*N*-acetylmuramyl-L-alanyl-D-isoglutamine). C R Acad Sci Paris Serie D 285:467–470

Bach M-A, Charreire J (1979) Role of a circulating thymic factor in self-recognition and self-tolerance. Ann NY Acad Sci 332:55–63

Bang EB, Warwick A (1960) Mouse macrophages as host cells for the mouse hepatitis virus and the genetic basis of their susceptibility. Proc Nacl Acad Sci USA 46:1065–1075

Banos Z, Anderlik P, Szeri I, Radnai B (1978) Course of lymphocytic choriomeningitis (LCM) virus infection in suckling mice treated with *Bordetella pertussis* vaccine. Acta Microbiol Acad Sci Hung 25:277–283

Barker AD, Dennis AJ, Moore VS, Rice JM (1979) Effects of thymosin on cytotoxicity and virus production in AKR mice. Ann N Y Acad Sci 332:70–80

Baron S, Brunell PA, Grosberg SE (1979) Mechanisms of action and pharmacology: The immune and interferon systems. In: Galasso GJ, Merigan TC, Buchanon RA (eds) Antiviral agents and viral disease of man. Raven Press, New York, p 151

Barot-Ciorbaru R, Wietzerbin J, Petit JF, Chedid L, Falcoff E, Lederer E (1978) Induction of interferon synthesis in mice by fractions from Nocardia. Infect Immun 19:353–356

Bast RC Jr, Zbar B, Borsos T, Rapp HJ (1973) BCG and cancer. In: Borsos T, Rapp HJ (eds) Conference on the Use of BCG in Therapy of Cancer, National Cancer Inst Monograph 39, DHEW Publication (NIH) 74–511

Baum M, Breese M (1976) Antitumor effect of *Corynebacterium parvum:* Possible mode of action. Brit J Cancer 33:468–473

Benjamin WR, Klein TW (1979) Alteration of macrophage function following *Bordetella pertussis* vaccine administration. Abstracts Annual Meeting Am Soc Microbiol, Washington DC p 57

Bennedsen J (1977) In vitro studies on normal, stimulated,and immunologically activated mouse macrophages. Acta Path Microbiol Scand Sect C 85:246–252

Bertrand J, Renoux G, Renoux M (1974) Lettre: Maladie de Crohn et levamisole. Nouv Presse Med 3:2265

Berry LJ (1977) Bacterial toxins. CRC Critical Rev Toxicol 5:239–318

Bierman SM (1976) BCG immunoprophylaxis of recurrent herpes genitalis. Arch Dermatol 112:1410–1415

Billiau A, Schonne E, Eyskmans L, De Somer P (1970) Interferon induction and resistance to virus infection in mice infected with *Brucella abortus*. Infect Immun 2:698–704

Blanden RV (1968) Modification of macrophage function.J Ret Endo Soc 5:179–202

Blanden RV (1969) Increased antibacterial resistance and immunodepression during graft-versus-host reactions in mice. Transplant 7:484–497

Blanden RV (1974) T cell response to viral and bacterial infection.Transplant Rev 19:56–88

Blanden RV, Gardner ID (1976) The cell-mediated immune response to ectromelia virus infection. Cell Immunol 22:271–279

Bliznakov EV, Adler AD (1972) Nonlinear response of the reticuloendothelial system upon stimulation. Path Microbiol 38:393–410

Borecky L, Lackovic V (1967) The cellular background of interferon production in vivo. Comparison of interferon induction by Newcastle disease virus and *B.pertussis*. Acta Virol 11:150–156

Breinig MC, Wright LL, McGeorge MB, Morahan PS (1978) Resistance to vaginal or system infection with herpes simplex virus type 2. Arch Virol 57:25–34

Brunell PA, Ross A, Miller LH, Kuo B (1969) Prevention of varicella by zoster immune globulin. N Engl J Med 280:1191–1194

Budzko DB, Casals J, Waksman BH (1978) Enhanced resistance against Junin virus infection induced by *Corynebacterium parvum*. Infect Immun 19:893–897

Burger DR, Wampler PA, Vanderbark AA, Regan DH (1979)A structural model for human transfer factor. Ann N Y Acad Sci 332:236–240

Butler RC, Friedman H (1979) Leukemia virus induced immunosuppression: Reversal by subcellular factors. Ann N Y Acad Sci 332:446–450

Cameron E, Pauling L, Leibovitz B (1979) Ascorbic acid and cancer: A review. Cancer Res 39:663–681

Cerutti I (1974) Proprietes antivirales du *C.parvum*. Compte rendu hebd Seanc Acad Sci Paris D279:963–966

Chang S-S, Hildemann WH (1964) Inheritance of susceptibility to polyoma virus in mice. J Natl Cancer Inst 33:303–313

Chany C, Cerutti I (1977) Effect stimulant de l'isoprinosine sur l'action antivirale de l'interferon. Compte Rend hebd Seanc Acad Sci Paris D 284:499–501

Chedid L, Audibert F, Johnson AG (1978) Biological activities of muramyl dipeptide, a synthetic glycopeptide analagous to bacterial ummunoregulating agents. Prog in Allergy 25:63–105

Chedid L, Parant M, Parant F, Audibert F, Lefrancier P, Choay J, Sela M (1979) Enhancement of certain biological activities of muramyl dipeptide derivatives after conjugation to a multi-poly (DL-alanine)--poly(L-lysine) carrier. Proc Natl Acad Sci USA 76:6557–6561

Chedid L, Parant M, Parant F, Lefrancier P (1977) Enhancement of non-specific immunity to *Klebsiella pneumoniae* infection by a synthetic immunoadjuvant (N-acetyl-muramyl-L-alanyl-D-isoglutamine) and several analogues. Proc Natl Acad Sci USA 74:2089–2093

Chesebro B, Wehrly K, Stimfling J (1974)Host genetic control of recovery from Friend leukemia virus-induced splenomegaly. J Exp Med 140:1457–1467

Ching C, Lopez C (1979) Natural killing of herpes simplex virus type 1-infected target cells: Normal human responses and influence of antiviral antibody. Infect Immun 26:49–56

Cluff LE (1970) Effects of endotoxins on susceptibility to infections. J Inf Dis 122:205–215

Cohn ZA, Benson B (1965) The differentiation of mononuclear phagocytes. Morphology, cytochemistry, and biochemistry. J Exp Med 121:153–169

Corey L, Reeves WC, Vontver LA, Alexander ER, Holmes KK (1976) Trial of BCG vaccine for the prevention of recurrent genital herpes. Abstract No 403, 16th ICAAC, Chicago

Cypress RK, BubinieckiAS, Hammon W McD (1973) Immunosuppression and increased susceptibility to Japanese B encephalitis virus in *Trichinella spiralis* infected mice. Proc Soc Exp Biol Med 143:469–473

DeClercq E (1974) Synthetic interferon inducers.Top Curr Chem 52:173–208

Djeu JY, Heinbaugh JA, Holden HT, Herberman RT (1979) Augmentation of mouse natural killer cell activity by interferon and interferon inducers. J Immunol 122:175–181

Doherty PC, Zinkernagel RM, Ramshaw IA (1974) Specificity and development of cytotoxic thymus-derived lymphocytes in lymphocytic choriomeningitis. J Immunol 112:1548–1559

du Buy H (1975) Effect of silica on virus infections in mice and mouse tissue culture. Infect Immun 11:996–1002

Dziarski R (1982) Effects of Staphylococcal cell wall products on immunity. In: Friedman H, Szentivanyi A (eds) Immunomodulation by bacteria and their products. Plenum Press, New York

Ellouz F, Ada A, Ciorbaru R, Lederer E (1974) Minimal structure requirements for adjuvant activity of peptidoglycan derivatives. Biochem Biophys Res Commun 59:1317–1325

England JF, Tait B (1977) HLA and herpes simplex. Med J Austral 2:464

Evans R, Alexander P (1972) Role of macrophages in tumor immunity. I. Co-operation between macrophages and lymphoid cells in syngeneic tumor immunity. Immunol 23:615–626

Feingold DS, Keleti C, Youngner JS (1976) Antiviral activity of *Brucella abortus* preparations: Separation of active components. Infect Immun 13:763–767

Feldman S, Hayes FA, Chaudhary S, Ossi M (1978) Inosiplex for localized herpes zoster in childhood cancer patients: Preliminary controlled study. Antimicrob Agents Chemother 14:495–497

Finger H, Emmerling P, Schmidt J (1967) Accelerated and prolonged multiplication of antibody-forming cells by *Bordetella pertussis* in mice immunized with sheep red blood cells. Experientia 23:591–592

Fink MA (1976) Editor – Immune RNA in Neoplasia. Academic Press, New York, p 1–316

Fischer GW, Balk MW, Crumrine MH, Bass JW (1976) Immunopotentiation and anti-viral chemotherapy in suckling rat model of herpesvirus encephalitis. J Infect Dis 133(A):217–220

Fischer GW, Podgore JK, Bass JW, Kelley JL, Kobayashi GY (1975) Enhanced host defense mechanisms with levamisole in suckling rats. J Infect Dis 132:578–581

Floc'h R, Werner GH (1976) Increased resistance to virus infections of mice inoculated with BCG (Bacillus Calmette-Guerin). Ann Immunol (Inst Pasteur) 127C:173–186

Floersheim GL (1965) Effect of pertussis vaccine on the tuberculin reaction. Int Archs Allergy Appl Immunol 26:340–344

Frank S, Specter S, Nowotny A, Friedman H (1977) Immunocyte stimulation in vitro by nontoxic bacterial lipopolysaccharide derivatives. J Immunol 119:855–860

Frankel JW, Horton EJ, Winters AL, Samis HWV, Ito Y (1980) Inhibition of viral tumorigenesis by a retinoic acid analogue. In: Nelson JD, Grassi C (eds) Current chemotherapy and infections disease. Am Soc Microbiol, Washington DC

Friedman H (1973) Editor – RNA in the immune response. Ann N Y Acad Sci 207:1–492

Friedman H (1979) Editor – RNA Subcellular factors in immunity. Ann N Y Acad Sci 332–625

Friedman SB, Grota LJ, Glasgow LA (1972) Differential susceptibility of male and female mice to encephalomyocarditis virus: Effects of castration, adrenalectomy, and the administration of sex hormones. Infect Immun 5:637–644

Galanos C, Freudenberg M, Hase S, Jay F, Ruschmann E, (1977) Biological activities and immunological properties of lipid A. In: Schlessinger D (ed) Microbiology 1977, American Society for Microbiology, Washington DC, p 269

Gershon AA, Steinberg S, Brunell PA (1974) Zoster immune globulin. A further assessment. N Engl J Med 290:243–245

Gidlund M, Orn A, Wigzell H, Senik A, Gresser I (1978) Enhanced NK cell activity in mice injected with interferon and interferon inducers. Nature 273:759–761

Ginsberg T, Glasky AJ (1977) Inosiplex: an immunomodulation model for the treatment of viral disease. Ann N Y Acad Sci 284:128–138

Glasgow LA, Galasso GJ (1972) Isoprinosine: lack of anti-viral activity in experimental model infections. J Infect Dis 126:162–169

Glasgow LA, Fischbach J, Bryant SM, Kern ER (1977) Immunomodulation of host resistance to experimental viral infections in mice. Effects of *Corynebacterium acnes, Corynebacterium parvum*, and Bacille Calmette-Guerin. J Inf Dis 135:763–770

Glasky AJ, Kestelyn J, Romero M (1978) Isoprinosine: a clinical overview of an antiviral/ immunomodulating agent. 7th Int Cong Pharmac, Paris, Abstract 2267

Gledhill AW (1959) The effect of bacterial endotoxin on resistance of mice to ectromelia. Brit J Exp Pathol 40:195–202

Goldstein G (1975) The isolation of thymopoietin. Ann N Y Acad Sci 249:177–185

Goodman GT, Koprowski H (1962a) Macrophages as a cellular expression of inherited natural resistance. Proc Natl Acad Sci USA 48:160–165

Goodman GT, Koprowski H (1962b) Study of the mechanism of innate resistance to virus infection. J Cell Comp Physiol 59:333–337

Gorke DS (1967) Inhibition of multiplication of foot and mouth disease virus in adult mice pretreated with Freund's complete adjuvant. Nature 216:1242–1244

Gorke DS, Asso J, Poraf A (1968) Effet du traitment prealable par les adjuvants de l'immunite sur la multiplication du virus de la fievre aphteuse chez le souris adulte. Ann Inst Pasteur 115:446–464

Grady GF, Lee VA (1975) Prevention of hepatitis from accidental exposure among medical workers. N Eng J Med 293:10–13

Hadden JW (1978) The action of immunopotentiators in vitro on lymphocyte and macrophage activation. In: Werner GH, Ploch F (eds) The pharmacology of immunoregulation. Academic Press, New York, p 369

Hadden JW, Hadden EM, Coffey EG (1976) Isoprinosine augmentation of phytohemagglutinin-induced lymphocyte proliferation. Infect Immun 13:382–388

Hadden JW, Lopez C, O'Reilly RJ, Hadden EM (1977) Levamisole and inosiplex antiviral agents with immunopotentiating action. Ann N Y Acad Sci 284:139–152

Haller O, Arnheiter H, Lindenmann J (1976) Genetically determined resistance to infection by hepatotropic influenza. A virus in mice: effect of immunosuppression. Infect Immun 13:844–854

Hamada S, Uetake H (1975) Mechanism of induction of cell-mediated immunity to virus infection: In vitro inhibition of intracellular multiplication of mouse adenovirus by immune spleen cells. Infect Immun 11:937–943

Hattwick MAW, Rubin RH, Music L, Sikes RK, Smith JS, Gregg MB (1974) Postexposure rabies prophylaxis with human rabies immune globulin. J Am Med Assoc 227:407–410

Helin, Bergh M (1974) Levamisole for warts. New Engl J Med 291:1311

Henson D, Smith RD, Gehrke (1966) Non-fatal mouse cytomegalovirus hepatitis. Combined morphologic, virology, and immunologic observations. Am J Pathol 49:871–888

Herberman RB, Holden HT (1979) Natural cell mediated immunity. Adv Cancer Res 27:305–377

Heymer B, Rietschel ET (1977) Biological properties of peptidoglycans. In: Schlessinger D (ed) Microbiology. American Society for Microbiology, Washington, p 344

Hibbs JB Jr, Lambert LH Jr, Remington JS (1971) Resistance to murine tumors conferred by chronic infection with intracellular protozoa, *Toxoplasma gondii* and *Besnoitia jellisoni*. J Infect Dis 124:587–592

Hibbs JB, Lambert LH, Remington JS (1972) Possible role of macrophage mediated nonspecific cytotoxicity in tumor resistance. Nature NB 235:48–50

Hirt HM, Becker H, Kirchner H (1978) Induction of interferon production in mouse spleen cell cultures by *Corynebacterium parvum*. Cell Immunol 38:168–175

Ho M-K, Kong AS, Morse SI (1980) The in vitro effects of *Bordetella pertussis* lymphocytosis-promoting factor on murine lymphocytes. V. Modulation of T cell proliferation by helper and suppressor lymphocytes. J Immunol 124:362–369

Huang KY, Donahoe RM, Gordon FB, Dressler HR (1971) Enhancement of phagocytosis by interferon-containing preparations. Infect Immun 4:581–588

Isaacs A, Lindemann J (1957) Virus interference-I. Interferon. Proc R Soc B147:258–267

Johnson AG, Audibert F, Chedid L (1978) Synthetic immunoregulating molecules: a potential bridge between cytostatic chemotherapy and immunotherapy of cancer. Cancer Immunol Immunother 3:219–227

Johnson RT (1964) The pathogenesis of herpes virus encephalitis. II. A cellular basis for the development of resistance with age. J Exp Med 120:359–374

Jungeblut CW (1935) Inactivation of poliomyelitis virus in vitro by crystalline vitamin C (ascorbic acid). J Exp Med 62:517–521

Jungeblut CW (1939) A further contribution to vitamin C therapy in experimental poliomyelitis. J Exp Med 70:315–322

Karnovsky ML, Lazdins J, Drath D, Harper A (1975) Biochemical characteristics of activated macrophages. J Exp Med 117:781–797

Kempe CH (1960) Studies on smallpox and complications of smallpox vaccination. Pediatrics 26:176–189

Kenyon AJ (1978) Treatment of Aleutian mink disease with levamisole. In: Siegenthaler W, Luthy R (eds) Current Chemotherapy, vol 1, Am Soc Microbiol, Washington DC p 357

Kern DH, Pilch YH (1979) Immune RNA in tumor immunology. Ann N Y Acad Sci 332:196–206

Kern ER, Glasgow LA, Overall JC (1976) Antiviral activity of an extract of *Brucella abortus:* Induction of interferon and immunopotentiation of host resistance. Proc Soc Exp Biol Med 152:372–376

Kierszenbaum F, Ferraresi RW (1979) Enhancement of host resistance against *Trypanosoma cruzi* infection by the immunoregulatory agent muramyl dipeptide. Infect Immun 25:273–278

Kilbourne ED, Horsfall FL (1961) Studies of herpes simplex virus in newborn mice. J Immunol 67:321–329

Kint A, Verlinden L (1974) Levamisole for recurrent herpes labialis. New Eng J Med 291:308

Kint A, Coucke C, Verlinden L (1974) The treatment of recurrent herpes infection with levamisole. Arch Belg Derm Syph 30:167–171

Kirchner H, Glaser M, Herberman RB (1975) Suppression of cell-mediated tumor immunity by *Corynebacterium parvum*. Nature 257:396–398

Kirchner H, Scott MT, Hirt HM, Munk K (1978) Protection of mice against viral infection by *Corynebacterium parvum* and *Bordetella pertussis*. J Gen Virol 41:97–104

Klein JJ, Goldstein AL, White A (1965) Enhancement of in vivo incorporation of labeled precursors into DNA and total protein of mouse lymph nodes after administration of thymic extracts. Proc Natl Acad Sci USA 53:812–817

Koff RS (1978) Viral hepatitis. John Wiley and Sons, New York

Kotani S, Konoshita F, Morisaki I, Shimono T, Okunaga T, Takada H, Tsujimoto M, Watanabe Y, Kato K, Shiba T, Kusumoto S, Okada S (1977) Immunoadjuvant activities of synthetic 6-*O*-acyl-*N*-acetylmuramyl-L-alanyl-D-isoglutamine with special reference to the effects of its administration with lysosomes. Biken J 20:95–103

Kotani S, Watanabe Y, Shimono T, Narita T, Kato K, Stewart-Tull DES, Kinoshita F, Yokogawa K, Kawata S, Shiba T, Kusumoto S, Tarumi Y (1975) Immunoadjuvant activities of cell walls, their water-soluble fractions and peptidoglycan subunits, prepared from various gram-positive bacteria, and of synthetic *N*-acetylmuramyl peptides. Z Immun-Forsch 149:302–319

Krueger RF, Mayer GD (1970) Tilorone hydrochloride: An orally active antiviral agent. Science 169:1213–1214

Krugman S (1963) The clinical use of gamma globulin. N Eng J Med 269:195–201

Kumar V, Luevano E, Bennett M (1979) Hybrid resistance to EL-4 lymphoma cells. I. Characterization of natural killer cells that lyse EL-4 cells and their distinction from bone marrow dependent natural killer cells. J Exp Med 150:531–547

Larson CL, Ushijima RN, Baker RE, Baker MB, Gillespie CA (1972) Effect of normal serum and antithymocyte serum on Friend disease in mice. J Natl Cancer Inst 48:1403–1407

Larson CL, Ushijima RN, Plorey MJ, Baker RE, Baker MB (1971) Effect of BCG on Friend Disease virus. Nature NB 229:243–244

Lawrence HS (1955) The transfer in humans of delayed skin sensitivity to Streptococcal M substance and to tuberculin with disrupted leukocytes. J Clin Invest 34:219–230

Lemonde P (1973) Protective effects of BCG and other bacteria against neoplasia in mice and hamsters. Natl Cancer Inst Monogr 39:21–29

Lennette EH, Koprowski H (1944) Influence of age on the susceptibility of mice to infection with certain neurotropic viruses. J Immunol 49:175–191

Lilly F, Pincus R (1973) Genetic control of murine leukemogenesis. Adv Cancer Res 17:231–277

Lindahl P, Gresser I, Leary P, Tovey M (1976) Interferon treatment of mice: Enhanced expression of histocompatibility antigens on lymphoid cells. Proc Natl Acad Sci USA 73:1284–1287

Lindahl P, Leary P, Gresser I (1972) Enhancement by interferon of the specific cytotoxicity of sensitized lymphocytes. Proc Natl Acad Sci USA 69:721–725

Lindenmann J, Deuel E, Franconi S, Haller O (1978) Inborn resistance of mice to myxoviruses: macrophages express phenotype in vitro. J Exp Med 147:531–540

Lods F (1976) Traitement de l'herpes corneen recidivant et des zonas ophtalmiques par le levamisole. Nouv Presse Med 5:148

Longley S, Dunning RL, Waldman RH (1973) Effect of isoprinosine against challenge with A (H3N2)/Hong Kong influenza virus in volunteers. Antimicrob Agents Chemotherap 3:506–509

Lopez C (1975) Genetics of natural resistance to herpesvirus infections in mice. Nature 258:152–153

Lopez C, Bennett (1978) Genetic resistance to HSV-1 in the mouse is mediated by a marrow (M)-dependent cell. Fourth Intl Congress Virol, p 82

Lopez C, Dudas G (1979) Replication of herpes simplex virus type 1 in macrophages from resistant and susceptible mice. Inf Immun 23:432–437

Low TLK, Thurman GB, Chincarini C, McClure JE, Marshall GD, Hu S-K, Goldstein AL (1979) Current status of thymosin research: Evidence for the existence of a family of thymic factors that control T-cell maturation. Ann N Y Acad Sci 332:23–32

McCord RS, Breinig MK, Morahan PS (199976) Antiviral effects of pyran against systemic infection of mice with herpes simplex virus type 2. Antimicrobial Agents Chemotherap 10:28–33

Macfarlan RI, Cereding R, White DO (1979) Comparison of natural killer cells induced by Kunjin virus and *Corynebacterium parvum* with those occurring naturally in nude mice. Infect Immun 26:832–836

Magrath IT, Ziegler JL (1976) Failure of BCG administration to alter the clinical course of Burkitt's lymphoma. Brit Med J 1:615–618

Mannini A, Medearis DN (1961) Mouse salivary gland virus infections. Am J Hyg 73:329–343

Manzella JP, Roberts NJ Jr (1979) Human macrophage and lymphocyte responses to mitogen stimulation after exposure to influenza virus, ascorbic acid, and hyperthermia. J Immunol 123:1940–1944

Mastrangelo MJ, Berd D, Bellet RE (1976) Critical review of previously reported clinical trials of cancer immunotherapy with non-specific immunostimulants. Ann N Y Acad Sci 277:94–123

Mazaheri MR, Hamblin AS, Zuckerman AJ (1977) Immunotherapy of viral infections with transfer factor. J Med Virol 1:209–217

Migliore-Samour D, Korontzes M, Jolles P, Maral P, Floc'h F, Werner GH (1974) Hydrosoluble immunopotentiating substances extracted from *Corynebacterium parvum*. Immunol Commun 3:593–603

Mims C (1964) Aspects of the pathogenesis of viral diseases. Bact Rev 28:30–71

Mogensen SC (1976) Biological conditions influencing the focal necrotic hepatitis test for differentiation between herpes simplex virus types 1 and 2. Acta Pathol Microbiol Scand Sect B 84:154–158

Mogensen SC (1977) Genetics of macrophage controlled resistance to hepatitis induced by herpes simplex virus type 2 in mice. Infect Immun 17:268–273

Mogensen SC (1978) Macrophages and age dependent resistance to hepatitis induced by herpes simplex type 2 virus in mice. Infect Immun 19:46–50

Mogensen SC (1979) Role of macrophages in natural resistance to virus infections. Microbiol Rev 43:1–26

Mogensen SC, Andersen HK (1977) Effect of silica on the pathogenic distinction between herpes simplex virus type 1 and 2 hepatitis in mice. Infect Immun 17:274–277

Mogensen SC, Andersen HK (1978) Role of activated macrophages in resistance of congenitally athymic nude mice to hepatitis induced by herpes simplex virus type 2. Infect Immun 19:792–798

Mogensen SC, Teisner B, Andersen HK (1974) Focal necrotic hepatitis in mice as a biological marker for differentiation of Herpesvirus hominis type 1 and 2. J Gen Virol 25:151–155

Moller-Larsen A, Haahr S (1978) Humoral and cell-mediated immune responses before and after revaccination with vaccinia virus. Infect Immun 19:34–39

Morahan PS, Kaplan AM (1977) Macrophage mediated tumor resistance. In: Chirigos MA (ed) Control of neoplasia by modulation of the immune system. Raven Press, New York, p 449

Morahan PS, McCord RS (1975) Resistance to herpes simplex type 2 virus induced by an immunopotentiator (Pyran) in immunosuppressed mice. J Immunol 115:311–313

Morahan PS, Kern ER, Glasgow LA (1977) Immunomodulator induced resistance against herpes simplex virus. Proc Soc Exp Biol Med 154:615–620

Morbidity and Mortality Weekly Report (1979) Varicella-Zoster Immune Globulin. 28:589

Morrison DC, Ulevitch RJ (1978) The effects of bacterial endotoxins on host mediation systems. Am J Pathol 93:527–617

Morse SI (1965) Studies on the lymphocytosis induced in mice by Bordetella pertussis. J Exp Med 121:49–68

Muldoon RL, Mezny L, Jackson GG (1972) Effects of isoprinosine against influenza and some other viruses causing respiratory diseases. Antimicrob Agents Chemotherap 2:224–228

Murgo AJ, Athanassiades TJ (1975) Studies on the adjuvant effect of Bordetella pertussis vaccine to sheep erythrocytes in the mouse. I. In vitro enhancement of antibody formation with normal spleen cells. J Immunol 115:928–931

Muyembe JJ, Billiau A, DeSomer P (1972) Mechanism of resistance to virus challenge in mice infected with Brucella abortus. Arch Ges Virusforsch 38:290–296

Nahmias AJ, Visintine AM, Reimer CB, DelBuono I, Shore SL, Starr SE (1975) Herpes simplex virus infection of the fetus and newborn. Prog Clin Biol Res 3:63–67

Nowotny A, Behling VH, Chang HL (1975) Relation of structure to function in bacterial endotoxins. VIII. Biological activities in a polysaccharide-rich fraction. J Immunol 115:199–203

Ojo E, Haller O, Kimura A, Wigzell H (1978) An analysis of conditions allowing *Corynebacterium parvum* to cause either augmentation or inhibition of natural killer cell activity against tumor cells in mice. Int J Cancer 21:444–452

Old LJ, Benacerraf B, Stockert E (1963) Increased resistance to Mengo virus following infection with bacillus Calmette-Guerin. In: Halpern BN (ed) Role du systeme reticuloendothelial dans l'immunite antibacterienne et anti-tumorale. CNRS Symp No 155, Paris, p 319

Oldstone MBA, Dixon FJ, Mitchell GF, McDevitt HO (1973) Histocompatibility-linked genetic control of disease susceptibility. J Exp Med 137:1201–1212

Oleske JM, Starr S, Kohl S, Shaban S, Nahmias A (1978) Clinical evaluation of transfer factor in patients with recurrent herpes simplex virus infections. In: Siegenthaler W, Luthy R (eds) Curr Chemotherapy Volume 1 Am Soc Microbiol, Washington, p 359

O'Reilly RJ, Chibbaro A, Wilmont R, Lopez C (1977) Correlation of clinical and virus specific immune responses following levamisole therapy of recurrent herpes progentalis. Ann N Y Acad Sci 284:161–170

Ortaldo JR, MacDermott RP, Bonnard GD, Kind PD, Herberman RB (1979) Cytotoxicity from cultured cells: Analysis of precursors involved in generation of human cells mediating natural and antibody-dependent cell-mediated cytotoxicity. Cell Immunol 48:356–368

Pachuta PM, Togo Y, Hornick RB, Schwartz AR, Tominaga S (1974) Evaluation of isoprinosine in experimental human rhinovirus infection. Antimicrob Agents Chemotherap 5:403–408

Papaevangelou G, Sparros L, Vissoulis C, Kyraukidoc A, Giokas G, Hadzimanolis J, Trichopoulos D (1977) The effect of intradermal administration of *Corynebacterium parvum* on the immune response to hepatitisB$_s$ antigen. J Med Virol 1:15–19

Par A, Barna K, Hollos I, Kovacs M, Miszlai Z, Patakfalvi A, Javor T (1977) Levamisole in viral hepatitis. Lancet 1:702

Perrin LH, Zinkernagel RM, Oldstone MBA (1977) Immune response in humans after vaccination with vaccinia virus. J Exp Med 146:949–968

Pierschbacher MD, Luckey TD, Kalden JR (1979) Biological activity of a pure thymus protein LSHr. Ann N Y Acad Sci 332:49–54

Rager-Zisman B, Allison AC (1973) The role of antibody and host cells in the resistance of mice against infection by Coxsackie B-3 virus. J Gen Virol 19:329–338

Rawls WE, Tompkins AF (1975) Desturction of virus-infected cells by antibody and complement. In: Notkins AL (ed) Viral immunology and immunopathology. Academic Press, New York, p 99

Reed D, Brown G, Merrick R, Sever J, Feltz E (1967) A mumps epidemic on St. George Island, Alaska. J Am Med Assoc 199:967–971

Regelson W (1975) Clinical immunoadjuvant studies with tilorone, DEAA fluorene (RML11, 002DA) and *Corynebacterium parvum* and some observations on the role of host resistance and herpes-like lesions in tumor growth. Ann N Y Acad Sci 277:269–287

Regelson W, Schneider BI, Colsky J, Olsen KB, Holland JF, Johnston CL Jr Dennis LH (1978) Clinical study of the synthetic polyanion pyran copolymen (NSC 46015, Dweems and its role in future clinical trials. In: Chirigos MA (ed) Immune modulation and control of neoplasia by adjuvant therapy. Raven Press, New York, p 469

Reid HW, Buxton D, Finlayson J, Holmes PH (1979) Effect of chronic *Trypanosoma brucei* infection on the course of louping-ill virus infection in mice. Infect Immun 23:192–196

Reikvam A, Gammeldvedt R, Hoiky EA (1975) Activated mouse macrophages: morphology. Lysosomal biochemistry, and microbicidal properties of in vivo and in vitro activated cells. Acta Pathol Microbiol Scand Sect C 83:129–138

Remington JS, Merigan TC (1969) Resistance to virus challenge in mice infected with protozoa or bacteria. Proc Soc Exp Biol Med 131:1184–1188

Renoux G (1978) Modulation of immunity by levamisole. J Pharm Ther 2:397–423

Renoux G, Renoux M (1971) Effect immunostimulant d'un imidazothiazole dans l'infection par Brucella abortus. Compte Rend Hebd Seanc Acad Sci Paris D272:349–350

Renoux G, Renoux M (1972) Levamisole inhibits and cures a solid malignant tumor and its pulmonary metastases in mice. Nature New Biol 240:217–218

Roder JC (1979) The beige mutation in the mouse. I. A stem cell predetermined impairment in natural killer cell function. J Immunol 123:2168–2173

Rojas A, Olivari AJ (1974) Levamisole: Effect in foot and mouth disease. Preliminary note. Rev Med Vet Argentina 55:263–265

Rolly H, Vertesy L, Neufarth A (1974) Studies on the chemotherapeutic actions of antiviral lipopolysaccharides. In: Daikos GK (ed) Progress in chemotherapy, vol 2. Hellenic Society of Chemotherapy, Athens, p 1013

Russell AS, Schlaut J (1977) Association of HLA-A1 antigen and susceptibility to recurrent cold scores. Arch Dermatol 113:1721–1722

Russell AS, Brisson E, Grace M (1978) A double blind controlled trial of levamisole in treatment of recurrent herpes labialis. J Infect Dis 137:597–600

Sabin AB (1952) Nature of inherited resistance to viruses affecting the nervous system. Proc Natl Acad Sci USA 38:540–546

Sadowski JM, Rapp F (1975) Inhibition by levamisole of metastases by cells transformed by herpes simplex type 1. Proc Soc Exp Biol Med 149:219–222

Schauf V, Falk L, Denhardt F (1975) Effect of bacillus Calmette-Guerin immunization in marmosets infected experimentally with herpesvirus saimiri. J Natl Cancer Inst 54:721–726

Schell K (1960) Studies on the innate resistance of mice to infection with mousepox. I. Resistance and antibody production. Aust J Exp Biol Med Sci 38:271–288

Schulman ST, Hutto JH, Scott B, Ayoub EM, McGuigan JE (1976) Transfer factor therapy of chronic active hepatitis. In: Ascher MS, Gottlieb AA, Kirkpatrick CH (eds). Academic Press, New York, p 439

Schwartz DB, Zbar B, Gibson WT, Chirigos MA (1971) Inhibition of murine sarcoma virus oncogenesis with living BCG. Int J Cancer 8:320–325

Schwerdt PR, Schwerdt CE (1975) Effect of ascorbic acid on rhinovirus replication in WI-38 cells. Proc Soc Exp Biol Med 148:1237–1243

Scott MT (1972) Biological effects of the adjuvant *Corynebacterium parvum*. I. Inhibition of PHA, mixed lymphocyte and GVH reactivity. Cell Immunol 5:459–468

Selgrade MK, Osborn JE (1974) Role of macrophages in resistance to murine cytomegalovirus. Infect Immun 10:1383–1390

Siegel BV, Morton JI (1977a) Vitamin C and the immune response. Experentia 33:393–395

Siegel BV, Morton JI (1977b) Vitamin C, interferon, and the immune response. Int J Vit Nutrit Res Suppl 16:245–265

Simon LN, Settineri R, Coats H, Glasky AJ (1978) Isoprinosine: integration of the anti-viral and immunoproliferative effects. In: Siegenthaler W, Luthy R (eds) Current chemotherapy, vol 1. Am Soc Microbiol, Washington DC, p 366

Soto AJ, Hall TS, Reed SE (1973) Trial of the antiviral action of isoprinosine against rhinovirus injection in volunteers. Antimicrob Agents Chemotherap 3:332–334

Specter S, Friedman H (1978) Viruses and the immune response. Pharmac Ther 2:595–622

Spencer JC, Ganguly R, Waldman RH (1977) Non-specific protection of mice against influenza infection by local or systemic immunization with bacille Calmette-Guerin. J Infect Dis 136:171–175

Spitler LE, Glogau RG, Nelms DC, Basch CM, Olson JA, Silverman S, Engleman EP (1975) Levamisole and lymphocyte response in herpes simplex virus infections. In: Symposium on antivirals with clinical potential. Stanford, California

Sporn MB (1978) Retinoid chemoprevention trial begins against bladder cancer. J Am Med Assoc 240:609–614

Starr SE, Visintine AM, Tomeh MO, Nahmias AJ (1976) Effects of immunostimulants on resistance of newborn mice to herpes simplex type 2 infection. Proc Soc Exp Biol Med 152:57–60

Steele RW (1980) Transfer factor and cellular reactivity to Varicella-Zoster antigen in childhood leukemia. Cell Immunol 50:282–289

Steele RW, Heberling RL, Eichberg JW, Eller JJ, Kalter SS, Kniker WT (1976) Prevention of herpes simplex virus type 1 fatal dissemination in primates with human transfer factor. In: Transfer factor, basis properties and clinical applications. Academic Press, New York, p 381

Stevens J, Cook M (1971) Restriction of herpes simplex virus by macrophages. J Exp Med 133:19–38

Stiffel C, Mouton D, Biozzi G (1970) Kinetics of the phagocytic function of reticuloendothelial macrophages in vivo. In: VanFurth R (ed) Mononuclear phagocytes. FA Davis Co., Philadelphia, p 335

Stineburg WR, Youngner JS (1964) Patterns of interferon appearance in mice injected with bacteria or bacterial endotoxin. Nature 204:712–713

Symoens J (1978) Treatment of the compromised hose with levamisole, a synthetic immunotherapeutic agent. In: Chirigos MA (ed) Immune modulation and control of neoplasia by adjuvant therapy. Raven Press, New York, p 1

Tagliabue A, Montavani A, Kilgallen M, Herbermann RB, McCoy JL (1979) Natural cytotoxicity of mouse monocytes and macrophages. J Immunol 122:2363–2369

Todaro GJ, DeLarco JE, Sporn MB (1978) Retinoids block phenotypic cell transformation produced by sarcoma growth factor. Nature 276:272–274

Trainin N, Rotter Y, Yakir V, Leve R, Handzel Z, Shohat B, Zaizov R (1979) Biochemical and biological properties of THF in animal and human models. Ann N Y Acad Sci 332:9–22

Turner GS, Ballard R (1976) Interaction of mouse peritoneal macrophages with fixed rabies virus in vivo and in vitro. J Gen Virol 30:223–231

Van Eygen M, Znamensky PY, Heck E, Raymaekers I (1976) Levamisole in prevention of recurrent upper respiratory tract infections in children. Lancet 1:382–385

Waldman RH, Canguly R (1977) Therapeutic efficacy of inosiplex (Isoprinosine) in rhinovirus infection. Ann N Y Acad Sci 284:153–160

Waldman RH, Khakoo RA, Watson G (1978) Isoprinosine: efficacy against influenza challenge infections in humans. In: Siegenthaler W, Luthy R (eds) Current chemotherapy, vol 1. Am Soc Microbiol, Washington DC, p 368

Webster RG, Glezen WP, Hannoun G, Laver WG (1977) Potentiation of the immune response to influenza subunit vaccines. J Immunol 119:2073–2077

Weiss DW, Yashphe DJ (1973) Nonspecific stimulation of antimicrobial and anti-tumor resistance and of immunological responsiveness by the MER fraction of tubercle bacilli. In: Zuckerman A, Weiss DW (eds) Dynamic aspects of host parasite relationships, vol 1. Academic Press, New York, p 163–223

Werner GH (1979) Immunopotentiating substances with antiviral activity. Pharmac Ther 6:235–273

White DO (1977) Antiviral immunity. In: Mandel TE (ed) Progress in immunology III, Proc 3rd Int Congr Immunol. Australian Academy of Science, Canberra, p 459

Wirth JJ, Levy MH, Wheelock EF (1976) Use of silica to identify host mechanisms involved in suppression of established Friend virus leukemia. J Immunol 117:2124–2130

Woodruff AW (1968) Helminths as vehicles and synergists of microbial infections. Trans Roy Soc Trop Med Hyg 62:446–452

Woodruff MFA, Warner NL (1977) Effect of *Corynebacterium parvum* on tumor growth on normal and athymic (nude) mice. J Natl Cancer Inst 58:111–116

Vap KL, Ada GL, McKenzie IFC (1978) Transfer of specific cytotoxic lymphocytes protects mice inoculated with influenza virus. Nature 273:238–239

Yoon J-W, Notkins AL (1976) Virus-induced diabetes mellitus. VI. Genetically determined host differences in the replication of encephalomyocarditis virus in pancreatic beta cells. J Exp Med 143:1170–1185

Youngner JS, Keleti G, Feingold DS (1974) Antiviral activity of an ether-extracted nonviable preparation of *Brucella abortus*. Infect Immun 10:1202–1206

Zaizov R, Vogel R, Wolach B, Cohen IJ, Varsano I, Shohat B, Handzel Z, Rotter V, Yakir Y, Trainin N (1979) The effect of THF in lymphoproliferative and myeloproliferative diseases in children. Ann N Y Acad Sci 332:172–183

Zinkernagel RM, Althage A (1977) Antiviral protection by virus immune cytotoxic T cells: infected target cells are lysed before infectious virus progeny is assembled. J Exp Med 145:644–651

Zinkernagel RM, Welsh RM (1976) H-2 compatibility requirement for virus specific T-cell mediated effector functions in vivo. I. Specificity of T cells conferring antiviral protection against lymphocytic choriomeningitis virus is associated with H-2K and H-2D. J Immunol 17:1495–1503

Zisblatt M, Goldstein AL, Lilly F, White A (1970) Acceleration by thymosin of the development of resistance to murine sarcoma virus induced tumor in mice. Proc Natl Acad Sci USA 66:1170–1174

Zisman B, Hirsch MS, Allison AC (1970) Selective effects of antimacrophage serum, silica, and antilymphocyte serum on pathogenesis of herpesvirus infection of young adult mice. J Immunol 104:1155–1159

Zisman B, Wheelock EF, Allison AC (1971) Role of macrophages and antibody in resistance of mice against yellow fever virus. J Immunol 107:236–243

Part B

CHAPTER 8

Guanidine

D. R. TERSHAK, F. H. YIN, and B. D. KORANT

A. Introduction and History

The earliest studies demonstrating inhibition of viral growth by guanidine were published approximately 20 years ago (RIGHTSEL et al. 1961). Soon after the initial discovery, mutants that were either resistant to or dependent upon guanidine were described (LODDO et al. 1963; NAKANO et al. 1963). In general, growth of many members of the Picornaviridae family, which comprises a large number of lipid-free animal viruses that contain single-stranded RNA genomes, is susceptible to inhibition by guanidine (CALIGUIRI and TAMM 1973). Included among the sensitive picornaviruses are the three strains of poliovirus, coxsackieviruses, echoviruses, rhinoviruses, and foot-and-mouth disease virus (FMDV). Echoviruses 6, 7, 8, 12, and coxsackievirus B6 are resistant to the compound (CROWTHER and MELNICK 1961). Orthomyxoviruses, paramyxoviruses, reoviruses, most togaviruses, and animal viruses that contain DNA are also naturally resistant to guanidine. Replication of Sindbis and Semliki Forest viruses of the *Alphavirus* genus of the togavirus family (FRIEDMAN 1970) and two plant viruses, tobacco necrosis (VARMA 1968) and tobacco mosaic virus (TMV; DAWSON 1975) are sensitive to the inhibitor.

An extensive review of the virus inhibitory activity of guanidine was published 9 years ago (CALIGUIRI and TAMM 1973). At that time, as well as presently, most studies were performed with the picornaviruses, particularly the enterovirus subgroup. The reader is referred to this previous discourse for a detailed bibliography. The intent of the present review is to summarize relevant background information, update our present knowledge of guanidine action, and interpret recent studies in light of current information about the molecular biology of viral development. Because studies with guanidine are slanted heavily toward the picornaviruses, a brief description of the molecular biology of picornavirus development is included.

B. Synthesis and Properties of Picornavirus Proteins

Picornaviruses have been among the most thoroughly studied of all animal viruses with regard to synthesis of virus-specific proteins. There are several reasons for this. The primary reason is that these viruses are able, rapidly and almost completely, to block host cell protein synthesis following infection, permitting identification of virus-specific proteins in infected cells. Also, they are resistant to actinomycin or other inhibitors of cellular messenger RNA transcription, permitting further artificial reductions in the background of cellular protein synthesis. In addition, the picornaviruses have a limited coding potential, and can specify approximately 2,500 amino acids, or about 5–10 proteins, so that the pattern of viral protein synthesis can be deciphered more easily than with larger viral genomes. They are positive-strand viruses, and the virion RNA is infectious when introduced into cells. The purified RNA is a reasonably efficient messenger in cell-free extracts, enabling the study of viral polypeptide synthesis under controlled biochemical conditions.

It is worth noting early in this review that there is no evidence for a direct effect of guanidine on the synthesis of viral proteins. The action of guanidine as an inhibitor is better explained by its interaction with one or more viral proteins to affect a configurational change, and alter protein–protein or protein–RNA associations. Guanidine, at millimolar levels, markedly reduces viral protein production only as a consequence of blocking viral RNA synthesis.

I. "Shutoff" of Host Cell Protein Synthesis

Inhibition of cellular protein synthesis occurs within 1.5–2.5 h after infection, depending on the multiplicity of infecting virus and cell type. If high multiplicities are used, the virus will accomplish the inhibition in the presence of guanidine (BABLANIAN et al. 1965; CALIGUIRI and TAMM 1973). The mechanism of inhibition of cell protein synthesis remains controversial. It is clear that cellular polyribosomes disaggregate soon after infection, and this appears to be a consequence of an inability to reinitiate translation of cellular messages. The cellular messenger RNAs are not detectably modified, and elongation and termination steps of cellular translation are also unaffected.

The mechanism of inhibition of host protein synthesis seems to require some expression of the viral genome, including synthesis and processing of viral protein (KORANT 1979). However, synthesis of a cellular protein or proteins may also be required for shutoff to occur. A summation of various proposed events involved in shutoff is made by LUCAS-LENARD (1979). These include: (1) competition of viral RNA with cellular mRNA for limiting initiation factors; (2) inactivation of initiation factors required by host cell messages; (3) inactivation of a ribosome-associated binding protein which affixes the methylated, inverted nucleotide caps of cellular messages to 40 S ribosomal subunits (picornavirus messengers have a novel peptide cap on their termini); (4) derangement following infection of ion balance, favoring viral translation; and (5) synthesis of double-stranded RNA, a potent inhibitor of protein synthesis in vitro.

Although the inhibition of cellular protein synthesis is fairly rapid, production is still sufficient up to 2 h after infection to obscure any viral protein synthesis which may occur. Thus far, no one has devised an approach for detecting picornavirus protein synthesis directed by the infecting virus. Until this can be done, it will be impossible to describe fully the intracellular events early in infection.

II. Synthesis of Viral Proteins

A current model that explains most of the data from infected cells is that initiation of protein synthesis occurs at a single site, at the NH_2 terminal of the structural protein, which is the 5′ coding region of viral RNA. There is no convincing evi-

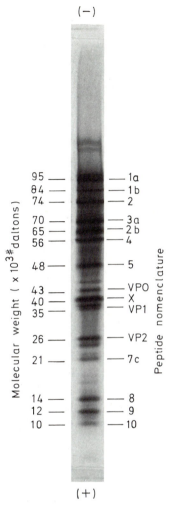

Fig. 1. Separation in a polyacrylamide gel containing sodium dodecyl sulfate (SDS) of poliovirus 2 polypeptides in the cytoplasm of infected cells (multiplicity 20 pfu/cell) were labeled with ^{14}C amino acids 3–4 h postinfection. The cells were then lysed in 1% SDS, and the proteins resolved in an 8%–18% slab of polyacrylamide gel containing 0.1% SDS. The dried gel was then placed in contact with Cronex 4 X-ray film for 1 week. (KORANT 1979)

dence for other initiation sites, although the possibility exists that such sites do occur, and are used early in infection when their products cannot be observed. There are reports from experiments with cell-free extracts that initiation may occur infrequently at secondary sites (EHRENFELD 1979).

The events that follow virus infection have been described in studies by several groups (reviewed by RUECKERT et al. 1979). The ribosomes proceed to translate the viral coat protein region. At the end of the coat protein, a cleavage signal is recognized, probably by a cellular protease, and the precursor is cleaved from the nascent protein. The ribosome continues translating the nonstructural polypeptides.

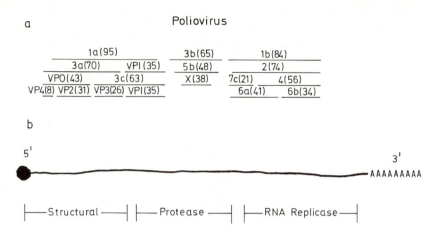

Fig. 2, a, b. Mapping of the poliovirus genome. **a** physical map, using pactamycin technique, and estimation of molecular weights of resolved polypeptides in an SDS polyacrylamide gel (adapted from Rueckert et al. 1979); **b** genetic and biochemical map

One or more additional cleavages occur, giving the primary cleavage products. Secondary cleavages of the structural precursor give rise to the coat proteins VP0, VP1, and VP3, with a reaction half-life of about 5 min. VP0 is the precursor of coat proteins VP4 and VP2. Most of the other proteolytic reactions take longer, up to 20 min or more (Butterworth and Rueckert 1972). The dynamics of the process can be readily assayed in polyacrylamide gels containing dodecyl sulfate. The polypeptides separate mainly according to size, migration of the larger species being more retarded (Fig. 1). Early experimenters were puzzled at resolving so many polypeptide species, since the combined molecular weights greatly exceeded the coding capacity. However, as it became apparent that precursor–product relationships existed for many of the components, the cleavage process became a suitable, and correct explanation.

As gel electrophoretic separations have improved, some additional picornavirus polypeptides have been identified in infected cells (Abraham and Cooper 1975). Peptide mapping studies have helped to assign these to cleavage pathways. To account for the origin of some of the minor species, the phenomenon of incomplete or alternative (ambiguous) cleavages has been proposed (Rueckert et al. 1979). Presumably, as even higher resolution techniques are applied, such as two-dimensional gels (O'Farrell 1975), additional minor species will be found to complicate the pattern further. A current cleavage map for poliovirus is given in Fig. 2.

The origin of the proteases is still under study, but several lines of evidence point to a virus-coded protease involved in the cleavage of the coat precursor to yield VP0, VP1, and VP3. A final cleavage of VP0 to VP4 and VP2 is of particular interest, since it occurs with high efficiency during maturation of the complete virus, and is blocked by guanidine (Jacobson and Baltimore 1968). Other cleavages of structural precursors are delayed by guanidine (Vande Woude and Ascione 1974). However, guanidine does not appear to block the reactions directly, but rather limits the availability of viral RNA for the maturation process (Caliguiri and Tamm 1973).

III. Mapping of the Viral Genome

Having a single initiation site on a viral message permits gene order to be determined by direct physical mapping. Using initiation inhibitors, e.g., pactamycin or hypertonic medium, means that in pulse labels with amino acids, polypeptides toward the 3′ end of the coding region will be more heavily labeled than those at the 5′ end. From comparisons of specific radioactivities for individual polypeptides before and after initiation is blocked, a physical map was obtained for several picornaviruses (TABER et al. 1971; SABORIO et al. 1974). The map positions are indicated in Fig. 2a. It was satisfying that maps so obtained could be readily fitted to earlier data for a genetic map, obtained by COOPER (1969) using recombination frequencies. The orientation of the genetic map could then be set by matching it to the physical map (see Fig. 2a). For purposes of this review, it is significant that the genetic map position for the guanidine sensitivity locus resides in the structural protein region and possibly an adjacent region, not in the RNA replicase gene.

The functions of many of the viral polypeptides present in the infected cytoplasm are not known. The capsid polypeptides have at least two functional roles; the protection of the viral genome RNA on its way from cell to cell, and the recognition of specific cell receptors present on the plasma membrane. Indirect evidence points to additional regulatory roles for the coat proteins, including shutoff of cellular metabolism (COOPER et al. 1973; STEINER-PRYOR and COOPER 1973) and participation in viral RNA synthesis (GHENDON 1972; KORANT 1977a; ADRIAN et al. 1979). Such roles have been more clearly defined for coat proteins of other RNA viruses, especially the RNA bacteriophages (SUGIYAMA et al. 1972). The finding with poliovirus deletion mutants that lack of coat proteins did not impair the mutants' ability to inhibit cellular protein synthesis or synthesize viral RNA (COLE and BALTIMORE 1973), would appear to eliminate a role for a complete complement of coat proteins in these processes, but this interpretation is in conflict with several reports already cited. Reconciliation of opposing views may not be possible until technical advances permit complete cell-free reconstructions of functional enzymatic systems from picornavirus-infected cells, so that synthesis of viral RNA strands can be initiated, completed, and assembled into virions. It would be premature at this stage to eliminate any viral protein from the process of RNA replication. Moreover, the role of cellular proteins or factors is also largely unknown (DMITRIEVA et al. 1979; DASGUPTA et al. 1980).

Assignment of functional roles to nonstructural picornaviral polypeptides is making slow but steady progress. Genetic and biochemical analyses have concurred in assigning a direct role in viral RNA synthesis to the polypeptides coded by the 3′ side of the viral genome. This includes a polypeptide of about 75,000 daltons molecular weight, and its cleavage products. A 56,000 daltons molecular weight cleavage product has been detected in numerous RNA replicase isolations, and has been implicated in elongation of viral RNA strands. Antibody which reacts with the replicase can precipitate this polypeptide (reviewed by PÉREZ-BERCOFF 1979). Recent experiments indicate template-free forms of the encephalomyocarditis (EMC) virus and poliovirus replicases are enriched in the 75,000 dalton molecular weight form (TRAUB et al. 1976; DASGUPTA et al. 1979). The most complete summary of current data is that the 75,000 dalton polypeptide is able to initiate RNA synthesis, and the cleaved form may play a role in elongation.

Other viral proteins have recently been associated with a proteolytic function, specific for the viral coat protein precursors. The assignments have been in the center of the physical map, to a 40,000 daltons molecular weight polypeptide for poliovirus (KORANT et al. 1979), and a 22,000 daltons molecular weight species for EMC (PALMENBERG et al. 1979; GORBALENYA et al. 1979).

As noted, there is no evidence for a direct effect on a viral protease of guanidine. It is not known presently how a protease generates the small RNA-linked peptides found on replicating RNA and genome RNA. Guanidine could exert an inhibitory effect on such a process, and thus affect viral RNA synthesis, but it is not possible at present to observe these reactions in infected cells. Pleiotropic effects of protease mutants have been observed to influence RNA synthesis functions (KORANT 1975, 1977a; KORANT et al. 1979; F. H. YIN, unpublished work 1979), but the mechanism is unclear.

IV. Isolation of Viral Polypeptides

It is difficult to isolate picornavirus polypeptides in purified, native states. They are not synthesized in abundance, and are often markedly contaminated with cellular proteins. An additional difficulty they offer is their tendency to be found in insoluble aggregates, bound to other viral proteins or RNA, or to lipid-containing vesicles in infected cells. They can be readily labeled and separated with denaturants, such as urea and high levels of guanidine (6 M), or with strong ionic detergents. However, such procedures tend to denature the proteins irreversibly, with respect to reconstitution of enzymatic functions.

The capsid polypeptides are particularly difficult to deal with. They are not obtainable in truly soluble form, although small, 6–14 S aggregates have been reported (KORANT 1973). The 14 S aggregates can assemble into empty capsids, but there are no detailed reports of further assembly in vitro of these capsids into mature virus particles (PHILLIPS et al. 1980). Soluble forms of the replicase family of polypeptides have been isolated in nondenaturing conditions using chromatography and zonal centrifugation; these are reported to retain some enzymatic functions (TRAUB et al. 1976; DASGUPTA et al. 1979). The majority of viral proteins are encountered in membrane-bound vesicles, where virus-specific processes seem to occur in cells. It is unclear what effects on the native protein structure isolation from such vesicles has. It is interesting that inhibitory levels of guanidine block the normal partitioning of poliovirus structural proteins to smooth membrane vesicles (YIN 1977a), disconnecting them from the sites of viral RNA synthesis (CALIGUIRI and COMPANS 1973).

C. Replication of Viral RNA

I. Viral RNA Structure

The general strategy for the replication of picornavirus RNA has been known for many years, although details of the replicative mechanism are being unfolded at a very slow rate. Very briefly, the RNA genome, upon entrance into a cell, is translated and a viral polymerase is made. Polymerase subsequently copies the incoming positive-stranded RNA via a structure called the replicative intermediate (RI) and synthesizes negative-stranded RNAs which in turn are templates for the synthesis of a series of positive-stranded RNAs. These positive-stranded RNAs can act as mRNA or be encapsidated into virions. A double-stranded RNA structure, sometimes called replicative form (RF) is found late in infection. It is probably an end product of replication and is commonly designated double-stranded RNA (dsRNA).

The 3′ end of all picornavirus genomic RNA contains a stretch of adenosine residue known as poly (A) (ARMSTRONG et al. 1972; YOGO and WIMMER 1972) which is of variable length, averaging 40–100 nucleotides. Studies with poliovirus have shown that complementary strands of RNA have poly (U) at their 5′ ends, and it appears that poly (U) encodes the poly (A) and vice versa (YOGO and WIM-MER 1973; DORSCH-HÄSLER et al. 1975). Thus the addition of poly (A) to picornavirus RNA differs from that of cellular mRNA in which the poly (A) is added by a posttranscriptional mechanism (BRAWERMAN 1974). The function of poly (A) is not clear; however, it is important for the infectivity of genomic RNA. Genomic RNA with naturally short regions of poly (A) (GOLDSTEIN et al. 1976; HRUBY and ROBERTS 1976) or artifically shortened poly (A) (SPECTOR and BALTIMORE 1974) has a lower specific infectivity than genomes with longer stretches of poly (A), although more recent studies with FMDV indicate that viral RNA with poly (A) regions of 10–12 residues has the same specific infectivity as RNA molecules with longer stretches of poly (A) (GRUBMAN et al. 1979). The nucleotide sequence of the 3′ region adjacent to poly (A), presumably involved in initiation of viral RNA replication, of ten picornaviruses has been determined recently. No sequence homology between subgroups is indicated while extensive sequence homologies are found among the viruses within a particular subgroup (PORTER et al. 1978).

The 5′ end of picornavirus RNA is unique; it is uncapped and covalently linked to a protein (reviews by WIMMER 1979; SANGAR 1979). Since eukaryotic mRNAs are all capped at the 5′ end (SHATKIN 1976), it was surprising that poliovirus mRNA terminates in pUp and does not contain a capping group (HEWLETT et al. 1976; NOMOTO et al. 1976). It was assumed for many years that poliovirus mRNA and poliovirus genomic RNA are identical because they have identical infectivities, sedimentation coefficients (35 S), and base composition (SUMMERS and LEVINTOW 1965; SUMMERS et al. 1967). Since de novo initiation of RNA synthesis usually occurs with purine rather than pyrimidine triphosphates, the questionable pUp terminus led to the further examination of the 5′ end of poliovirus genomic RNA. It was found not to terminate with a capping group, pppNp, ppNp, or even pNp (FERNANDEZ-MUNOZ and DARNELL 1976; LEE et al. 1976). Furthermore, it does not possess a free hydroxyl group (WIMMER 1972).Instead, the 5′ end of genomic RNA of poliovirus differs from poliovirus mRNA, and is covalently linked to a small protein, VPg (LEE et al. 1977; FLANEGAN et al. 1977). A comparable protein has been found on several other picornavirus RNAs including FMDV (SANGAR et al. 1977), EMC (HRUBY and ROBERTS 1978), and rhinovirus (F. GOLINI, E. WIMMER, and B. D. KORANT, unpublished work 1979), and also on cowpea mosaic virus (DAUBERT et al. 1978) and adenovirus (REKOSH et al. 1977). The protein VPg has a molecular weight of 6–12,000 daltons as estimated by SDS–acrylamide gel electrophoresis and chromatography; it is basic and hydrophobic (LEE et al. 1976,

1977; Nomoto et al. 1977 a). However, partial amino acid sequencing and mapping provides estimates of 3,296–2,732 daltons for VPg of poliovirus (Kitamura et al. 1980). VPg is linked to the 5′ terminal sequence pU-U-AAAA-CAG through a tyrosine-O^4-U linkage (Ambros and Baltimore 1978; Rothberg et al. 1978). VPg can be labeled with amino acids when host cell protein synthesis is severely depressed (Lee et al. 1977). Also, the physical properties of VPgs of different picornaviruses depend upon the infective virus rather than the host cell (Golini et al. 1978). Heterogeneity of VPg of FMDV (King et al. 1980) and poliovirus (Richards et al. 1981) has been demonstrated by nonequilibrium electrofocusing, suggesting either several distinct genetic sequences or posttranslational modifications. Whether different species of VPg perform distinct functions remains an open question. Thus, VPg is most probably encoded by the viral genome.

The functional significance of VPg is largely unknown. Genomic RNA without VPg is infectious (Nomoto et al. 1977 b; Sangar et al. 1977). Mengo virus RNA lacking VPg directs the synthesis of the same set of polypeptides in vitro as the untreated Mengo virus RNA (Pérez-Bercoff and Gander 1978). Thus, VPg does not seem to be involved in early steps of penetration and protein synthesis. On the other hand, VPg is found on RNA species that are involved in RNA synthesis; the nascent strands of the RI structure (Nomoto et al. 1977 a; Petterson et al. 1978), 5′ end of negative-stranded RNA as well as double-stranded RNA (Nomoto et al. 1977 a). A small portion of mRNA of FMDV might also contain VPg (for review see Sanger 1979). Based on these findings, it has been proposed that VPg may function as a primer for the initiation of viral RNA synthesis and be covalently bound to the first nucleotide of the nascent strand. Another possible function of VPg may be in a regulatory role (Wimmer 1979; Palmenberg et al. 1979). An enzyme which is able to cleave the tyrosine-O^4-U linkage specifically is found in infected and uninfected cells (Ambros et al. 1978). This enzyme may be involved in cleavage of VPg from genome RNA before it can function as a mRNA.

Cardioviruses and FMDVs, but not the enteroviruses or rhinoviruses, contain a region of cytosine residues (Brown et al. 1974; Harris and Brown 1976) which is located within 400–1,000 nucleotides of the 5′ end (Rowlands et al. 1978). Again the functional significance is not known. Recently, Lundquist et al. (1979) studied the viral genome of defective interfering (DI) particles of poliovirus and observed that the deleted regions begin about 6%–7% from the 5′ end and extend to 45%–52% of the viral genome, implying that a complete complement of capsid proteins plays no essential role during synthesis of viral RNA. The sharp boundary at the 5′ end of the deleted region coincides with the 3′ end of the poly (C) tract of the cardioviruses, suggesting that the first 450–525 nucleotides of the picornavirus genome play a critical role in replication. Hewlett and Florkiewicz (1980) reported that the first ten nucleotides at the 5′ end of the genomic RNA adjacent to VPg are identical for poliovirus 1 and 2 and coxsackievirus B1. The next 10 nucleotides show a difference of one base between poliovirus 1 and 2 and 50% homology between poliovirus 1 and coxsackievirus B1. This remarkable conservation of the 5′ region may signify a recognition site between viral mRNA and the cellular translation system.

The degree of conservation of nucleotide sequences at the 5′ end of nine different strains of FMDV has also been examined (Harris 1980). The first 27 nucleotides from the 5′ end of the RNA (S fragment) from the 5′ side of the poly (C) tract were highly conserved. Since this region of the viral genome does not appear to be involved in translation (SANGAR et al. 1980), the function of a highly conserved region remains unknown. Speculatively, it might serve as a signal for attachment or removal of VPg.

II. Viral Polymerase

The poliovirus RNA-dependent RNA polymerase was first isolated from infected cells as a complex with its endogeneous RNA template (BALTIMORE et al. 1963). Polymerase activity is measured as elongation of preexisting nascent chains. Viral polymerase in the complex was later identified as the 56,000 daltons molecular weight polypeptide encoded by the extreme 3′ end of the genome (LUNDQUIST et

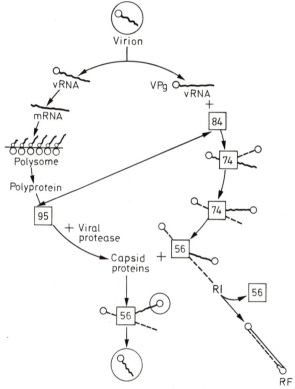

Fig. 3. Proposed replication scheme of picornavirus RNA. Incoming viral RNA is first translated into polyprotein which is cleaved into 95,000 and 84,000 dalton fragments. The 84,000 dalton fragment binds viral RNA and is cleaved by viral protease into a 74,000 dalton fragment and VPg which together are responsible for the transcription of positive-stranded as well as negative-stranded RNA. Positive-stranded RNA, with VPg cleaved off then becomes mRNA; the 74,000 dalton fragment is later cleaved into a 56,000 dalton fragment which can elongate RNA, but is incapable of reinitiating new viral strands. The viral RNA in replicative intermediate (RI) can combine with capsid protein to become a virion or become replicative form. (After PALMENBURG et al. 1979)

al. 1974). A poliovirus specific, poly(A), oligo(U)-dependent poly(U) polymerase was later purified from infected cell cytoplasm (Flanegan and Baltimore 1977) and the enzyme can also copy poliovirus RNA to make complementary, negative strands in the presence (Flanegan and van Dyke 1979) or in the absence of a primer (Dasgupta et al. 1979), depending upon the purification procedure. One or more viral polypeptides identified in the partially purified preparations are encoded by the 3' end of the genome. Similar results have been found with EMC (Traub et al. 1976; Lund and Scraba 1979), and FMDV (Newman et al. 1979; Lowe and Brown 1981). How the polymerase initiates polynucleotide chain synthesis in vitro remains obscure. It is possible that VPg, with its close association to viral RNA, might be in the primary sequence of the polymerase before proteolysis occurs (Palmenberg et al. 1979). Röder and Koschel (1974), Korant (1975, 1977 a), and Bowles and Tershak (1978) have described the regulation of the in vivo function of viral polymerase; the initiation of RNA synthesis is probably regulated by limited proteolysis. A current appraisal of the connection between viral protein synthesis and cleavage and the synthesis of viral RNA is shown in Fig. 3.

D. Chemistry of Guanidine

Guanidine is a basic compound with a pK_a of about 12.5. At physiologic pH the molecule gains a proton and exists as a positively charged ion, as shown below.

$$\underset{\substack{\| \\ \mathrm{NH}}}{\mathrm{H_2N} \diagdown \underset{C}{} \diagup \mathrm{NH_2}} + \mathrm{H^+} \rightarrow \left[\underset{\substack{\| \\ \mathrm{NH_2}}}{\mathrm{H_2N} \diagdown \underset{C}{} \diagup \mathrm{NH_2}} \right]^{\oplus}$$

Whether some of the biologic properties are determined by the uncharged fraction of molecules in solution has not been ascertained. The protonated molecule is planar and symmetric with bond distances of 1.32 Å between carbon and nitrogen (Haas et al. 1965), and is probably much smaller than hydrated sodium or potassium ion (Davidoff 1973). The guanidino group is a component of arginine, creatine, creatinine, methylguanidine, dimethylguanidine, guanidinosuccinic acid, and guanidinoacetic acid; metabolites commonly isolated from animal tissue and serum. The phosphorylated derivative, phosphocreatine, is a well-known high energy compound.

E. Effects of Guanidine on Virus Replication

I. Spectrum of Inhibited Viruses

Guanidine has been used at molar concentrations to establish molecular weights of proteins by gel filtration, to dissociate proteins, to dissociate avidin–biotin complexes, and to extract nucleic acids from cellular constituents. However, the use of guanidine as a protein denaturant is probably not relevant to a discussion of its selective, suppressive effects on viral growth. At virus-inhibitory concentrations of

0.2–3 mM, slight changes in tertiary structure of viral proteins undoubtedly occur, and such conformational alterations are probably the basis for interference with viral growth (KORANT 1977b). This mechanism of action is inferred from the chemical nature of guanidine. The modifications generated by low levels of the compound must be unique because of the limited spectrum of viruses inhibited and its innocuous effects on host cells.

Since the last exhaustive review (CALIGUIRI and TAMM 1973), relatively few studies have been performed with guanidine that change our overall perspective of its mode of action and little work has been done with viruses other than the picornaviruses. As noted in the previous sections, in addition to picornaviruses, two togaviruses, Sindbis and Semliki Forest viruses (FRIEDMAN 1970), and two plant viruses, tobacco necrosis virus (VARMA 1968), and TMV (DAWSON 1975) have demonstrable sensitivity to guanidine. High concentrations of 30 mM were used to inhibit togaviruses; concentrations in the range of 10–50 mM were responsible for inhibition of tobacco necrosis virus and 10–40 mM were tested with TMV. Permeation of plant tissues could be inefficient in comparison with animal cells, thus necessitating higher levels of guanidine to achieve inhibition. In the study with togaviruses, the level of inhibitor employed was 10–30-fold higher than that generally used with picornaviruses. Although the effects of guanidine on replication of numerous viruses have been examined, it appears that DNA viruses such as vaccinia, polyoma, adenoviruses, and herpesviruses as well as RNA viruses such as influenza, parainfluenza, and reoviruses are resistant.

Substituted guanidines have also be examined for virus-inhibitory activity with positive results (CALIGUIRI and TAMM 1973). Whether repression of virus growth is due to the positively charged guanidine base, the substituent group, or both remains an open question. The site of inhibition during viral replication has not been studied in any detail with the guanidinium compounds.

II. Effects on Cells

Guanidine is a natural constituent of animal serum and, along with several other guanidinium compounds, has been suspected of contributing to toxemia during uremic poisoning. However, clinical studies have not confirmed this view (STEIN and MICKLUS 1973). The effects of guanidine in animals will be discussed later in Sect. G. Since most virologic experiments have been concerned with the effects of guanidine on viral growth in tissue culture cells, it is pertinent to evaluate its effects on host cells in vitro. At virus-inhibitory concentrations such as 1 mM, guanidine has a negligible effect on the division of HeLa cells over approximately 3 days (CALIGUIRI and TAMM 1973) and has only slight effects on monkey kidney cells at 2 mM after 7 days (CROWTHER and MELNICK 1961). Concentrations of approximately 10 mM have no detectable adverse effects on HeLa cells or primary cattle cells (LODDO et al. 1962). The compound reversibly penetrates cells in culture, since it can be rapidly depleted by several cycles of rinsing with guanidine-free solution (EGGERS et al. 1965a; TERSHAK 1974). Cells that have been pretreated with guanidine for 8 h prior to infection still support viral growth (LODDO et al. 1962), indicating that only interference with virus-specific metabolic processes occurs in infected cells.

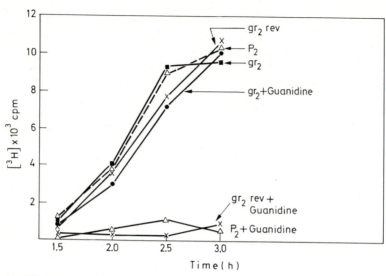

Fig. 4. Effect of guanidine on poliovirus RNA synthesis. Cultures of HeLa cells were infected with 20 pfu/cell of poliovirus 2 (P_2), a guanidine-resistant mutant (gr_2), or a sensitive revertant (gr_2 rev). To those cultures receiving guanidine (2 mM), the compound was added 1 h postinfection. Uridine, labeled with ^{3}H, was added to all cultures at 1.5 h postinfection, and then samples were taken at 0.5-h intervals, precipitated with trichloroacetic acid, and counted in a liquid scintillation counter. (Korant 1977 b)

III. Stage of Viral Growth Inhibited by Guanidine

Guanidine has no direct effect on virions (Loddo et al. 1962), and attachment as well as penetration of virus are not inhibited in its presence (Carp 1964). In fact, guanidine has no inhibitory effect on guanidine-sensitive virus up to about 1 h postinfection and is not essential for dependent variants during the early latent period (Eggers et al. 1965a). The inhibitory effects (with sensitive virus) and virus-stimulatory effects (dependent virus) begin approximately midway through the latent phase and continue throughout the remainder of the reproduction cycle. Studies establishing this point have been performed with poliovirus 1 and coxsackievirus A9 (Eggers et al. 1965a). When added during mid-log growth, guanidine rapidly retards synthesis of poliovirus RNA (Caliguiri and Tamm 1968a; Koschel and Wecker 1971; Fig. 4), and blocks development of UV resistance by infective centers (Eggers et al. 1965b), the latter phenomenon being dependent upon viral RNA synthesis (Tershak 1964). Interestingly, in one study, the addition of guanidine to poliovirus-infected cells for 15 min 1–2 h postinfection caused a 1.5–2-h delay in growth of guanidine-sensitive virus after removal of the inhibitor (Tershak 1974). Although the basis for this observation remains undetermined, protease inhibitors such as L-1-tosylamide-2-phenylethylchloromethylketone (TPCK) and N-α-p-tosyl-L-lysinechloromethylketone (TLCK) partially shortened the lag period after removal of guanidine, suggesting that guanidine might stimulate turnover of viral proteins through conformational changes in substrate, protease, or both.

A more recent report also suggests that guanidine might alter cleavage of several viral proteins, in particular enhanced cleavage of poliovirus protein NCVP1a into 3a and 3c was observed (KOCH et al. 1980). The effect was noted under conditions where cells were exposed to hypertonic medium and suggested that guanidine might alter viral proteins, interfere with interactions between viral proteins and cellular components, or inhibit proteases. Because guanidine retarded virus-induced blockage of host protein synthesis, the possibility that limited levels of viral protease were present owing to delayed viral growth must be considered. Modifications in cleavage could then result from preferential binding of limited enzyme to several viral proteins that have high affinities for protease. Under conditions where protease is not limited, a different pattern of protein processing might ensue.

Data obtained with FMDV also suggest a role for a 34 Kd protein in regulating the antiviral action of guanidine (SAUNDERS et al. 1981). Of twenty guanidine-sensitive mutants of FMDV, one exhibited a shift in isoelectric focusing point in a coat protein, while four mutants induced synthesis of a modified 34Kd protein that is probably the counterpart of poliovirus NCVPX. Because coat proteins of poliovirus covary with the guanidine marker (COOPER et al. 1970; KORANT 1977b), it is not surprising that mutations in substrates or protease modify the guanidine marker. The properties of guanidine suggest that its capacity to block viral growth depends upon conformational changes in macromolecules, and data suggesting altered proteolytic processing in the presence of guanidine, are in concert with this mode of action. The ideal experimental system for examining guanidine-induced changes might be cell-free extracts that synthesize and process authentic viral proteins.

Even though guanidine appears to manifest no inhibitory effects on the growth of sensitive strains of virus up to 1 h postinfection, it can partially interfere with the capacity of virus to block cellular protein synthesis with low input multiplicities of infection of ten infectious particles per cell (HOLLAND 1964; KOSCHEL and WECKER 1971). Possibly, a by-product of early replication that is not essential for growth of virus is responsible for turnoff of host protein synthesis. The dependence of the phenomenon upon input levels of virus would imply that a minimal number of translation products is required for interference with synthesis of cellular proteins.

A unique observation was made during investigations with TMV and systemically inoculated leaves of tobacco plants (DAWSON 1975). Depending upon concentration of guanidine tested, a biphasic activity of inhibition of viral growth was observed. A concentration of 10 mM guanidine restricted virus replication when present 2–12 h postinfection, a time when viral RNA synthesis is not detectable; 12 h postinfection, when viral RNA synthesis is generally in progress, higher concentrations of 25–40 mM inhibitor were necessary for blockage of virus growth. At the present time there is no explanation for this biphasic type of inhibition. Possibly, less inhibitor is needed during the early stages of infection when newly synthesized viral RNA is present at very low levels. As the pool of RNA-replicating structures expands, more guanidine might be essential for inhibition. In a sense, this would be analogous to studies already cited, where interference with poliovirus-induced blockage of host protein synthesis by guanidine was shown to depend upon the input level of infectious particles (HOLLAND 1964; KOSCHEL and WECKER 1971). However, permeability changes or the involvement of two viral replicases cannot be ruled out as contributors to the biphasic inhibition observed with TMV.

It was shown in one series of experiments that synthesis of poliovirus RNA is quantitatively the same up to 2 h postinfection in HeLa cells during all stages of the cell cycle (KOCH et al. 1974); 2 h postinfection, when the major portion of viral RNA is being synthesized, S-phase cells were the most active producers of viral RNA. Guanidine apparently blocked viral RNA synthesis 2–4.5 h postinfection in S-phase cells and had a limited effect on early viral RNA synthesis in cells during any phase of the mitotic cycle. The authors suggested that two different viral replicases participate during viral growth, or alternatively, two different conformations of one enzyme; the enzyme that functions during the latent period would be resistant to guanidine (KOCH et al. 1974). The possibility that poliovirus RNA synthesized during early stages of replication is predominantly complementary to virion RNA and the product of a polymerase distinct from the enzyme responsible for synthesis of virion RNA during maximum synthesis has been considered, but seems unlikely. Hybridization experiments with poliovirus RNA indicate that about 17% of the RNA in the replicative intermediate is complementary (negative-stranded) while only 1%–5% of the single-stranded viral RNA is complementary type 1–5 h postinfection (MITCHELL and TERSHAK 1973). If two polymerases are involved during poliovirus growth, their synthetic activities remain proportionally unaltered throughout the growth cycle.

Several investigations with Mengo virus, a cardiovirus, indicate that the infectivity of viral dsRNA is suppressed by treating host cells with actinomycin D, α-amanitin, or cordycepin (PÉREZ-BERCOFF et al. 1974), compounds that are known to disrupt cellular transcription. A host cell factor is probably responsible for the infectivity of picornavirus dsRNA. Cells infected with dsRNA ^{3}H of Mengo virus contain RNA ^{3}H, sedimenting in sucrose gradients with characteristics of RI molecules; pulse-labeling cells with uridine ^{14}C 3 h postinfection with dsRNA ^{3}H results in cytoplasmic RI with both ^{3}H and ^{14}C isotopes (PÉREZ-BERCOFF et al. 1979). In addition to these findings, it was shown that suppression of cellular transcription with actinomycin D resulted in coordinate loss of the capacity of host cells to convert dsRNA to RI, indicating that a cellular process is essential for conversion. From kinetic studies in vivo it can also be inferred that viral dsRNA participates in the replication cycle late in infection (NOBLE and LEVINTOW 1970).

To summarize, guanidine seems to have little, if any, effect on picornavirus growth during early stages of the latent period, although at low input virus:cell ratios guanidine can delay virus-induced inhibition of host protein synthesis. Several studies directly and indirectly indicate that one or more host factors might participate in the replication cycle.

IV. Guanidine-Suppressive Compounds

LWOFF (1965) made the observation that L-arginine, L-ornithine, carbazide, and citrulline, compounds which contain amino groups, inhibit poliovirus growth at concentrations ranging from 5 to 25 mM. These substances appear to share a common mode of action with guanidine, because poliovirus mutants that are resistant to guanidine also exhibit a coordinated decrease in sensitivity to them. Nonetheless, many compounds with amino groups, such as glutamine, do not hinder poliovirus growth.In addition, urea retards poliovirus growth, but urea-resistant mutants do not exhibit cross-resistance to guanidine, suggesting distinct, nonoverlapping sites of action. In his original study, Lwoff also showed that methionine, valine, and choline, at low concentrations, partially reversed the inhibitory effects of guanidine on drug-sensitive strains of poliovirus; an observation in agreement with earlier experiments showing rescue of foot-and-mouth disease virus in the presence of guanidine by amino acids (DINTER and BENGSTON 1964). Amino acids capable of reversing guanidine action are methionine, valine, leucine, and threonine, in decreasing order of effectiveness. Serine and alanine were only slightly effective. Subsequent studies showed that methylated and ethylated compounds could similarly prevent the inhibition of poliovirus growth by guanidine (LODDO et al. 1966; PHILIPSON et al. 1966; MOSSER et al. 1971). In order of effectiveness, dimethylpropanolamine, ethanolamine, and choline were antagonists of guanidine with guanidine-sensitive virus, but could not replace guanidine as a metabolite for guanidine-dependent poliovirus in HeLa cells (PHILIPSON et al. 1966). Choline, methionine, and dimethylethanolamine in fact inhibited growth of guanidine-dependent poliovirus in the presence of guanidine (MOSSER et al. 1971). Effectiveness of the various metabolites depended upon cell type; choline blocked guanidine action best in KB (human nasopharyngeal carcinoma) cells while dimethylethanolamine was most active in HeLa cells (PHILIPSON et al. 1966).

Although the mechanism of action of guanidine-suppressive agents remains an enigma, they do not appear to methylate guanidine (LWOFF 1966; PHILIPSON et al. 1966). The observation that amino acids act synergistically with choline and dimethylethanolamine led to the hypothesis that two nonidentical sites of action of anti-guanidine substances were involved intracellularly. One plausible suggestion was that binding of guanidine antagonists to sites adjacent to the site of guanidine action could modify the microenvironment and displace guanidine (MOSSER et al. 1971). Guanidine has several effects during viral replication, one being reduction in choline incorporation into membranes that proliferate during viral growth (PENMAN and SUMMERS 1965). However, it is doubtful that the anti-guanidine metabolites function through restoration of choline incorporation and inferentially, synthesis of cellular membranes, because they inhibit growth of drug-dependent strains of virus in the presence of guanidine (MOSSER et al. 1971).

Genetic (COOPER 1969) and biochemical (COOPER et al. 1970; KORANT 1977b) data suggest that capsid proteins (or their precursor) are at least one determinant of guanidine sensitivity and resistance with poliovirus. Whether guanidine suppressive compounds modify, directly or indirectly, viral structural proteins, a second product of translation that interacts with structural proteins, or a complex of proteins and membranes remains undetermined. Nor have data been published establishing association of these substances with distinct sites on a single translational product. Since the precise mode of action of guanidine is not presently understood, it is impossible to evaluate accurately compounds that negate its activity. In addition, data referred to earlier suggest a role for viral proteases in regulating guanidine sensitivity-resistance with picornaviruses (KOCH et al. 1980; SAUNDERS et al. 1981). The capacity for molar concentrations of guanidine to disrupt tertiary structure of proteins implies that low levels cause subtle changes in the conformation of proteins. These changes could be rendered harmless by allosteric effects induced by anti-guanidine metabolites.

V. Site of Action of Guanidine

Although guanidine has been shown to block the development of several viruses specifically (RIGHTSEL et al. 1961; LODDO et al. 1963; CROWTHER and MELNICK 1961), the exact mechanism of inhibition has not been elucidated. A plethora of effects has been noted during viral replication and assuredly many of these reflect polarity changes in a complex growth cycle, involving synthesis and processing of viral proteins, synthesis of viral RNA, maturation of virions, and translocation of virus-specific macromolecules. Guanidine causes depression in choline incorporation into membranes (PENMAN and SUMMERS 1965), blocks morphogenesis of virions (JACOBSON and BALTIMORE 1968), and prevents the association of procapsid with smooth membranes (YIN 1977a). The restriction on choline incorporation elicited by guanidine is probably not the basis of interference with viral growth. In the previous section, the inhibitory effects of choline, methionine, and ethanolamine on growth of guanidine-dependent poliovirus in the presence of guanidine was mentioned. Clearly, metabolites that counteract guanidine under one set of conditions and prove to be inhibitory under a second set of experimental conditions add another level of complexity to our understanding of guanidine action.

Published literature indicates that the major and most rapid effect of guanidine is inhibition of viral RNA synthesis, particularly the production of single-stranded RNA (CALIGUIRI and TAMM 1968b; NOBLE and LEVINTOW 1970; KOSCHEL and WECKER 1971). This leads secondarily to inhibition of viral protein synthesis and maturation of virions (JACOBSON and BALTIMORE 1968), a process that cannot occur in the absence of viral RNA. In the presence of guanidine, infected cells accumulate procapsid particles (80 S) which lack viral RNA, and prelabeled procapsid can be chased into mature virions following removal of the guanidine block (JACOBSON and BALTIMORE 1968). Procapsids of poliovirus have been found in association with the viral replication complex in smooth membrane fractions obtained after rupturing cells and banding membranous structures in discontinuous, isopycnic sucrose gradients (YIN 1977a). Since synthesis of viral proteins occurs in association with rough membranes (CALIGUIRI and TAMM 1970), translocation of coat proteins to the region of viral RNA synthesis is a likely requisite for virion morphogenesis. Intracellular arrangements of the cytoskeletal framework of poliovirus-infected cells suggest that viral polysomes are situated at the cell periphery while the viral replication complex, empty capsids, and mature virions occupy the central region of the cytoplasm (LENK and PENMAN 1979). Possibly smooth membranes, which are the sites of viral RNA synthesis, and rough membranes, which are the sites of viral protein synthesis, are physically divorced rather than in close proximity. Transport of virion precursors would then be a critical function necessary for assembly of virions.

The capacity of guanidine to restrict association of procapsids with the replication complex has been interpreted to indicate an essential role for capsid proteins for continual synthesis of viral RNA (YIN 1977a). This hypothesis is in concert with data establishing a function for capsid subunits in regulating the growth response of poliovirus to guanidine (COOPER et al. 1970; KORANT 1977b). Genetic studies of guanidine sensitivity of poliovirus indicated that a viral protein is the site of guanidine action, and placed the guanidine sensitivity locus within the coat protein "cistron" (COOPER et al. 1970). Independent of these studies, physicochemical and biologic characterizations of viral mutants with altered guanidine sensitivities indicated changes in capsid polypeptides. Differences between mutants included electrophoretic mobilities of virions and capsid subunits, chromatographic behavior of individual capsid polypeptides (KORANT 1977b) and changes in isoelectric focusing mobilities of a 34 Kd protein of undefined function (SAUNDERS 1981). A comparison of two polioviruses, differing in guanidine sensitivity, is shown in Fig. 5.

In apparent conflict is the observation that DI particles of poliovirus that have lost about one-third of the capsid locus through deletion mutations still produce DI-specific RNA, and synthesis of this RNA is as sensitive to guanidine as parent virus (COLE and BALTIMORE 1973). However, cells infected with DI particles produce an unstable precursor of capsid proteins and it is contestable whether low levels of this transient parent molecule or oligopeptide fragments of this precursor affect the growth response of DI particles to guanidine. An alternative, trivial explanation for the interference with translocation of procapsid by guanidine is that migration of these proteins to sites of virion maturation requires a critical level of single-stranded viral RNA. Inhibition of viral RNA synthesis by guanidine would then indirectly depress transport of capsid proteins. How inhibition of viral RNA synthesis could modulate translocation of capsid peptides in conjectural, but partitioning of viral RNA among smooth and rough membranes is well established. The signals that control this distribution as well as translocation of proteins remain undefined.

VI. Mechanism of Action of Guanidine

1. Previous Studies

Although the principal site of guanidine action appears to be synthesis of viral RNA, more than one step may be affected. Studies by CALIGUIRI and TAMM (1968a, 1973) demonstrated that elongation and completion of synthesis of single-stranded viral RNA continue briefly in the presence of guanidine, and these investigators suggested that the inhibitor blocked the initiation step of polynucleotide synthesis. Inhibition of synthesis of viral RNA by guanidine and actidione in the middle of the viral replication cycle led KOSCHEL and WECKER (1971) to conclude that guanidine might prevent assembly of polymerase precursors. The outcome would be failure to initiate new RNA strands.

Poliovirus polymerase was shown to be insusceptible to the inhibitory effects of guanidine in vitro, even at concentrations 50–100-fold higher than employed during in vivo expriments (BALTIMORE et al. 1963). The interpretation generally accepted for this observation is that initiation of viral RNA synthesis does not occur in cell-free extracts, only completion of RNA chains in the process of synthesis during the extraction of crude enzyme (CALIGUIRI and TAMM 1973). The poliovirus

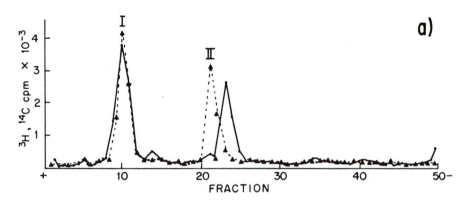

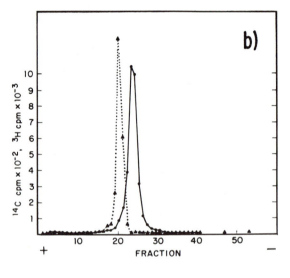

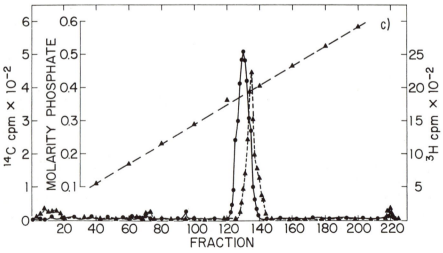

polymerase from infected cells is a complex mixture of viral proteins (CALIGUIRI and COMPANS 1973; RÖDER and KOSCHEL 1975) and endogenous RNA, particularly RI (GIRARD et al. 1967; LUNDQUIST and MAIZEL 1978). In vitro experiments with poliovirus polymerase and guanidine are difficult to interpret because the predominant types of RNA synthesized are RI and dsRNA (BALTIMORE 1964; McDONNELL and LEVINTOW 1970; YIN 1977b), species that comprise only about 10% of the viral RNA produced in vivo. In one study, the in vitro product of the viral enzyme mimicked that observed in vivo, but the effects of guanidine were not determined (GIRARD 1969). More recently, relatively pure preparations of picornavirus polymerase that utilize exogenous viral RNA or polyadenylic acid as template and oligouridylic acid as primer have been obtained, but the effects of guanidine on these enzymes have not been examined (FLANEGAN and BALTIMORE 1977; FLANEGAN and VAN DYKE 1979; LUND and SCRABA 1979). In one study, the viral enzyme appeared to initiate synthesis of new RNA chains, but experiments with guanidine were not reported (DASGUPTA et al. 1979).

Although a detailed product analysis has not been undertaken, hybridization of the in vitro product with virion RNA in two studies showed the product to be complementary to template RNA (FLANEGAN and VAN DYKE 1979; DASGUPTA et al. 1979). If crude preparations of viral polymerase fail to initiate synthesis of virus RNA in vitro, the inability of guanidine to inhibit enzyme activity in cell-free extracts would suggest that template-bound enzyme in the process of RNA synthesis is refractory to the inhibitor. Only one investigation is at variance with this hypothesis. Exposure of infected cells to guanidine was shown to cause an increase in size of the viral replication complex, a result that is anticipated if release of mature RNA chains is retarded by guanidine (HUANG and BALTIMORE 1970). In this study, nascent viral RNA that was synthesized in the absence of guanidine was released from the viral replication complex in the presence of guanidine and the suggestion by others (CALIGUIRI and TAMM 1973) that RNA produced only in the presence of guanidine might not be processed properly merits consideration. Overall, published data to date indicate that initiation of synthesis of viral RNA is depressed by guanidine while release of completed RNA chains is restricted under certain conditions. Drug-dependent mutants would require guanidine for assembly of active enzyme or for association of an enzyme aggregate with its RNA template. New data regarding this point is presented in Sect. E.VI.2.

2. Effects on Poliovirus Polymerase in Vitro

To date, only one study has been published showing inhibition of viral polymerase by guanidine in an in vitro assay. The failures of past experiments

---

◄ **Fig. 5, a–c.** Comparison of poliovirus 2 and a guanidine-resistant mutant selected after passage of the virus in $2 \, \text{m}M$ guanidine. **a** cytoplasmic polypeptide aggregates of the two viruses, compared according to charge in an electric field, applied to a sucrose gradient containing the proteins (KORANT 1973); aggregate I contains the nonstructural polypeptides; aggregate II the 6 S structural proteins, VP0, VP1, and VP3, **b** same comparison as **a**, except with purified virions of the two viruses; **c** chromatography of VP2 of the two viruses on a SDS hydroxyapatite column (KORANT 1977). In all data shown, poliovirus 2 was labeled with ^{3}H *(circles)* and gr_1 with ^{14}C *(triangles)*

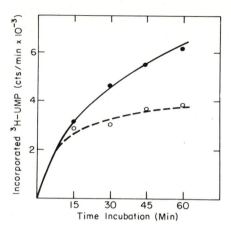

Fig. 6. Effect of guanidine on poliovirus polymerase in vitro. Enzyme was incubated with 70 µCi/ml UTP ^{3}H in the absence *(full circles)* and presence of 2 mM guanidine *(open circles)*. Inhibitor was added at the start of incubation and at intervals 25 µl samples were mixed with 3 ml cold 5% trichoroacetic acid (TCA). Precipitates were collected on Whatman GF/A glass fiber filters, washed five times with 15 ml volumes of 2% TCA, and radioactivity was measured in vials containing 5 ml Econofluor (New England Nuclear Corporation) scintillation fluid. Polymerase was prepared by the procedure of CELMA and EHRENFELD (1975). To assay enzyme activity, equal volumes of polymerase extract were combined with equal volumes of a reaction mixture that contained 230 mM Tris-HCl pH 7.4, 18 mM Mg(OAc)$_2$, 56 mM KCl, 29.7 mM phosphocreatine, 667 µg/ml creatine phosphokinase, 136–170 µM, adenosine-5′-triphosphate, cytidine-5′-triphosphate, guanosine-5′-triphosphate, 100 µg/ml actinomycin D, and 2 µM uridine-5′-triphosphate (UTP). Reactions were carried out at 36 °C in tightly sealed vials (TERSHAK, 1982)

might be attributed to several characteristics of enzyme preparations such as a deficiency in RNA chain initiation and possibly limited synthesis of 35 S viral RNA. As noted earlier, the majority of crude enzyme extracts produce predominantly RI and dsRNA. However, recent published observations with cell-free extracts from poliovirus-infected HeLa cells indicate that guanidine is capable of inhibiting viral RNA synthesis in vitro and that the most likely step affected is initiation of new RNA molecules. These experiments are more fully described in this section.

To examine the effects of guanidine in vitro, preparations of viral polymerase were incubated at 36 °C and incorporation of UMP ^{3}H into acid-insoluble polynucleotide was measured in the absence and presence of 2 mM guanidine (Fig. 6). Incorporation in the absence of inhibitor was linear for approximately 10 min, them decreased. Although incorporation of UMP ^{3}H decreased about 50% after 15 min incubation, linear synthesis continued for another 60 min. Six separate enzyme preparations were examined and in all cases synthesis of RNA continued for at least 2.5 h, which was the maximum period tested. In the presence of 2 mM guanidine, polymerization was equivalent to the control for 10–15 min, thereafter severe inhibition occurred. In several similar studies, inhibition of RNA synthesis by guanidine averaged approximately 75% between 15 and 90 min incubation. Although data are not shown on the graph, extracts from uninfected cells incorporated only background levels of radioactivity.

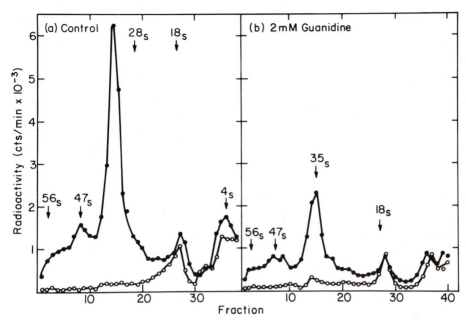

Fig. 7, a, b. In vitro product of poliovirus polymerase; Polymerase (1 ml reaction volumes) was incubated at 36 °C with 25 µCi UTP ³H for 90 min in the absence **a** or presence **b** of 2 mM guanidine. Equal volumes of TEN buffer (1.0% SDS, 100 mM NaCl, 1 mM EDTA, 10 mM Tris-HCl, pH 7.2) were added to terminate the reactions and samples were immediately layered over 36 ml 30%–15% sucrose gradients and centrifuged 18.5 h, 18,000 rpm, 20 °C in a Beckman SW27 rotor. After fractionation, each gradient sample was divided in half. Radioactivity was measured in one set without RNAse treatment *(full circles)* and after incubation with 20 µg/ml RNAse in 0.5 M NaCl *(open circles)*. The 28 and 18 S regions were determined by measuring UV absorbance at a wavelength of 254 nm with an ISCO UA-5 absorbance unit (Tershak, 1982)

During intracellular growth of poliovirus, about 90% of the viral RNA produced is virion type RNA with a sedimentation coefficient of 35 S. The RI and dsRNA species of RNA comprise approximately 10% of the intracellular virus-specific RNA (Caliguiri and Tamm 1968a). To determine whether the crude polymerase synthesized the same proportions of RNA species that are observed in vivo, products of the in vitro reaction were examined with linear sucrose gradients. RNA produced by the extracts resembled that observed in vivo (Fig. 7a). The RI, a large heterogeneous molecule, sedimented from approximately 56 to 16 S; the ribonuclease-resistant 16 S component represents dsRNA. In this investigation the sedimentation coefficient of the latter ranged from 16 to 18 S. This variation was probably due to mixtures of dsRNA and RI containing short segments of nascent, single-stranded RNA. RNA that sedimented at approximately 4 S and exhibited resistance to RNAse is generally not found in vivo. It could represent fragmented backbone of RI or an abnormal product of in vitro synthesis. Addition of 2 mM guanidine to the assay mixture caused 65% inhibition of synthesis of 35 S viral RNA after 90 min incubation (Fig. 7b). In other studies inhibition was as high as 75%. Production of RI and dsRNA were reduced to about 50% of control levels.

This finding is similar to data obtained in vivo that show synthesis of RI and dsRNA to be more refractory to guanidine than synthesis of 35 S RNA (CALIGUIRI and TAMM 1968a).

To determine which stage of viral RNA synthesis is blocked by guanidine in vitro, reaction mixtures were incubated with UTP ^{3}H and following a short incubation, a chase was performed with a 200-fold excess of nonradioactive UTP. In the first series of experiments, cell-free extracts were administered UTP ^{3}H during the initial 7 min incubation, then radioactivity was chased with unlabeled UTP for 15 min in the absence or presence of 2 mM guanidine. Products of the reaction were analyzed by sucrose gradient centrifugation and the results of one representative study are presented in Fig. 8a. During the pulse a heterogeneous population of RNA molecules, sedimenting from approximately 60 to 18 S, incorporated precursor. A portion of RNA in the 35 S region of the gradients is probably completed, single-stranded RNA. Following the chase, in the absence of guanidine, 58% of the radioactivity in the small replicative intermediate (fractions 20–30) shifted to both the 35 S region of the gradient and the larger replicative intermediate. On the average 24%–32% of the radioactivity that was lost from fractions 20–30 appeared in fractions 5–15. After the chase in the presence of guanidine 60% of the small replicative intermediate disappeared from fractions 20–30 and radioactivity was redistributed to the 35 S and large replicative intermediate regions of the gradient. The data suggest that about 15% more 35 S RNA was present in untreated control sample compared with the guanidine-treated sample following the chase. However, in several identical experiments this was not a reproducible observation. It appears that radioactive RNA was chased from the smaller RI into large RI and 35 S viral RNA with equal efficiency in the absence or presence of guanidine, a finding in agreement with data obtained in vivo (CALIGUIRI and TAMM 1968a).

Because synthesis of viral RNA decreased after 10–15 min incubation in the in vitro reaction, and because guanidine manifested inhibitory effects in vitro during the second stage of synthesis (see Fig. 6), pulse-chase studies were also conducted during the latter period. Enzyme was incubated with a complete reaction mixture at 36 °C and 10 min later UTP ^{3}H was added. Following a 7-min pulse, a chase was effected with unlabeled UTP, with or without guanidine. Sucrose gradient centrifugation of the products of the reaction show that, again, after the chase period 60% of the radioactivity in the small RI was depleted with simultaneous appearance of increased radioactivity in the large RI and 35 S viral RNA (Fig. 8b). The chase was equally effective in the presence or absence of guanidine. In this particular study, guanidine was present only during the chase period, but other studies produced analogous results when guanidine was present throughout the entire experiment. Also, the distribution of RNA throughout the gradient differs from the distribution in Fig. 8b because a longer centrifugation time was employed.

There appears to be a less effective chase of radioactivity into 35 S viral RNA in comparison with pulse-chase studies performed during the early stages of the in vitro reaction (compare Fig. 8a with Fig. 8b). This might merely reflect a proportionally larger amount of 35 S prior to the chase presented in Fig. 8b. The overall results indicate that guanidine does not noticeably restrict elongation or release of polynucleotide chains from the viral replication complex during early or later

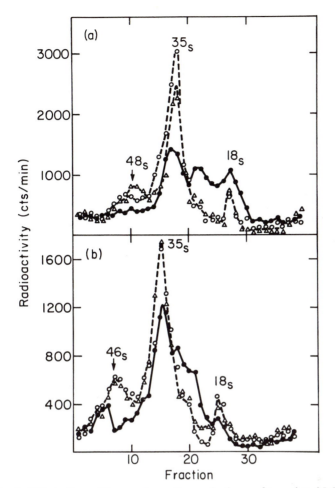

Fig. 8, a, b. Effect of guanidine on elongation and release of complete 35 S viral RNA from the viral replication complex. **a** an enzyme reaction mixture of 2.4 ml was incubated 7 min, 36 °C with 50 µCi UTP ^{3}H; one-third of the mixture was mixed with an equal volume of TEN buffer containing 1% SDS and placed on ice *(solid circles)*, one-third was incubated an additional 15 min with a 200-fold excess of unlabeled UTP then combined with an equal volume of TEN buffer *(open circles)*, and one-third was incubated an additional 15 min in the presence of a 200-fold excess of unlabeled UTP and 2 mM guanidine *(triangles)*; samples were centrifuged 17 h, 18,000 rpm, 20 °C in a Beckman SW27 rotor, fractionated, and incorporated UMP ^{3}H was measured; **b** the experiment was similar to that of **a** with several modifications. UTP ^{3}H was added to the enzyme mixture after 10 min at 36 °C and the chase was performed 7 min later in the absence *(open circles)* or presence *(triangles)* of 2 mM guanidine. *Full circles* represent the pulse. Centrifugation was 18.5 h, 18,000 rpm, 20 °C in a Beckman SW27 rotor (TERSHAK, 1982)

stages of incubation in vitro. This implies that guanidine retards polynucleotide chain initiation.

The data indirectly point to the initiation step of RNA synthesis as the probable site of guanidine action. If initiation of viral RNA synthesis is inhibited by guanidine, a short pulse with UTP ^{3}H should provide information that would di-

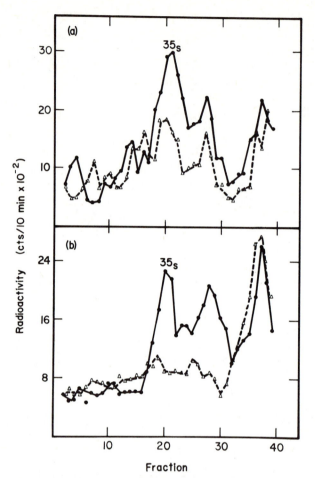

Fig. 9, a, b. Effect of guanidine on initiation of synthesis of viral RNA. Two enzyme reaction mixtures of 1 ml were incubated for 25 min at 36 °C in the absence *(full circles)* or presence *(triangles)* of 2 m*M* guanidine; 25 µCi UTP ³H were added to each reaction mixture for 4 min. An equal volume of TEN buffer was then added and the samples were centrifuged 18 h, 18,000 rpm, 20 °C on 30%–15% sucrose gradients. **a** and **b** represent experiments with two different enzyme preparations (Tershak, 1982)

rectly support this hypothesis. In an untreated control, UMP ³H should be incorporated into large RI, small RI, and 35 *S* RNA. If initiation were restricted by guanidine, proportionally less of the small RI would incorporate UMP ³H compared with controls incubated without guanidine. This assumption was tested by pulse-labeling viral RNA in vitro for 4 min following 25 min preincubation at 36 °C. The enzyme in the treated sample was incubated with guanidine at the start of incubation. The data from two experiments with separate enzyme preparations are shown in Fig. 9. In the control samples, a short pulse with precursor resulted in incorporation of precursor into RNA that was distributed from 56 to 16 *S* in sucrose gradients (fractions 5–30). A similar pulse with enzyme incubated with guanidine showed a reduced level of incorporation of UMP ^{3}H into the small RI (fractions 20–30); a result that is anticipated if RNA chain initiation were hindered by the inhibitor. The synthesis of 35 *S* viral RNA appears to be severly blocked in the experiment in Fig. 9 b. However, the 35 *S* region of sucrose gradients contains RI molecules and the overall drop in radioactivity in this area of the gradients in the presence of guanidine probably reflects decreased synthesis of RI. This is supported by the lack of buildup of large RI molecules (fractions 5–15) which would be expected if release of mature RNA chains were inhibited. Overall the data presented in this section strongly point to the initiation step of viral RNA synthesis as the site of guanidine inhibition.

3. Probable Mode of Action of Guanidine

One can only surmise that guanidine elicits mild conformational changes in viral proteins. Such postulated alterations would not occur with cellular proteins or proteins of most viruses because of the absence of specific amino acid sequences that lead to unique protein conformations. In support of this thesis is the observation that guanidine manifests a thermomimetic effect on the production of foot-and-mouth disease virus (NICK and AHL 1976). The optimal temperature for growth of FMDV ranges from approximately 32° to 37 °C in secondary calf kidney cells. This temperature range is shifted down by 3° to 5 °C in the presence of 1–2 m*M* guanidine and with some virus strains the yield of virus at infraoptimal temperatures in the presence of guanidine surpassed that observed in control experiments by a factor of ten. Although data were not presented, the investigators indicated that the growth enhancing effect of guanidine could be negated by D_2O. These experiments do not necessarily parallel studies with guanidine antagonists and guanidine-dependent virus noted earlier because substances such as choline, methionine, and dimethylethanolamine inhibit growth of drug-dependent virus in the presence of guanidine (MOSSER et al. 1971). The collective data with temperature, D_2O, metabolites, and guanidine lead to the conclusion that viral proteins contain numerous regions that are susceptible to conformational modifications. Depending upon the particular effector and site or combination of sites of action, the outcome could be potentiation of guanidine inhibition or reversal of inhibition.

During the past several years the 5′ end of poliovirus RNA was shown to contain a small covalently linked protein termed VPg (genome-linked virus protein; LEE et al. 1977; AMBROS and BALTIMORE 1977). Since the discovery of VPg, other picornaviruses such as FMDV, encephalomyocarditis, and rhinoviruses have proved to contain similar proteins (reviewed by SANGAR 1979). Because VPg is found on nascent strands of the poliovirus RI, it was suggested that it acts as a primer for synthesis of viral RNA (NOMOTO et al. 1977 a) and possibly serves a role during maturation of virions. The hypothesis that VPg is part of the enzyme responsible for initiation of RNA synthesis and is cleaved from the enzyme to produce VPg and the elongation enzyme is an interesting idea that should be evaluated in the near future (PALMENBERG et al. 1979). Whether this unique protein or its precursor is essential for the action of guanidine during viral growth remains to be determined.

As noted earlier, genetic (Cooper 1969) and biochemical (Cooper et al. 1970; Korant 1977 b) data suggest that capsid proteins and proteases are determinants of guanidine sensitivity and resistance to poliovirus. Perhaps synthesis and encapsidation of viral RNA are closely regulated processes that require both capsid subunits (or their precursor) and VPg. Interaction of guanidine with either of these components could simultaneously cause multiple aberrations such as inhibition of RNA synthesis (Caliguiri and Tamm 1968 b; Noble and Levintow 1970; Koschel and Wecker 1971), or inhibition of maturation (Jacobson and Baltimore 1968) and also prevent capsid proteins from associating with smooth membranes (Yin 1977 a). Although this hypothesis might be appealing on the surface, one minor drawback must be taken into account. Viruses that are naturally resistant to the compound must either contain no VPg or a protein characteristic of laboratory-generated, drug-resistant mutants. DNA-containing viruses such as adenovirus and herpesvirus pose no conceptual problem, but picornaviruses such as echoviruses 6, 7, 8, and coxsackievirus B6, which are naturally resistant to guanidine, should contain VPg units structurally different from those of sensitive viruses. In due course, this prediction should be amenable to experimental evaluation.

A recent study concerning guanidine action deserves mention. During the late stages of infection, a four-fold influx of sodium ion was found to occur in HeLa S_3 cells infected with poliovirus type 2. The accumulation of sodium ion was blocked by guanidine but restored by choline (Nair et al. 1979). Because choline is commonly used to replace sodium ions during transport studies, the investigators suggested that guanidine functions at the level of a cation-dependent viral function such as folding and processing of viral macromolecules. As noted earlier, guanidine is probably a smaller molecule than hydrated sodium or potassium ion (Davidoff 1973) and the likelihood that it affects protein conformations at low concentrations is inferential; at molar concentrations its protein denaturing properties are well documented.

F. Guanidine as a Therapeutic Agent in Animals

Until 1976, studies with animals showed guanidine to be an ineffective chemotherapeutic compound. The outcome of these investigations could have been due to excretion of guanidine and/or the selection of drug-resistant variants during therapy. However, Eggers (1979) successfully treated echovirus 9 and coxsackievirus A9 infections in newborn mice with a combination of guanidine and 2-(α-hyroxybenzyl)-benzimidazole (HBB). Mice (age 24 h) injected with echovirus 9, about 2×10^6 pfu/animal developed paralysis and died, while mice injected with guanidine and HBB subcutaneously with two doses per day showed marked survival. Although sample numbers were not large, the findings are significant because either compound alone proved to be ineffective and measurement of virus in the animals showed several days' delay in detectable virus growth along with 50%–90% reduction in virus yield. Except for one instance with coxsackievirus A9, isolates from treated animals remained as sensitive to inhibitors as the parent virus. Projected, not measured, levels of inhibitor were $200 \, \mu M$ HBB and $2 \, mM$

guanidine with one injection. These doses, which were not toxic to animals, are comparable to those employed during in vitro studies, although actual blood levels following several days of multiple doses are uncertain. Several puzzling observations were made during the investigation. HBB alone, but not guanidine alone, blocked paralysis induced by coxsackievirus A9 in animals. Why HBB alone was effective with coxsackievirus A9 but not echovirus 9 in vivo is not known. In vitro, both viruses are equally sensitive to HBB, indicating that other complex factors come into play in vivo. Since skeletal muscle is affected by both viruses, the likelihood of several unique target sites was suggested. Access to specific sites by drugs might determine chemotherapeutic value. At the moment, the efficacy of guanidine in the treatment of virus infections of animals deserves further testing. Chapter 9 more clearly addresses the effectiveness of treatment of infected animals with HBB and guanidine.

G. Clinical Nonvirologic Studies

Guanidine and guanidine derivatives have been employed extensively in both investigational and therapeutic studies. Guanidine and various substituted guanidines have served as antihypertensives, hypoglycemics, diuretics, and have also been used with partial success for treatment of botulism, myasthenia gravis, and malaria (see DAVIDOFF 1973, for a brief review). As early as 1876, guanidine was shown to elicit muscle spasms in frogs following injection. Subsequent investigations led to the hypothesis that guanidine and its derivatives specifically react with metal ion receptor sites on membranes. The effects of guanidine on neuromuscular excitability can be alleviated by calcium ions, a finding that eventually led to the development of biguanides as antidiabetic agents in concert with insulin. In neurobiologic studies it was shown that guanidine functioned like sodium and could replace sodium for maintaining action potential in the nerve axon. This effect is probably not specific because positively charged, quaternary ammonium compounds manifest analogous pharmacologic behavior.

It has been inferred that derivatives of guanidine, such as biguanides, bind to membrane sites, displace divalent metals such as calcium, and enhance the effects of insulin. In mitochondria, octylguanidine inhibits oxidative phosphorylation by blocking sodium-stimulated uptake of oxygen and sodium-stimulated release of potassium (GOMEZ-PUYOU et al. 1973). However, respiratory inhibition appears to occur with abnormally high, nontherapeutic doses of guanidine derivatives, while low doses appear to amplify peripheral action of insulin.

The earlier studies demonstrating enhanced nerve excitability after injection with guanidine pointed to a possible role for guanidine and its naturally occurring derivatives in determining the pathologic picture during uremic poisoning. However, serum levels of guanidine and methylguanidine are similar in control groups and uremic patients, although excretion of methylguanidine is significantly enhanced among individuals in renal failure (STEIN and MICKLUS 1973). At the present time, it appears doubtful that guanidine, methylguanidine, or dimethylguanidine contribute to uremic toxicity. The role of guanidinosuccinic acid is this pathologic condition remains uncertain.

In addition to the investigations noted, guanidine has found questionable use for treatment of paralyses caused by botulinus toxin. In experimental animals, guanidine was shown to effect a partial reversal of the neuromuscular block without noticeable side effects and changes in both nerve excitability and clinical symptoms were observed (Cherington et al. 1973). In a clinical trial with a single human patient, similar results were obtained (Cherington and Schultz 1977). Although the patient was administered 10,000 U bivalent botulinus antitoxin A and B along with germine monoacetate, it was found that a guanidine dose of 51 mg/kg daily, followed later by twice that dose was needed to produce beneficial effects. However, most reports with laboratory animals indicate that guanidine has minimal usefulness for the treatment of botulism.

References

Abraham G, Cooper P (1975) Poliovirus polypeptides examined in more detail. J Gen Virol 29:199–213

Adrian T, Rosenwirth B, Eggers H (1979) Isolation and characterization of temperature-sensitive mutants of echovirus 12. Virology 99:329–339

Ambros V, Baltimore D (1978) Protein is linked to the 5′ end of poliovirus RNA by a phosphodiester linkage to tyrosine. J Biol Chem 253:5263–5266

Ambros V, Petterson RF, Baltimore D (1978) An enzymatic activity in uninfected cells that cleaves the linkage between polio virion RNA and the 5′ terminal protein. Cell 15:1439–1446

Armstrong JA, Edmonds M, Nakazato H, Phillips BA, Vaughan MH (1972) Polyadenylic acid sequences in the virion RNA of poliovirus and Eastern Equine Encephalitis virus. Science 176:526–528

Bablanian R, Eggers H, Tamm I (1965) Studies on the mechanism of poliovirus-induced cell damage. II. The relation between poliovirus growth and virus-induced morphological changes in cells. Virology 26:114–121

Baltimore D (1964) In vitro synthesis of viral RNA by the poliovirus RNA polymerase. Proc Natl Acad Sci USA 51:450–456

Baltimore D, Franklin RM, Eggers HJ, Tamm I (1963) Poliovirus induced RNA polymerase and the effects of virus-specific inhibitors on its production. Proc Natl Acad Sci USA 49:843–849

Bowles S, Tershak D (1978) Proteolysis of non-capsid protein 2 of type 3 poliovirus at the restrictive temperature: breakdown of non-capsid protein 2 correlates with loss of RNA synthesis. J Virol 27:443–448

Brawerman G (1974) Eukaryotic messenger RNA. Annu Rev Biochem 43:621–642

Brown F, Newman JFE, Stott J, Porter A, Frisby D, Newton C, Carey N, Fellner P (1974) Poly C in animal viral RNAs. Nature 251:342–344

Butterworth B, Rueckert R (1972) Kinetics of synthesis and cleavage of EMC virus-specific proteins. Virology 50:535–549

Caliguiri LA, Compans RW (1973) The formation of poliovirus particles in association with the RNA replication complexes. J Gen Virol 21:99–108

Caliguiri LA, Tamm I (1968a) Action of guanidine on the replication of poliovirus RNA. Virology 35:408–417

Caliguiri LA, Tamm I (1968b) Distribution and translation of poliovirus RNA in guanidine treated cell. Virology 36:223–231

Caliguiri LA, Tamm I (1970) The role of cytoplasmic membranes in polio biosynthesis. Virology 42:100–111

Caliguiri LA, Tamm I (1973) Guanidine and 2-(α-hydroxybenzyl)-bensimidazole (HBB): selective inhibitors of picornavirus multiplication. In: Carter W (ed) Selective inhibitors of viral function. CRC Press, Cleveland, pp 257–294

Carp RI (1964)Studies on the guanidine character of poliovirus. Virology 22:270–279

Celma ML, Ehrenfeld E (1975) Translation of poliovirus RNA in vitro: detection of two different initiation sites. J Mol Biol 98:761–780

Cherington H, Greenberg H, Soyer A (1973) Guanidine and germine in botulism. Clin Toxicol 6:83–89

Cherington M, Schultz D (1977) Effect of guanidine, germine, and steroids in a case of botulism. Clin Toxicol 11:19–25

Cole CN, Baltimore D (1973) Defective interfering particles of poliovirus. II. Nature of the defect. J Mol Biol 76:325–343

Cooper PD (1969) The genetic analysis of poliovirus. In: Levy HB (ed) The biochemistry of viruses. Dekker, New York, pp 177–218

Cooper PD, Wentworth BB, McCahon D (1970) Guanidine inhibition of poliovirus: a dependence of viral RNA synthesis on the configuration of structural protein. Virology 40:486–493

Cooper PD, Steiner-Pryor A, Wright P (1973) A proposed regulator for poliovirus: the equestron. Intervirology 1:1–10

Crowther D, Melnick JL (1961) Studies of the inhibitory action of guanidine on poliovirus multiplication in cell culture. Virology 15:65–74

Dasgupta A, Baron M, Baltimore D (1979) Poliovirus replicase: a soluble enzyme able to initiate copying of polioviral RNA. Proc Natl Acad Sci USA 76:2679–2683

Dasgupta A, Zabel P, Baltimore D (1980) Dependence of the activity of poliovirus replicase on a host cell protein. Cell 19:423–429

Daubert SD, Bruening G, Najarian RC (1978) Protein bound to the genome RNAs of Cowpea mosaic virus. Eur J Biochem 92:45–51

Davidoff F (1973) Guanidine derivatives in medicine. N Engl J Med 289:141–146

Dawson WO (1975) Guanidine inhibits tobacco mosaic virus RNA synthesis at two stages. Intervirology 6:83–89

Dinter Z, Bengston Z (1964) Suppression of the inhibitory action of guanidine on virus multiplication by some amino acids. Virology 24:254–261

Dmitrieva T, Shcheglova M, Agol V (1979) Inhibition of activity of EMC virus-induced RNA polymerase by antibodies against cellular components. Virology 92:271–277

Dorsch-Häsler K, Yogo Y, Wimmer E (1975) Replication of picornaviruses. I. Evidence from in vitro RNA synthesis that poly (A) of the poliovirus genome is genetically coded. J Virol 16:1512–1527

Eggers HJ (1979) Successful treatment of enterovirus-infected mice by 2-(α-hydroxybenzyl)-benzimidazole and guanidine. J Exp Med 143:1367–1381

Eggers HJ, Ikegami N, Tamm I (1965a) Comparative studies with selective inhibitors of picornavirus reproduction. Ann NY Acad Sci 130:267–281

Eggers HJ, Ikegami N, Tamm I (1965b) The development of ultravioletirradiation resistance by poliovirus infective centers and its inhibition by guanidine. Virology 25:475–478

Ehrenfeld E (1979) In vitro translation of picornavirus RNA in cell-free extracts. In: Pérez-Bercoff R (ed) Molecular biology of picornaviruses. Plenum, New York, p 223

Fernandez-Munoz R, Darnell J (1976) Structural differences between the 5′ termini of viral and cellular mRNA in poliovirus infected cells: possible basis for the inhibition of host protein synthesis. J Virol 18:719–726

Flanegan JB, Baltimore D (1977) Poliovirus-specific primerdependent RNA polymerase able to copy poly (A). Proc Natl Acad Sci USA 74:3677–3680

Flanegan JB, van Dyke T (1979) Isolation of a soluble and template dependent poliovirus RNA polymerase that copies virion RNA in vitro. J Virol 32:155–166

Flanegan JB, Pettersson RF, Ambros V, Hewlett MJ, Baltimore D (1977) Covalent linkage of a protein to a defined nucleotide sequence at the 5′-terminus of a virion and replicative intermediate RNAs of poliovirus. Proc Natl Acad Sci USA 74:961–965

Friedman RM (1970) Basis for variable response of arboviruses to guanidine treatment. J Virol 6:628–636

Ghendon Y (1972) Conditional lethal mutants of animal viruses. Prog Med Virol 14:68–122

Girard M (1969) In vitro synthesis of poliovirus ribonucleic acid: role of the replicative intermediate. J Virol 3:376–384

Girard M, Baltimore D, Darnell JE (1967) The poliovirus replication complex: site for synthesis of poliovirus RNA. J Mol Biol 24:59–74

Goldstein NO, Pardoe IU, Burness A (1976) Requirement of an adenylic acid rich segment for the infectivity of EMC RNA. J Gen Virol 31:271–278

Golini F, Nomoto A, Wimmer E (1978) The genome-linked protein of picornavirus. IV. Difference in the VPgs of EMC virus and poliovirus as evidence that the genome linked proteins are virus coded. Virology 89:112–118

Gomez-Puyou A, Sandoval F, Lotina B, Gomez-Puyou T (1973) Guanidine sensitive transport of Na$^+$ and K$^+$ in mitochondria. Biochem Biophys Res Commun 52:74–78

Gorbalenya A, Svitkin Y, Kazachkou Y, Agol V (1979) EMC virus-specific polypeptide p22 is involved in the processing of the viral precursor polypeptides. FEBS Lett 108:1–5

Grubman M, Barth B, Bachrach HL (1979) Foot-and-mouth disease virion RNA: studies on the relation between length of its 3′ (A) segment and infectivity. Virology 97:22–31

Haas DJ, Harris DR, Mills HH (1965) The crystal structure of guanidinium chloride. Acta Crystallogr (Copenh) 19:676–679

Harris TJR (1980) Comparison of the nucleotide sequence at the 5′ end of RNAs from nine aphthoviruses, including representatives of the seven serotypes. J Virol 36:659–664

Harris TJR (1976) The location of the poly (C) tract in the RNA of foot-and-mouth disease virus. J Gen Virol 33:493–501

Hewlett M, Florkiewicz R (1980) Sequence of picornavirus RNAs containing a radioiodinated 5′-linked peptide reveals a conserved 5′ sequence. Proc Natl Acad Sci USA 77:303–307

Hewlett MJ, Rose JK, Baltimore D (1976) 5′-Terminal structure of poliovirus polyribosomal RNA is pUp. Proc Natl Acad Sci USA 73:327–330

Holland JJ (1964) Inhibition of host macromolecular synthesis by high multiplicities of poliovirus under conditions preventing virus synthesis. J Mol Biol 8:574–581

Hruby DE, Roberts WK (1976) Encephalomyocarditis virus RNA: Variations in polyadenylic acid content and biological activity. J Virol 19:325–330

Hruby DE, Roberts WK (1978) Encephalomyocarditis virus RNA. III. Presence of a genome associated protein. J Virol 25:413–415

Huang AS, Baltimore D (1970) Initiation of polysome formation in poliovirus-infected HeLa cells. J Mol Biol 47:275–291

Jacobson MF, Baltimore D (1968) Morphogenesis of poliovirus. I. Association of the viral RNA with coat protein. J Mol Biol 33:369–378

King AMQ, Sangar DV, Harris TJR, Brown F (1980) Heterogeneity of the genome-linked protein of foot-and-mouth disease virus. J Virol 34:627–634

Kitamura N, Adler C, Wimmer E (1980) Structure and expression of the picornavirus genome. Ann NY Acad Sci 354:183–201

Koch AS, Eremenko T, Benedetto A, Volpe P (1974) A guanidine-sensitive step of the poliovirus RNA replication cycle. Intervirology 4:221–225

Koch G, Hiller E, Scharli C (1980) Influence of medium hyperosmolarity and guanidine on the synthesis and processing of poliovirus proteins. In: Koch G, Richter G (eds) Biosynthesis, modification, and processing of cellular and viral proteins. Academic Press, New York London, pp 246–262

Korant B (1973) Cleavage of poliovirus-specific polypeptide aggregates. J Virol 12:556–563

Korant B (1975) Regulation of animal virus replication by protein cleavage. In: Reich E, Rifkin D, Shaw E (eds) Proteases and biological control. Cold Spring Harbor Lab Press, New York, p 621

Korant B (1977a) Protein cleavage in virus-infected cells. Acta Biol Med Ger 36:1565–1573

Korant BD (1977b) Poliovirus coat protein as the site of guanidine action. Virology 81:17–28

Korant B (1979) Role of cellular and viral proteases in the processing of picornavirus proteins. In: Pérez-Bercoff R (ed) Molecular biology of picornaviruses. Plenum, New York, p 149

Korant B, Chow N, Lively M, Powers J (1979) Virus-specified protease in poliovirus-infected HeLa cells. Proc Natl Acad Sci USA 76:2992–2995

Koschel K, Wecker E (1971) Early functions of poliovirus. III. The effect of guanidine on early functions. Z Naturforsch 26b:940–944

Lee YF, Nomoto A, Wimmer E (1976) The genome of poliovirus is an exceptional eukaryotic mRNA. Prog Nucleic Acid Res Mol Biol 19:89–96

Lee YF, Nomoto A, Detjen BM, Wimmer E (1977) A protein covalently linked to poliovirus genome RNA. Proc Natl Acad Sci USA 74:59–63

Lenk R, Penman S (1979) The cytoskeletal framework and poliovirus metabolism. Cell 16:289–301

Loddo B, Ferrari W, Brotzu G, Spanedda A (1962) In vitro inhibition of infectivity of poliovirus by guanidine. Nature 193:97–98

Loddo B, Mutoni S, Spanedda A, Brotzu G, Ferrari W (1963) Guanidine conditional infectivity of ribonucleic acid extracted from a strain of guanidine-dependent polio-1 virus. Nature 197:315

Loddo B, Gressa GL, Schivo ML, Spanedda A, Brotzu G, Ferrari W (1966) Antagonism of the guanidine interference with poliovirus replication by simple methylated and ethylated compounds. Virology 28:707–712

Lowe PA, Brown F (1981) Isolation of a soluble and template dependent foot-and-mouth disease virus RNA polymerase. Virology 111:23–32

Lucas-Lenard J (1979) Inhibition of cellular protein synthesis after virus infection. In: Pérez-Bercoff R (ed) Molecular biology of picornaviruses. Plenum, New York, p 73

Lund GA, Scraba DC (1979) The isolation of mengo virus stable non-capsid polypeptides from infected L cells and preliminary characterization of an RNA polymerase activity associated with polypeptide E. J Gen Virol 44:391–403

Lundquist RE, Maizel JV (1978) Structural studies on the RNA component of the poliovirus replication complex. I. Purification and biochemical characterization. Virology 85:434–444

Lundquist RE, Ehrenfeld E, Maizel JV (1974) Isolation of a viral polypeptide associated with the poliovirus replication complex. Proc Natl Acad Sci USA 71:4773–4777

Lundquist R, Sullivan M, Maizel JV (1979) Characterization of a new isolate of poliovirus defective interfering particles. Cell 18:759–769

Lwoff A (1965) The specific effectors of viral development. Biochem J 96:289–302

McDonnel JP, Levintow L (1970) Kinetics of appearance of poliovirus-induced RNA polymerase. Virology 42:999–1006

Mitchell W, Tershak DR (1973) The synthesis of complementary ribonucleic acid during infection with LSc poliovirus. Virology 54:290–293

Mosser AG, Caliguiri LA, Tamm I (1971) Blocking action of guanidine on poliovirus multiplication. Virology 45:653–663

Nair CN, Stowers JW, Singfield B (1979) Guanidine-sensitive Na$^+$ accumulation by poliovirus-infected HeLa cells. J Virol 31:184–189

Nakano M, Iwami S, Tagawa I (1963) A guanidine-dependent variant of poliovirus. Virology 21:264–266

Newman JFE, Cartwright B, Doel TR, Brown F (1979) Purification and identification of the RNA dependent RNA polymerase of foot-and-mouth disease virus. J Gen Virol 45:497–507

Nick H, Ahl R (1976) Inhibitors of foot-and-mouth disease virus. II. Temperature-dependence of the effect of guanidine on virus growth. Arch Virol 52:71–83

Noble J, Levintow L (1970) Dynamics of poliovirus-specific RNA synthesis and the effects of inhibitors of virus replication. Virology 40:634–642

Nomoto A, Lee YF, Wimmer E (1976) The 5′ end of poliovirus mRNA is not capped with m^{7}G(5′)ppp(5′)-Np. Proc Natl Acad Sci USA 73:375–380

Nomoto A, Detjen B, Pozzatti R, Wimmer E (1977a) The location of the polio genome protein in viral RNAs and its implication for RNA synthesis. Nature 268:208–213

Nomoto A, Kitamura N, Golini F, Wimmer E (1977b) The 5′ terminal structure of polio virion RNA and poliovirus mRNA differ only in the genome linked protein VPg. Proc Natl Acad Sci USA 74:5345–5349

O'Farrell P (1975) High resolution two-dimensional electrophoresis of proteins. J Biol Chem 250:4007–4021

Palmenberg A, Pallansch M, Rueckert R (1979) Protease required for processing picornaviral coat protein resides in the viral replicase gene. J Virol 32:770–778

Penman S, Summers D (1965) Effects on host metabolism following synchronous infection with poliovirus. Virology 27:614–620

Pérez-Bercoff R (1979) Replication of picornavirus RNA. In: Pérez-Bercoff R (ed) Molecular biology of picornaviruses. Plenum, New York, p 293

Pérez-Bercoff R, Gander M (1978) In vitro translation of mengovirus RNA deprived of the terminally-linked (capping?) protein. FEBS Lett 96:306–312

Pérez-Bercoff R, Cioé L, Degener AM, Meo P, Rita G (1979) Infectivity of mengovirus replicative form. IV. Intracellular conversion into replicative intermediate. Virology 96:307–310

Pérez-Bercoff R, Cioé L, Meo P, Carra G, Mechali M, Falcoff E, Rita G (1974) Infectivity of mengovirus replicative form. Relationship to cellular transcription. J Gen Virol 25:53–62

Petterson RF, Ambros V, Baltimore D (1978) Identification of a protein linked to nascent poliovirus RNA and to the polyuridylic acid of negative-strand RNA. J Virol 27:357–365

Philipson L, Bengston S, Barbera-Oro J (1966) The reversion of guanidine inhibition of poliovirus synthesis. Virology 29:317–329

Phillips B, Lundquist R, Maizel J (1980) Absence of subviral particles and assembly activity in HeLa cells infected with defective-interfering particles of poliovirus. Virology 100:116–124

Porter A, Fellner P, Black D, Rowlands D, Harris T, Brown F (1978) 3-Terminal nucleotide sequences in the genome RNA of picornavirus. Nature 276:298–300

Rekosh DM, Russell WC, Bellett AJD (1977) Identification of a protein linked to the ends of adenovirus DNA. Cell 11:283–295

Richards OG, Hey TD, Ehrenfeld E (1981) Two forms of VPg on poliovirus RNAs. J Virol 38:863–871

Rightsel WA, Dice JR, McAlpine RJ, Timm EA, McLean IW, Dixon GJ, Schabel FM (1961) Antiviral effect of guanidine. Science 134:558–559

Röder A, Koschel K (1974) Reversible inhibition of poliovirus RNA synthesis in vivo and in vitro by viral products. J Virol 14:846–852

Röder A, Koschel A (1975) Virus-specific proteins associated with the replication complex of poliovirus RNA. J Gen Virol 28:85–98

Rothberg P, Harris T, Nomoto A, Wimmer E (1978) O⁴-(5′uridylyl)tyrosine is the bond between the genome-linked protein and the RNA of poliovirus. Proc Natl Acad Sci USA 75:4868–4872

Rowlands DJ, Harris TJR, Brown F (1978) More precise location of the polycytidylic acid tract in foot-and-mouth disease virus RNA. J Virol 26:335–343

Rueckert R, Mathews T, Kew O, Pallausch M, McLean C, Omilianowski D (1979) Synthesis and processing of picornaviral polyprotein. In: Pérez-Bercoff R (ed) Molecular biology of picornaviruses. Plenum, New York, p 113

Saborio J, Pong S, Koch G (1974) Selective and reversible inhibition of initiation of protein synthesis in mammalian cells. J Mol Biol 85:195–211

Sangar DV (1979) The replication of picornaviruses. J Gen Virol 45:1–13

Sangar DV, Rowlands DJ, Harris TJR, Brown F (1977) A protein covalently linked to foot-and-mouth disease virus RNA. Nature 268:648–650

Sangar DV, Black DN, Rowlands DJ, Harris TJR, Brown F (1980) Location of the initiation site for protein synthesis on foot-and-mouth disease virus RNA by in vitro translation of defined fragments of RNA. J Virol 33:59–68

Saunders K, King AMQ, Slade WR, Newman JWI, McCahon D (1981) Coding arrangements of polypeptides in the middle of the FMDV genome: A possible site of action of guanidine. 5th Int Congress of Virology, Strasbourg, p 357

Shatkin AJ (1976) Capping of eucaryotic mRNAs. Cell 9:645–653

Spector DH, Baltimore D (1974) Requirement of 3′-terminal poly (adenylic acid) for the infectivity of poliovirus RNA. Proc Natl Acad Sci USA 71:2983–2987

Stein IM, Micklus MJ (1973) Concentrations in serum and urinary excretion of guanidine, 1-methylguanidine, and 1,1-dimethylguanidine in renal failure. Clin Chem 19:583–585

Steiner-Pryor A, Cooper P (1973) Temperature-sensitive poliovirus mutants defective in repression of host protein synthesis are also defective in structural protein. J Gen Virol 21:215–225

Sugiyama T, Korant B, Lonberg-Holm K (1972) RNA virus gene expression and its control. Annu Rev Microbiol 26:467–502

Summers DF, Levintow L (1965) Constitution and function of polysomes of poliovirus-infected HeLa cells. Virology 27:44–53

Summers DF, Maizel JV, Darnell JE (1967) The decrease in size and synthetic activity of poliovirus polysomeslate in the infectious cycle. Virology 31:427–435

Taber R, Rekosh D, Baltimore D (1971) Effect of pactamycin on synthesis of poliovirus protein: a method of genetic mapping. J Virol 8:395–401

Tershak DR (1964) Effect of 5-fluorouracil on poliovirus growth. Virology 24:264–269

Tershak DR (1974) Guanidine inhibition of poliovirus growth. Partial elimination by protease antagonists and low temperature. Can J Microbiol 20:817–824

Tershak DR (1982) Inhibition of poliovirus polymerase by guanidine in vitro. J Virol 41:313–318

Traub A, Diskin B, Rosenberg H, Kalmar E (1976) Isolation and properties of the replicase of EMC virus. J Virol 18:375–382

Vande Woude G, Ascione R (1974) Translation products of foot-and-mouth disease virus-infected baby hamster kidney cells. Archiv Ges Virusforsch 45:259–271

Varma JP (1968) Inhibition of tobacco necrosis virus by guanidine carbonate. Virology 36:305–308

Wimmer E (1972) Sequence studies of poliovirus RNA. I. Characterization of the 5'-terminus. J Mol Biol 68:537–540

Wimmer E (1979) The genome-linked protein of picornaviruses: discovery, properties, and possible functions. In: Pérez-Bercoff R (ed) Molecular biology of picornaviruses. Plenum, New York, p 175

Yin FH (1977a) Involvement of viral procapsid in the RNA synthesis and maturation of poliovirus. Virology 82:299–307

Yin FH (1977b) Possible in vitro repair of viral RNA by ligase-like enzyme(s) in poliovirus-infected cells. J Virol 21:61–68

Yogo Y, Wimmer E (1972) Polyadenylic acid at the 3' terminus of poliovirus RNA. Proc Natl Acad Sci USA 69:1877–1882

Yogo Y, Wimmer E (1973) Poly (A) and poly (U) in poliovirus double stranded RNA. Nature 242:171–174

CHAPTER 9

Benzimidazoles*

Selective Inhibitors of Picornavirus Replication in Cell Culture and in the Organism

H. J. EGGERS

A. Introduction and Historical Remarks

In the present discussion I shall focus on recent developments in the field of the virus-inhibitory action of benzimidazoles. Special emphasis will be placed on the effects of these compounds in the virus-infected and uninfected organism. Several reviews on the subject have appeared in the last two decades (TAMM and EGGERS 1963 a; EGGERS and TAMM 1966; TAMM and CALIGUIRI 1972; CALIGUIRI and TAMM 1973). I shall not deal in any detail with the effects of halogenated ribofuranosylbenzimidazoles on cellular and viral biosynthesis, since they have been summarized recently by TAMM and SEHGAL (1978).

Since 1952, benzimidazoles have been studied intensely as inhibitors of virus multiplication (TAMM et al. 1952). Extensive investigations on the relation between chemical structure and virus-inhibitory activity led to the key recognition that virus-inhibiting activity and cell toxicity of benzimidazole derivatives can vary independently (TAMM 1955, 1956a, b). These findings fitted well with the then growing concept that the biologic specificity of viruses resides in specific nucleoproteins, though at that time the precise basis of selective action could not be obvious. It was noted, however, that vitamins played a role in nucleic acid synthesis, and a benzimidazole nucleoside moiety, 5,6-dimethyl-1-α-D-ribofuranosylbenzimidazole, was known to be a structural part of vitamin B_{12}.

Starting with the central finding that benzimidazole derivatives did vary in selectivity, it was hoped that, upon appropriate chemical modification, highly virus-selective inhibitors might be found. The experimental studies developed in different directions.

1. Various halogenated ribofuranosylbenzimidazoles were found to inhibit multiplication of RNA and DNA viruses of different major groups as well as the synthesis of cellular DNA. The significance of these findings for the understanding of cellular and viral biosynthesis has been reviewed by TAMM and SEHGAL (1978), as indicated.

2. 5-Methyl-2-D-ribobenzimidazole (MRB) was shown to increase the yield of influenza virus (types A and B) in the chorioallantoic membrane from embryonated chicken eggs (TAMM 1956c). The compound had no enhancing effect on the multiplication of poliovirus or vaccinia virus; it did not increase measurably the metabolic activities of the host cells. At the time, this finding strengthened the view

---

* To JSB for enheartening consolation and reassurance during the long months of summer and fall 1980

that compounds with virus-selective action could be found. Subsequently, it was demonstrated (Tamm 1973), that MRB, in fact, restores the ability of chorioallantoic membranes from older chick embryos (e.g., 13-day-old) to produce larger yields of virus after infection with a low virus dose; untreated membranes from 13-day-old chick embryos produce only a fraction of virus compared with membranes from 7-day-old embryos in which MRB has no effect on the influenza virus yields. Thus, after all, MRB in this system seems to operate at the cellular level. Apparently, this effect is unrelated to the interferon system. The enhancing effect of MRB on influenza virus multiplication and structural requirements of benzimidazoles to obtain these effects are discussed by Tamm and Sehgal (1978).

3. Further support for the thesis that benzimidazoles might exhibit virus-specific activities came from the report by Hollinshead and Smith (1958) that 2-(α-hydroxybenzyl)-benzimidazole (HBB), given orally at the time of virus inoculation delayed or prevented death from poliovirus 2 infection in mice. Various other benzimidazole and purine derivatives were also reported to inhibit in tissue culture poliovirus, influenza A virus, and an adenovirus. In another study, Tamm and Nemes (1959) had found that HBB inhibits multiplication of poliovirus 2 in monkey kidney cell culture at concentrations which caused no microscopic changes in the cells. HBB had no direct inactivating activity on the infectivity of poliovirus 2. Influenza virus multiplication remained unaffected.

Thus, it was quite apparent that, contrary to common belief at the time, virus multiplication could be selectively inhibited. Subsequently, this thesis was amply substantiated; HBB was shown to inhibit members of the picornavirus group selectively (with significant exceptions), whereas representatives of other virus families remained unaffected. Mutants of HBB-sensitive picornaviruses were isolated which are resistant to or dependent on the drug. On the other hand, at concentrations inhibitory for picornavirus reprouction, HBB did not inhibit vital cellular metabolic activities. Morphological alterations in cells were not detectable and, most important, cell multiplication remained unaffected (Eggers and Tamm 1961 a). All these findings clearly demonstrated the virus-selective action of HBB. In further studies, it was shown that HBB inhibits the synthesis of picornavirus RNA (Eggers and Tamm 1962 a, 1963 a), the first demonstration of specific chemical inhibition of the synthesis of viral nucleic acid.

B. 2-(α-Hydroxybenzyl)-Benzimidazole

2-(α-Hydroxybenzyl)-benzimidazole (HBB; Fig. 1) and its antiviral activity has been studied in greater detail. The essential features are summarized in Sects. B.I–VII.

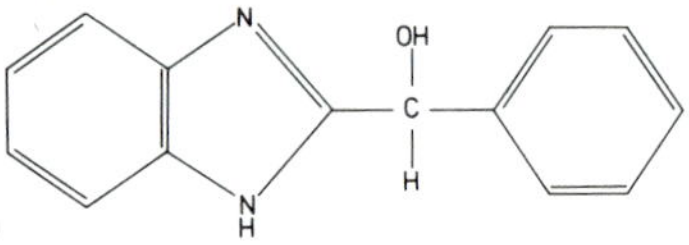

Fig. 1. 2-(α-Hydroxybenzyl)-benzimidazole (HBB)

I. Virus-Inhibitory Spectrum

As to be expected a priori for any inhibitor, the susceptibility of various viruses to HBB varies considerably. However, as already indicated, very soon after initiation of these studies (EGGERS and TAMM 1961 a, b), a remarkable pattern emerged. At concentrations of HBB nontoxic to cells, viz., 220 μM, the multiplication of many members of the genus *Enterovirus* was found to be inhibited, whereas members of other virus families were found insusceptible.

Inhibition of virus multiplication was determined in multiple cycle experiments in cell culture, whereby the development of viral cytopathic effects (CPE) was taken as indicative of virus multiplication. Cultures containing HBB, or control cultures with no HBB, were infected with about 100 median infective doses (ID_{50}) of virus and the development of CPE quantitated (percentage cells affected). Characteristic examples for HBB-susceptible and HBB-insusceptible viruses are shown in Fig. 2. This method has proven to be simple and to yield reproducible results. They correlate well with results obtained in single-cycle virus multiplication studies in the presence of various concentrations of HBB.

In many cases, it is not difficult to classify a virus as HBB-susceptible or not. Details are found in the excellent summary tables by TAMM and CALIGUIRI (1972). As an index of susceptibility one may take $\geq$ 75% inhibition of CPE by 220 μM HBB in comparison with untreated control cultures at any day of observation. Accordingly, many human enteroviruses were found to be susceptible: poliovirus 1–3, coxsackievirus B1–6, coxsackievirus A9, echovirus1–9, 11–21, and 24–27. HBB was also found to inhibit the multiplication of various porcine (DARDIRI et al. 1964) and bovine enteroviruses (DINTER 1964). There was, however, considerable variation in HBB sensitivity. Representative members of various other virus families were found to be insusceptible. Noteworthy were exceptions within the Picornavirus family (EGGERS and TAMM 1961 a). Echovirus 22 and 23 were found to be HBB insusceptible, thus confirming the distinct character of these types within the enterovirus group (SHAVER et al. 1961).

All type A coxsackieviruses other than A9 were found to be HBB insusceptible. It has been known for a long time that coxsackievirus A9 behaves more like an echovirus in that it replicates better in monkey kidney cell culture than in newborn mice (MELNICK and SABIN 1959). Rhinoviruses present a more complicated picture. However, it is fair to say that, despite some conflicting and inconsistent results, the majority of the types tested was found to be HBB insusceptible (EGGERS and TAMM 1961 a, b; TAMM and EGGERS 1962; HAMPARIAN et al. 1963; HAMRE et al. 1964; CONNELLY and HAMRE 1964; KISCH et al. 1964; WEBB et al. 1964; GWALTNEY 1968). Foot-and-mouth disease virus strains (aphthoviruses) were found to be HBB insusceptible (DINTER 1964; DARDIRI et al. 1964), a finding consistent with the fact that aphthoviruses differ in a number of characteristics from enteroviruses.

A so far unexplained result is the finding that members of the arenavirus family (three strains of lymphocytic choriomeningitis virus) are moderately HBB sensitive (PFAU and CAMYRE 1968). Whether this inhibition, like that seen with enteroviruses, is due to an effect on viral RNA synthesis is not known. It remains to be seen whether or not the effects of HBB are the same in apparently completely different virus families. In contrast to previous observations, inhibition of lympho-

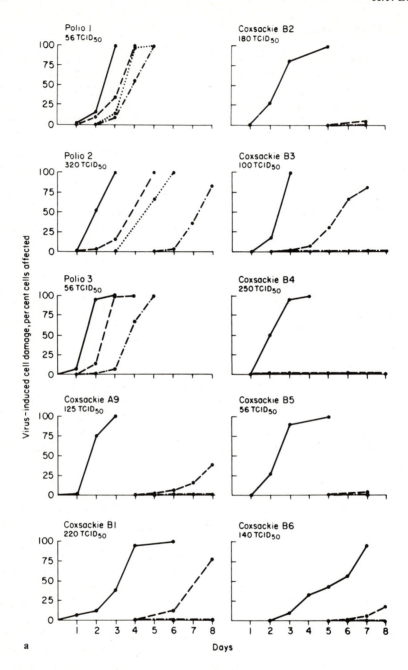

Fig. 2. a Inhibition by HBB of the cytopathic effects of HBB-susceptible enteroviruses in monkey kidney cell cultures. $TCID_{50}$ = median infective dose in tissue culture. Concentrations of HBB (μM): *full curve* 0; *dashed curve* (98); *dotted curve* (219); *dashed-dotted curve* (493). (EGGERS and TAMM 1961 a) **b** Lack of inhibitory effect of HBB on the virus-induced cell damage by HBB-insusceptible viruses. Concentrations of HBB as in a. (EGGERS and TAMM 1961 a)

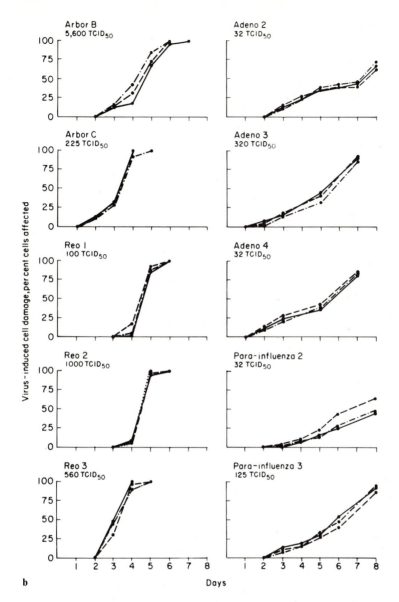

cytic choriomeningitis virus multiplication appears to be host cell dependent, i.e., inhibition is observed in HeLa cells, but not in L cells (PFAU 1975).

II. Effects of HBB on Uninfected Cells

The fact that concentrations of HBB highly inhibitory to susceptible enteroviruses (219 μM HBB) did not affect the virus yields of insusceptible viruses already suggested that essential metabolic pathways of cells might not be disturbed by HBB.

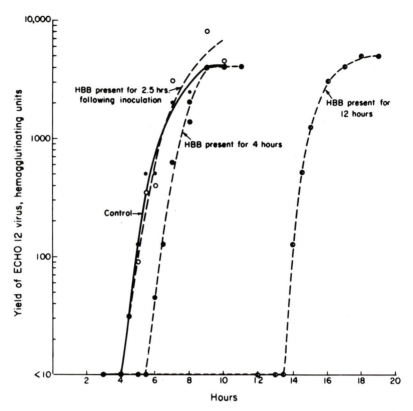

Fig. 3. Time course of echovirus 12 multiplication with 219 μM HBB present for 2.5, 4, or 12 h after virus inoculation. (Eggers and Tamm 1962a)

This conclusion turned out to be correct in further studies on the effects of HBB on metabolic reactions of uninfected primary monkey kidney cells.

Extensive morphological observations of HBB-treated primary monkey kidney cells for 5–7 days (up to 219 μM) had demonstrated no significant differences from untreated cultures (Eggers and Tamm 1961a). Only at 493 μM were minimal to moderate morphological changes seen after 3–5 days of incubation (granular appearance of the cytoplasm of the cells, particularly in batches of cultures of lesser quality). But even at 876 μM, only moderate changes were seen (Tamm et al. 1961, 1969; Eggers and Tamm 1961a; Tamm and Eggers 1962).

Concentrations of up to 493 μM HBB caused no effects on the following metabolic activities of monkey kidney cells (up to 3 h): cumulative O_2 uptake, glucose utilization, lactic acid production, adenosine ^{14}C uptake into RNA, and L-alanine uptake into proteins (Eggers and Tamm 1961a). At 219 μM, the uridine ^3H uptake into RNA was also unaffected during the duration of the experiment (6.5 h; Eggers and Tamm 1962a).

As a more complex activity, cell multiplication was also found to be unaffected in the presence of 219 μM HBB (Eggers and Tamm 1962a). Lack of effect on cell multiplication was also demonstrated for HeLa cells (Eggers and Tamm 1961a).

The nature of toxicity of HBB on cells at higher concentrations has not yet been defined, yet the essential point is the lack of demonstrable toxicity at concentrations of HBB (up to 219 μ*M*) which are highly virus inhibitory, a further strong argument in favor of the virus selectivity of HBB.

In the Ames test (AMES et al. 1977) D-HBB·HCl in concentrations of 1–5,000 μg/plate exhibited no mutagenic activity on five test strains (TA 98, TA 100, TA 1,535, TA 1,537, TA 1,538), independent of the presence or absence of liver homogenate (A. GRAFE, unpublished work 1980). D-HBB·HCl also proved nonmutagenic in the *Saccharomyces cerevisiae* test in a range of concentrations between 0.001 and 10 mg/ml (A. GRAFE unpublished work 1980).

III. Kinetics of Antiviral Action, Effects on Viral Replication, and Mechanism of Action

1. Kinetic Aspects of Action

The time course of the HBB-sensitive process on the viral replicative cycle has been well defined (EGGERS and TAMM 1962a). It was determined by removing or adding the compound at various times during the replication cycle. Figure 3 demonstrates that no HBB-inhibitable process takes place during the first 2.5 h of the latent period, but that during the last 1.5 h of this period an HBB-inhibitable process does occur. It can also be seen in this experiment that the activity of HBB is fully reversible. Once the HBB-inhibitable process has started, HBB has a prompt inhibitory effect on the production of *infectious* virus: within 15 min at most, when infectious virus production comes to a complete stop. This interval extends beyond the latent period until the latest rapid increase phase (H. J. EGGERS, unpublished work 1974; HALPEREN et al. 1964). This has been shown, not only for echovirus 12, but also for coxsackievirus A9 (EGGERS et al. 1963b). The observed effects in mass cultures are not due to asynchrony of infection, since HBB also stops ongoing virus replication in single cells (CALIGUIRI et al. 1965).

2. Effects on the Virus Replication Cycle

It was obvious from the kinetics of the antiviral action of HBB that early steps of viral multiplication might not be affected by the compound. This was in fact shown to be the case; adsorption and virus penetration, measured as cell-adsorbed virus no longer neutralizable by virus-specific antibody, remained unaffected (EGGERS and TAMM 1962a); also uncoating of the virus proceeded normally (EGGERS and WAIDNER 1970). Uncoating was measured as the acquisition of light resistance by virus sensitized to neutral red in infected cells. Furthermore, sequential treatment of cells infected with echovirus 12, first with HBB and subsequently with 2-thio-4-oxothiazolidine (rhodanine), a specific inhibitor of virus uncoating, had no effect on virus replication, again confirming the lack of effect of HBB on uncoating (EGGERS 1977).

In picornavirus-infected cells, viral RNA and viral protein synthesis are continuing throughout the rapid-increase phase of virus production (LURIA et al. 1978). The kinetics of the HBB-inhibitable process, therefore, suggested an effect

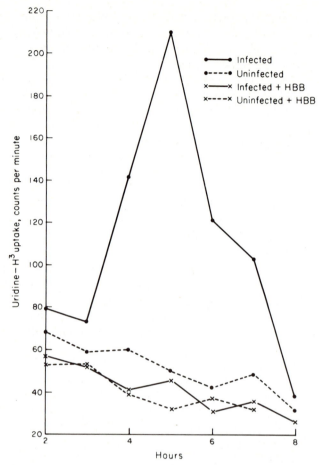

Fig. 4. Coxsackievirus A9 stimulation of RNA synthesis in actinomycin-treated monkey kidney cells, and its inhibition by 219 μ*M* HBB. Curves are indicated by: *circles and full curve* (infected); *circles and broken curve* (uninfected); *crosses and full curve* (infected plus HBB); *crosses and broken curve* (uninfected plus HBB). (Eggers and Tamm 1963a)

on virus macromolecular synthesis. This was in fact shown to be the case; synthesis of infectious viral RNA was demonstrated to be inhibited by HBB in cells infected with echovirus 12, coxsackievirus A9, and coxsackievirus B4 (Eggers and Tamm 1962a). Inhibition of synthesis of viral RNA by HBB has also been demonstrated through measurements of the rates of incorporation of uridine ³H into virus-specific RNA in actinomycin-treated cells (Figs. 4 and 5), thus excluding the possibility that HBB might in some way inhibit only the acquisition of infectivity of viral RNA which has already been synthesized (Eggers and Tamm 1963a; B. Rosenwirth and H. J. Eggers, unpublished work 1977).

Dose–response curves, describing inhibition of infectious virus and viral RNA, ran an essentially similar course, though some deviations were apparent (Eggers and Tamm 1962a). Whether these were exclusively due to the relatively crude

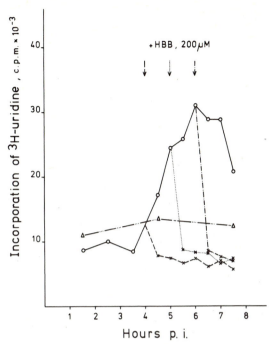

Fig. 5. Rapid stop of echovirus 12 stimulation of RNA synthesis in actinomycin-treated GMK cells by 200 μ*M* D-HBB·HCl at various times during the exponential-increase period of the virus. Curves are indicated by: *circles* (infected); *triangles* (uninfected); *crosses* indicate HBB at the following times: *dashed curve* (4 h); *dotted curve* (5 h); *dashed-dotted curve* (6 h). (B. Rosenwirth and H. J. Eggers, unpublished work 1976)

methods used and/or the more complex system (free and encapsidated viral RNA in infected cells) remains undecided. Yet, the dichotomy might also signal some differential effect on viral RNA synthesis and virus production.

In kinetic experiments with a relatively high concentration of HBB (200 μ*M*), however, there was no indication of a differential effect on viral RNA and virion synthesis. Within 30 min after addition of HBB to cells infected with echovirus 12 during various times of the rapid-increase phase of virus, no viral RNA synthesis was detectable in uridine ³H pulses (Fig. 5). As already indicated, virus production has also been shown to come to a complete stop within 15 min after addition of the compound. Only experiments with lower concentrations of HBB might settle the point of whether there is a differential effect of HBB on production of infectious virus and viral RNA.

Cessation of viral RNA synthesis eventually stops viral protein synthesis. The use of the hemagglutinating echovirus 12, however, clearly demonstrated a differential effect of HBB on viral protein and virion synthesis. It could be shown that the increase in virus hemagglutinin for a period of approximately 1–1.5 h after addition of HBB (Fig. 6) was exclusively due to formation of empty capsids, whereas synthesis of the RNA-containing virions had come to an immediate stop (Fig. 7; Eggers and Tamm 1962a; Halperen et al. 1964), a result in complete agreement with the rapid stop of infectious virus after addition of HBB. Furthermore, it was

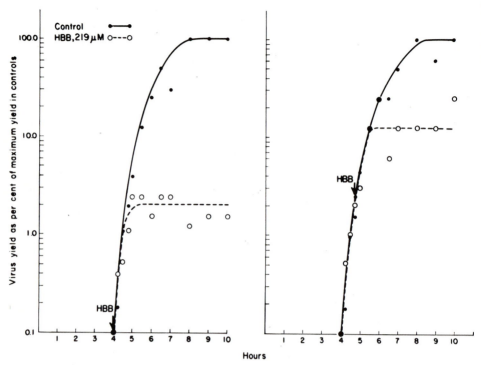

Fig. 6. Effects of HBB on production of echovirus 12 hemagglutinin when the compound is added during the exponential increase in virus. (EGGERS and TAMM 1962a)

shown that the empty capsids produced after addition of HBB were comprised of polypeptides, synthesized after addition of the compound (HALPEREN et al. 1964). This experiment demonstrates that HBB does not directly inhibit synthesis of viral capsid proteins. It may also give some indication of the lifetime of enterovirus messenger RNA, although we are aware of the fact that by the addition of HBB to the cultures, a highly regulated system has been severely disturbed.

It thus appears that some aspects of the virus-inhibitory activity of HBB can be explained by its inhibiting effects on viral RNA synthesis. Therefore, a study was indicated to determine the effects of HBB on the appearance in enterovirus-infected cells of virus RNA polymerase activity (BALTIMORE et al. 1963). This was done in poliovirus-infected HeLa cells. Addition of HBB to infected cells during the early rapid-increase phase of virus multiplication caused a marked decrease in viral polymerase activity to almost background level, as demonstrated in an assay in cell extracts. On the other hand, the compound had no apparent effect on the activity of the viral enzyme preparation when added to the cell-free RNA polymerase assay.

At first glance, these findings might be interpreted as follows: HBB inhibits the synthesis of a virus-directed RNA polymerase, the enzyme responsible for the replication of viral RNA. With inhibition of synthesis of the RNA polymerase the replication of viral RNA also comes to a halt which, in turn, finally leads to inhibition of synthesis of viral capsid polypeptides. This straightforward interpretation, how-

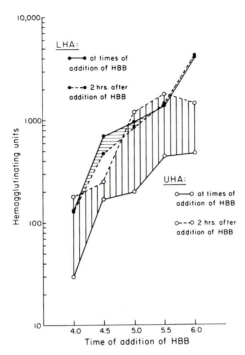

Fig. 7. Changes in UHA (upper hemagglutinin; empty capsids) and LHA (lower hemagglutinin; complete infectious virus) in a 2-h period of incubation with 219 μM HBB, added at various times in the viral replication cycle. Curves are indicated by: *full circles* (LHA); *open circles* (UHA); *full curves* (at time of addition of HBB); *broken curves* (2 h after addition of HBB). HALPEREN et al. 1964)

ever, raises difficulties. It would imply a differential effect on viral protein synthesis, since capsid protein synthesis continues for at least 1 h after addition of HBB. Does synthesis of viral capsid proteins also mean synthesis of the enterovirus polyprotein including noncapsid proteins such as viral RNA polymerase?

After addition of HBB to enterovirus-infected cells, a central finding is the rapid halt, not only of production of infectious virus, but also of viral RNA synthesis. This observation makes it unlikely that inhibition of viral RNA synthesis by HBB is mediated directly through inhibition of synthesis of viral RNA polymerase. Though the latter appears unstable during the viral replication cycle (EGGERS et al. 1963 a), the rapid and complete stop of viral RNA synthesis after addition of HBB cannot be explained by this mechanism. Rather, a direct effect of HBB on viral RNA synthesis appears much more plausible.

This interpretation might appear to be in conflict with the observation that the in vitro enzyme activity is apparently unimpaired by the inhibitor. However, it must be kept in mind that the preparation used is very crude, consisting of template and enzymes probably under nonoptimal conditions. The incorporation of precursors into RNA in this system may, in a large part, be due to a completion of nascent RNA chains rather than initiation of new chains (CALIGUIRI and TAMM 1968 a, b). In fact, the RNA products synthesized under these conditions in the presence of HBB have not been sufficiently characterized and may be quite different from those synthesized in the infected cell (see Chap. 8; Dmitrieva and Agol 1974). Thus, a reasonable working hypothesis suggests that HBB in some way inhibits viral RNA synthesis, thereby inhibiting multiplication of infectious virus (see also Sect. B.V).

3. Mechanism of Action

In molecular terms, the precise site of action of HBB is not known. As to guanidine, various speculations have been presented in Chap. 8. Though the virus-inhibitory mechanisms of action of guanidine and HBB (including its derivatives) are not identical, similar systems may by involved. The complexity of the replication processes of the picornaviruses makes a precise analysis very difficult. One of many facets we may point out again is the interrelationships between viral capsid proteins and viral RNA synthesis (Cooper et al. 1970; Korant 1977; Adrian et al. 1979). A most fruitful approach seems to us to be a study of conformational modifications of the viral proteins by various effectors (Eggers and Tamm 1966). It should be stressed, however, that in contrast to guanidine, the virus-inhibitory activity of HBB appears to be unaffected by temperature and metabolites (antiguanidines).

IV. HBB Resistance and Dependence: Genetics of the System

After prolonged incubation of cells infected with a drug-sensitive virus in the presence of not-too-high concentrations of HBB, resistant virus populations commonly emerge (Eggers and Tamm 1961 a). This is illustrated in Fig. 8. Clonal populations of susceptible and resistant virus particles were prepared by the plaque isolation technique. Clones of varying degrees of HBB resistance were obtained. Upon repeated passage of the various cloned populations in the absence of HBB, the original degree of HBB susceptibility or resistance did not change, indicating that sensitivity to HBB is a genetic property of the virion (Tamm and Eggers 1963 b).

An HBB-resistant mutant exhibits only a slight increase in resistance to guanidine·HCl, another specific inhibitor of picornavirus replication, and vice versa (Tamm and Eggers 1962). Other differences between HBB and guanidine will be discussed in Sect. B.VI. However, it should be noted that combined treatment with both HBB and guanidine has a superadditive effect (Eggers and Tamm 1963 c) besides the suppressive effects on the emergence of the resistant mutants, a consequence of the limited cross-resistance between HBB and guanidine.

It has not been determined whether HBB only selects preexisting HBB-resistant mutants or whether mutations to HBB resistance are also drug induced. Some difficulty in doing such experiments comes from the fact that there exist in any virus population virus particles that exhibit differing degrees of HBB resistance, and altogether represent a continuous spectrum of varying HBB sensitivities. This situation may also account for the observation that resistant virus often emerges from treated cultures infected with low doses of infective virus (Eggers and Tamm 1961 a). HBB has no direct inactivating effects on the infectivity of virus (Eggers and Tamm 1961 a) or on the viral RNA (Eggers and Tamm 1962 a).

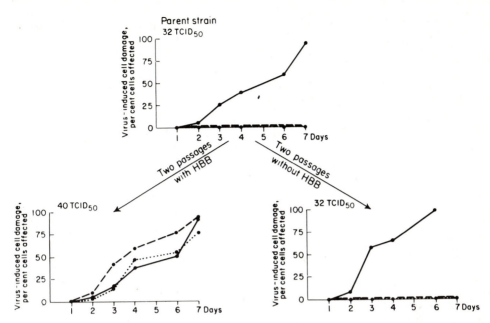

Fig. 8. Emergence of an HBB-resistant variant of coxsackievirus A9 after two passages in the presence of 98 μM HBB. Concentrations of HBB (μM) *full curve* (0); *dashed curve* (98); *dotted curve* (219). (EGGERS and TAMM 1961 a)

In addition to HBB-resistant mutants, HBB-dependent mutants of various enteroviruses have been isolated (EGGERS 1962; EGGERS and TAMM 1962 b, 1963 b). This represented the first demonstration of drug dependence in viruses. It was discovered when HBB-sensitive coxsackievirus A9 was plaqued with HBB in the overlay. A single plaque developed, and the virus contained in it could only be passaged optimally with HBB in the culture medium.

Apparently HBB dependence is genetically determined; infective RNA extracted from the HBB-dependent virus is unable to induce production of new virus without HBB. HBB-dependent virus does adsorb and undergo early virus–cell interactions in the absence of compound. HBB is required for the RNA synthesis of HBB-dependent virus. This has been demonstrated by measuring the replication of infectious RNA of dependent virus and by determining the incorporation of uridine ^{3}H into viral RNA in actinomycin-treated cells infected with HBB-dependent coxsackievirus A9 (EGGERS et al. 1963 b). During the exponential-increase period of HBB-dependent virus, the continued presence of compound is required. The data presented and the results of kinetic experiments suggest that the drug-dependent and drug-sensitive processes may be biochemically analogous, since dependence and sensitivity are the apparent opposites of one another (EGGERS et al. 1963 b).

Nevertheless, regarding the compounds, the structural requirements for the processes of dependence and inhibition are not the same, in that the requirements for the selective virus-inhibitory activity are more stringent. For replication of dependent mutants, HBB can be substituted by 2-(*o*-hydroxybenzyl)-benzimidazole, by 5-methyl-2-D-ribobenzimidazole and unsubstituted bezimidazole, but these compounds exhibit little or no selective virus-inhibitory activity. Adenosine (1 mM), imidazole (2 mM), arginine (60 mM), histidine (20 mM), and creatinine (2 mM) were without effect (EGGERS and TAMM 1963 b).

Surprisingly, guanidine·HCl fully supports the multiplication of HBB-dependent enteroviruses at concentrations which are required for marked inhibition of the drug-sensitive parent virus (EGGERS and TAMM 1963 b). The guanidine-requiring process of HBB-dependent coxsackievirus A9 also begins during the second half of the latent period (EGGERS et al. 1965 b). Its duration has not been exactly determined, since, despite repeated washings, guanidine is retained in monkey kidney cells (EGGERS et al. 1965 b).

HBB-dependent mutants give rise among their progeny to HBB-independent virus particles with considerable frequency. Even after repeated cloning in the presence of HBB, no clones were obtained consisting entirely of HBB-dependent particles, i.e., there was always a proportion (in the range of 0.2%–1% for coxsackievirus A9) of HBB-independent virus (EGGERS and TAMM 1963 b). Back mutation is either to drug resistance or sensitivity. However, in the presence of HBB, resistant mutants are more commonly observed, probably a consequence of selection due to the presence of the virus-inhibitory compound.

To avoid this difficulty, use was made of the unsubstituted benzimidazole which permits optimum multiplication of HBB-dependent coxsackievirus A9 at concentrations which do not inhibit the reproduction of sensitive virus (EGGERS and TAMM 1963 b, 1965). The virus was plaqued in the presence of 1 mM benzimidazole. Three plaques that developed at high dilution of virus were picked and replaqued in the presence or absence of HBB to ascertain that HBB-dependent virus had been obtained. Revertants from HBB dependence were isolated by picking random plaques from these subclones, which had been plaqued in the absence of HBB. After one passage of the individual clones in monkey kidney tube cultures in the absence of compound (to eliminate possible residual HBB-dependent virus), the drug-independent clones were tested for HBB sensitivity or resistance. The 79 clones tested revealed a whole spectrum of sensitivities to HBB. At one extreme, highly sensitive clones were found; at the other, there were some clones completely resistant to 100 μM HBB. Over this wide range all degrees of sensitivity were almost evenly distributed (EGGERS and TAMM 1965). Samples of clones of these revertant HBB-independent virus particles proved genetically stable. On the basis of these experiments, it is not possible to determine precisely the mutation frequency from HBB dependence to independence. However, the mutation indices for the three plaques tested indicate a frequency in the order of 10^{-4} mutations per replication.

As already discussed, passage of HBB-sensitive wild-type virus in the presence of HBB readily permits the isolation of HBB-resistant mutants of varying degrees of resistance. The simplest explanation – particularly in conjunction with the results obtained in the studies on mutation from HBB dependence to independence – is to assume that, during replication of HBB-sensitive virus, mutants of varying degrees of resistance to HBB arise which are then selected by the presence of the compounds. Similar studies have been carried out with guanidine-resistant and guanidine-dependent mutants (MELNICK et al. 1961; LODDO et al. 1962; LEDINKO

1963; EGGERS and TAMM 1965). On the basis of all of the available results, it can be proposed that picornaviruses may occur in any state of drug sensitivity, drug resistance, or drug dependence, and may mutate directly to any other state.

V. Rescue

Rescue phenomena have been demonstrated with guanidine-sensitive, guanidine-resistant, and guanidine-dependent polioviruses (CORDS and HOLLAND 1964; HOLLAND and CORDS 1964; WECKER and LEDERHILGER 1964; AGOL and SHIRMAN 1964; IKEGAMI et al. 1964). In particular, it was shown that either guanidine-sensitive or guanidine-resistant poliovirus, replicating in HeLa cells, permit the simultaneous multiplication of guanidine-dependent mutants of poliovirus in the absence of the drug. Conversely, guanidine-dependent or guanidine-resistant poliovirus can rescue guanidine-sensitive poliovirus strains in HeLa cells treated with guanidine. The genotype of the rescued virus is that of the parent virus, though, phenotypically, the rescued virus has acquired (at least in part) the capsid of the assisting virus. The results support the hypothesis that the assisting virus supplies a function for the rescued one. A likely candidate for supplying such a function is the viral RNA polymerase.

In analogous experiments, it has been demonstrated that HBB-dependent coxsackievirus A9 can be rescued in monkey kidney cells by HBB-sensitive echovirus 7 in the absence of HBB. Conversely, no significant rescue of HBB-sensitive echovirus 7 by HBB-dependent coxsackievirus A9 could be demonstrated in cultures treated with 100 μM HBB. This phenomenon may be due to inhibitory effects of HBB on processes other than synthesis of viral RNA polymerase which the assisting virus would not be expected to alter.

As indicated in Sect. B.III.2, a direct effect of HBB on viral RNA synthesis, not mediated by the viral RNA polymerase, appears plausible. Thus, rescue of an HBB-sensitive virus in the presence of HBB may not be possible. The relation to the guanidine system is not clear at present. However, in this connection it should be mentioned that not all combinations in the guanidine system resulted in rescue. For example, a guanidine-resistant poliovirus 1 (derived from the drug-sensitive Brunhilde strain) did not rescue the drug-sensitive poliovirus 2 (P 712-ch-2ab) in guanidine-treated cultures (IKEGAMI et al. 1964). Lastly, technical problems may sometimes play a role also, since primary monkey kidney cultures are infected by echovirus 7 and coxsackievirus A9 with only low efficiency (IKEGAMI et al. 1964).

VI. Superadditive Antiviral Effects of HBB and Guanidine

As indicated, an HBB-resistant mutant exhibits only a slight increase in resistance to guanidine, and vice versa. In multiple-cycle experiments, combined treatment with HBB and guanidine has proven much more effective than treatment with either compound alone in suppressing the multiplication of susceptible enteroviruses (TAMM and EGGERS 1962).

The basis for this increased effectiveness appears to be two-fold. First, it is to be assumed to be due to the limited cross-resistance between HBB and guanidine, whereby resistant mutants do have a reduced probability of replication. Second,

Table 1. Superadditive effects of HBB, 1-propyl-HBB, and guanidine on the multiplication of coxsackievirus A9, strain 530. (H.J. Eggers, unpublished work 1976)

Compound	Concentration (μM)	Virus yield	
		PFU/0.2 ml	% of untreated control
None		1.1×10^8	100
D-HBB · HCl	10	7.2×10^7	65.5
	20	1.6×10^7	14.5
	40	7.7×10^3	0.0070
Guanidine · HCl	200	8.9×10^7	80.9
	400	7.8×10^7	70.9
	800	2.5×10^6	2.3
1-Propyl-HBB · HCl	2	6.2×10^7	56.4
	4	3.0×10^4	0.027
	8	$< 10^1$	$<$ 0.00001
D-HBB · HCl:guanidine · HCl	10:100	1.2×10^7	10.9
	20:100	5.6×10^3	0.0051
	10:200	9.0×10^4	0.082
	20:200	1.4×10^2	0.00013
1-Propyl-HBB · HCl:guanidine · HCl	1:100	8.5×10^7	77.2
	2:100	1.7×10^6	1.6
	1:200	2.7×10^7	24.5
	2:200	1.9×10^4	0.018

however, there is evidence for a superadditive virus-inhibitory action of the two compounds on enterovirus multiplication (Eggers and Tamm 1963c). This is clearly shown in Table 1. Coxsackievirus A9, strain 530, was grown in GMK cells (a continuous line derived from kidney cells of the green monkey, *Cercopithecus aethiops*) in a single infectious cycle. D-HBB·HCl and guanidine·HCl, either alone or in combination, were added to the cultures at the end of the viral adsorption period. The cultures were harvested 8 h after virus inoculation and virus yields were determined by plaque assay. D-HBB, 10 μM, or guanidine, up to 400 μM, had no significant effect on virus reproduction when given alone. Two-fold higher concentrations of D-HBB or guanidine reduced the virus yields 7–50-fold. On the other hand, 10 μM D-HBB plus 200 μM guanidine, given in combination, inhibited virus reproduction by a factor of more than 1,000, 20 μM D-HBB plus 200 μM guanidine reduced the virus yield to 10^{-6} of the control value. Thus, the superadditive (synergistic) effects of D-HBB (or HBB) and guanidine are quite apparent.

The molecular basis of the synergism between HBB and guanidine is not known. Both are inhibitors of picornavirus replication, both inhibit the synthesis of viral RNA and functional viral RNA polymerase, and both apparently do not directly affect viral protein syntheses (Halperen et al. 1964). However, some differences should be noted. The virus-inhibitory spectrum of both compounds is different (Tamm and Caliguiri 1972; Caliguiri and Tamm 1972). Drug-resistant mutants exhibit only limited cross-resistance, as already indicated. The virus-inhibi-

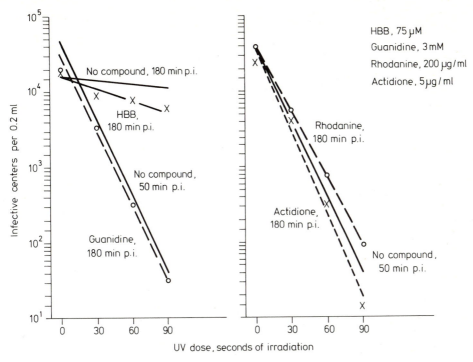

Fig. 9. Acquisition of UV irradiation resistance by echovirus 12 in GMK cell-infective centers with time after infection. Effects of D-HBB·HCl, guanidine·HCl, rhodanine, or actidione. (H. J. EGGERS, unpublished work 1976). (Method according to EGGERS et al. 1965 a)

tory action of HBB could not be blocked by uridine, cytidine, adenosine, or guanosine (EGGERS and TAMM 1962a). On the other hand, certain amino acids, choline, and certain other compounds containing methyl or ethyl groups are able to block the antiviral effect of guanidine (DINTER and BENGTSSON 1964; LWOFF and LWOFF 1964; PHILIPSON et al. 1966; LODDO et al. 1966).

On the basis of kinetic experiments it seems very likely that virus multiplication becomes sensitive to guanidine 1–2 h after virus inoculation (EGGERS et al. 1963 b, 1965 b), somewhat earlier in the latent period than has been determined for HBB (EGGERS and TAMM 1962a). Some support for this view is provided by results of UV irradiation experiments, using the infective center technique (EGGERS et al. 1965a). The capability of infective centers to produce virus is readily destroyed by UV irradiation if the cells are irradiated shortly after infection. However, the infective centers become resistant to UV irradiation between 50 and 110 min after virus inoculation. This resistance to UV irradiation does not develop if the infected cells are treated with guanidine or actidione (Fig. 9). However, infective centers treated with concentrations of D-HBB which inhibit echovirus 12 multiplication to the same degree as guanidine, do acquire resistance to UV irradiation with time after infection (Fig. 9; H. J. EGGERS, unpublished work 1976). This finding seems to support further the thesis that HBB acts somewhat later in the replication cycle than guanidine. However, a straightforward interpretation of these findings is limited

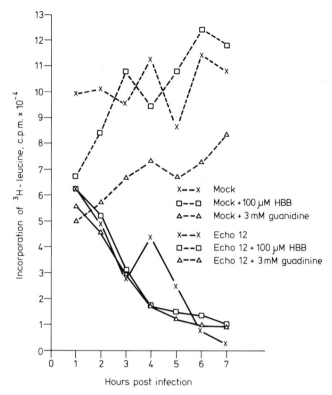

Fig. 10. Host cell protein synthesis shutoff in GMK cells infected with echovirus 12. Lack of effect on shutoff by D-HBB·HCl or guanidine·HCl. Curves are indicated by: *broken curves* (control); *full curves* (echovirus 12); *crosses* (no treatment); *squares* (plus 100 μM HBB); *triangles* (plus 3 mM guanidine). (B. ROSENWIRTH and EGGERS, unpublished work 1978). (Methods according to ROSENWIRTH and EGGERS 1977, 1978)

by the observation that higher concentrations of HBB (100–200 μM) also increasingly tend to prevent the acquisition of UV irradiation resistance with time after virus infection (H. J. EGGERS, unpublished work 1976). As expected, 2-thio-4-oxothiazolidine (rhodanine), a selective inhibitor of uncoating of echovirus 12 (EGGERS 1977) also prevents the acquisition of UV irradiation resistance (Fig. 9).

VII. Effects of HBB on Enterovirus-Infected Cells

HBB markedly delays the development of enterovirus-induced morphological changes in monkey kidney cells, though the ultimate degeneration of the infected cells cannot be prevented, even in the absence of detectable virus replication (BABLANIAN et al. 1966). The virus-induced morphological changes are quite different from those observed in infected, untreated cells. A likely hypothesis to explain the ultimate degeneration of infected, HBB-treated cells consists of the following (see also Fig. 10). In GMK cells infected with echovirus 12 and treated with D-HBB (under conditions where more than 99% of the cells are infected) cellular protein and RNA shutoff occurs with kinetics indistinguishable from that of infected, untreated cells. Under these circumstances it seems unlikely that the cell can survive for any length of time, though cytopathic effects are not visible before 24 h postinfection (in infected, untreated cells cytopathic effects are complete by 6–8 h postinfection).

Virus-induced, cellular shutoff has also been observed in poliovirus-infected cells treated with guanidine (BABLANIAN et al. 1965 a, b). A difficulty in interpreting the results of those studies resides in the fact that the kinetics of cellular shutoff in treated cells have been somewhat slower than in untreated infected cells. The results already mentioned, obtained with HBB and also with guanidine, however, (Fig. 10) clearly demonstrate that the conventional virus-induced morphological alterations cannot be due to the phenomenon of cellular shutoff, but may be due to the synthesis of virus-specific proteins, perhaps capsid proteins (BABLANIAN et al. 1965 a, b; see also BIENZ et al. 1980).

HBB prevents the development in LLC-MK2 cells (a continuous line of rhesus monkey kidney cells), infected with echovirus 12, of cytoplasmic membrane-bound bodies (SKINNER et al. 1968); this phenomenon is also seen with guanidine in poliovirus-infected HeLa cells (DALES et al. 1965). Further studies are needed to analyze in sequence the complex events leading ultimately to virus-induced cell death.

C. HBB and Guanidine Chemotherapy in Animals

I. Description of the Mouse System: Successful Treatment of Enterovirus-Infected Animals

HBB is a very potent inhibitor of enterovirus multiplication in cell culture, preventing any detectable virus replication in cell culture (less than 10^{-8} infectious units compared with the untreated control group; EGGERS and WAIDNER 1970), but only recently has information appeared about its protective effects in virus-infected animals. Experiments with HBB or its derivatives in mice or cynomolgus monkeys yielded only marginal effects; in fact, in most cases – despite assertions to the contrary – a striking antiviral activity was not observed (HOLLINSHEAD and SMITH 1958; FARA and COCHRAN 1963; O'SULLIVAN et al. 1969). The discrepancy between the results in cell culture systems and in animals has been explained on the basis of rapid emergence of drug-resistant mutants, which can readily be isolated in cell culture, as described in Sect. C.IV.

In view of the high antiviral potency of HBB and also that of guanidine, a systematic reinvestigation of the problem was initiated first in newborn mice infected with echovirus 9 (EGGERS 1976). This system has the advantage that even a modest inhibition of virus multiplication would become clinically apparent, since, for paralysis to occur in this system, virus multiplication has to lead to a critical level of virus concentrations within 4–5 days after birth (EGGERS and SABIN 1959).

In the first experiments, an attempt was made to work under optimum conditions to achieve clinical improvements. D-HBB·HCl, either alone or in combination with guanidine·HCl, was injected subcutaneously twice daily into mice, starting at the time of virus inoculation. The dose injected was calculated to achieve a

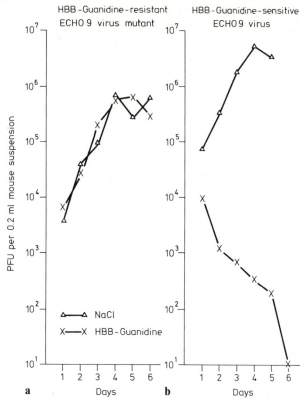

Fig. 11a, b. Uninhibited multiplication of an HBB plus guanidine-resistant echovirus 9 mutant **a** in mice treated with HBB plus guanidine twice daily for 10.5 days. **b** Effects of treatment on the multiplication of the drug-sensitive parent virus. Curves are indicated by: *triangles* (saline); *crosses* (HBB plus guanidine). (Eggers 1976)

concentration of 200 μM D-HBB·HCl (and 2 mM guanidine·HCl), assuming an even distribution of the compounds in the body. Drugs were inoculated every 12 h. Newborn mice infected with echovirus 9 or coxsackievirus A9 were protected from paralysis and death by combined treatment with such concentrations of D-HBB and guanidine. D-HBB alone also protected animals infected with coxsackievirus A9 animals, but not – in the first series of experiments – those infected with echovirus 9, whereas guanidine alone was found to be ineffective in both cases.

In order to demonstrate that the protective effects of treatment are in fact due to the virus-selective activity of the compounds, the following experiments were carried out. First, it was shown in drug-treated and protected animals that virus multiplication was inhibited (Eggers 1976). Second, an echovirus 9 mutant, doubly resistant to HBB and guanidine, was prepared in cell culture and used to infect other animals. The multiplication of this mutant was unaffected in treated mice which did not respond to treatment (Fig. 11). For comparison, the multiplication of a drug-sensitive echovirus 9 in mice treated either with saline or D-HBB plus guanidine under standard conditions is shown. The treated mice, in this case, did not exhibit any clinical signs and virus multiplication was inhibited.

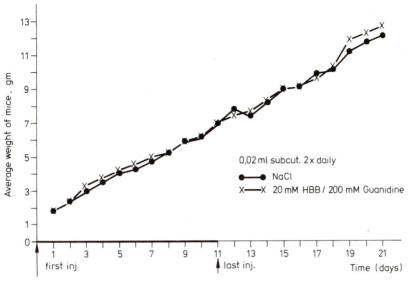

Fig. 12. Weight gain of newborn mice inoculated subcutaneously twice daily for 11 days with 20 mM D-HBB·HCl plus 200 mM guanidine·HCl compared with saline controls. Curves are indicated by: *circles* (saline); *crosses* (200 mM HBB plus 200 mM guanidine). (EGGERS 1976)

Toxicity experiments were carried out by treating mice from single litters with saline or test substances and their weights were recorded daily. Under these conditions, 20 mM D-HBB·HCl or 100 mM guanidine (0.02 ml inoculated subcutaneously, twice daily) did not prove toxic, nor, in most cases, did the combined injection of 20 mM HBB plus 200 mM guanidine (Fig. 12). Higher doses of guanidine were toxic. Subcutaneous inoculation of 0.02 ml 20 mM D-HBB·HCl three times daily, was the maximum tolerated regimen.

In Chinese hamsters *(Cricetulus griseus)* the effect of D-HBB·HCl on sister chromatid exchange in bone marrow cells has been tested. The experiments were performed in male and female animals, 18 weeks old (weight about 40 g). D-HBB·HCl at a single dose of 1,000 mg/kg exhibited no mutagenic effects (A. GRAFE, unpublished work 1980).

II. Failure of Drug-Resistant Mutants to Emerge in Animals

The hypothesis that failure of treatment may be due to emergence of drug-resistant mutants has been tested. Echovirus 9 or coxsackievirus A9 recovered from animals which had been treated with either saline, D-HBB, or guanidine twice daily for 7 days or longer, and had not responded to treatment, was tested for HBB and guanidine sensitivity, respectively. No difference in drug sensitivity between the various isolates could be detected. Also, no change in sensitivity was apparent in comparison with the virus originally inoculated into the mice. Since studies of this kind have been carried out with very large numbers of animals (EGGERS 1976, H. J. EGGERS, unpublished work 1977), it is concluded that failure of treatment

Table 2. Effects of D-HBB · HCl treatment[a] on echovirus 9 disease in newborn mice. (H.J. Eggers and G. Federmann, unpublished work 1976)

Saline	20 mM D-HBB · HCl
21/21	3/10
(14/21 died)	(0/10 died)

[a] 0.02 ml drug administered subcutaneously three times daily for 10 days, beginning at time of virus inoculation. Figures show number of mice paralyzed as a fraction of total number of mice

with D-HBB or guanidine alone must not be a result of development of drug-resistant mutants. O'Sullivan et al. (1969) in a study with 1-propyl-HBB in mice infected with coxsackievirus A9, also found no evidence of emergence of resistant virus (see also Sect. C.III). On the other hand, Fara and Cochran (1963) reported the development of HBB resistance in poliovirus isolated from the central nervous system of HBB-treated, paralyzed cynomolgus monkeys.

If, at least in most cases, drug-resistant virus does not emerge, why then should only combined treatment of infected mice with HBB plus guanidine be successful? All available evidence today is in favor of the thesis that the synergistic effects of HBB plus guanidine play a decisive role in achieving good protective effects.

III. The Importance of Drug Distribution, Metabolism, and Elimination on Therapeutic Efficacy

1. Introduction

In a reinvestigation of the effects of D-HBB alone on mice infected with echovirus 9, it could be shown that application of 20 mM D-HBB·HCl three times daily has definite protective activity (Table 2). This is in line with previous results obtained with mice infected with coxsackievirus A9, where marginal, though definite, protective effects could be achieved with D-HBB·HCl alone (Eggers 1976). The interpretation of these findings is as follows. A concentration of D-HBB·HCl is reached in the target organ (striated muscle) which is just capable of inhibiting virus multiplication. This delicate balance can be shifted easily in either direction. It is shown below that, for pharmacologic reasons, it is difficult to achieve high concentrations of HBB in the target organs. By combined treatment with D-HBB plus guanidine, the synergistic effects of the compounds come into play and lower concentrations of each compound suffice to inhibit virus multiplication.

Parenthetically, it should be mentioned that, in contrast to our previous results (Eggers 1976), coxsackievirus A9 (strain Woods) proved very slightly more sensitive to HBB than echovirus 9 (strain A. Barty). Thus, mice infected with coxsackievirus A9 are afforded protection by somewhat lower doses of D-HBB, as experimentally verified.

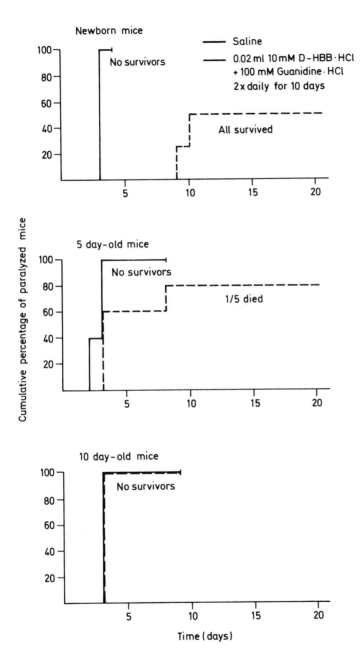

Fig. 13. Effect of age of mice infected with coxsackievirus A9 on the efficacy of treatment with D-HBB · HCl plus guanidine · HCl. Curves are indicated by: *full curves* (saline); *broken curves* (0.02 ml 10 m*M* D-HBB · HCl plus 100 m*M* guanidine · HCl, twice daily for 10 days). (H. J. EGGERS and G. FEDERMANN, unpublished work 1976)

Table 3. Distribution of D-HBB · HCl in various organs of mice after injection of compound

Organ	D-HBB · HCl (μg/g organ)[a] Time postinjection (h)				
	0[b]	4	10	20	27
Muscle					
Left forelimb	120.0	37.3	22.3	5.1	0.66
Right hindlimb	39.5	33.8	20.2	5.5	0.63
Liver	76.4	51.0	34.9	6.7	0.40
Brain	46.6	28.1	15.4	3.0	0.33

[a] Concentration of D-HBB · HCl in the various organs determined fluorimetrically (H. J. EGGERS and J. HENGSTMANN, unpublished work 1975)
[b] At zero time, 0.011 ml 10 mM D-HBB · HCl per g body weight injected into the left forelimb of 5-day-old mice

2. Distribution and Excretion of HBB in the Mouse: Effects of Age

The thesis that the pharmacology of HBB might be the decisive determinant for the outcome of the antiviral activity of the compound in the organism, and be responsible for the different results obtained in cell culture and in animals, was further supported in the following experiments (H. J. EGGERS and G. FEDERMANN, unpublished work 1976; FEDERMANN 1980). A strain of coxsackievirus A9, strain 530, which is also pathogenic for 15-day-old mice was used. It was injected into newborn, 5-day-old or 10-day-old mice. The animals received combined treatment with D-HBB·HCl and guanidine·HCl twice daily (Fig. 13). As can be seen, treatment was successful in the newborn mice, significantly less in 5-day-old mice, and without beneficial effects in 10-day-old mice. Similar results were obtained when treatment was carried out with D-HBB alone. An interpretation of these results is that, with increasing age of the mice, there is an increasing capacity to metabolize HBB.

This has been borne out directly in pharmacologic experiments. Using a highly sensitive fluorimetric method, the concentration of benzimidazoles in various organs and in the whole mouse has been determined at various times after injection of D-HBB·HCl (H. J. EGGERS and J. HENGSTMANN, unpublished work 1975). As can be seen from Table 3, HBB is readily found in substantial concentrations in the skeletal muscle, in the liver, and also in the brain; 20 h after injection, only marginal concentrations were detected. The half-life of HBB is about 10 h (Fig. 14) in the intact mouse.

A shortcoming of the fluorimetric method stems from the fact that it detects not only HBB but also other benzimidazole derivatives and unsubstituted benzimidazole. On the other hand, only very few benzimidazoles are potent and selective inhibitors of enterovirus multiplication (TAMM et al. 1969). It was thus of the utmost importance to determine the actual concentrations of HBB. This was achieved by using ^{14}C-labeled DL-HBB · HCl or D-HBB · HCl. HBB and its metabolic products were characterized by thin layer chromatography (H. J. EGGERS and K. OETTE, unpublished work 1978).

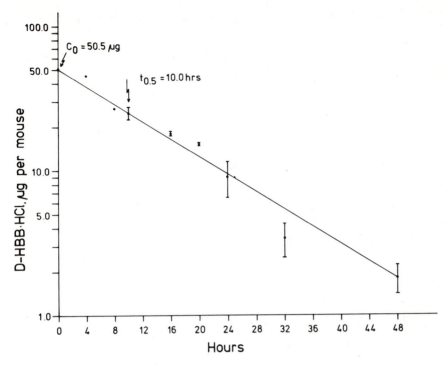

Fig. 14. Concentration of benzimidazole in the whole mouse at various times after inoculation of D-HBB · HCl into 5-day-old mice. Initial concentration 50.5 µg, half-life 10.0 h. For methods see Table 3. (H.J. EGGERS and J. HENGSTMANN unpublished work 1975)

Table 4. Effect of age on excretion and metabolism of HBB in suckling mice. (H.J. EGGERS and K. OETTE, unpublished work 1978)

Age[a] (days)	Total counts	Counts HBB	Counts HBB (%)	Mean HBB left after 20 h (%)
3	134,900	88,494	65.6	21.1
	107,100	67,580	63.1	
6	91,300	47,293	51.8	12.5
	77,800	45,357	58.3	
10	13,553	2,047	15.1	1.1
	25,507	5,918	23.2	
13	14,552	2,808	19.3	0.7
	10,189	2,659	26.1	

[a] At indicated age, mice were inoculated subcutaneously with 20 µl 30 mM DL-HBB · HCl ^{14}C (370,000 dpm); 20 h later, mice were assayed for total radioactivity and the radioactivity due to unaltered HBB; all mice were from the same litter

Table 5. Distribution of radioactivity in adult mice[a] after administration of HBB · HCl ^{14}C. (K. OETTE and H. J. EGGERS, unpublished work 1978)

Time (min)	Right hindlimb	Left forelimb	Liver	Brain	Residual animal
10	23,371[b] (26,588)	22,372 (26,608)	28,241 (39,388)	19,638 (20,350)	(17,350)
30	8,288 (14,988)	8,289 (14,645)	11,991 (21,963)	3,549 (10,111)	(20,701)
120	n. d.[c] (2,202)	n. d. (2,813)	91 (5,672)	n. d. (1,547)	(5,339)
240	n. d. (412)	n. d. (597)	n. d. (1,253)	n. d. (340)	(2,138)

[a] Mice ($\sim$ 30 g) were injected with 0.02 ml 10 mM HBB (3.75 parts D-HBB · HCl plus 1 part DL-HBB · HCl ^{14}C (specific activity 0.3 µCi/µM)) per g body weight subcutaneously into the right hindlimb (32,280 dpm/g body weight)
[b] Figures refer to dpm/g organ due to HBB, figures in parenthesis to total dpm/g organ
[c] n. d. = not detectable

Table 6. Effect of pretreatment with HBB on excretion and metabolism of the compound in suckling mice. (H. J. EGGERS and K. OETTE, unpublished work 1978)

Time (h)	Untreated mice			Pretreated mice[a]		
	Total counts	Counts HBB	Counts HBB (%)	Total counts	Counts HBB	Counts HBB (%)
0.5	298,700	276,297	74.7	319,600	297,228	80.3
6	266,900	207,915	56.2	254,200	157,604	42.6
8	244,600	188,097	50.8	121,900	52,660	14.2
10	252,050	171,898	46.5	150,350	53,825	14.5
12	184,100	132,367	35.8	110,000	39,820	10.8
24	52,200	18,739	5.1	12,400	< 5,000	< 1.4
48				2,860		

[a] 2-day-old mice were inoculated subcutaneously with 0.02 ml 10 mM D-HBB · HCl, twice daily for 5 days. Subsequently, pretreated and untreated mice (from same litter) were inoculated with 20 µl 30 mM DL-HBB · HCl ^{14}C (370,000 dpm). At indicated times, mice were assayed for total radioactivity and the radioactivity due to unaltered HBB

The effect of age on the excretion and metabolism of DL-HBB·HCl is shown in Table 4. With increasing age, HBB was excreted and metabolized at an increased rate. The effect of age on excretion and metabolism of HBB is also apparent in Table 5. Table 5 also confirms the rapid distribution of HBB into the various organs. The data agree well with the results depicted in Fig. 13, where it is shown that HBB exhibited a decreasing antiviral effect in mice as age increased.

In some experiments, there were also suggestions that, with extended duration of treatment with HBB, its antiviral effects diminished. The results presented in Table 6 clearly confirm that pretreatment of mice with D-HBB · HCl causes more

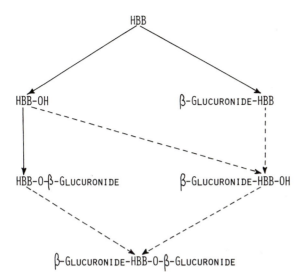

Fig. 15. Metabolic pathways of HBB in mice and isolated rat hepatocytes. *Arrows with uninterrupted lines* indicate proven pathways, those with *broken lines* indicate possible pathways which, however, have not yet been experimentally verified. (K. OETTE and H. J. EGGERS, unpublished work 1978)

rapid excretion and metabolism of the compound. It is thus evident that, with increasing age of the mice and extended duration of treatment, HBB is metabolized and excreted at an increasing rate. The results obtained so far may fully explain the discrepancy in the degree of antiviral effects obtained in cell culture and the reduced protection seen in mice.

3. Metabolic Pathway of HBB in the Mouse and in Isolated Hepatocytes

One main site of the metabolism of HBB in the mouse appears to be the liver. After addition of HBB to cultures of hepatocytes, three main products of HBB metabolism detected in the mouse have been obtained: 2-(α-hydroxybenzyl-β-glucuronide)-benzimidazole (β-glucuronide-HBB), 2-(α-hydroxybenzyl)-hydroxybenzimidazole (HBB-OH), and 2-(α-hydroxybenzyl)-hydroxybenzimidazole-β-glucuronide (HBB-O-β-glucuronide) (Fig. 15; EGGERS et al. 1978; K. OETTE and H. J. EGGERS, unpublished work 1978). These three metabolic products of HBB have been shown to be devoid of antiviral activity (Table 7; H. J. EGGERS and K. OETTE, unpublished work 1979).

4. Distribution and Excretion of Guanidine·HCl in the Mouse

D-HBB·HCl is frequently injected in combination with guanidine·HCl and it seemed of interest to follow the distribution and excretion of guanidine·HCl in mice. As seen in Table 8, guanidine·HCl reaches various organs (including the brain, though in lower concentrations); 9 h after application substantial concentrations of guanidine·HCl were still measurable in the striated muscle and in the

Table 7. Virus-inhibitory activity of metabolites of HBB in the organism. (H. J. EGGERS and K. OETTE, unpublished work 1980)

Treatment of cultures in single cycle growth curve		Yield of echovirus 12 (PFU/0.2 ml)
Untreated control		1.6×10^8
HBB-O-glucuronide[a]	$100 \ \mu M$[b]	1.6×10^8
Glucuronide-HBB	$100 \ \mu M$[b]	1.9×10^8
HBB-OH	$100 \ \mu M$[b]	1.5×10^8
HBB from urine	$75 \ \mu M$[b]	2.8×10^3
D-HBB · HCl (standard)	$75 \ \mu M$	1.9×10^2

[a] Or glucuronide-HBB-O-glucuronide
[b] The various fractions were isolated from urine of rats which had been injected with ^{14}C-labeled HBB. The indicated molarities are based on the radioactivity of the isolated and highly purified material

Table 8. Distribution of radioactivity in suckling mice after inoculation[a] of guanidine · HCl ^{14}C. (K. OETTE and H. J. EGGERS, unpublished work 1980)

Time (h)	Left forelimb	Right hindlimb	Liver	Brain	Residual animal
0.033	6,609[b]	88	148	59	2,527
1	3,037	2,499	4,186	754	2,501
3	2,640	2,145	3,251	654	2,065
5	1,762	1,674	1,524	1,057	1,607
7	1,055	1,391	884	407	968
9	1,003	1,079	902	353	950
24	38	56	31	15	48

[a] Mice (~ 2.3 g) were injected with 0.02 ml 100 mM guanidine · HCl ^{14}C (specific activity 1.55 mCi/mmol^{-1} g^{-1} subcutaneously into the left forelimb
[b] Figures refer to μmol/kg (tissue), mean of two measurements

liver; after 24 h the concentrations had fallen to background levels. No evidence for metabolic products of guanidine was found in mice and rats (K. OETTE and H. J. EGGERS, unpublished work 1980).

5. Experiments to Define Optimum Treatment

Optimum treatment of mice infected with various enteroviruses has been established (H. J. EGGERS, G. FEDERMANN and C. HECKER, unpublished work 1976–1980; FEDERMANN 1980; HECKER 1981), but the many details of the experiments cannot be presented here. Suffice it to say that success of the treatment depends to a large extent on the pathogenesis of the disease, in particular the sites and speed of virus multiplication and the age of the animals. In the case of newborn mice infected with echovirus 9, a 3-day treatment beginning at the time of virus inoculation renders protection, since under these conditions, virus multiplication will be sufficiently delayed for the animals to reach a refractory state (EGGERS 1976). On the other hand, the aforementioned strain 530 of coxsackievirus A9 is still pathogenic when inoculated into 15-day-old mice. Thus, extended treatment over 10–15 days, whether with D-HBB·HCl alone or in combination with guanidine·HCl, yields better results than treatment for only 5–6 days.

6. Treatment of Mice Infected with Coxsackievirus B4 and Poliovirus 2

Partial protection by D-HBB·HCl alone (20%) or by D-HBB plus guanidine (60%) is achieved in newborn mice, inoculated with 200 median paralytic doses (PD_{50}) of the neurotropic coxsackievirus B4, when treatment is begun 24 h after virus inoculation (H. J. EGGERS and C. HECKER, unpublished work 1978; HECKER 1981). All control animals die within 2–4 days after virus inoculation.

Poliovirus-infected newborn mice (200 PD_{50}, intracerebral inoculation) were also partially protected by combined treatment with D-HBB·HCl plus guanidine·HCl, when treatment was begun immediately after virus inoculation (H. J. EGGERS and C. HECKER, unpublished work 1978; HECKER 1981). Treatment with either D-HBB or guanidine alone delayed onset of symptoms compared with the saline control.

Subcutaneous or intraperitoneal injections yield similar results. Even after inoculation of large virus doses (10^4–10^6 PD_{50}), at least in the case of echovirus 9 and coxsackievirus A9, protection is offered by D-HBB · HCl alone or by combined treatment with D-HBB plus guanidine.

7. Late Treatment When First Symptoms Have Appeared: Combined Effects of D-HBB, Guanidine, and Virus-Specific Antiserum

An important aspect of chemotherapy is whether treatment is still efficient when first symptoms of disease become manifest. Therefore, newborn mice were infected with 200 PD_{50} of echovirus 9. At the time when paresis was first apparent in one or several mice, the animals were subdivided at random into various groups which were subjected to the following treatments: (1) saline; (2) D-HBB · HCl plus guanidine · HCl; (3) specific antiserum; (4) D-HBB · HCl plus guanidine·HCl plus antiserum. As can be seen in Fig. 16, each treatment yielded some positive results. The best results were obtained by combined chemotherapy plus specific antiserum. It can also be seen that animals recovered which had already been paralysed. Similar experiments have been carried out with newborn mice infected with coxsackievirus B4 (data not shown) and poliovirus 2 (Fig. 17; Table 9). Again, in each case the best results were achieved by the combination of chemotherapy and treatment with specific antiserum. Table 9 also demonstrates the importance of early treatment after infection.

In summary, the recent extensive studies with D-HBB·HCl (plus guanidine·HCl) in enterovirus-infected mice have yielded highly encouraging results, results at least as good as with other antiviral substances including interferons. The combination of D-HBB plus guanidine plus specific antiserum appears to be a very promising approach. The discrepancy between results obtained in cell culture and in intact animals can be explained by the pharmacodynamics of HBB and guanidine in the animal.

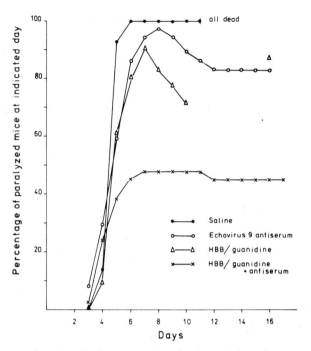

Fig. 16. Percentage of paralyzed mice at any day after inoculation of 200 PD_{50} echovirus 9 (strain A. Barty). Effect of indicated treatments which have been started at first onset of paresis (see text): *full circles* (saline); *open circles* (human antiserum diluted 1:5, 0.1 ml intraperitoneally, on two occasions 24 h apart); *triangles* (10 mM D-HBB·HCl plus 100 mM guanidine·HCl, 0.02 ml subcutaneously, twice daily for 5 days); *crosses* (treatments combined). Note: in the HBB plus guanidine group, beyond day 10, mice became ill owing to death of the nursing mother, unrelated to echovirus 9 infection or treatment. (H. J. Eggers and C. Hecker, unpublished work 1978)

Table 9. Early and late treatment of mice infected with poliovirus 2 (200 PD_{50}). (H. J. Eggers and C. Hecker, unpublished work 1978)

Start of therapy (h postinfection)	Saline	Poliovirus 2 antiserum	D-HBB·HCl +guani-dine·HCl	D-HBB·HCl +guanidine +antiserum
0	26/26[a]	6/16	19/31	7/23
24	27/27	10/23	30/32	10/24
48	25/25	21/24	21/22	13/24
72	19/19	15/15	22/23	13/22
96	15/15		22/23	12/16
Onset of paralysis[b]	30/30	32/32	24/25	24/30
Sum[c]	142/142 (100)	84/110 (76.3)	138/156 (88.5)	79/139 (56.8)

[a] Number of mice dead as a fraction of the total
[b] At least one mouse in group exhibits paralysis
[c] Figures in parentheses are percentages

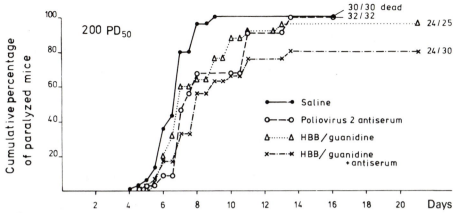

Fig. 17. Percentage of paralyzed mice after inoculation of 200 PD_{50} of poliovirus 2 (strain MEF 1). Effect of indicated treatments which have been started at first onset of paralysis (see text); *full circles* (saline); *open circles* (human antiserum diluted 1:5, 0.05 ml intraperitoneally, on two occasions 24 h apart); *triangles* (10 mM D-HBB·HCl plus 100 mM guanidine·HCl, 0.02 ml subcutaneously, twice daily for 15 days); *crosses* (treatments combined). (H. J. EGGERS and C. HECKER, unpublished work 1978)

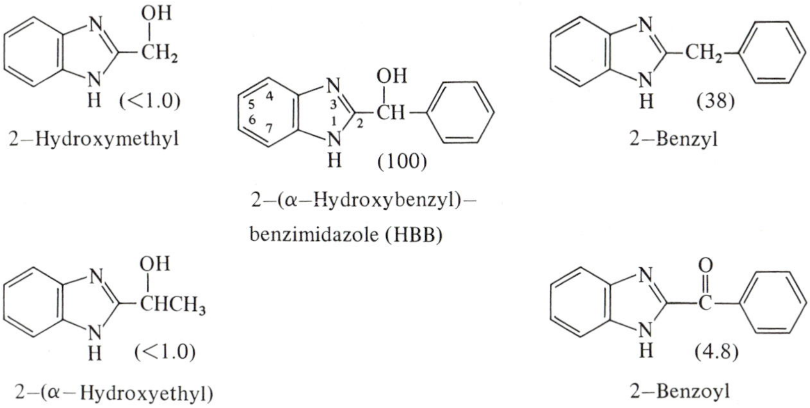

2−Hydroxymethyl   (<1.0)

2−(α−Hydroxybenzyl)−

benzimidazole (HBB)   (100)

2−Benzyl   (38)

2−(α−Hydroxyethyl)   (<1.0)

2−Benzoyl   (4.8)

Fig. 18. The structural basis of picornavirus-inhibitory activity of HBB. The activities are expressed relative to the poliovirus-inhibitory activity of HBB. (TAMM and EGGERS 1963 b)

D. Chemical Derivatives of HBB and Their Antiviral Activity in Cell Culture and in the Organism

I. Structure–Activity Studies

In view of the virus-selective activity of HBB, it was desirable to search for even more active substances by chemical modifications of HBB. Despite extensive studies in this field, only very few compounds with activity comparable to HBB have been found. The results of studies on structure–activity relationships with compounds related to HBB can be summarized as follows. The hydroxybenzyl grouping at position 2 of the benzimidazole ring is of critical importance, since the 2-hydroxymethyl and the 2-(α-hydroxyethyl) derivatives are inactive (Fig. 18; TAMM et al. 1961; TAMM and EGGERS 1963 b). Also the 2-benzyl and the 2-benzoyl compounds are less active and selective than HBB (Fig. 18). On the other hand, both 2-(α-methoxybenzyl)-benzimidazole and 2-(α-acetoxybenzyl)-benzimidazole are about as active and selective as HBB (TAMM et al. 1969; O'SULLIVAN et al. 1965). It follows that intramolecular hydrogen bonding involving the hydroxyl group is not essential for virus-inhibitory activity, since, in these derivatives, such bonding cannot occur. The replacement of the benzimidazole nucleus of HBB by, for example, an imidazole ring, results in complete loss of activity (TAMM et al. 1969).

Of the two optical isomers of HBB, the D-(−)-HBB·HCl is 2–3 times more effective than L-(+)-HBB·HCl (KADIN et al. 1964). The molecular basis of this finding is at present unknown. Certain 1-substituted derivatives, such as 1-propyl-, 1-β-methylpropyl-, and 1-phenyl-HBB (O'SULLIVAN and WALLIS 1963; O'SULLIVAN et al. 1967) are more active and selective in cell culture systems than HBB. This observation and the pharmacologic studies already described make it unlikely that HBB, in order to be active, is being converted to a nucleoside at position 1 of the bezimidazole ring.

All in all, it appears that the selective virus-inhibitory activity of HBB is dependent on the overall geometry of the molecule and that most structural modifications lead to loss of virus activity and/or selectivity. As already indicated, only few chemical derivatives of HBB have been found with activity similar to that of HBB. The following ones have been studied in some detail.

II. 1-Propyl-2-(α-Hydroxybenzyl)-Benzimidazole (1-Propyl-HBB) and Its Hydrochloride Salt

1-Propyl-HBB (Fig. 19) has been shown to be a highly active inhibitor of multiplication of polioviruses (O'SULLIVAN and WALLIS 1963). In our hands, the compound was about 1.5–2 times more selective than D-HBB in cell cultures infected with either echovirus 9 or coxsackievirus A9 (strain 530) (H.J. EGGERS and G. FEDERMANN, unpublished work 1976; FEDERMANN 1980).

O'SULLIVAN et al. (1969) also studied the activity of 1-propyl-HBB in newborn or 3-day-old mice inoculated with low doses of coxsackievirus A9. The compound, given up to doses of 1.6 mg/day, at best delayed the time of death. In similar experiments with coxsackievirus A9 (strain 530), we were able to confirm these results; while the mortality could not be reduced by 1-propyl-HBB·HCl (Table 10), a slight delay in the time of death was seen (H.J. EGGERS and G. FEDERMANN, unpublished work 1976; FEDERMANN 1980). Upon combined treatment with guanidine·HCl, however, a significant reduction in the occurrence of paresis and death could be achieved. This effect, in all probability, is due to the synergistic action of 1-propyl-HBB·HCl and guanidine·HCl (see Table 1).

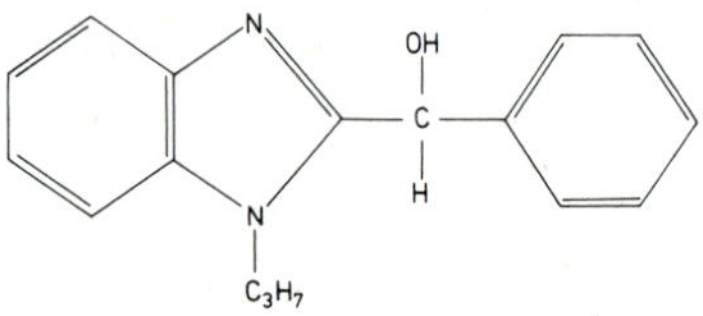

Fig. 19. 1-Propyl-2-(α-hydroxybenzyl)-benzimidazole (1-propyl-HBB)

Table 10. Effect of treatment[a] by D-HBB · HCl or structural derivatives on coxsackievirus A9 disease in newborn mice. (H.J. EGGERS and G. FEDERMANN, unpublished work 1976)

Saline	D-HBB · HCl 20 mM	α-Methyl-HBB · HCl 20 mM	1-Propyl-HBB or 1-Propyl-HBB · HCl 20 mM
88/88[b]	23/25	19/25	27/27
(88/88)	(7/25)	(5/25)	(27/27)

[a] 0.02 ml indicated drugs were inoculated (s.c. or i.p.) three times daily for 10 days. Dose of coxsackievirus A9, strain 530: 3.500–4.650 PD_{50} s.c.

[b] Number of paralyzed mice as a fraction of the total. Figures in parentheses: number of dead mice as a fraction of the total

Table 11. Effect of combined treatment[a] of benzimidazole derivatives with guanidine · HCl on coxsackievirus A9 disease in newborn mice. (H.J. EGGERS and G. FEDERMANN, unpublished work 1976)

Saline	10 mM D-HBB · HCl + 100 mM guanidine · HCl	10 mM α-Methyl-HBB · HCl + 100 mM guanidine · HCl
34/34[b]	20/28	6/17
(34/34)	(2/28)	(1/17)

[a] 0.02 ml indicated drugs were inoculated (s.c. or i.p.) three times daily for 10 days. Dose of coxsackievirus A9, strain 530: 3.500–4.650 PD_{50} s.c.

[b] See Table 10

The relative inactivity of 1-propyl-HBB and 1-propyl-HBB·HCl in the mouse system is remarkable; in cell culture the compound (and its hydrochloride salt) is active at a concentration one-sixth to one-eighth of that of D-HBB·HCl (FEDERMANN 1980), whereas in newborn mice at molar concentrations similar to that of D-HBB·HCl it is almost inactive. The pharmacologic basis of this observation is being studied.

III. 2-(α-Methyl-α-Hydroxybenzyl)-Benzimidazole Hydrochloride (α-Methyl-HBB · HCl)

α-Methyl-HBB (Fig. 20) has been shown in cell culture to be somewhat more active and selective than HBB (TAMM et al. 1969). Studies on its antiviral activity in mice infected with coxsackievirus A9 were, therefore, of interest. As can be seen in Table 10, the compound exhibited an activity similar to that of D-HBB. In addi-

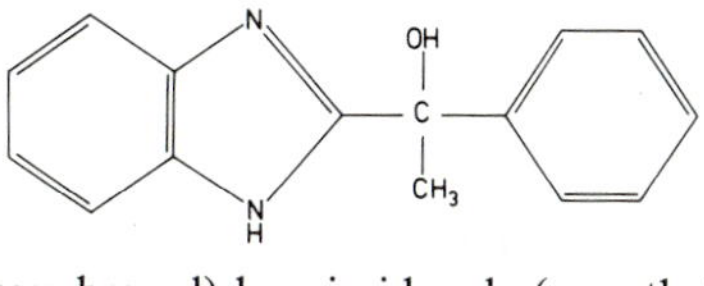

Fig. 20. 2-(α-Methyl-α-hydroxybenzyl)-benzimidazole (α-methyl-HBB)

tion, combined treatment with guanidine·HCl further improved the results of treatment (see Table 11). In mice, a striking superiority of α-methyl-HBB·HCl compared with D-HBB·HCl has not been observed (H. J. Eggers and G. Federmann, unpublished work 1976; Federmann 1980).

IV. 1,2-bis-(5-Methoxy-2-Benzimidazolyl)-1,2-Ethanediol (1,2-bis-Benzimidazole)

In 1963 O'Sullivan and Wallis reported slight antipoliovirus activity of 1,2-bis-(2-benzimidazolyl)-1,2-ethanediol, a derivative of HBB. Upon chemical modification of this compound, it was shown by Akihama et al. (1968) that 1,2-bis-(5-methoxy-2-benzimidazolyl)-1,2-ethanediol (Fig. 21) was even more effective against poliovirus 1. In cell culture experiments with coxsackievirus A9, the R,R-1,2-bis-benzimidazole was demonstrated to be virus inhibitory at 1–10 μM. Compared with D-HBB it was about 12.5–15 times more selective (H. J. Eggers and G. Federmann, unpublished work 1976; Federmann 1980).

In an analysis of the mechanism of action of R-R-1,2-bis-benzimidazole (H. J. Eggers, unpublished work 1974), we could show that the compound did not inhibit processes of early virus–cell interactions. In particular, adsorption, penetration, and uncoating of echovirus 9 proceeded undisturbed in the presence of highly inhibitory concentrations of the compound, a result compatible with that of Schleicher et al. (1972). Infective viral RNA, however, is not being synthesized in cells infected with echovirus 9 in the presence of the compound. Also, viral RNA synthesis is being inhibited by the compound in cells infected with echovirus 9, as measured by uptake of uridine ^{3}H into acid-insoluble RNA.

At first glance, the mechanism of action of 1,2-bis-benzimidazole appears similar to that of HBB. However, some remarkable differences can be observed, e.g., the virus-inhibitory spectrum of both compounds is different. Whereas poliovirus 1–3, coxsackievirus A9, coxsackievirus B 1–6, and a large number of echovirus types are found to be susceptible in tissue culture to 1,2-bis-benzimidazole (Schleicher et al. 1972; H. J. Eggers, unpublished work 1974), some 55 rhinovirus serotypes – in contrast to HBB – were also found to be susceptible to the compound (Schleicher et al. 1972). On the other hand, various representatives belonging to virus groups other than picornaviruses were found to be insusceptible to 1,2-bis-benzimidazole, as also seen with HBB. Pfau and his co-workers (Stella et al. 1974) reported susceptibility of arenaviruses (lymphocytic choriomeningitis, Parana, and Pichinde viruses) to S,S-1,2-bis-benzimidazole. It is remarkable, however, that the observed virus-inhibitory activity was host cell dependent in that it appeared restricted to infected L cells and was not noticed in HeLa cells. (See also

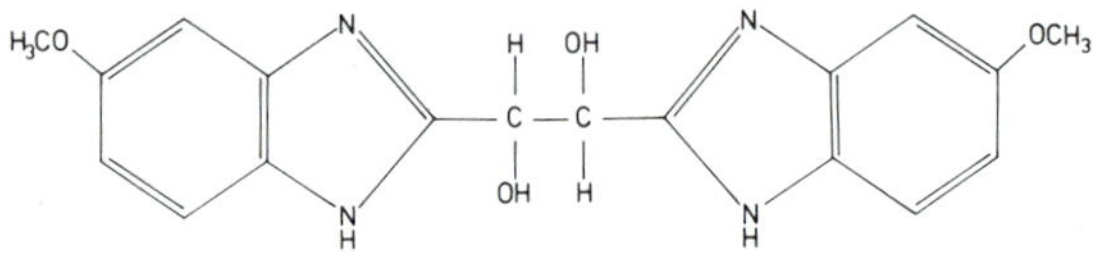

Fig. 21. S,S-1,2-bis-(5-Methoxy-2-benzimidazolyl)-1,2-ethanediol (S,S-1,2-bis-benzimidazole)

Table 12. Effect of 1,2-bis-benzimidazole treatment[a] on echovirus 9 disease in newborn mice. (H.J. EGGERS and C. HECKER, unpublished work 1978)

Saline	10 mM R,R-1,2-bis-Benzimidazole	10 mM R,R-1,2-bis-Benzimidazole + 100 mM guanidine · HCl
5/5[b]	25/25	7/15
(5/5)	(20/25)	(4/15)

[a] 0.02 ml indicated drugs were inoculated s.c. twice daily for 5 days, beginning 24 h post-infection. Dose of echovirus 9, strain A. Barty: 200 PD$_{50}$ s.c.
[b] See Table 10

the host-cell-dependent effects of HBB on lymphocytic choriomeningitis virus which, however, are restricted to HeLa cells.) Another remarkable difference between HBB and 1,2-bis-benzimidazole consists of the total lack of cross-resistance between virus mutants resistant to either one of the compounds (H. J. EGGERS, unpublished work 1975). Also noteworthy is the fact that it is more difficult to obtain 1,2-bis-benzimidazole-resistant mutants, whereas HBB-resistant mutants are readily obtained, as described above.

RODERICK et al. (1972) synthesized various chemical derivatives of 1,2-bis-benzimidazole. Several of those derivatives were also active against rhinoviruses 1A and 42. However, none of those derivatives appeared more active than 1,2-bis-benzimidazole. All three stereoisomers of 1,2-bis-benzimidazole (S,S; S,R; R,R) exhibited similar virus inhibitory activity (however, the test system was rather crude). The structure–activity relations of the bis-benzimidazoles have been delineated for the tested rhinoviruses.

S,S-1-2-bis-Benzimidazole appeared to be active in rhinovirus type 30 infections in chimpanzees (SHIPKOWITZ et al. 1972); animals treated for 4 consecutive days with a dose of 100 mg kg^{-1} day^{-1} (given in three divided doses per day) shed no virus on days 1–8 postinfection compared with the untreated animals. Treatment was begun prior to infection. Virus, however, could be recovered from two of three treated animals on day 10 postinfection. All three treated animals exhibited a seroconversion to rhinovirus 30. The chimpanzees given 100 mg/kg for 4 days developed diarrhea 3 days after their final medication. Within 1 week they recovered. Chimpanzees treated with lower doses of the drug exhibited no side effects, but the antiviral efficacy was at best marginal (SHIPKOWITZ et al. 1972).

After oral application of the compound to mice, antiviral drug levels were found in various organs (SHIPKOWITZ et al. 1972). In mice infected with echovirus 9 and treated under various regimens with R,R-1,2-bis-benzimidazole in doses comparable to those applied to chimpanzees, a slight improvement in the death rate could be achieved, but development of paralysis could not be inhibited (see Table 12) (H. J. EGGERS and C. HECKER, unpublished work 1979; HECKER 1981). Treatment of mice infected with coxsackievirus B4 was without success (H. J. EGGERS and C. HECKER, unpublished work 1978; HECKER 1981). These results, like those with 1-propyl-HBB, have been unexpected in view of the remarkable antiviral and selective activity of 1,2-bis-benzimidazole in cell culture. The basis of this phenomenon is being intensively studied in our laboratory.

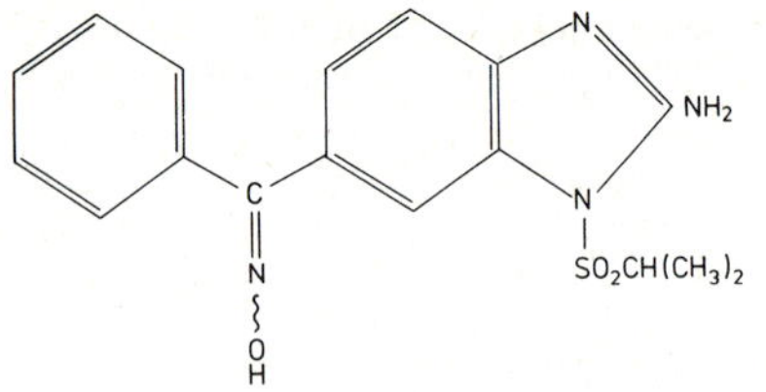

Fig. 22. 2-Amino-1-(isopropylsulfonyl)-6-benzimidazole phenyl ketone oxime (LY 122 771-72)

Contrary to treatment of mice infected with echovirus 9 with 1,2-bis-benzimidazole alone, combined application of 1,2-bis-benzimidazole (10 mM) plus guanidine (100 µM) twice daily (0.02 ml each subcutaneously) saved about two-thirds of the infected mice (Table 12). In mice infected with coxsackievirus B4, this combined treatment has been without success (H. J. Eggers and C. Hecker, unpublished work 1978; Hecker 1981).

V. 2-Amino-1-(Isopropylsulfonyl)-6-Benzimidazole Phenyl Ketone Oxime

Replication of rhinovirus type 31 in human embryonic nasal organ cultures was shown to be inhibited by the compound LY 122 771-72 [2-amino-1-(isopropylsulfonyl)-6-benzimidazole phenyl ketone oxime; Fig. 22] at a concentration of 0.2 µg/ml, though ciliary activity of uninfected cultures was unimpaired at a concentration of 25 µg/ml. Inhibition of virus multiplication, as measured by lack of development of cytopathic effects or reduction in plaque formation, was also obtained in Hela cells; besides rhinovirus type 31, many other rhinovirus types as well as representatives of other picornaviruses appear susceptible (DeLong and Reed 1980; Wikel et al. 1980). The anti-oxime isomer (LY 122 772, enviroxime) appears to exhibit consistently more antiviral potency than the syn-oxime isomer (LY 122771) (Wikel et al. 1980).

In view of the broad spectrum of antiviral activity in vitro against rhinoviruses, the high virus selectivity in vitro, and absorption of the drug to produce effective blood and lung levels of compound in mice and dogs after oral administration, the activity of enviroxime against rhinovirus type 9 infection in humans has been studied (Phillpotts et al. 1981). In this study, a group of 18 volunteers was given oral plus intranasal enviroxime for one day before and five days after challenge with a small dose of human rhinovirus type 9. A placebo group also consisted of 18 individuals. Medication was given four times daily. The daily dose of enviroxime was 102 mg per person. The clinical effects were monitored by an observer blind to the allocations of the groups.

The investigators conclude that in the enviroxime group as compared with the control group, there occurred reductions in the number and severity of colds, clinical scores, rhinorrhea and quantity of virus shed. However, these results cannot be considered statistically significant, and the virus challenge dose was very low.

As to toxicity, there were no clinically significant changes in hematology, biochemistry, or urinanalysis results after treatment with enviroxime. But almost 60%

of the volunteers in the enviroxime group complained of side effects, in particular nausea, vomiting and abdominal pain. It remains to be seen whether in another study enviroxime dosage can be restricted to nasal administration which is expected to be better tolerated.

E. Conclusions

Until now, there have been very few antiviral substances at hand for the treatment of virus infections of humans or animals. Today, however, it is clearly established on theoretical grounds and by practical experience that antiviral chemotherapy is feasible. The detailed investigations on the virus-selective activity of benzimidazoles have contributed to the present-day achievements in this area and also to basic virology. The demonstration of the enterovirus-selective action of HBB and the specific effects of HBB on enterovirus nucleic acid synthesis strengthened the view of the existence of virus specificity, despite the intimate dependence of virus multiplication on host cell functions. The phenomena of drug resistance and dependence have been studied early and extensively with HBB-resistant and HBB-dependent enterovirus mutants.

The animal experiments on the pharmacology of HBB provide a rational basis to understand the quantitatively different virus-inhibitory effects of HBB in cell culture and in the animal. Nevertheless, considerable success can be reported in the treatment of enterovirus-infected animals, even when treatment is initiated late in infection. Combined treatment with various drugs and antiserum has been particularly effective. It appears that more intensive studies on antiviral substances are badly needed at various levels: the screening systems, the mechanism of action of lead compounds, and the pharmacologic behavior of such substances in the organism in relation to cell cultures. Such systematic and thorough work will eventually invite the touch of good luck.

Acknowledgment. Part of the experimental work of the author was supported by grants from Der Minister für Wissenschaft und Forschung des Landes Nordrhein-Westfalen and Der Bundesminister für Forschung und Technologie.

References

Adrian Th, Rosenwirth B, Eggers HJ (1979) Isolation and characterization of temperature-sensitive mutants of echovirus 12. Virology 99:329–339

Agol VI, Shirman GA (1964) Interaction of guanidine-sensitive and guanidine-dependent variants of poliovirus in mixedly infected cells. Biochem Biophys Res Commun 17:28–33

Akihama S, Okude M, Sato K, Iwabuchi S (1968) Inhibitory effect of 1,2-bis(2-benzimidazolyl)1,2-ethanediol derivatives of poliovirus. Nature 217:562–563

Ames BN, McCann J, Yamasaki E (1977) Methods for detecting carcinogens and mutagens with the salmonella/mammalian-microsome mutagenicity test. In: Handbook of mutagenicity test procedures. Elsevier, Amsterdam New York Oxford, pp 1–17

Bablanian R, Eggers HJ, Tamm I (1965a) Studies on the mechanism of poliovirus-induced cell damage. I. The relation between poliovirus-induced metabolic and morphological alterations in cultured cells. Virology 26:100–113

Bablanian R, Eggers HJ, Tamm I (1965b) Studies on the mechanism of poliovirus-induced cell damage. II. The relation between poliovirus growth and virus-induced morphological changes in the cells. Virology 26:114–121

Bablanian R, Eggers HJ, Tamm I (1966) Inhibition of enterovirus cytopathic effects by 2-(α-hydroxybenzyl)-benzimidazole. J Bacteriol 91:1289–1294

Baltimore D, Eggers HJ, Franklin RM, Tamm I (1963) Poliovirus-induced RNA polymerase and the effects of virus-specific inhibitors on its production. Proc Natl Acad Sci USA 49:843–849

Bienz K, Egger D, Rasser Y, Bossart W (1980) Kinetics and location of poliovirus macromolecular synthesis in correlation to virus-induced cytopathology. Virology 100:390–399

Caliguiri LA, Tamm I (1968a) Action of guanidine on the replication of poliovirus RNA. Virology 35:408–417

Caliguiri LA, Tamm I (1968b) Distribution and translation of poliovirus RNA in guanidine-treated cells. Virology 36:223–231

Caliguiri LA, Tamm I (1972) Guanidine. In: Bauer DJ (ed) The international encyclopedia of pharmacology and therapeutics, vol 1. Pergamon, Oxford New York, pp 181–230

Caliguiri LA, Tamm I (1973) Guanidine and 2-(α-hydroxybenzyl)-benzimidazole(HBB): selective inhibitors of picornavirus multiplication. In: Carter W (ed) Selective inhibitors of viral functions. CRC Press, Cleveland, pp 257–293

Caliguiri LA, Eggers HJ, Ikegami N, Tamm I (1965) A single-cell study of chemical inhibition of enterovirus multiplication. Virology 27:551–558

Connelly AP Jr, Hamre D (1964) Virologic studies on acute respiratory disease in young adults. II. Characteristics and serologic studies of three new rhinoviruses. J Lab Clin Med 63:30–43

Cooper PD, Wentworth BB, McCahon D (1970) Guanidine inhibition of poliovirus: a dependence of viral RNA synthesis on the configuration of structural protein. Virology 40:486–493

Cords CE, Holland JJ (1964) Replication of poliovirus RNA induced by heterologous virus. Proc Natl Acad Sci USA 51:1080–1082

Dales S, Eggers HJ, Tamm I, Palade GE (1965) Electron microscopic study of the formation of poliovirus. Virology 26:379–389

Dardiri AH, DeLay PD, Bachrach HL (1964) Effect of 2-(α-hydroxybenzyl) benzimidazole on Teschen disease virus, pig enteric viruses, and foot-and-mouth disease virus in kidney cell cultures. Can J Comp Med 28:161–168

De Long DC, Reed SE (1980) Inhibition of rhinovirus replication in organ culture by a potential antiviral drug. J Infect Dis 141:87–91

Dinter Z (1964) Differenzierung einiger boviner Picorna-Viren mittels Guanidin and 2-(Alpha-Hydroxybenzyl)-Benzimidazol (HBB). Wien Tierärztl Monatsschr 51:70–73

Dinter Z, Bengtsson S (1964) Suppression of the inhibitory action of guanidine on virus multiplication by some amino acids. Virology 24:254–261

Dmitrieva TM, Agol VI (1974) Selective inhibition of the synthesis of single-stranded RNA of encephalomyocarditis virus by 2-(α-hydroxybenzyl)-benzimidazole in cell-free systems. Arch Ges Virusforsch 45:17–26

Eggers HJ (1962) Discussion to: Genetic recombination with Newcastle disease virus, poliovirus, and influenza (by G. K. Hirst). Cold Spring Harbor Symp Quant Biol 27:309

Eggers HJ (1976) Successful treatment of enterovirus-infected mice by 2-(α-hydroxybenzyl)-benzimidazole and guanidine. J Exp Med 143:1367–1381

Eggers HJ (1977) Selective inhibition of uncoating of echovirus 12 by rhodanine. Virology 78:241–252

Eggers HJ, Sabin AB (1959) Factors determining pathogenicity of variants of ECHO 9 virus for newborn mice. J Exp Med 110:951–967

Eggers HJ, Tamm I (1961a) Spectrum and characteristics of the virus inhibitory action of 2-(α-hydroxybenzyl)-benzimidazole. J Exp Med 113:657–682

Eggers HJ, Tamm I (1961b) 2-(α-Hydroxybenzyl)-benzimidazole (HBB) as an aid in virus classification. Virology 13:545–546

Eggers HJ, Tamm I (1962a) On the mechanism of selective inhibition of enterovirus multiplication by 2-(α-hydroxybenzyl)-benzimidazole. Virology 18:426–438

Eggers HJ, Tamm I (1962 b) A variant of coxsackie A9 virus which requires 2-(α-hydroxy-benzyl)-benzimidazole (HBB) for optimal growth (Abstr). VIII th Int Congr Microbiol, p 85

Eggers HJ, Tamm I (1963 a) Inhibition of enterovirus ribonucleic acid synthesis by 2-(α-hy-droxybenzyl)-benzimidazole. Nature 197:1327–1328

Eggers HJ, Tamm I (1963 b) Drug dependence of enteroviruses: variants of coxsackie A9 and ECHO 13 viruses that require 2-(α-hydroxybenzyl)-benzimidazole for growth. Virology 20:62–74

Eggers HJ, Tamm I (1963 c) Synergistic effect of 2-(α-hydroxybenzyl)-benzimidazole and guanidine on picornavirus reproduction. Nature 199:513–514

Eggers HJ, Tamm I (1965) Coxsackie A9 virus: mutation from drug dependence to drug in-dependence. Science 148:97–98

Eggers HJ, Tamm I (1966) Antiviral chemotherapy. Annu Rev Pharmacol 6:231–250

Eggers HJ, Waidner E (1970) Effect of 2-(α-hydroxybenzyl)-benzimidazole and guanidine on the uncoating of echovirus 12. Nature 227:952–953

Eggers HJ, Baltimore D, Tamm I (1963 a) The relation of protein synthesis to formation of poliovirus RNA polymerase. Virology 21:281–282

Eggers HJ, Reich E, Tamm I (1963 b) The drug-requiring phase in the growth of drug-de-pendent enteroviruses. Proc Natl Acad Sci USA 50:183–190

Eggers HJ, Ikegami N, Tamm I (1965 a) The development of ultraviolet-irradiation resis-tance by poliovirus infective centers and its inhibition by guanidine. Virology 25:475–478

Eggers HJ, Ikegami N, Tamm I (1965 b) Comparative studies with selective inhibitors of picornavirus reproduction. Ann NY Acad Sci 130:267–281

Eggers HJ, Oette K, Tschung TS (1978) Chemotherapy of enterovirus-infected animals. Fourth International Congress for Virology, The Hague. Centre for Agricultural Pub-lishing and Documentation, Wageningen, p 124

Fara GM, Cochran KW (1963) Antiviral activity of selected benzimidazoles. Boll Ist Sieroter Milan 42:630–637

Federmann G (1980) Behandlung von Enterovirus-Infektionen der saugenden Maus mit D-HBB·HCl und chemischen Derivaten. Dissertation, Universität Köln

Gwaltney JM Jr (1968) The spectrum of rhinovirus inhibition by 2-(α-hydroxybenzyl)-benz-imidazole and D-(−)-2-(α-hydroxybenzyl)-benzimidazole HCl, Proc Soc Exp Biol Med 129:665–673

Halperen S, Eggers HJ, Tamm I (1964) Evidence for uncoupled synthesis of viral RNA and viral capsids. Virology 24:36–46

Hamparian VV, Hilleman MR, Kettler A (1963) Contributions to characterization and clas-sification of animal viruses. Proc Soc Exp Biol Med 112:1040–1050

Hamre D, Connelly AP Jr, Procknow JJ (1964) Virologic studies of acute respiratory disease in young adults. III. Some biologic and serologic characteristics of seventeen rhinovirus serotypes isolated October, 1960, to June, 1961. J Lab Clin Med 64:450–460

Hecker C (1981) Therapieversuche bei Enterovirusinfektionen in neugeborenen Mäusen. Dissertation, Universität Köln

Holland JJ, Cords CE (1964) Maturation of poliovirus RNA with capsid protein coded by heterologous enteroviruses. Proc Natl Acad Sci USA 51:1082–1085

Hollinshead AC, Smith PK (1958) Effects of certain purines and related compounds on virus propagation. J Pharmacol Exp Ther 123:54–62

Ikegami N, Eggers HJ, Tamm I (1964) Rescue of drug-requiring and drug-inhibited en-teroviruses. Proc Natl Acad Sci USA 52:1419–1426

Kadin SB, Eggers HJ, Tamm I (1964) Synthesis and virus-inhibitory activity of D- and L-isomers of 2-(α-hydroxybenzyl)-benzimidazole. Nature 201:639–640

Kisch AL, Webb PA, Johnson KM (1964) Further properties of five newly recognized picor-naviruses (rhinoviruses). Am J Hyg 79:125–133

Korant DB (1977) Poliovirus coat protein as the site of guanidine action. Virology 81:17–28

Ledinko N (1963) Genetic recombination with poliovirus type 1. Studies of crosses between a normal horse serum-resistant mutant and several guanidine-resistant mutants of the same strain. Virology 20:107–119

Loddo B, Ferrari W, Spanedda A, Brotzu G (1962) In vitro guanidine-resistance and guanidine-dependence of poliovirus. Experientia 18:518–519

Loddo B, Gessa GL, Schivo ML, Spanedda A, Brutzu G, Ferrari W (1966) Antagonism of the guanidine interference with poliovirus replication by simple methylated and ethylated compounds. Virology 28:707–712

Luria SE, Darnell JE Jr, Baltimore D, Campbell A (1978) General virology. Wiley, New York

Lwoff A, Lwoff M (1964) Neutralisation par divers métabolites de l'effet inhibiteur de la guanidine sur le développement du poliovirus. C R Acad Sci Paris 259:949–952

Melnick JL, Sabin AB (1959) The ECHO virus group. In: Rivers TM, Horsfall FL (eds) Viral and rickettsial infections of man. Lippincott, Philadelphia Montreal, p 548

Melnick JL, Crowther D, Barrera-Oro J (1961) Rapid development of drug-resistant mutants of poliovirus. Science 134:557

O'Sullivan DG, Wallis AK (1963) New benzimidazole derivatives with powerful protective action on tissue-culture cells infected with types 1, 2, and 3 poliovirus. Nature 198:1270–1273

O'Sullivan DG, Pantic D, Wallis AK (1965) Protection offered to poliovirus-infected tissue-culture cells by methoxy- and hydroxy-methyl compounds related to 2-benzylbenzimidazole. Nature 205:262–264

O'Sullivan DG, Pantic D, Wallis AK (1967) New 1,2-disubstituted benzimidazoles with high inhibiting effects on poliovirus replication. Experientia 23:704–706

O'Sullivan DG, Pantic D, Dane DS, Briggs M (1969) Protective action of benzimidazole derivatives against virus infections in tissue culture and in vivo. Lancet I:446–448

Pfau CJ (1975) Arenavirus chemotherapy-retrospect and prospect. Bull WHO 52:737–744

Pfau CJ, Camyre KP (1968) Inhibition of lymphocytic choriomeningitis virus multiplication by 2-(α-hydroxybenzyl)-benzimidazole. Virology 35:375–380

Philipson L, Bengtsson S, Dinter Z (1966) The reversion of guanidine inhibition of poliovirus synthesis. Virology 29:317–329

Phillpotts RJ, DeLong DC, Wallace J, Jones RW, Reed SE, Tyrrell DAJ (1981) The activity of enviroxime against rhinovirus infection in man. Lancet I:1342–1344

Roderick WR, Nordeen CW Jr, von Esch AM, Appell RN (1972) Bisbenzimidazoles. Potent inhibitors of rhinoviruses. J Med Chem 15:655–658

Rosenwirth B, Eggers HJ (1977) Echovirus 12-induced host cell shutoff is prevented by rhodanine. Nature 267:370–371

Rosenwirth B, Eggers HJ (1978) Structure and replication of echovirus type 12. 2. Viral polypeptides synthesized in the infected cell. Eur J Biochem 92:61–67

Schleicher JB, Aquino F, Rueter A, Roderick WR, Appell RN (1972) Antiviral activity in tissue culture systems of bis-benzimidazoles, potent inhibitors of rhinoviruses. Appl Microbiol 23:113–116

Shaver DN, Barron AL, Karzon DT (1961) Distinctive cytopathology of ECHO viruses types 22 and 23. Proc Soc Exp Biol Med 106:648–652

Shipkowitz NL, Bower RR, Schleicher JB, Aquino F, Appell RN (1972) Antiviral activity of a bis-benzimidazole against experimental rhinovirus infections in chimpanzees. Appl Microbiol 23:117–122

Skinner MS, Halperen S, Harkin JC (1968) Cytoplasmic membrane-bound vesicles in echovirus 12-infected cells. Virology 36:241–253

Stella JP, Yankaskas KD, Morgan JH, Fox MP, Pfau CJ (1974) Characteristics of the in vitro inhibition of arenavirus synthesis by bis-benzimidazoles. Antimicrob Agents Chemother 6:747–753

Tamm I (1955) Selective inhibition of virus multiplication by synthetic chemicals. Bull NY Acad Med 31:537–540

Tamm I (1956a) Selective chemical inhibition of influenza B virus multiplication. J Bacteriol 72:42–53

Tamm I (1956b) Antiviral chemotherapy. Yale J Biol Med 29:33–49

Tamm I (1956c) Enhancement of influenza virus multiplication by 5-methyl-2-D-ribobenzimidazole. Virology 2:517–531

Tamm I (1973) Kinetics and quantitative aspects of enhancement of influenza virus multiplication by 5-methyl-2-D-ribobenzimidazole (MRB). Virology 51:138–148

Tamm I, Caliguiri LA (1972) 2-(α-Hydroxybenzyl) benzimidazole and related compounds. In: Bauer DJ (ed) The international encyclopedia of pharmacology and therapeutics, vol 1. Pergamon, Oxford New York, pp 115–179

Tamm I, Eggers HJ (1962) Differences in the selective virus inhibitory action of 2-(α-hydroxybenzyl)-benzimidazole and guanidine·HCl. Virology 18:439–447

Tamm I, Eggers HJ (1963 a) Specific inhibition of replication of animal viruses. Science 142:24–33

Tamm I, Eggers HJ (1963 b) Unique susceptibility of enteroviruses to inhibition by 2-(α-hydroxybenzyl)-benzimidazole and derivatives. In: Kuemmerle HP, Preziosi P, Rentchnick P (eds) 2nd International Symposium of Chemotherapy, Naples 1961, Part II. Karger, Basel New York, pp 88–118

Tamm I, Nemes MM (1959) Selective inhibition of poliovirus multiplication. J Clin Invest 38:1047

Tamm I, Sehgal PB (1978) Halobenzimidazole ribosides and RNA synthesis of cells and viruses. Adv Virus Res 22:187–258

Tamm I, Folkers K, Horsfall FL Jr (1952) Inhibition of influenza virus multiplication by 2,5-dimethylbenzimidazole. Yale J Biol Med 24:559–567

Tamm I, Bablanian R, Nemes MM, Shunk CH, Robinson FM, Folkers K (1961) Relationship between structure of benzimidazole derivatives and selective virus inhibitory activity. J Exp Med 113:625–656

Tamm I, Eggers HJ, Bablanian R, Wagner AF, Folkers K (1969) Structural requirements of selective inhibition of enteroviruses by 2-(α-hydroxybenzyl)-benzimidazole and related compounds. Nature 223:785–788

Webb PA, Johnson KM, Mufson MA (1964) A description of two newly-recognized rhinoviruses of human origin. Proc Soc Exp Biol Med 116:845–852

Wecker E, Lederhilger G (1964) Curtailment of the latent period by double-infection with polioviruses. Proc Natl Acad Sci USA 52:246–251

Wikel JH, Paget CJ, DeLong DC, Nelson JD, Wu CYE, Paschal JW, Dinner A, Templeton RJ, Chaney MO, Jones ND, Chamberlin JW (1980) Synthesis of syn and anti isomers of 6-[[(hydroxyimino)phenyl]-methyl]-1-[(1-methylethyl)sulfonyl]-1H-benzimidazol-2-amine. Inhibitors of rhinovirus multiplication. J Med Chem 23:368–372

Arildone: A β-Diketone

J. J. McSharry and F. Pancic

A. Introduction

A new class of antiviral compounds, the aryl β-diketones, was recently discovered. A few members of this group of compounds have been tested for antiviral activity with promising results. One of these compounds, arildone, was extensively studied and shown to be active against a wide variety of DNA and RNA viruses in vitro. In addition, arildone was shown to be effective against herpesvirus infections in vivo. Arildone and its metabolites were well tolerated in animal toxicity studies and they were not mutagenic. This drug shows promise as an effective antiviral agent for use in the treatment of cutaneous herpetic infections in humans. Currently, arildone is undergoing clinical trials for herpesvirus infections in the United States, Asia, and Europe. This review summarizes the current state of knowledge concerning the antiviral activity and possible mode of action of arildone.

B. Chemical Structure and Synthesis

During the course of routine screening of compounds for antiviral activity at the Sterling-Winthrop Research Institute, it was observed that several acyclic β-diketones of the general structure 1 (Fig. 1) inhibited the replication of equine rhinovirus in vitro (Diana et al. 1977a, b, 1978a, b). This observation was unusual in that acyclic β-diketones had not previously been shown to have antiviral activity, and thus represented a new class of antiviral drugs. In an effort to establish a structure–activity relationship, a substantial number of homologs were synthesized. The methylenedioxy diketone, structure 2 (Fig. 1), was the original compound. In order to maximize its antiviral activity, this compound was modified. The approach for chemical modification was to examine five parameters with respect to in vitro antiviral activity: (1) the size of the diketone moiety; (2) the necessity of the ethyl side chain; (3) the necessity of the double bond in the alkyl bridge; (4) the length of the alkyl bridge; and (5) the effect of various substituents on the ring structure. Following an aggressive synthetic effort, structure 3 (Fig. 1) emerged as the most promising candidate in this series, exhibiting in vitro antiviral activity against both equine rhinovirus and herpes simplex virus.

The activity against herpes simplex virus was of particular interest and prompted the synthesis of a related series of compounds similar to structure 4 (Fig. 1). This latter series of compounds offered two advantages in that they were simple to prepare and more amenable to chemical modification. The general scheme for their

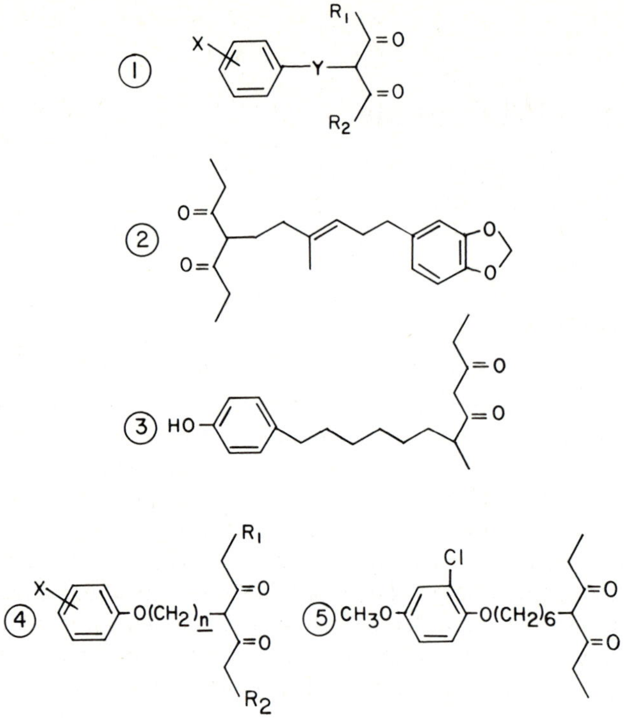

Fig. 1. Structure of arildone and some related compounds

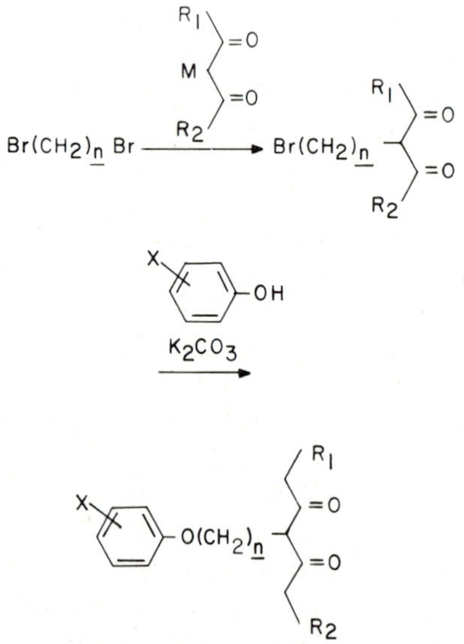

Fig. 2. Reactions involved in the synthesis of arildone and related arylalkyl diketones. R_1 and $R_2 = H$, CH_3 or C_2H_5; $M = Li$ or Na; $N = 3$ to 10

synthesis is outlined in Fig. 2. Several homologs were prepared and tested for in vitro and in vivo antiviral activity against herpes simplex virus types 1 and 2 (HSV-1 and HSV-2). The compound with the best in vitro and in vivo antiviral activity was structure 5 (Fig. 1). This compound, 4-[6-(2-chloro-4-methoxy)phenoxy]hexyl-3,5-heptanedione, was given the name arildone. The compound was composed of a β-diketone separated from a substituted benzene ring by an alkyl chain of six carbons. Substituents of the benzene ring contributed to lipophilicity and substitution or addition of more hydrophilic substituents decreased the antiviral activity of the compound. An alkyl chain of six to eight carbon atoms had maximum activity, whereas shorter or longer alkyl chains decreased antiviral activity. Changes in the diketone portion of the molecule had less predictable effects on its antiviral activity. Arildone is a white solid in the form of irregular rod-shaped crystals. The compound is stable to light and heat, non-hydroscopic, and virtually insoluble in water (54 μM).

C. Antiviral Effects

Arildone inhibited virus replication in vitro and in vivo. For in vitro testing, arildone was dissolved in dimethylsulfoxide (DMSO) followed by dilution in appropriate medium. For in vivo studies, arildone was usually prepared as a 4% or 8% solution in 90% DMSO, 10% polyethylene glycol 400, or in a cream base consisting of an oil in water emulsion.

I. In Vitro Studies

1. Inhibition of Cytopathic Effects in Cell Culture

The ability of arildone to inhibit viral multiplication, as determined by inhibition of cytopathic effects (CPE), was tested for two groups of DNA viruses and eight groups of RNA viruses (DIANA et al. 1977 a, b, 1978 a, b). Virus was added to tube cultures of cell monolayers and allowed to adsorb at 37 °C for 60 min. Then medium containing varying concentrations of arildone was added and CPE determined microscopically. The results showed that the minimum inhibitory concentrations (MIC) ranged from 0.8 μM for poliovirus to 16.2 μM for HSV-1 and HSV-2 (Table 1). The maximum tolerated concentrations of arildone for the various cells ranged from 32.4 to 67.5 μM. Higher concentrations caused intracellular granulation after 3 days of continuous exposure.

2. Plaque Reduction Tests

Because of the clinical importance of infections associated with herpesviruses and picornaviruses, further studies were conducted on the antiviral effect of arildone against members of these two groups of viruses.

a) Poliovirus 2

The effect of arildone on poliovirus plaque formation has been reported (MCSHARRY et al. 1979; KIM et al. 1980). Virus was diluted in varying concentrations of arildone, adsorbed to monolayer cultures of HeLa cells at 37 °C for 60 min, the inoculum was aspirated and agar overlay medium containing appropriate concentrations of arildone was added. The results showed that the MIC of arildone for poliovirus 2 is less than 0.27 µM (Table 1). This is considerably lower than that reported for the inhibition of CPE (0.8 µM) and is due most likely to the fact that arildone was added at the same time as virus in the plaque reduction assay, whereas it was added after adsorption in the CPE assay.

b) Herpes Simplex Virus 1 and 2

Plaque reduction assays were performed on monolayer cultures of BSC_1 cells with various concentrations of arildone present both during the adsorption period and in the agar overlay medium (McSharry and Caliguiri 1979). The data showed that under these conditions the MIC of arildone for HSV-1 was less than 1.35 µM (Table 1). Similar results (MIC of approximately 2.4 µM) have been reported for HSV-1 and HSV-2 (Kim et al. 1980). Plaque reduction assays on 15 strains of HSV-1 and HSV-2 in which the arildone was added only in the agar overlay gave an MIC of less than 5.4 µM (Pancic et al., unpublished work 1980). The MIC for some of the HSV isolates are presented in Table 1. The slight difference in the MIC (< 1.35 to < 5.4 µM) could be due to strains of virus as well as to the time of addition of arildone.

c) Varicella Zoster Virus

The effect of arildone on the plaque forming ability of varicella zoster virus was tested in monolayer cultures of human melanoma cells (C. Grose, personal communication 1980). Various concentrations of arildone were added to the carboxymethylcellulose overlay; arildone was not present during the adsorption period. Arildone (2.7 µM) reduced the number of plaques and, at higher concentrations, also reduced the size of the remaining plaques. The MIC is less than 2.7 µM (Table 1). The results of these experiments show that arildone inhibited plaque formation by HSV-1, HSV-2, varicella zoster virus, and poliovirus 2 at concentrations that were well tolerated by the cell monolayer (Sects. F.I.2, F.I.3.a).

d) Other Viruses

Plaque reduction assays have been performed to determine the MIC of arildone for vaccinia virus, coronavirus, Sindbis virus, adenovirus, vesicular stomatitis virus (VSV), and influenza A_o/WSN (H_oN_1) virus. In these assays, arildone was present only after virus infection and did not prevent plaque formation by these viruses (Table 1). Kim et al. (1980) demonstrated a 50% plaque reduction of VSV by 13.5 µM arildone using Liebowitz L-15 medium which contains galactose in place of glucose for the agar overlay, and Vero (monkey kidney) cells for the plaque assay. On the other hand, no reduction in pfu occurred in the presence of 27 µM arildone when VSV was plaqued in MDBK (bovine kidney) cells in Dulbecco's medium containing 4,000 mg/l glucose in the overlay (J. J. McSharry, unpublished work 1980). This difference in susceptibility of VSV to arildone may be due to the use of different cells and overlay media in these experiments. The replication of VSV and HSV-1 in MDBK cells was poorly inhibited by arildone irrespective of

Table 1. Effect of arildone on virus infectivity

Virus	MIC (μM)[a]	
	CPE	Plaque reduction
Poliovirus 2	0.8	< 0.27
Murine cytomegalovirus		10.8
Herpes simplex virus 1		
Sheely strain	16.2	< 1.35
Robinson strain		< 5.4
McKrae strain		< 5.4
Herpes simplex virus 2		
Curtis strain	16.2	< 5.4
75-1000 strain		< 5.4
Varicella zoster virus		< 2.7
Corona virus A 59		> 27
Vesicular stomatitis virus		
Indiana serotype	1.9	> 27
Influenza A_0/WSN/(H_0N_1) virus		> 27
Vaccinia virus	8.1	> 13.5
Adeno virus		> 27
Sindbis virus		> 27

[a] Minimal inhibitory concentration expressed as μM arildone required to reduce CPE or plaque formation by 50%

the media used, suggesting that MDBK cells are resistant to the antiviral effects of arildone (J. J. MCSHARRY, unpublished work 1980). In addition, it was shown that media containing high concentrations of glucose (4,000–10,000 mg/l) reduced the antiviral activity of arildone against HSV-1 and HSV-2 (F. PANCIC, unpublished work 1980). Currently, L-15 medium is routinely used for studies on the effect of arildone on HSV replication. Interestingly, there is no effect of glucose on the ability of arildone to inhibit poliovirus replication in HeLa or Vero cells (MCSHARRY et al. 1979). Thus, the different results on effects of arildone against VSV were due to differences in cells and media. Table 1 presents a complete list of viruses tested by plaque reduction assays for arildone. Picornaviruses and herpesviruses were very sensitive to the drug, whereas other viruses were less sensitive. Concentrations of arildone in the range 13.5–27 μM were toxic to some cultures and plaque assays could not be performed adequately at these higher concentrations.

3. Effect on Virus Yield

The effect of arildone on the yield of virus was determined for poliovirus 2, HSV-1 and HSV-2, VSV, murine cytomegalovirus virus (MCMV), Semliki Forest virus (SFV), and coxsackievirus A9 (KIM et al. 1980). Multiplicity of infection (m.o.i.) was between 0.1 and 1 pfu/cell and arildone was present from the time of adsorption throughout the entire virus growth cycle. Virus yield was determined by plaque assay 24 h after infection, except for MCMV which was assayed 72 h after

Table 2. Effect of arildone on virus replication

Virus	MIC (μM)[a]
Murine cytomegalovirus	<8.1
Semliki forest virus	<8.1
Vesicular stomatitis virus	2.7
Poliovirus 2	<2.7
Herpes simplex virus 1	2.7
Herpes simplex virus 2	<2.7
Coxsackievirus A9	<5.4

[a] Minimal inhibitory concentration expressed as μM arildone required to reduce the yield of virus by 50%

infection. The results (Table 2) showed: MIC for MCMV and SFV < 8.1 μM; VSV and HSV-1 2.7 μM; poliovirus 2 and HSV-2< 2.7 μM; and coxsackievirus < 5.4 μM. Similar results have been presented for HSV-2 (Kuhrt et al. 1979). At m.o.i. 50, arildone (5.4 μM) inhibited the yield of poliovirus by 3 log units (McSharry et al. 1979). At m.o.i. 1–10, 5.8 μM arildone inhibited the yield of VSV by 50% (J. J. McSharry and L. A. Caliguiri, unpublished work 1979). The replication of Epstein–Barr virus lymphoblastoid cells was reduced by 50% in the presence of ≥ 27 μM arildone (Sumaya and Ench 1980). These results show that arildone inhibited the replication of a wide variety of DNA and RNA viruses in vitro at concentrations which did not inhibit cellular macromolecular synthesis (Sect. F.I.2). As in the plaque reduction tests, the yield of herpesviruses and picornaviruses were more sensitive to arildone than that of some other viruses.

II. In Vivo Studies Against Herpes Simplex Virus

The effect of arildone on HSV infection in the guinea pig has been extensively studied (Steinberg and Pancic 1976; F. Pancic, unpublished work 1980).

1. Arildone in DMSO
a) Effect on the Development of Lesions

In vivo studies have demonstrated that arildone is effective topically in a guinea pig skin infection produced by HSV-1 and HSV-2. Application of 8% arildone in cream formulation or 8% arildone in 90% DMSO five times daily starting 24 h postinfection suppressed the formation and progression of herpetic vesicles and significantly reduced virus titer in the lesion sites. Guinea pigs were infected intradermally with HSV-1 and 24 h later arildone was applied to the infected area. The effect of arildone on the development of herpetic vesicles was evaluated daily and the lesion was assigned a score based on severity (Steinberg and Pancic 1976; F. Pancic, unpublished work 1980). The effect of 4% and 8% arildone in DMSO on the development of herpetic vesicles was evident after 1 day therapy (Fig. 3). The growth of vesicles was arrested at the stage at which the therapy was initiated, and no new vesicles formed after that time. During the next 24 h therapy, drying, and

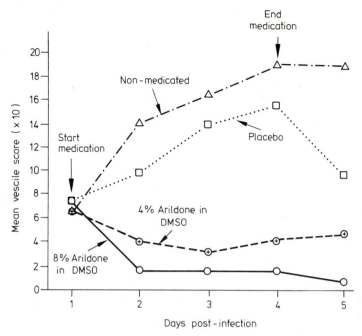

Fig. 3. The effect of 8% and 4% arildone in 90% DMSO on the development of herpetic vesicles in guinea pigs. Animals were infected intradermally with HSV-1. Medication was applied topically five times daily for 4 days. Scoring was as follows: 0 = no vesicles, no erythema; 0.5 = 1–4 small vesicles, barely raised; 1.0 = 1–4 raised vesicles, slight erythema; 1.5 = 1–4 large vesicles, pronounced erythema; 2.0 = 4–10 large vesicles, edematous tissue; 2.5 = > 10 large vesicles, partly coalescent, edematous tissue; 3.0 = coalescent vesicles, edematous tissue

crusting began in all arildone-treated sites, while in placebo DMSO-treated animals, drying of the skin was observed around existing vesicles, but not on the vesicles themselves. In those animals as well as in untreated ones, vesicles were moist and continued to increase in size. New vesicles were still in the process of forming in the placebo-treated animals. On the fourth and fifth days, the infection sites in the arildone-treated animals' skin was dry, smooth, slightly thickened, and showed no evidence of active infection. In placebo-treated animals, some crusting was observed at that time; however, each vesicle site was marked with a scab which, upon removal, revealed serous fluid under the crust.

Statistical analysis showed a significant difference between lesion scores of animals treated with 4% or 8% arildone and those of placebo-treated controls after 24 h treatment. The healing and drying of vesicles was observed after 24 h treatment in both groups treated with 4% and 8% arildone. The 8% arildone treated group showed a trend in the score that was significantly different from the placebo-treated group ($P=0.01$); the drug treatment results showed a decrease of score whereas the placebo score increased over time. Similar results were obtained with 4% arildone but to a lesser degree. Both drug concentrations showed overall mean scores that were significantly different from the placebo-treated group ($P=0.01$). There was no significant difference between 4% and 8% arildone in terms of

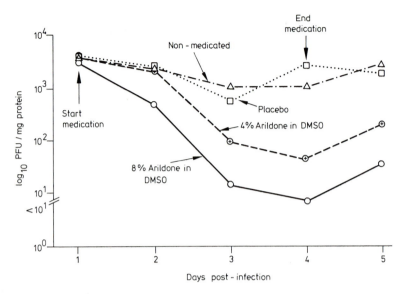

Fig. 4. The effect of 8% and 4% arildone in 90% DMSO on the virus content of herpetic lesions in guinea pigs. Animals were infected and medication applied as described in Fig. 3. The infected site was scraped into balanced salt solution with a sterile scalpel, virus was released by sonication, and large debris was removed by low speed centrifugation. The virus in the supernatant was quantitated by plaque formation and protein analysis

trends; however, the means were significantly different ($P = 0.01$). There was a significant difference between the nonmedicated and placebo-treated groups in terms of trend over time ($P = 0.01$), the latter having a flatter curve than the former. The overall means were comparable.

b) Effect on Virus Growth

For the purpose of determining virus titers in the lesion sites, guinea pigs were infected intradermally with HSV-1 and, from day 1 (24 h postinfection) through day 5, animals were killed daily. Virus was recovered from the skin by scraping the site with a sterile disposable scalpel and the amount of infectious virus was determined by plaque assay. Results showed that 4% and 8% arildone in 90% DMSO, applied to the skin of guinea pigs infected with HSV-1 starting 24 h postinfection, reduced the virus content in the lesions compared with virus content in placebo-treated and infected nonmedicated animals (Fig. 4); 4% and 8% arildone showed linear trends with time that were significantly different from placebo ($P = 0.01$). Based on comparison between treatment means within a time period, the time–response curves diverged starting on day 3 (Fig. 4). There was no significant difference in trend between 4% and 8% arildone; however, within the time period comparison suggested a difference between the two starting on day 3 ($P = 0.05$). There was no significant difference between the nonmedicated and placebo-treated groups, either in terms of trends with time or comparisons between treatment means within a time period.

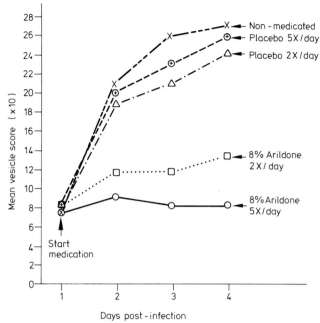

Fig. 5. The effect of 8% arildone in a cream base on the development of herpetic vesicles in guinea pigs. Animals were infected and medicated, and the results were scored as described in the legend for Fig. 3. Medication was applied either twice or five times daily for 4 days

2. Arildone in Cream

a) Effect on the Development of Lesions

The effect of the 8% arildone in cream preparation was also studied using the guinea pig skin infection model with HSV-1; 8% arildone in cream was effective in controlling the development of herpetic lesions in which the drug was applied either twice or five times daily, with the latter showing an overall greater effect (Fig. 5). The therapeutic effect was not as rapid and marked as that produced by arildone prepared in DMSO. The clinical process of the infection was arrested after 24 or 48 h therapy. The size of the herpetic vesicles remained constant and new ones failed to develop. The difference in the appearance of vesicles in arildone-treated and placebo-treated or untreated animals was even more evident on the third and fourth days of therapy when progressively larger and coalescing vesicles were observed in placebo-treated and untreated animals, while the vesicles in aril-done-treated sites became smaller and crust formation began.

Statistical analysis of data showed a significant difference ($P=0.01$) between lesion scores of animals treated five times daily with arildone and those treated five times daily with placebo cream on days 2, 3, and 4 postinfection. The difference between lesion scores in animals treated twice daily with arildone compared with those treated twice daily with placebo was also statistically significant ($P=0.01$) on days 2, 3, and 4 postinfection. However, the scores were consistently lower for the group treated five times daily on all days compared with the group treated twice daily. There were no significant differences between the groups treated with place-bo twice of five times daily and the nonmediated groups.

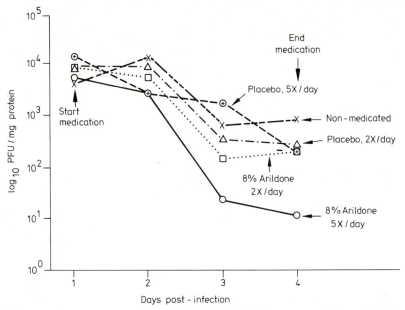

Fig. 6. The effect of 8% arildone in cream base on the virus content of herpetic lesions in guinea pigs. Animals were infected and virus was assayed as described in Fig. 4. Medication was applied to the infected area either twice or five times daily for 4 days

b) Effect on Virus Growth

Comparison of the effect of 8% arildone in cream on the virus growth in skin lesion after treatments twice or five times daily showed that virus titers were more significantly effected in animals treated five times daily with arildone, than in those treated only twice daily (Fig. 6). Arildone (8%) applied five times daily to the skin had a greater effect on the virus titer than when the compound was applied only twice daily. The statistically significant difference between virus titers in the skin scrapings of animals treated five times daily and corresponding placebo-treated animals was $P = 0.01$ on days 3 and 4 postinfection. The virus titers in groups treated twice daily with arildone were not statistically different from the corresponding placebo-treated groups. There were no significant differences between either of the two placebo-treated groups (those treated twice or five times) daily and the nonmedicated animals. Similar results were obtained when other strains of HSV-1 and HSV-2 were used and 8% arildone applied topically either in DMSO or in a cream preparation. These results indicate that topical application of arildone may be useful in the treatment of cutaneous herpetic infection in humans.

D. Mode of Action

I. Herpes Simplex Virus

In a preliminary report, it was shown that 8.1 μM arildone prevented HSV-2 replication and the synthesis of HSV-2-specific DNA and proteins (Kuhrt et al.

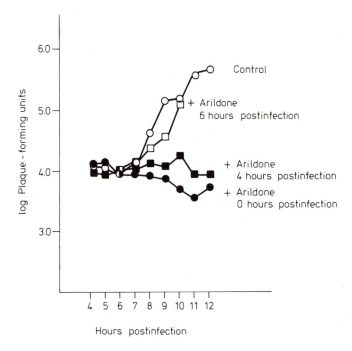

Fig. 7. Effect of adding arildone at various times after infection. BSC₁ cell monolayers were infected with HSV-2 at m.o.i. ∼ 1. After the adsorption period, virus growth medium was added. At various times postinfection arildone (8.1 μM) was added to the growth medium. The yield of virus 24 h postinfection was determined by plaque assay. (KUHRT et al. 1979)

1979). Addition of the drug during the first 6 h postinfection at low m.o.i. reduced the yield of virus, whereas addition of the drug after 6 h postinfection did not reduce virus yield (Fig. 7). These results showed that at low m.o.i. (1.0 pfu/cell), the sensitive step in HSV-2 replication was between 0 and 6 h postinfection. If arildone was removed from HSV-2-infected cells between 0 and 6 h postinfection, the yield of virus was not reduced, suggesting that the antiviral effect of arildone was reversible.

Arildone inhibited HSV replication by an unknown process, but it seemed to inhibit an early event since addition of the drug after 6 h postinfection did not change the course of the infection. One early event is the uncoating of HSV in the cytoplasm which occurs over a period of time and may not be complete until the virus enters the nucleus. The preliminary data on the arildone-sensitive stage in herpesvirus-infected cells are consistent with the idea that arildone prevents herpesvirus replication by inhibiting the uncoating of HSV in the cytoplasm of infected cells. Further studies with herpesviruses will be required to determine if arildone inhibits HSV uncoating. If arildone blocks uncoating during HSV infections, as it does in poliovirus infections (Sect. D.II), it will be very suggestive that the mechanism of action is the same for other viruses.

Table 3. Effect of arildone on early events in poliovirus replication[a]

Addition of compound $(2.7\,\mu M)$		PFU (% of control)
Adsorption at 0 °C	Incubation at 37 °C	
−	−	100
+	+	0
+	−	97
−	+	22

[a] HeLa cell monolayers were inoculated with poliovirus in the presence (+) or absence (−) of arildone $(2.7\,\mu M)$ at 0 °C for 1 h. The inoculum was removed, the monolayers washed twice with ice-cold Eagle's MEM and the cells were incubated in the presence (+) or absence (−) of arildone at 37 °C for 1 h. The medium was aspirated and replaced with an agar overlay without arildone. Plaques were counted 48 h after incubation at 37 °C under an atmosphere of 5% CO_2. (McSharry et al. 1979)

Table 4. Effect of arildone on penetration of poliovirus[a]

Treatment	Infective centers per plate[b]	
	Untreated	Arildone $(2.7\,\mu M)$
End adsorption at 4 °C	4.6×10^4	5.1×10^4
Antibody added after incubation at 37 °C for:		
0 min	4.0×10^3	1.6×10^3
30 min	5.8×10^4	5.0×10^4
60 min	5.7×10^4	4.2×10^4

[a] Poliovirus was adsorbed by cells for 1 h at 4 °C in the presence or absence of $2.7\,\mu M$ arildone, and one set of cultures was assayed for infective centers without exposure to poliovirus-specific antibody. Other sets of cultures were exposed to poliovirus-specific antibody after additional incubation at 37 °C for various periods. (McSharry et al. 1979)
[b] Penetration was measured as infective centers no longer sensitive to poliovirus 2 antibody. Arildone was present in the treated cultures from the time of inoculation at 4 °C until the end of antibody treatment (30 min at 20 °C)

II. Poliovirus

The mode of action of arildone against poliovirus has recently been elucidated. Arildone inhibited poliovirus replication by preventing intracellular uncoating of the virion (McSharry et al. 1979). More recent studies suggested that arildone prevented intracellular uncoating of poliovirus by stabilizing the capsid proteins in such a way that these proteins cannot undergo the conformational changes required for uncoating and release of virion RNA (Caliguiri et al. 1980).

Table 5. Effects of arildone on photoinactivation of neutral red poliovirus[a]

Time (h)	Irradiation	Infectious centers	
		No arildone	Arildone (2.7 μM)
0	−	2.8×10^4	1.6×10^4
	+	$<0.3 \times 10^0$	$<0.3 \times 10^0$
3	−	2.8×10^4	2.5×10^4
	+	2.0×10^4	1.3×10^1

[a] Virus grown in the presence of neutral red is photosensitive as long as the dye remains within the viral capsid. Neutral red poliovirus was adsorbed by GMK cell monolayers in the dark at 0 °C in the presence or absence of arildone (2.7 μM). One set of cultures was irridated at the end of adsorption at 0 °C, or 3 h after transfer of cultures to 37 °C. The cells were detached from the monolayer, diluted and assayed for infective centers. (McSHARRY et al. 1979)

Previous experiments with plaque reduction assays suggested that arildone inhibited an early event in poliovirus replication, possibly adsorption, penetration, or uncoating. Arildone did not inhibit adsorption to or penetration of poliovirus into HeLa cells (McSHARRY et al. 1979). The data are presented in Table 3. When the drug was present only during incubation at 0 °C, poliovirus adsorbed to HeLa cells and formed plaques. When the drug was present during incubation at 0° and 37 °C or only during incubation at 37 °C, the number of plaques was reduced by 100% and 78%, respectively. The results of this experiment showed that arildone blocked an event which occured at 37 °C, after the adsorption period. The data (Table 4) showed that arildone did not prevent penetration of poliovirus into African green monkey kidney (GMK) cells after incubation at 37 °C for 30 or 60 min. In this experiment, poliovirus was adsorbed to GMK cells at 4 °C in the presence or absence of arildone. After the adsorption period, the plates were incubated at 37 °C and poliovirus-specific antibody was added at various times. Arildone did not prevent adsorption at 4 °C. Antibody did not reduce infectivity when added (immediately) after incubation at 37 °C, indicating that virus was still at the cell surface and susceptible to neutralization by antibody. After 30 and 60 min at 37 °C, antibody did not neutralize virus, indicating that the virus had penetrated the cell. The results of this experiment showed that arildone did not inhibit penetration of poliovirus into GMK cells. Arildone did prevent uncoating of poliovirus in GMK cells (McSHARRY et al. 1979). The data showed that, in the absence of arildone, virus was not sensitive to photoinactivation, indicating that it had undergone intracellular uncoating (Table 5).

The results of these experiments showed that arildone inhibited poliovirus replication by blocking uncoating of the virus after it had entered the cell and it was postulated that arildone inhibited the intracellular uncoating of poliovirus by a direct interaction of the drug with the viral capsid proteins. The isolation of drug-resistant mutants of poliovirus also suggested a direct interaction between arildone and the viral capsid proteins (L. A. CALIGUIRI, J. A. LAFFIN, M. SCHROM, and

Table 6. Effect of arildone on thermal inactivation of poliovirus

Time (min)[a]	Poliovirus titer (pfu/ml)		
	Eagle's MEM	Eagle's MEM +0.01% DMSO	Eagle's MEM +2.7 μM arildone +0.01% DMSO
0	3.4×10^9	4.3×10^9	4.0×10^9
2.5	2.5×10^9	2.3×10^9	4.5×10^9
5	2.2×10^8	2.4×10^8	2.3×10^9
10	2.3×10^7	6.1×10^7	2.5×10^9
20	1.3×10^6	3.4×10^6	2.2×10^9

[a] Time of incubation of poliovirus 2 at 47 °C. (Caliguiri et al. 1980)

Table 7. Effect of arildone on alkaline inactivation of poliovirus

Time (min)[a]	Poliovirus titer (pfu/ml)			
	Eagle's MEM	pH 10.5	0.01% DMSO pH 10.5	2.7 μM arildone pH 10.5
0	9.2×10^7	7.3×10^7	9.1×10^7	8.5×10^7
15	3.0×10^7	2.7×10^7	3.0×10^7	6.4×10^7
30	8.4×10^6	1.4×10^7	1.1×10^7	8.1×10^7
60	8.1×10^6	5.1×10^4	1.6×10^4	5.4×10^7

[a] Time of incubation of poliovirus 2 at 40 °C at pH 10.5. (Caliguiri et al. 1980)

J. J. McSharry, unpublished work 1980; H. J. Eggers, personal communication 1979). To test this hypothesis, the effect of arildone on the thermal and alkaline degradation of poliovirus in vitro was studied (Caliguiri et al. 1980).

The results of these experiments showed that arildone prevented the loss of infectivity and the change in sedimentation due to heating poliovirus at 47 °C for various periods of time (Table 6, Fig. 8) and the loss of infectivity of poliovirus incubated at 40 °C at pH 10.5 (Table 7). The results presented in Fig. 9 show that arildone prevented the change in sedimentation profile of poliovirus incubated at 40 °C at pH 10.5 up to 20 min. However, after 60 min incubation under these conditions, arildone failed to protect poliovirus from changes in sedimentation rate. The fact that arildone protected poliovirus infectivity for 60 min incubation at 40 °C at pH 10.5, but did not completely stabilize the virus particle, suggests that heat and alkali inactivation of poliovirus occur via different mechanisms.

The results of these inactivation studies on the poliovirus showed that arildone stabilized poliovirus in the presence of heat and alkali. These results are in agreement with the previous studies, which showed that arildone stabilized the viral capsid in such a way that it can not uncoat after penetrating HeLa or GMK cells. Thus, the mode of action of arildone against poliovirus replication is to prevent uncoating by stabilizing the virion capsid proteins in such a manner as to prevent the conformational changes required for uncoating and release of viral RNA in the cytoplasm of host cells.

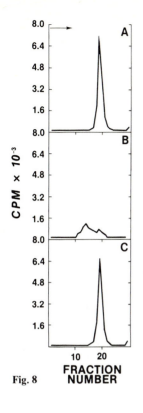

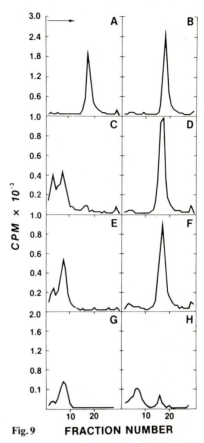

Fig. 8 a–c. Sedimentation of poliovirus in sucrose gradients. Purified methionine ^{35}S labeled poliovirus 2 was sedimented in preformed linear 15%–30% sucrose reticulocyte standard buffer (w/w) gradients: **a** native, unheated poliovirus, **b** poliovirus incubated at 47 °C for 20 min in Eagle's MEM; **c** poliovirus incubated at 47 °C for 20 min in Eagle's MEM containing 2.7 µM arildone and 0.01% DMSO. The arrow indicates the direction of sedimentation. (CALIGUIRI et al. 1980)

Fig. 9 a–h. Sedimentation of poliovirus in sucrose gradients after incubation at alkaline pH. Purified, methionine ^{35}S labeled poliovirus 2 was sedimented in preformed, linear 15%–30% sucrose reticulocyte standard buffer (w/w) gradients. Poliovirus incubated in glycine buffer, pH 10.5 at 40 °C for: **a** 5 min; **c** 10 min; **e** 20 min; and **g** 60 min. Poliovirus incubated in glycine buffer, pH 10.5 containing 2.7 µM arildone at 40 °C for: **b** 5 min; **d** 10 min; **f** 20 min; and **h** 60 min. The *arrow* indicates the direction of sedimentation. (CALIGUIRI et al. 1980)

E. Metabolism

The following studies were performed at the Sterling-Winthrop Research Institute and the data, while not published, are on file. Because of space limitations, only a small portion of the studies are presented with accompanying data. Similar results were obtained from studies in other systems.

WIN 40848   HO—⟨ring, Cl⟩—O(CH₂)₆ CH with C=O, C₂H₅ groups

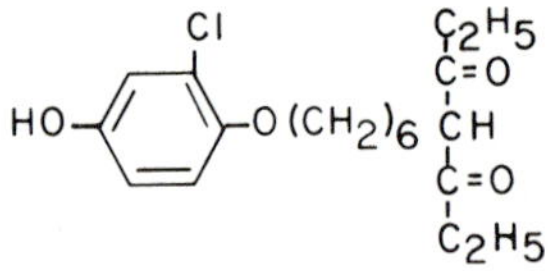

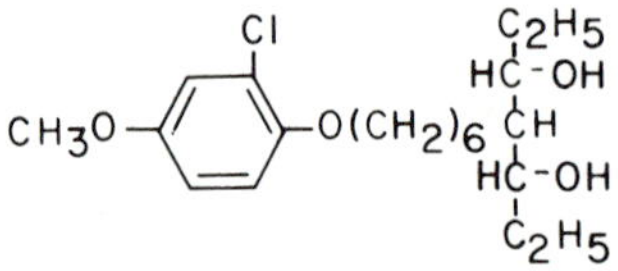

WIN 42162   CH₃O—⟨ring, Cl⟩—O(CH₂)₆ CH with HC-OH, C₂H₅ groups

WIN 42209   CH₃O—⟨ring, Cl⟩—O(CH₂)₆ CH with C=O, HC-OH, C₂H₅ groups

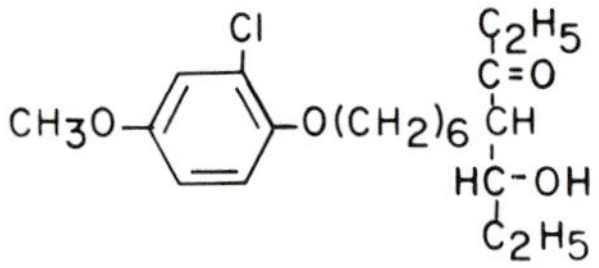

Fig. 10. Structures of some of the in vivo and in vitro metabolites of arildone

I. In Vitro Studies

1. Metabolism by CATR Cells

The metabolism of arildone ³H was studied in normal human amnion (CATR) cells in tissue culture. CATR cells were incubated in medium containing 8.1 μM arildone ³H for 24 h. After incubation, the media were pooled and sequentially extracted. The cells remaining affixed to the inside of the bottles were also extracted. Aliquots of each extract were spotted on thin layer chromatography (TLC) plates, along with arildone as a reference and the plates were developed. Large quantities of metabolites designated WIN 42162 and WIN 42209 were detected as well as a compound which matches the R_F of arildone. Their structures are shown in Fig. 10. In the extract of the medium, only metabolite WIN 42209 and the suspected arildone were present in significant amounts. In the extracts of the cells, metabolites WIN 42162, WIN 42209, and arildone were detected.

Mass spectral analysis of metabolites WIN 42162 and WIN 42209 identified these compounds as 4 [6-(2-chloro-4-methoxy)phenoxyl]hexyl 3,5-heptanediol and 4- [6-(2-chloro-4-methoxy)phenoxyl]hexyl -5-hydroxy-3-heptanone, respectively. Metabolite WIN 42162 was synthesized and chromatographed by TLC along with a CATR extract. A radioscan of the TLC plate showed metabolite WIN 42162 to have an identical R_F with the synthesized material. WIN 40848 (Sect. E.II.2) and WIN 42209 were active in vitro against HSV-1 and HSV-2. These two compounds inhibited virus-induced CPE at concentrations of 32.4 μM while WIN 42162 was inactive.

Table 8. Disposition of radioactivity following oral administration[a] of arildone [14]C

Specimen	Killing time					
	0.75 h			24 h		
	dpm/g[b]	(µg/g)	(% dose)	dpm/g[b]	(µg/g)	(% dose)
GI tract	1910	550	88.2	572	170	35.5
Liver	129	37	3.94	28.7	8.3	1.39
Adrenal glands	37.1	11	< 0.01	16.2	4.7	< 0.01
Spleen	35.7	10	0.05	14.0	4.1	0.03
Kidneys	29.7	8.7	0.16	18.0	5.3	0.12
Heart	16.7	4.7	0.03	8.67	2.3	0.02
Lungs	12.3	3.5	0.07	6.67	1.9	0.04
Carcass	9.53	2.8	4.41	26.0	7.5	33.4
Muscle	3.60	1.0		2.69	0.8	
Testes	3.33	1.0	0.02	18.0	5.2	0.09
Brain	3.33	1.0	0.02	0.57	0.6	< 0.01
Urine			1.83			25.6
Feces			0			3.17
Total recovery			98.7			99.4

[a] DMSO solution, 50 mg/kg; three animals
[b] dpm in thousands

II. In Vivo Studies

1. Disposition in Laboratory Animals

The adsorption and disposition of arildone ^{14}C were studied in rats after oral administration. Rats were given an oral dose of arildone ^{14}C in DMSO (50 mg/kg). The animals were killed at 0.75 or 24 h postmedication and disposition of radioactivity in various tissues, feces, and urine was determined. The results are presented in Table 8. Radioactivity in the gastrointestinal tract decreased from 88.2% of the dose at 0.75 h to 35.5% at 24 h. Liver radioactivity was equivalent to 37 and 8.3 µg/g of arildone at 0.75 and 24 h, respectively. Other tissues with high levels of arildone radioactivity at 24 h were kidney (5.3 µg/g), testes (5.2 µg/g), and carcass (7.5 µg/g). At 24 h, 25.6% of the dose was excreted in the urine, whereas only 3.2% appeared in the feces. The major repository for radioactivity at 24 h was the carcass which contained 33% of the dose.

The disposition of arildone after intravenous inoculation was also determined. Rats were inoculated intravenously with arildone [14]C (5 mg/kg) in DMSO. Blood samples were collected at various intervals after inoculation and radioactivity determined. The results are presented in Fig. 11. After intravenous administration of arildone ^{14}C, a biphasic decline in radioactivity was observed. The graphically determined half-lives were about 0.5 (α) and 5.5 h (β). The mean equivalent blood concentrations of arildone were 2.4 µg/ml at 3 min and 0.01 µg/ml at 24 h. The data, presented in Table 9, showed that, at 72 h postmedication, feces contained 57% of dose, urine 34.5%, gastrointestinal tract 2.7%, and remainder of animal

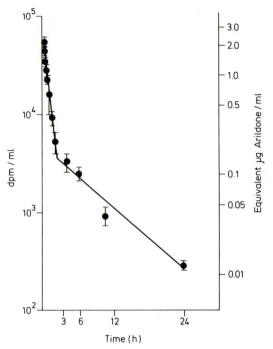

Fig. 11. Blood radioactivity after intravenous administration of arildone ^{14}C to rats. Arildone (5 mg/kg) in DMSO was injected into the external jugular vein of four rats. At various times postmedication, blood was withdrawn from the tail vein and radioactivity was determined

Table 9. Disposition of radioactivity following intravenous administration[a] of arildone [14]C

Specimen	% dose				
	Animal[b]				
	1	2	3	4	Mean ± standard error
Feces	51.0	69.4	49.2	58.5	57.0 ± 4.6
Urine	38.1	33.9	31.1	34.9	34.5 ± 1.4
GI tract	3.3	2.9	2.9	1.6	2.7 ± 0.4
Body[c]	1.5	1.7	2.4	1.4	1.8 ± 0.2
Total recovery	93.9	108	85.6	96.4	96.0 ± 4.6

[a] DMSO solution, 5 mg/kg
[b] Animals killed 72 h postmedication
[c] All tissues except GI tract

1.8%. Thus, after intravenous administration, arildone was rapidly removed from the blood and excreted in the feces and urine.

Similar studies of the disposition of radioactively labeled arildone administered to mice, rats, rabbits, and monkeys by various routes including intravenous inoculation in 70% ethanol, oral administration in gum tragacanth, or topical applica-

Table 10. Identification of fecal radioactivity following oral administration[a] of arildone [14]C

Fraction	% dose			
	Animal[b]			
	A	B	C	Mean ± standard error
Arildone	51.6	53.0	59.3	54.6 ± 2.4
WIN 40848	7.8	10.9	11.1	9.9 ± 1.1
Unidentified	10.0	15.4	11.6	12.3 ± 1.6
Nonextractable	27.8	4.2	4.3	12.1 ± 7.8
Total radioactivity	97.2	83.5	86.3	88.9 ± 4.0

[a] Gum tragacanth, 50 mg/kg
[b] Fecal samples, 0–24 h

tion in 8% cream to skin or vagina showed that arildone rapidly entered the various compartments of the body and was removed from the body quickly. Between 50% and 70% of the radioactivity was excreted in the feces and 20%–30% was excreted in the urine.

2. Metabolism in Laboratory Animals

Metabolic derivatives of arildone were isolated from the feces of rats fed arildone ^{14}C in gum tragacanth. Feces collected 10–24 h postmedication were extracted with hexane and then with ethyl acetate and the organic phases analyzed by thin layer chromatography. The data showed that approximately 55% of the radioactivity was recovered in the feces as arildone (Table 10). The desmethyl metabolite, WIN 40848 (Fig. 10), represented 10% of the dose. An unidentified polar component constituted 12% of the dose. The balance of the fecal radioactivity was not extractable with either hexane or ethyl acetate.

Mice, rats, and dogs were injected intravenously with arildone ^{14}C in DMSO. Blood was collected, the plasma separated and extracted with acetone and methanol. Urine from the dogs was assayed directly. The samples were analyzed for arildone and its various metabolites by high pressure liquid chromatography (HPLC). Arildone rapidly disappeared from the plasma of dog, mouse, and rat after intravenous administration of arildone [14]C. The rapid metabolism of arildone in the dogs was evidenced by the rapid decrease in the plasma concentrations of intact drug and the concomitant increase in the plasma concentration of two polar metabolites, chlorohydroquinone sulfate and 2-chloro-4-methoxyphenyl sulfate. Arildone had a graphically determined (from 5 to 60 min) half-life of approximately 20 min in the dog. The same pattern of metabolism was evident in the rat and mouse, although the mouse plasma contains an additional radioactive peak. All species showed evidence of WIN 40848 (Fig. 10); however the concentrations of this desmethyl metabolite were, in general, significantly lower than arildone. In the two dogs, the plasma concentrations of free chloromethoxyphenol were significantly lower than those of the conjugated chloromethoxyphenyl sulfate. However,

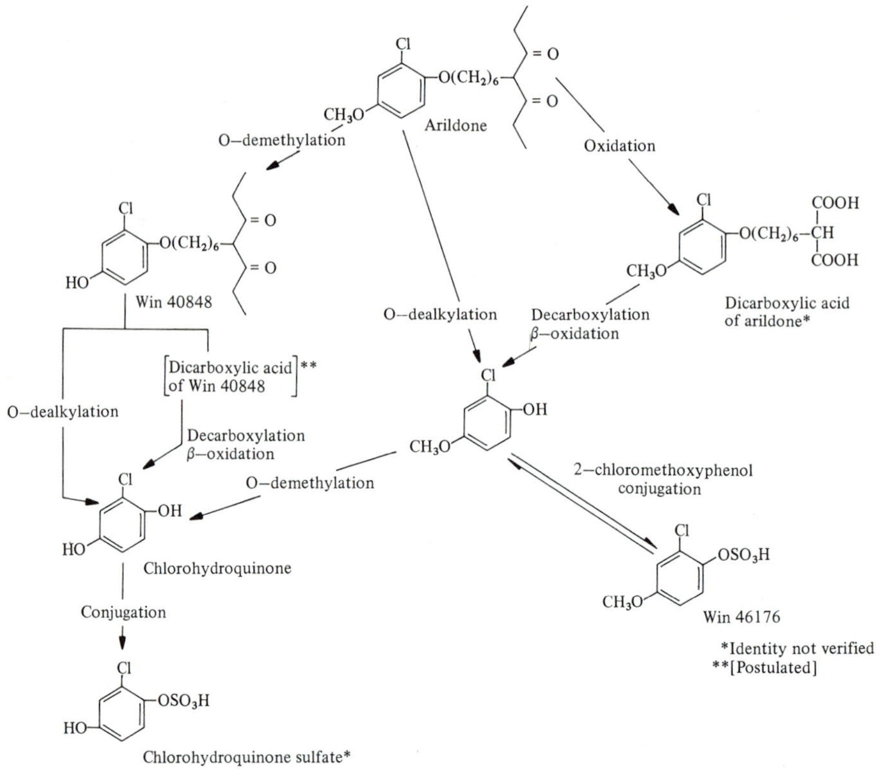

Fig. 12. Proposed pathway for arildone metabolism. * Identity not verified; ** postulated

in the rat and mouse, the concentrations of the free and conjugated chloromethoxyphenol were similar. The dog urine samples analyzed by HPLC had high concentrations of 2-chloro-4-methoxyphenyl sulfate (11.9%–12.2% of the dose), chloromethoxyphenol (4.4%–5.9% of the dose) and chlorohydroquinone sulfate (3.5%–8.1%) of the dose). Only trace amounts of arildone and WIN 40848 were present.

The proposed pathways for arildone metabolism are shown in Fig. 12. There are two possible metabolic routes that would yield phenolic end products. First, the entire side chain could be removed intact by O-dealkylation. Second, the branched chain could be oxidized to the corresponding dicarboxylic acid. This malonate type derivative could then undergo decarboxylation (as does malonic acid); the remaining chain could then be degraded by β-oxidation like a fatty acid. In either case, the free phenols are then conjugated and excreted.

F. Toxicology

Toxicologic studies necessary to assure the tolerance and safety of arildone in humans were performed at the Sterling-Winthrop Research Institute and are summarized here to give the reader an overview of the benign effects of arildone and some of its metabolites in various in vivo and in vitro model systems.

Table 11. Effect of arildone on HeLa cell macromolecular synthesis

Arildone (μM)	Activity ($10^3 \times$ cpm)[a]					
	Leucine ³H		Thymidine ³H		Uridine ³H	
	Acid soluble	Acid insoluble	Acid soluble	Acid insoluble	Acid soluble	Acid insoluble
0	2.0	7.2	6.2	40.3	48.0	119.3
	(100)	(100)	(100)	(100)	(100)	(100)
2.7	2.1	7.2	4.9	32.3	54.0	101.4
	(105)	(100)	(82)	(80)	(113)	(85)
27.0	2.1	6.8	5.2	26.5	33.0	70.9
	(105)	(94)	(87)	(66)	(69)	(59)

[a] Average of four determinations; numbers in parentheses give the percentage of untreated control sample

I. In Vitro Studies

1. Mutagenic Evaluation of Arildone

Arildone was evaluated for mutagenic activity in the presence and absence of microsomal activation enzymes by the microbial assays developed by AMES et al. (1975) and at concentrations between 0.05 μg/plate and 2,000 μg/plate, arildone was not mutagenic. Arildone was not mutagenic in a mouse lymphoma assay, did not induce genetic damage in germ cells of rats fed up to 250 μg kg^{-1} day^{-1} for 5 days, nor did it cause any chromosomal abnormalities in bone marrow cells when rats were fed up to 250 μg kg^{-1} day^{-1}. The results of these tests showed that arildone was not mutagenic in vitro and did not cause chromosomal abnormalities or measurable genetic defects in vivo.

2. Effect of Arildone on Cellular Macromolecular Synthesis

A number of permanent cell lines were treated with various concentrations of arildone; 24 h after the addition of arildone to the cell monolayers, the cells were labeled with uridine ³H, thymidine ³H, or leucine ³H to label RNA, DNA, or protein, respectively. At the end of the 30-min pulse, the medium was removed, the monolayers were washed thoroughly in cold PBS, extracted with 5% TCA, and TCA-insoluble material was solubilized with 0.1 M NaOH. TCA-soluble and TCA-insoluble radioactivity was measured by liquid scintillation counting in Biofluor (New England Nuclear Corporation). The results, presented in Tables 11 and 12 showed that 2.7 μM arildone did not inhibit the transport of leucine ³H or uridine ³H into HeLa cells, whereas the transport of thymidine ³H was inhibited by 18%. At the same concentration, the incorporation of leucine ³H into protein was not affected, whereas the incorporation of thymidine ³H into DNA was inhibited by approximately 20% and that of uridine ³H was inhibited by 15%. At 1.4 μM, arildone had little effect on the transport of precursors into acid-soluble

Table 12. Effect of arildone on BSC_1 cell macromolecular synthesis

Arildone (μM)	Activity ($10^3 \times$ cpm)[a]					
	Leucine ^{3}H		Thymidine ^{3}H		Uridine ^{3}H	
	Acid soluble	Acid insoluble	Acid soluble	Acid insoluble	Acid soluble	Acid insoluble
0	0.76 (100)	3.4 (100)	2.43 (100)	12.40 (100)	67.28 (100)	64.14 (100)
1.4	0.73 (96)	3.2 (94)	2.44 (100)	12.25 (99)	61.18 (91)	54.33 (85)
14.0	0.66 (87)	2.8 (82)	1.81 (74)	10.13 (82)	34.20 (51)	32.08 (50)

[a] Average of four determinations; numbers in parentheses give the percentage of untreated control sample

pools of BSC_1 cells (monkey kidney cell cultures) and only a slight effect on the incorporation of one of the precursors (uridine ^{3}H) into acid-insoluble material. Similar results have been obtained with MDBK, BHK21-F, CV1, and HKCC cells. The results of these experiments showed that arildone, at concentrations which were near or greater than the MIC of HSV and poliovirus (Sects. C.I.2a, C.I.2b), has only minimal inhibitory effects on cellular macromolecular synthesis.

3. Effect of Arildone and Its Metabolites on Cell Growth

a) Cell Culture Studies

The cytotoxicity and tolerance of arildone and its in vivo and in vitro metabolites WIN 42162, WIN 40848, and WIN 42209 (Sects. E.I, E.II) were studied in monkey kidney cell cultures (BSC_1). Cultivation of cells for 4 days in the presence of 5.4–21.6 μM arildone or its metabolites had no effect on the viability of BSC_1 cells. Higher concentrations of arildone or its metabolites inhibited growth. Cells treated with arildone (5.4–21.6 μM) could be passed in the presence of identical concentrations of the drug with no significant loss of viability. Arildone (32.4 μM) inhibited the viability of cells passed in its presence. Similar results were obtained after growth of primary rabbit kidney cells in arildone or its metabolic products. These results showed that arildone, at concentrations near or greater than the MIC for poliovirus and herpesviruses, did not inhibit cell growth.

b) Organ Culture Studies

Arildone was evaluated for cytotoxicity on ciliary cells of ferret and rhesus monkey trachea organ cultures. Cell viability was measured by observation of ciliary movement and vital dye staining. The maximum nontoxic concentration of arildone was 270–540 μM in ferret trachea organ culture and 540 μM in rhesus monkey trachea organ culture, indicating that arildone was 10–20 times less cytotoxic for tracheal organ cultures than for monolayer cultures of BSC_1 cells.

II. In Vivo Studies

Arildone was tested for acute oral toxicity in mice and rats. Studies were performed in young adult male mice and rats with suspensions of arildone in 1% gum tragacanth. The 7-day LD_{50} was > 8,000 mg/kg in both species. There were no deaths or overt symptoms at 2,000, 4,000, or 8,000 mg/kg. Arildone (8%) cream was studied in young adult male albino mice and rats. The arildone cream was administered by intubation. The 7-day LD_{50} was > 40 ml/kg in both species. There were no deaths in mice given 40 ml/kg and only two (of ten) deaths at that dose level in the rats.

Arildone (8%) cream was also studied topically on abraded and nonabraded sites on the backs of New Zealand White rabbits. No overt or adverse effects on the skin or the healing time, attributable to medication, were observed. No adverse effect on body weight occurred, and the results of hematologic studies and blood analyses were normal at the end of the 3-week treatment period. Gross and microscopic tissue evaluation of other organs revealed no drug-related changes in any of the medicated rabbits, and organ weights of liver, kidneys, and adrenal glands were normal. Plasma levels of arildone were determined on days 2, 9, and 22, about 2 h after the second daily application. There was no evidence of accumulation of the drug over the 3-week period.

In additional studies, arildone (8%) cream was studied for tolerance by intravaginal instillation in rabbits and dogs, three times a day over a 3-week period. No systemic or local adverse effects were observed when responses were compared with those seen in rabbits or dogs similarly medicated with the vehicle cream or in a control group (treated with water). No gross or microscopic tissue changes attributable to arildone medication were observed. Plasma levels of arildone determined on or about days 2, 8, and 21 were below detectable limits (25 ng/ml) in most samples. There was no evidence of drug accumulation over the 3-week period. Gross and microscopic examination of the external genitalia and vaginal tracts did not indicate any changes attributable to medication with arildone cream or its vehicle.

To assess the systemic toxicity, arildone was administered orally to rats and monkeys. Drug was administered to male and female albino rats in single daily doses of 40, 200, or 1,000 mg/kg for 1 month. The compound was very well tolerated at all dose levels. Growth, food consumption, and the results of hematologic studies and blood and urine analyses were normal. No gross or microscopic tissue changes were observed. Teratogenic potential of arildone was studied in rats and rabbits. Arildone was administered orally to pregnant albino rats in single daily doses of 200, 500, or 1,200 mg/kg from the 6th through the 15th day of gestation. No drug-induced gross skeletal or visceral teratogenic effects were observed at any dose level. There was no effect on litter size, number of resorptions, fetal weight, sex ratio, or pre- and postimplantation loss. Pregnancy rate, number of implantations, and number of corpora lutea were also normal.

The results of these toxicity studies showed that arildone and its metabolic derivatives are well tolerated in cellular and animal experimental models. From these results it has been suggested that arildone should be well tolerated in humans and hence a promising antiviral agent for the control of human viral diseases.

G. Summary and Perspectives

In vitro studies have shown that arildone inhibits cytopathic effect of a number of RNA and DNA viruses at concentrations ranging from 0.8 to 16.2 μM. Plaque formation of 15 strains of HSV-1 and HSV-2 was inhibited in tissue culture with less than 5.4 μM arildone. In addition, arildone at concentrations of 2.7 μM inhibits the CPE of varicella zoster virus (C. Grose, personal communication). Other studies have shown that arildone is active against other herpesviruses such as murine cytomegalovirus (Kim et al. 1980) and Epstein–Barr virus (Sumaya and Ench 1980). Arildone was effective at drug concentrations which did not significantly inhibit cellular metabolism.

This potent activity against members of the herpesvirus group prompted animal studies and the therapeutic effect of arildone has been demonstrated in an experimental HSV-1 and HSV-2 skin infection in guinea pigs. Topical application of a solution of 4% or 8% arildone in 90% DMSO and 10% polyethylene glycol 400 as well as in an 8% arildone cream preparation suppressed development of vesicles when the treatment was initiated 24 h postinfection. Virus titers in the treated lesions were statistically lower in animals treated with both preparations. The 8% arildone DMSO preparation afforded the most rapid effect on the herpetic vesicles, aborting their development after only 24 h of five applications or less. Arildone in DMSO produced a greater reduction of virus replication in skin lesions than did the cream preparation. Both arildone preparations suppressed vesicles and reduced the virus titer of HSV-2 in the skin of guinea pigs; the DMSO formulation produced a significantly more rapid effect on vesicle suppression and a greater magnitude of virus reduction.

The most potent activity of arildone was against poliovirus; thus, the mode of action of the drug was studied first against this virus. Data indicate that arildone inhibits poliovirus replication by preventing intracellular uncoating of the virion (McSharry et al. 1979). Studies on purified poliovirus suggested that arildone prevents uncoating of the virion by stabilizing the protein–protein interactions of the capsid proteins (Caliguiri et al. 1980). Herpesvirus replication was inhibited by arildone by blocking an early step, one that occurs during the first 6 h after HSV infections, preventing virus replication. Although the mode of action of arildone against HSV is unknown, one possibility is that it blocks uncoating of the HSV nucleocapsid, either in the cytoplasm or in the nucleoplasm.

There are a number of analogs of arildone which possess antiviral activity in vivo and in vitro and are more soluble than arildone. WIN 41258-3, (4-[6-(2-chloro-4-methoxyphenoxy)hexyl]-3-diethyl-1-H-pyrazole methane sulfonate), and WIN 42202, an aryloxyalkyl phosphonate, are two compounds which are more soluble than arildone and have been shown to be effective against HSV-1 and HSV-2 infections of the mouse genital tract and guinea pig skin (Pancic et al. 1978, 1980 a, b). Preliminary results indicated that these two compounds were no more toxic to cells than arildone (J. J. McSharry and L. A. Caliguiri, unpublished work 1980). In addition, these various modifications of the parent compound have led to changes in the antiviral spectrum of the drug. WIN 41258-3 does not inhibit poliovirus replication whereas it does inhibit HSV-1 and HSV-2 replication (L. A. Caliguiri, J. A. Laffin, and J. J. McSharry, unpublished work 1980). By correlating the chemical change of the drug with the antiviral spectrum of these drugs it may be possible to elucidate the means for rational modification to enhance their clinical effectiveness.

Presently, a concerted effort is being made to determine the mode of action of arildone on HSV replication. The working hypothesis is that arildone inhibits HSV replication by blocking uncoating of the HSV nucleocapsid in a manner similar to that demonstrated for poliovirus. If arildone blocks HSV replication by preventing uncoating, then a single mechanism would be involved in the antiviral activity of the drug.

Arildone appears to be tolerated very well in experimental animals and may prove to be a useful drug in the treatment of cutaneous herpetic disease, especially herpes labialis, herpes genitalis, and varicella zoster in humans. The suppression of development of vesicles in the early phase, particularly with the DMSO preparation, may be a very significant achievement. The superior activity of arildone in a DMSO preparation is probably the result of deeper and more effective penetration of the drug, which may be of particular importance in varicella zoster patients. Currently, other vehicles and formulations are being studied which may provide a suitable delivery of arildone by the systemic route in herpetic and other viral infections. Clinical studies are under way to assess the effectiveness of arildone against herpesvirus infections in humans.

Acknowledgments. We wish to thank Jerome Edelson, Director, and David Benziger, Staff Member, of the Department of Drug Metabolism and Disposition, and Hans Peter Drobeck, Director of Toxicology at Sterling-Winthrop Research Institute for the use of unpublished data.

References

Ames BN, McCann J, Yamasaki E (1975) Methods for detecting carcinogens and mutagens with salmonella/mammalian microsome mutagenicity test. Mutat Res 31:347–363

Caliguiri LA, McSharry JJ, Lawrence GW (1980) Effect of arildone on modifications of poliovirus in vitro. Virology 105:86–93

Diana GD, Salvador UJ, Zalay ES, Johnson RE, Collins JE, Johnson D, Hinshaw WB, Lorenz RR, Thielking WH, Pancic F (1977a) Antiviral activity of some β-diketones. 1. Aryl alkyl diketones. In vitro activity against both RNA and DNA viruses. J Med Chem 20:750–756

Diana GD, Salvador UH, Zalay ES, Carabataes PM, Williams GL, Collins JE, Pancic F (1977b) Antiviral activity of some β-diketones. 2. Aryloxyl alkyl diketones. In vitro activity against both RNA and DNA viruses. J Med Chem 20:757–761

Diana GD, Carabateas PM, Salvador UJ, Williams GL, Zalay ES, Pancic F, Steinberg BA, Collins JC (1978a) Antiviral activity of some β-diketones 3. Aryl Bis (β-diketones). Antiherpetic activity. J Med Chem 21:689–692

Diana GD, Carabateas PM, Johnson RE, Williams GL, Pancic F, Collins JC (1978b) Antiviral activity of some β-diketones. 4. Benzyl diketones. In vitro activity against both RNA and DNA viruses. J Med Chem 21:889–894

Kim KS, Sapienza VJ, Carp RI (1980) Antiviral activity of arildone on deoxyribonucleic acid and ribonucleic viruses. Antimicrob Agents Chemother 18:276–280

Kuhrt M, Fancher MJ, Jasty V, Pancic F, Came P (1979) Preliminary studies on the mode of action of arildone, a novel antiviral agent. Antimicrob Agents Chemother 15:813–819

McSharry JJ, Caliguiri LA (1979) Inhibition of herpes simplex virus type 1 replication by arildone. In: Abstracts of the annual meeting of the American Society for Microbiology. American Society for Microbiology, Washington D.C., p 275

McSharry JJ, Caliguiri LA, Eggers HJ (1979) Inhibition of uncoating of poliovirus by aril-
    done, a new antiviral drug. Virology 97:307–315
Pancic F, Steinberg BA, Diana GD, Came PE (1978) In vivo antiviral activity of a pyrazole
    compound WIN 41528-3. In: Abstracts of annual meeting of the American Society for
    Microbiology. American Society for Microbiology, Washington, D.C., p 302
Pancic F, Steinberg BA, Diana GD, Gorman WG, Came PE (1980a) Topical activity of
    WIN 41528-3, a pyrazole compound, against herpes simplex type 1 in guinea pig skin
    infection. In: Abstracts of annual meeting of the American Society for Microbiology.
    American Society for Microbiology, Washington, D.C., p 5
Pancic F, Steinberg BA, Diana GD, Gorman WG, Came PE (1980b) Topical activity of
    WIN 42202, an aryl-oxy-alkyl phosphonate compound, against herpes simplex virus
    types 1 and 2 in guinea pig skin infections. In: Abs. of Interscience conference of
    antimicrobial agents and chemotherapy. American Society for Microbiology, Washing-
    ton D.C., p 310
Steinberg BA, Pancic F (1976) Aryldiketones, a new class of compounds active against her-
    pes simplex: In vivo activity in guinea pig skin. In: Abstr. of Interscience conference on
    antimicrobial agents and chemotherapy. American Society for Microbiology, Washing-
    ton D.C., p 418
Sumaya CV, Ench Y (1980) Inhibition of Epstein-Barr virus by arildone. In: Abstr. of In-
    terscience conference on antimicrobial agents and chemotherapy. American Society for
    Microbiology, Washington D.C., p 312

CHAPTER 11

Phosphonoacetic Acid

L. R. Overby

A. Introduction and History

Viruses carry within their genomes the necessary information to program their own replication within a susceptible host cell, using many of the preexisting cellular enzymes, substrates, and energy generating systems. In principle, a DNA virus in a cellular universe of double-stranded DNA with existing functional transcription, translation, and DNA replication systems needs only to divert these to its own use for replication. The simplest double-stranded DNA viruses would therefore need only structural genes and their promotors for synthesis of capsid proteins in order to protect progeny viral DNA in the external environment. In this simplistic example, specific interference with viral replication within the cell, without affecting essential cellular events, would not be possible. However, many viruses carry additional genes for enzyme subunits or regulatory molecules that do not preexist in normal cells, and these functions serve to give the virus a selective advantage for replication. These virus-specific molecules can provide a target for selective attack on a virus-infected cell since they are absent in normal cells. The herpesviruses induce a new DNA polymerase in infected cells, and the preceding rationale could have led to the discovery of phosphonoacetic acid, a unique and highly selective inhibitor of the viral polymerase. However, SHIPKOWITZ et al. (1973) discovered the drug through random screening of herpesvirus-infected W1-38 tissue culture cells. The initial results were not particularly exciting from a chemotherapeutic standpoint. First, the simple chemical structure (Fig. 1) suggested little opportunity

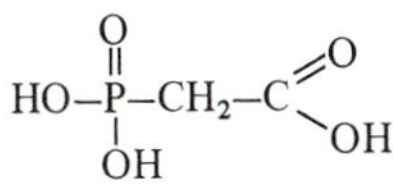

$$HO-\overset{\overset{O}{\|}}{\underset{\underset{OH}{|}}{P}}-CH_2-C\overset{\nearrow O}{\searrow_{OH}}$$

Fig. 1. Phosphonoacetic acid

for chemical manipulations to optimize activity or therapeutic index. In chemotherapy screening it is not usual that a first random discovery represents the most active compound. Second, a concentration of about 100 µg/ml was required to maintain consistent antiviral activity in cell culture. This would be comparable to a dose in animals approximating 5 g/kg. Third, only herpes simplex virus (HSV) appeared to be susceptible to phosphonoacetate. Other DNA and RNA viruses were resistant. A "broad spectrum" antiviral agent is the goal of many programs. However, alternate reasoning suggested further study of these original observations.

The drug showed little or no toxicity to human diploid fibroblast cells at levels several times the HSV-inhibitory level, and it was specific for herpesviruses only. This suggested an inhibitory activity directed toward a *virus-specific* event in infected cells. SHIPKOWITZ et al. (1973) demonstrated a potential clinical efficacy of phosphonoacetic acid by showing that topical application was therapeutic for experimental HSV skin infections in mice and for corneal infections in rabbits. The skin-infected mice were also protected when the compound was administered orally at a dosage of 800–1,400 mg/kg/day. Normal control animals tolerated the drug without obvious toxicity.

These in vivo studies suggested further investigations on the effects of phosphonoacetic acid on molecular events in normal and HSV-infected human cells. Growth and cell division of W1-38 cells were not affected by phosphonoacetate at levels of 100 µg/ml. OVERBY et al. (1974) found no significant changes in the rate of normal cell RNA, DNA, and protein synthesis in the presence of phosphonoacetic acid. In HSV-infected cells, synthesis of virus-specific DNA was completely inhibited by phosphonoacetic acid. MAO et al. (1975) isolated the virus-induced DNA polymerase from infected cells and confirmed the virus specificity by showing direct inhibition of the partially purified HSV-induced enzyme.

The original discoveries of antiviral activity of phosphonoacetate have been confirmed and extended by numerous other investigators. It is an effective inhibitor of all herpesviruses studied in cell culture and in animal laboratory models, and for several naturally occurring herpesviruses diseases. The drug has not been investigated in human disease, but the in vitro and animal studies suggest a potential for therapy of human herpesvirus infections. Since there are no reported clinical studies, this review will emphasize the mechanism of action and efficacy in cell and animal models. BOEZI (1979) has recently published a similar review.

B. DNA Polymerases

Numerous investigators have confirmed that phosphonoacetate reversibly inhibits herpesvirus-induced DNA polymerase. A comparative understanding of the normal mammalian cell DNA polymerases, and the herpesvirus-induced enzyme, is useful in clarifying the antiviral role of phosphonoacetic acid. The cellular polymerases are required for cell division and DNA repair, while the viral enzyme is necessary for virus replication. The drug is highly selective for the viral polymerase, but does inhibit to a lesser extent at least one of the cellular enzymes.

I. Cellular DNA Polymerases

Three physically and biochemically distinct DNA polymerases have been characterized for mammalian cells. These are designated α, β, and γ in the order of their discovery. WEISSBACH (1979) has reviewed the nature of and the functional roles of these polymerases. A summary of their general biochemical properties compared with herpesvirus polymerases is shown in Table 1.

DNA polymerase α is the major enzyme of this class in vertebrate cells. During cell division, the enzyme rises to high levels, and there is much evidence that en-

Table 1. Comparative properties and functions of herpesvirus and mammalian cell DNA polymerases

Property	Polymerase			
	HSV	α	β	γ
Function	Virus DNA replication	Cell DNA replication	DNA repair	Mitochondrial DNA synthesis
Molecular weight (daltons)	1.5×10^4	$1.1–1.8 \times 10^5$	$3–5 \times 10^4$	$1.6–3.3 \times 10^5$
pH optimum	8.0–8.5	7.3	7.9	8.5
Mg^{2+} concentration (mM)	3	5–10	5–10	5
Phosphonoacetic acid inhibitory concentration (μM)	1–2	25–30	>100	>100
Reference	Powell and Purifoy (1977)	Weissbach et al. (1971)	Wang et al. (1975)	Knopf et al. (1976)

zyme α plays a specialized role in replication of chromosomal DNA. Spadari and Weissbach (1975) found that, of the three cellular polymerases, only the α form was active in initiating DNA replication with an RNA primer base-paired to the template DNA. Papovaviruses do not require a virus-induced enzyme for replication. Edenberg et al. (1978) have proposed a role for the cellular α polymerase in SV40 DNA replication.

Chemical or physical damage of cellular DNA can be repaired by nucleotide excision in single strands of DNA, followed by replacement of the nucleotides through base pairing with the intact strand. The β polymerase of mammalian cells is thought to be the polymerase responsible for excision repair, although there is no direct evidence for this activity. The level of DNA polymerase β remains constant throughout the cell cycle, and in vitro it has been shown to catalyze repair of breaks in template DNA. The participation of the β enzyme in normal chromosomal DNA replication cannot be excluded.

Mitochondria contain a circular DNA genome and its mode of replication is different from the more complex nuclear chromosomal DNA. Purified mitochondria contain only DNA polymerase γ (Bolden et al. 1977); therefore, this enzyme most likely catalyzes mitochondrial DNA replication by a strand displacement model as proposed by Robberson et al. (1972).

The three known normal cellular DNA polymerases differ biophysically, and have different functions. They can be selectively inhibited, which supports further their biochemical specificity. Dideoxythymidine triphosphate selectively inhibits the β and γ polymerase, but not the α polymerase (Edenberg et al. 1978). Aphidicolin is a selective inhibitor of the α polymerase (Ohashi et al. 1978).

Thus, the preexisting cellular DNA polymerases have very highly specialized functions for the cell's own economy; therefore a virus, carrying genes for its own enzyme, could have a selective advantage for replication. Such a gene product could also offer a selective target for inhibiting viral replication.

II. Herpesvirus DNA Polymerase

The herpesviruses have a complex linear genome of $80-100 \times 10^6$ daltons molecular weight. Thus, they have genetic information for many gene products. The virus-specific proteins (α, β, γ) are synthesized at different times during the infectious cycle and are not to be confused with the α, β, and γ polymerases of normal cells. α Proteins appear first and are associated with regulatory functions for the host cells and for viral transcription. The β proteins appear next and function for replication of viral DNA. A DNA polymerase is included in the β proteins. The γ proteins arise late in infection and serve as capsid and maturation virion proteins.

A new herpesvirus-specific DNA polymerase in infected cells was first recognized by KIER and GOLD in 1963. KIER et al. (1966) later showed that the enzyme was antigenically distinct from cellular polymerases. A similar induced polymerase has been identified for all herpesviruses studied. The enzyme has been purified and characterized from herpes simplex virus (POWELL and PURIFOY 1977), Epstein-Barr Virus (OOKA et al. 1979), cytomegalovirus (HIRAI and WATANABE 1976), varicella zoster virus (MAR et al. 1978), Marek's disease virus (BOEZI et al. 1974) and equine herpesvirus (ALLEN et al. 1977). The partially purified enzymes have several properties that distinguish them from normal cell enzymes (MAR and HUANG 1979). They are separable from cellular enzymes by phosphocellulose chromatography, have different ionic requirements for optimal activity and are inhibited completely by 50 µg/ml phosphonoacetate. The cellular DNA polymerases are less sensitive to phosphonoacetate.

Purified HSV DNA polymerase has a molecular weight of about 150,000 daltons (POWELL and PURIFOY 1977), and the biochemical similarity of the enzymes to other herpesviruses suggests a genetic relatedness of the virus class. The isolation of phosphonoacetic acid-resistant herpesvirus strains by HONESS and WATSON (1977), and temperature-sensitive mutants by PURIFOY et al. (1977) and PURIFOY and POWELL (1977) clearly established that the DNA polymerase was encoded by the viral genome. Phosphonoacetate resistance as a specific genetic marker has been a useful tool in classifying and clarifying the molecular biology of herpesviruses.

C. Chemistry

I. Structure

Phosphonoacetic acid was first reported in 1924 by NYLEN. Compounds with carbon-phosphorous bonds are rare in nature (CROFTS 1958) and have not been extensively investigated for biologic activity. The simple compound can be obtained by hydrolysis of 2-(diethylphosphono)-ethylacetate, which is prepared by condensing ethylchloroacetate and triethylphosphite (NYLEN 1924).

Phosphonoacetic acid is structurally similar to pyrophosphoric acid and methylene diphosphonate (Fig. 2). Pyrophosphate is a normal substrate in many biochemical reactions in living systems, particularly the biosynthesis of nucleotides and polyribo- and deoxyribonucleotides. Methylene diphosphonate has been found to be a competitive inhibitor of pyrophosphate in pyrophorolysis reactions

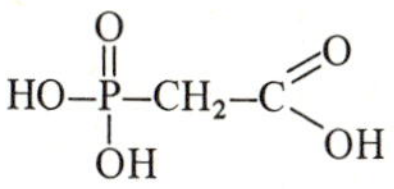

$$HO-\overset{\overset{\displaystyle O}{\|}}{\underset{\underset{\displaystyle OH}{|}}{P}}-CH_2-C\overset{\diagup O}{\diagdown OH}$$

Phosphonoacetic acid

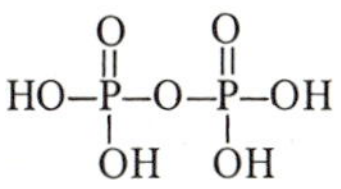

$$HO-\overset{\overset{\displaystyle O}{\|}}{\underset{\underset{\displaystyle OH}{|}}{P}}-O-\overset{\overset{\displaystyle O}{\|}}{\underset{\underset{\displaystyle OH}{|}}{P}}-OH$$

Pyrophosphoric acid

$$HO-\overset{\overset{\displaystyle O}{\|}}{\underset{\underset{\displaystyle OH}{|}}{P}}-CH_2-\overset{\overset{\displaystyle O}{\|}}{\underset{\underset{\displaystyle OH}{|}}{P}}-OH$$

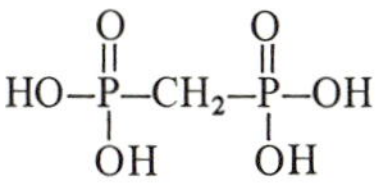

Methylene diphosphonate

Fig. 2. Structurally related analogs of pyrophosphate

(LEINBACH et al. 1976). Of the three structurally similar compounds, only phosphonoacetate inhibits herpesvirus DNA polymerase at biochemically significant concentrations.

The chemistry of phosphonoacetic acid is uncomplicated, but the biochemical specificity of this simple compound is surprising and challenging. It is a highly charged and highly soluble compound, and one must wonder how it transits the cellular membrane. 'BOEZI (1979) reported the pK_a values at zero ionic strength as: $pK_1 = 2.30$ (P–OH); $pK_2 = 5.40$ (COOH); and $pK_3 = 8.60$ (P–OH). It is a physically and chemically stable molecule. The anion can form stable salts with divalent and trivalent cations, but is otherwise chemically unreactive.

II. Structure–Activity Relationships

The structural requirements for activity of phosphonoacetic acid are rigorous. A number of analogs have been synthesized and tested as inhibitors of isolated viral DNA polymerase in vitro, viral replication in cell culture, and in infected animal model systems. Only the parent compound and the formate analog have shown consistent activity.

1. Analogs

A compilation of analogs studied is shown in Table 2, with the appropriate reference for the evaluations. All of the compounds except the formate analog are considerably less active than phosphonoacetate. However, it is difficult to assess whether all three levels of evaluation were used in each case; i.e., enzyme inhibition, viral replication in tissue culture, and animal infectivity. Full assessment would require both in vitro and in vivo evaluations because: (1) an analog inactive in vitro could conceivably be converted to the original or another active form by cellular or organ biochemical systems; or (2) observed in vitro activity could be enhanced by preferential transport into cells with increased effective concentration at the site of viral replication.

Table 2. Analogs of phosphonoacetate tested for antiherpesvirus activity

Analog	Activity	Reference
I. Carboxyl esters		
Ethyl; propyl; *t*-butyl	Yes (ethyl)	Herrin et al. (1977)
Cyclohexyl; octyl; benzyl	Yes (octyl)	Herrin et al. (1977)
II. Monophosphate esters		
Methyl; propyl; hexyl	No	Herrin et al. (1977)
III. Triesters		
Trimethyl	No	Lee et al. (1976)
Triethyl	No	Shipkowitz et al. (1973)
IV. Monophosphinic acids		
Phenyl; 4-methoxyphenyl; methyl	No	Herrin et al. (1977)
V. Phosphono analogs		
Sulfoacetate	No	Leinbach et al. (1976)
Malonate	No	Leinbach et al. (1976)
Arsenoacetate	Yes	Newton (1979)
VI. Carboxyl analogs		
Phosphonoacetaldehyde	No	Boezi (1979)
Phosphonoacetamide	No	Boezi (1979)
N-Methylphosphonoacetamide	No	Boezi (1979)
N-Propyl-; *N*-butyl-; *N*-cyclohexyl-; •*N*-amantylphosphonoacetamide	Yes	von Esch (1978)
Acetonylphosphate	No	Boezi (1979)
Aminomethylphosphonate	No	Lee et al. (1976)
α-Amino ethyl phosphonate	No	Lee et al. (1976)
N-(phosphonoacetyl)-L-aspartate	No	Boezi (1979)
Methylene diphosphonate	No	Lee et al. (1976)
Methylene diarsonate	Yes	Newton (1979)
Arsonomethylphosphonate	Yes	Newton (1979)
VII. Methylene analogs		
Phosphonoformate	Yes	Reno et al. (1978)
Phosphonopropionate	No	Shipkowitz et al. (1973)
Phosphonobutyrate	No	Shipkowitz et al. (1973)
α-Phosphonopropionate	No	Leinbach et al. (1976)
α-Methyl-2-phosphonopropionate	No	Leinbach et al. (1976)
α-Phenylphosphonoacetate	No	Leinbach et al. (1976)
α-Aminophosphonoacetate	No	Leinbach et al. (1976)
VIII. Other related compounds		
Phosphoglycolate	No	Leinbach et al. (1976)
Imidodiphosphonate	No	Boezi (1979)
Carbamyl phosphate	No	Boezi (1979)
2'-Deoxyribothymidine-5'-phosphorophosphonoacetate	No	Boezi (1979)
Purine-5'-mono-carboxymethyl-phosphonate	Yes	Heimer and Nussbaum (1977)
Pyrimidine-5'-mono-carboxymethyl-phosphonate	Yes	Heimer and Nussbaum (1977)

a) Ester Derivatives

HERRIN et al. (1977) prepared a series of carboxyl and phosphate esters, and three monophosphinic analogs of phosphonoacetic acid. Each compound was tested for inhibition of purified herpes simplex virus DNA polymerase in vitro, and in a mouse animal model. The compounds tested are indicated as groups I, II, and IV of Table 2. The trimethyl ester was evaluated by LEE et al. (1976), and the triethyl ester by SHIPKOWITZ et al. (1973), as indicated in group III of Table 2.

Generally, esters were found to be inactive. However, HERRIN et al. (1977) reported that ethylphosphonoacetate and octylphosphonoacetate were equivalent to phosphonoacetic acid in inhibiting the DNA polymerase in vitro. The octyl ester was inactive in vivo, but the ethyl ester was equivalent to the free acid in the mouse model test. BOEZI (1979) found that low molecular weight carboxyl esters were *inactive*. The discrepancy between these two studies has not been rectified.

The ester analogs do not appear to have potential for improved therapeutic index; however, there have been no reports on their cellular toxicity properties. Since the esters are less acidic, local toxicity for tissues could be reduced compared with the free acids. Ideally, an ester with increased transport into the cell and susceptible to hydrolysis to the parent compound at the site of action would have, theoretically, highly desirable properties.

b) Phosphono Analogs

The phosphoric acid group appears to be indispensable for activity. LEINBACH et al. (1976) reported that the sulfo and carboxy (malonate) analogs were inactive and that the free phosphono group was required for inhibition of herpesvirus of turkeys. NEWTON (1979) reported the synthesis of analogs based on the replacement of phosphorous by arsenic. He reported that arseno analogs, including methylene diarsonate and arsonomethyl phosphonate (Table 2, group VI), were effective in a plaque reduction assay of HSV-1 in L cells or BHK cells at molarities equivalent to phosphonoacetate. He reported that reduction of plaques by the drug was effective at 24 h after infection, but was less effective afterwards. He suggested that the compounds were not stable, and that accounted for the lack of persistence of inhibitory activity. Unfortunately the compounds were not tested against DNA polymerases in vitro or in animal models, and no primary laboratory results were given in the report. Organic arsenicals are generally very stable compounds, but may exhibit cellular toxicity, and it seems likely that this also could account for a short-term inhibition of HSV replication in tissue culture. The chemical similarity of phosphorous and arsenic suggests that further study of arseno analogs of phosphonoacetate, particularly as regards therapeutic index for antiherpesvirus activity, could be a useful and needed study.

c) Carboxyl Analogs

Substitution of the carboxyl group of phosphonoacetic acid by other acidic, basic or neutral moieties (Table 2, group VI) generally yields inactive compounds. The only exceptions are certain amide derivatives and the arseno analogs. As already discussed, NEWTON (1979) reported that arsonomethyl phosphonate and methylene diarsonate were active in a plaque reduction assay of HSV-1. LEE et al. (1976)

reported that the corresponding methylene diphosphonate was inactive. The arseno derivatives require further studies. In the case of the amide derivatives, von Esch (1978) reported the activity of seven derivatives as inhibitors of DNA polymerase in vitro and in the mouse test. The butamide derivative showed good activity in both tests and, like the ester derivatives, caused less local irritation. However, it is clear that a free carboxyl group confers optimal antiviral activity.

d) Methylene Analogs

An unsubstituted methylene group is required for antiviral activity of phosphonoacetic acid (Table 2, group VIII). The propionate and butyrate analogs are inactive, and substitutions of methyl, amino, or phenyl on the methylene carbon also yield inactive compounds. Separation of the acidic groups by a methylene carbon is not essential. Reno et al. (1978) found that phosphonoformate had activity comparable to phosphonoacetate when tested against several herpesviruses in cell culture, and also selectively inhibited the cell-free DNA polymerases. This is the only analog of phosphonoacetate with comparable activity and will be discussed fully in Sect. C.II.2.

e) Nucleoside Analogs

Phosphonoacetic acid is structurally analogous to inorganic pyrophosphate, which plays a key role in nucleic acid biosynthesis. Heimer and Nussbaum (1977) reported the synthesis of purine and prymidine nucleoside analogs of phosphonoacetate and evaluated their activity as antiviral and anticancer agents. The adenosine, guanosine, thymidine, and uridine analogs were about equally active in protecting mice against lethal intraperitoneal injections of herpes simplex virus. The drugs were injected three times: 24 h before virus inoculation, at the time of virus inoculation, and 24 h after inoculation. The protective doses for 50% survival were 180, 144, 185, and 127 mg/kg for the adenosine, guanosine, thymidine, and uridine analogs, respectively.

The drugs were also tested in tissue culture against herpes simplex virus and the concentrations required for 99% reduction in virus yield were determined. The values were: 250 µg/ml for the adenosine analog; 500 µg/ml for guanosine and thymidine analogs; and 125 µg/ml for the uridine analog. Several halogenated base derivatives were evaluated and the activity was not markedly different from the unsubstituted base analogs.

The mechanism of action of the nucleoside derivatives was not investigated by Heimer and Nussbaum. Since esters generally are inactive as DNA polymerase inhibitors, it does not seem likely that nucleoside esters could inhibit virus replication via this mechanism. The relatively low antiviral activity of the nucleoside analogs compared with phosphonoacetate suggests little potential for eventual clinical usefulness.

2. Phosphonoformic Acid

Reno et al. (1978) first investigated the analog, phosphonoformate as an inhibitor of the DNA polymerase of herpesvirus of turkeys. The compound on a concentration basis was essentially identical to phosphonoacetate; the apparent inhibition constants for both compounds were about 1–3 μM. In tissue culture, virus replication was inhibited 50% by 60–70 μM of either compound. The mechanism of action of the two compounds were shown to be identical by kinetic analyses and by showing that an enzyme from a phosphonoacetate-resistant virus was also equally resistant to phosphonoformate.

Later, HELGSTRAND et al. (1978) reported similar results of phosphonoformate with herpes simplex virus DNA polymerase and a somewhat broader inhibitory spectrum. The two compounds had comparable activities against several herpesvirus polymerases, but the formate analog also inhibited influenza virus RNA polymerase 50% at 50 μM.

The compounds were equally active in inhibiting virus replication in cell culture (HELGSTRAND et al. 1979). Further parallel activities of the two compounds were demonstrated in experimental herpesvirus infections in animals. KERN et al. (1978) reported that the formate was effective in mice and guinea pigs inoculated intravaginally with herpes simplex virus. The drug was also administered intravaginally and was equal to the acetate in reducing viral titers and preventing external lesions. KLEIN et al. (1979) studied skin infections with herpes simplex virus in hairless mice. The formate, like the acetate, reduced the severity of lesions, but did not prevent the establishment of latency in the sensory ganglia. Therapeutic efficacy of phosphonoformate for cutaneous infections in guinea pigs was shown by ALENIUS et al. (1978).

WAHREN and OBERG (1979, 1980) studied the appearance of cytomegalovirus antigens in the presence of phosphonoformic acid. Only the early viral antigens were expressed and no viral DNA or infectious virus was produced. The inhibitions were reversible because late antigens and infectious virus appeared in cultures after removal of the drug. This suggested that the viral information persisted during the phosphonoformate treatment in many and probably all originally infected cells. Similar effects on Epstein–Barr virus (EBV) infections were reported by MARGALITH et al. (1980 b). Viral capsid antigens (VCA) were inhibited but Epstein–Barr nuclear antigens (EBNA) were not inhibited by phosphonoformate. The drug also inhibited transformation of human cord blood lymphocytes by EBV, suggesting that viral DNA synthesis was prevented. An interesting aspect of phosphonoformate is that it is a general inhibitor of reverse transcriptase (SUNDQUIST and OBERG 1979). In this respect it is different from phosphonoacetate. SHANNON (1976) reported that the acetate inhibited reverse transcriptase, but it required concentrations of 350–1,500 μM. In contrast, SUNDQUIST and OBERG (1979) found that the formate acted on the enzyme of both avian and mammalian retroviruses at much lower concentrations. Table 3 lists the comparative inhibitory activity of the acetate and formate analogs with different reverse transcriptases. Phosphonoformate at 10 μM gave significant inhibition of all the retrovirus polymerases, except for avian myeloblastosis virus (AMV) with the endogenous primer. At 100 μM, all enzymes were completely inhibited except the endogenous AMV activity. In contrast, phosphonoacetate at 10 μM did not inhibit any of the polymerases. At doses of 100 and 500 μM, Rauscher leukemia virus (RLV), baboon endogenous virus (BEV), and simian sarcoma virus (SSV) reverse transcriptases were partially inhibited. The stimulatory effect of phosphonoacetate for the AMV enzyme was reproducible and an explanation is currently unavailable.

Table 3. Inhibition of various reverse transcriptase activities by phosphonoformic acid and phosphonoacetic acid (Sundquist and Oberg 1975)

Enzyme, source[a]	Template/ primer	dTMP³H (cpm) incorporated without inhibitor	Inhibition (%)[c]					
			(μM) Phosphonoformate			(μM) Phosphonoacetate		
			10	100	500	10	100	500
RLV	$(rA)_n \cdot (dT)_{10}$	169,600	90	96	99	0	10	35
VV	$(rA)_n \cdot (dT)_{10}$	6,585	ND[d]	95	99	ND	3	25
BLV	$(rA)_n \cdot (dT)_{10}$	5,076	ND	88	93	ND	0	10
BEV	$(rA)_n \cdot (dT)_{10}$	46,400	96	>99	>99	5	58	71
SSV	$(rA)_n \cdot (dT)_{10}$	60,860	92	>99	>99	0	44	58
AMV	$(rA)_n \cdot (dT)_{10}$	72,700	43	94	99	0	−34	−86
AMV	Endogenous	4,340	15	49	70	0	−2	−3
AMV[b]	$(rA)_n \cdot (dT)_{10}$	106,950	45	96	>99	0	0	19

[a] RLV: Rauscher leukemia virus; VV: Visna virus; BLV: bovine leukemia virus; BEV: baboon endogeneous virus; SSV: simian sarcoma virus; AMV: avian myeloblastosis virus. Virion polymerases were assayed at a final concentration of about 150 µg/ml
[b] Purified AMV polymerase assayed at 0.1 µg/ml
[c] dTMP³H incorporated as percentage of control without drug. Negative values indicate stimulation over control value
[d] Not determined

The hepatitis B virus has a virion DNA polymerase (Kaplan et al. 1973). The virus has not been grown in culture. Nordenfelt et al. (1979) found that the virion enzyme was inhibited 50% by 20 μM phosphonoformate. At the same concentration, phosphonoacetate was stimulatory for the virion enzyme. Hess et al. (1980) confirmed these observations and established that the mode of action was similar to that of phosphonoacetate. Their studies also suggested that the formate and acetate analogs have different affinities for the hepatitis B polymerase, or alternately, they bind to different sites.

In summary, the formic acid analog and phosphonoacetic acid have the same spectrum of activity as antiherpesvirus agents. Herpesviruses in culture and in infected animals are inhibited to the same extent by equimolar concentrations of the two compounds. Both also inhibit eukaryotic cell DNA polymerases equally (Sabourin et al. 1978). The mechanism of action for inhibition of herpesvirus polymerases is identical for both analogs; however, the formate is less specific since it also inhibits influenza virus RNA polymerase, hepatitis virus B virion DNA polymerase, and avian and mammalian oncornavirus reverse transcriptases.

D. Spectrum of Activity

The original reports from Abbott Laboratories indicated that phosphonoacetic acid was a specific inhibitor of herpesviruses (Shipkowitz et al. 1973; Overby et al. 1974; Mao et al. 1975). Subsequent reports from a large number of laboratories have verified and extended the original observations. Every herpesvirus tested has been shown to be sensitive. In addition, vaccinia virus, African swine fever virus,

Table 4. Viruses sensitive to inhibition of replication by phosphonoacetic acid in cell culture

Virus	References
Herpes simplex virus 1 and 2	SHIPKOWITZ et al. (1973)
	OVERBY et al. (1977)
Equine rhinopneumonitis virus	OVERBY et al. (1977)
Varicella zoster virus	OVERBY et al. (1977)
	MAY et al. (1977)
Cytomegalovirus	
Human	HUANG (1975)
Murine	OVERALL et al. (1976)
Simian	HUANG et al. (1976)
Marek's disease virus	LEE et al. (1976)
	NAZERIAN and LEE (1976)
Herpesvirus of turkeys	LEE et al. (1976)
Owl herpesvirus	LEE et al. (1976)
Herpesvirus saimiri	HUANG et al. (1976)
	BARAHONA et al. (1977)
	PEARSON and BENEKE (1977)
Channel catfish herpesvirus	KOMMENT and HAINES (1978)
Subacute myelo-opticoneuropathy virus (SMON)	NISHIBE and INOUE (1978)
Epstein-Barr virus	NYORMOI et al. (1976)
	SUMMERS and KLEIN (1976)
	YAJIMA et al. (1976)
Vaccinia virus	OVERBY et al. (1977)
	BOLDEN et al. (1975)
	BERGER et al. (1978)
African swine fever virus	GIL-FERNANDEZ et al. (1979)
	MORENO et al. (1978)
Frog virus 3	ELLIOTT et al. (1980)

and frog virus 3 have been shown to be sensitive to this compound (Table 4). Four approaches have been used to study the activity: inhibition of isolated viral DNA polymerases, inhibition of normal cell DNA synthesis, inhibition of viral replication in cell culture, and therapy in herpesvirus-infected animal models. The latter three subjects will be covered in this section, and studies on purified enzymes will be discussed in Sect. F.

I. Virus Replication in Tissue Culture

Phosphonoacetic acid reduced the growth of the entire group of herpesviruses in cell cultures. Investigators have used numerous cell types and a variety of measurements for inhibition of viral replication including: decreased cytopathology, plaque formation, and virus yields.

1. Productive Infections

Typically, 10–20 µg/ml phosphonoacetate in culture medium has given a 50% inhibition of virus yield. Complete inhibition occurs in the presence of 25–100 µg/ml.

Table 4 lists the viruses shown to be sensitive and indicates the highly specific nature of this antiviral compound. Except for three, all viruses shown in Table 4 are well-characterized herpesviruses. Vaccinia virus is a poxvirus and is characterized by a virus-induced DNA polymerase. It is inhibited, but is much less sensitive to the drug than herpesviruses. African swine fever virus and frog virus 3 are large icosohedral deoxyriboviruses which replicate in the cytoplasm of infected cells and induce a DNA polymerase activity. Some features of their replication resemble herpesviruses, and in complexity, these viruses are between herpesviruses and poxviruses.

It is of interest that cytolytic viruses (herpes simplex, equine rhinopneumonitis) and noncytolytic viruses (Epstein–Barr) are similarly affected. The compound does not inhibit replication of the papovoviruses, picornaviruses, myxoviruses, or parvoviruses.

2. Transformed Cells

Phosphonoacetic acid sensitivity has been a useful genetic marker for herpesviruses since it can identify a viral gene product, the DNA polymerase. Its use with the Epstein–Barr virus system has provided new insights into the molecular biology and gene expression in transformed cells carrying the virus genome. Epstein–Barr virus is associated with infectious mononucleosis. Considerable epidemiologic and molecular genetic evidence suggests that the virus is also associated with transformed lymphocytes in human Burkitt's lymphoma and nasopharyngeal carcinoma (KLEIN 1972; ZUR HAUSEN 1975). Cell lines initiated from these tumors express a virus-specific, Epstein–Barr nuclear antigen (EBNA) and a nonvirion early antigen (EA). The transformed cells may have an average of 50–300 virus genomes per cell (YAJIMA et al. 1976). Some of the transformed cells synthesize viral DNA and VCA and produce infectious virus. Nonproducing cells can be induced to become producer cells. Therefore, the *complete* viral genome must be present in transformed cells either as an integrated or extrachromosomal entity.

Most of the viral DNA copies in producer cell are present as free circular plasmids (ADAMS and LINDAHL 1975; LINDAHL et al. 1976). Following the reports on inhibition of herpes simplex virus by phosphonoacetate, NYORMOI et al. (1976), SUMMERS and KLEIN (1976), and MENEZES et al. (1978) found that synthesis of VCA, but not EA or EBNA, was inhibited by concentrations of phosphonoacetate that had no measurable effects on cellular growth. PATEL and MENEZES (1979) found that in some nonproducer cell lines EA was not inhibited and suggested that EA could arise by two pathways, one sensitive and one resistant to phosphonoacetate. YAJIMA et al. (1976) showed that Epstein–Barr viral DNA synthesis was inhibited by phosphonoacetate in superinfected lymphoid tumor cells, but the synthesis of viral DNA in transformed cells was not. SEEBECK et al. (1977) used isolated nuclei from superinfected transformed Raji cells and showed that viral DNA synthesis was inhibited by phosphonoacetate. Similarly, the number of copies of viral DNA in producer cells decreased from the equivalent of 150 to about 65 after treatment with phosphonoacetate (SUMMERS and KLEIN 1976). These results support the idea that in producer cells transformed by Epstein–Barr virus, the DNA for progeny virus is replicated by the herpesvirus polymerase, while the integrated viral

DNA is maintained by the host cell DNA replication apparatus. The molecular mechanism of transformation of normal peripheral B-lymphocytes by Epstein–Barr virus is not known. At the time of transformation and proliferation of the lymphocytes, there is an increase in DNA synthesis and appearance of EBNA in the cell nucleus. THORLEY-LAWSON and STROMINGER (1976) showed that phosphonoacetate prevented DNA synthesis by lymphocytes in the presence of transforming virus. The cells treated with phosphonoacetate did not transform and proliferate, thus identifying a phosphonoacetate-sensitive event in the transformation mechanism. Mitogen-stimulated lymphocytes used as controls were insensitive to the drug. The authors suggest that amplification of the viral genome is a prerequisite for stable transformation. If the virus-induced DNA polymerase is required for gene amplification, it follows that phosphonoacetate would interrupt the transformation sequence.

RICKINSON and EPSTEIN (1978) argued against the existence of a phosphonoacetate-sensitive event unique to Epstein–Barr virus transformation. They confirmed that levels of drug that allowed growth of transformed cells would inhibit VCA and virus particle synthesis. However, the same concentrations did not prevent transformation of fetal cord blood lymphocytes.

MARGALITH et al. (1980a) attempted to inhibit EBV production in a transformed lymphoblastoid cell line with various levels of phosphonoacetate. The percentage of cells producing VCA was similar in the treated and untreated cultures. However, there was ten times less transforming virus in the treated cultures. The authors suggested that either virus assembly or infectious DNA synthesis was decreased in the presence of phosphonoacetate. MARGALITH et al. (1980c) and MANOR and MARGALITH (1979) extended these observations by studying the effects of phosphonoacetate on transformation of human cord blood lymphocytes by EBV. The drug completely inhibited transformation at a concentration of 100 μg/ml.

II. Normal Cells

SHIPKOWITZ et al. (1973) discovered antiviral activity of phosphonoacetate based on inhibition of herpes simplex virus replication in W1-38 human fibroblast cells at concentrations that did not interfere with growth of uninfected cells. MAO et al. (1975) partially purified DNA polymerase activity from W1-38 cells and reported that the enzymes were relatively insensitive to the drug. The specific enzyme (α, β, γ) was not characterized in these studies. Subsequent studies by BOLDEN et al. (1975) showed that the α polymerase from HeLa cells was sensitive to phosphonoacetate, but the β and γ enzymes were insensitive. HUANG (1975) and HIRAI and WATANABE (1976) also reported that the γ and β polymerases of W1-38 cells were not inhibited. These discrepancies were clarified by SABOURIN et al. (1978) who isolated the polymerases from HeLa cells, W1-38, phytohemagglutinin-stimulated human lymphocytes, and Chinese hamster ovary cells, and determined the apparent phosphonoacetate inhibition constant for each of the enzymes. The double-reciprocal plots with the four nucleoside triphosphates and phosphonoacetate as inhibitor for the HeLa α polymerase are shown in Fig. 3. The apparent inhibition constants K_i for the several polymerases are shown in Table 5.

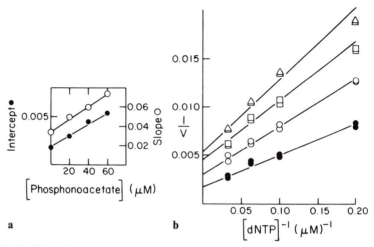

Fig. 3 a, b. Double-reciprocal plots with the four dNTPs as the variable substrate and phosphonoacetate as inhibitor of the purified HeLa α polymerase. Activated DNA was at 200 μg/ml. The initial velocities **b** were expressed as pmol ^{3}H-labeled dTMP incorporated into DNA per 30 min. Phosphonoacetate concentrations were 0 *(full circles)*, 20 *(open circles)*, 40 *(squares)*, and 60 μM *(triangles)*. Equimolar concentrations of each of the four dNTPs were present in the different reaction mixtures. The replots **a** of the slopes *(open circles)* and intercepts *(full circles)* as a function of phosphonoacetate concentration are also shown. (Sabourin et al. 1978)

Table 5. Inhibition constants K_i of polymerases (Sabourin et al. 1978)

Polymerase source	K_i (μM)
Herpesvirus	1–2
HeLa	29
W 1–38	15
Human lymphocyte	30
Chinese hamster ovary	30

Thus, the α polymerases of some eukaryotic cells are sensitive to phosphonoacetate, but they are 15–30 times less sensitive than herpesvirus DNA plymerases. Similar results were reported for duck embryo fibroblasts (Leinbach et al. 1976) and horse tumor cells (Allen et al. 1977).

These generalizations are not absolute, because Allaudeen and Bertino (1978), found that the α polymerase from L1210 cells was just as sensitive to phosphonoacetate as was herpesvirus polymerase. L1210 is a murine leukemia cell line and produces C-type virus particles. The authors compared four different DNA polymerases from this cell and its virus with herpes simplex virus DNA polymerase, simian sarcoma virus (SSV) reverse transcriptase, and terminal deoxynucleotidyl transferase from human acute lymphocytic leukemia peripheral leukocytes. The comparative inhibition of the purified enzymes at four levels of phosphonoacetate is shown in Table 6. DNA polymerase α was the most sensitive of the

Table 6. Inhibition of DNA polymerases by phosphonoacetic acid

Phosphono-acetic acid $\times 10^{-4}$ M	Inhibition of DNA polymerase activity (%)						
	α	β	γ	HSV	SSV RT	L1210 RT	TdT
0.5	61.1	31.0	24.5	69.5	47.3	32.0	29.0
1	74.2	45.0	46.2	81.0	64.0	62.0	57.1
2	81.7	46.0	47.0	82.3	73.0	61.4	59.1
10	94.5	87.0	75.0	98.0	82.2	79.0	62.0

The enzyme unit represents pmol of the corresponding dNMP incorporated at 37 °C for 60 min under optimum assay conditions. The 100% activity of the DNA polymerases α, β, and γ from L1210 cells were 53, 42, and 11 units, respectively; 100% activity of herpesvirus polymerase (HSV), simian sarcoma virus (SSV) reverse transcriptase. L1210 reverse transcriptase and terminal deoxynucleotidyl transferase (TdT) represent 9, 27, 31, and 7 units of activity, respectively (ALLAUDEEN and BERTINO 1978)

cellular polymerases. The concentration of phosphonoacetate required for 50% inhibition of HSV DNA polymerase was 2.5×10^{-5} M. Corresponding values for SSV reverse transcriptase and deoxynucleotidyl transferase (TdT) of acute lymphocytic leukemia leukocytes were 7×10^{-4} and 8×10^{-4} M, respectively. Kinetic analyses for the various enzymic reactions indicated a similar mechanism of action in each case. For all enzymes, the inhibition was noncompetitive with substrates and uncompetitive with DNA template. The inhibitory effects of phosphonoacetate on isolated polymerases reported by ALLAUDEEN and BERTINO (1978) were not observed with L1210 cells in culture. At 50 µg/ml, the compound did not have any noticeable effect on cell growth, but the oncornavirus production (requiring reverse transcriptase) was inhibited more than 50%.

Regardless of the specific effects on cellular DNA polymerases, concentrations of phosphonoacetate several times higher than antiviral levels may inhibit growth of some cells and be cytotoxic, apparenty by other mechanisms. NEWTON (1979) reported that cell division of L cells in culture was completely inhibited by concentrations higher than 100 µg/ml, but DNA synthesis in the arrested cells was not inhibited. The DNA content reached twice the normal value and the cells appeared grossly abnormal. The changes were irreversible when the drug was removed after 24 h. NEWTON (1979) did not explain the observed cytotoxicity, but invoked a speculation that adenyl cyclase could be involved.

It is clear that cell types differ in their sensitivity and resistance to phosphonoacetate. BERGER et al. (1979) explained a basis for these differences after a careful and complete study of L cells, the transformed L1210 line, and phytohemagglutinin-stimulated normal human peripheral lympocytes. The three cell types showed striking differences in sensitivity to phosphonoaceate. As shown in Fig. 4, DNA synthesis in L cells was quite sensitive to phosphonoacetate, and human lymphocytes were relatively insensitive. This difference in sensitivity was accounted for by differences in the rate of uptake of phosphonoacetate ^{14}C by intact cells. The intracellular levels of the compound at periods up to 24 h in the three cells are shown in Fig. 5. To confirm that the intrinsic cellular DNA polymerases, with their existing templates, were equally sensitive to similar concentrations of phospho-

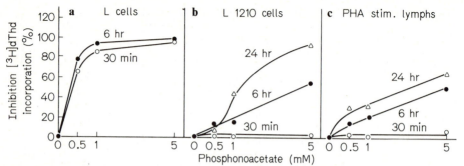

Fig. 4 a–c. Effects of phosphonoacetate on DNA synthesis in intact cells. L cells **(a)**, L1210 cells **(b)**, or phytohemagglutinin-stimulated human lymphocytes **(c)** were incubated with phosphonoacetate at the indicated concentrations for 30 min *(open circles)*, 6 h *(full circles)*, or 24 h *(triangles)*. At the end of each incubation period, 2-ml aliquots of treated and untreated cell suspensions were pulsed with 1 µCi thymidine ^{3}H for 30 min at 37 °C. Cell pellets were prepared to determine incorporation of thymidine ^{3}H into acid-precipitable counts. Percentage inhibition is calculated relative to control, untreated cultures performed at each time point. The amount of thymidine ^{3}H incorporated during the first 30 min pulse by the control cells was 129×10^3 dpm/10^5 L cells, 115×10^3 dpm/10^5 L1210 cells, and 23×10^3 dpm/10^5 lymphocytes. (Berger et al. 1979)

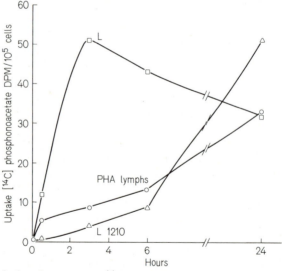

Fig. 5. Uptake of phosphonoacetate ^{14}C by intact cells. L cells *(squares)*, L1210 cells *(triangles)* in mid log phase growth, or phytohemagglutinin-stimulated human lymphocytes *(circles)* on day 3 of culture were suspended in fresh media containing 0.5 mM phosphonoacetate ^{14}C. Duplicate aliquots were removed from each suspension at the indicated times and assayed for intracellular phosphonoacetate ^{14}C. (Berger et al. 1979)

noacetic acid, the cells were made permeable to exogenous small molecules. The kinetics of DNA synthesis in the permeabilized cells indicated that the compound had direct access to the replication complexes within the cell. As shown in Fig. 6, the permeabilized cells were virtually identical in their DNA synthesis in the presence of increasing concentrations of phosphonoacetate.

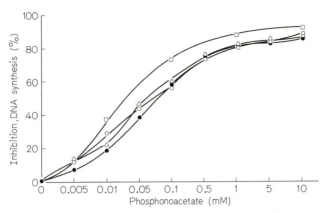

Fig. 6. Concentration dependence of phosphonoacetate inhibition of DNA synthesis in permeabilized cells. L cells *(squares)*, L1210 cells *(triangles)*, and phytohemagglutinin-stimulated human lymphocytes from two different donors *(open and full circles)* were permeabilized and incubated in complete DNA synthesis mix including dTTP ^{3}H and varying concentrations of phosphonoacetate. Reactions were incubated for 30 min at 37 °C and incorporation of radioactivity into acid-precipitable material was determined. Percentage inhibition was calculated relative to the DNA synthesized by untreated cells in the same permeabilization and incubation. (BERGER et al. 1979)

Phosphonoacetate selectively inhibits herpesvirus-induced DNA polymerases and, at concentrations 10–20 times higher, inhibits cellular polymerases. Some uninfected cells are relatively resistant and others are more sensitive. The differences in inhibition of DNA synthesis in uninfected cells can be accounted for by differences in drug uptake rather than intrinsic differences in the cellular replication complexes. A wide variety of herpesvirus-infected cells appears to have almost the same level of sensitivity to the drug for inhibiting virus replication. It is an interesting speculation that the virus infection itself could change the permeability of the cells for phosphonoacetate. An increased permeability of only the infected cell would further select this cell as a target and amplify the therapeutic index.

III. Animal Models

Numerous investigations have proved the antiviral efficacy of phosphonoacetic acid in laboratory animal models. Frequently used models for herpesviruses are skin or eye infections where the drug can be applied directly to the lesions, but systemic administration of the drug has also been efficacious for skin and eye infections in some animals. A summary of animal studies with herpes and related viruses is given in Table 7.

1. Cutaneous Herpesvirus Infections

The original studies of SHIPKOWITZ et al. (1973) showed that orally or topically administered phosphonoacetate reduced the mortality associated with HSV-2 infection of hairless skin in mice. In the mouse, herpes simplex virus dermal infections initially produce a skin vesicle which spreads and leads to a posterior paralysis; and without treatment death follows. For topical application, beginning early after infection, SHIPKOWITZ et al. (1973) showed that preparations of phosphonoacetate (0.5%–5.0%) were efficacious. An aqueous solution given orally at dosage 800–1,400 mg/kg/day for 6 days also prolonged survival of the infected mice. Similar antiviral activity in herpesvirus-infected mice was reported by KLEIN and FRIEDMAN-KIEN (1975), HARRIS and BOYD (1977), and DESCAMPS et al. (1979). KLEIN and FRIEDMAN-KIEN reported that phosphonoacetate and adenine arabinoside (Ara-A) were about equally effective. In similar comparisons, HARRIS and BOYD found that phosphonoacetate was more effective than ara-A. The latter study included a comparison of five established antiherpes compounds in hairless mice with herpetic skin lesions. The comparative results with the various compounds are shown in Table 8. The authors reported that phosphonoacetic acid, E-5-(2-bromovinly)-2′-deoxyuridine, acycloguanosine, and trisodium phosphonoformate were the most active agents.

Primary herpes simplex virus infections of hairless skin of guinea pigs were also susceptible to therapy by phosphonoacetic acid (McCARTY and JARRATT 1979; ALENIUS and OBERG 1978). Topical applications of the drug reduced the severity of primary lesions, even when applied 48 h after inoculation. At 3, 12, or 24 h after inoculation, lesion formation was completely suppressed.

The major negative comments by these investigators for topical application of phosphonoacetate in rodents and guinea pigs were based on skin irritations and erythema at aqueous concentrations of 2% and higher. In most cases, marked suppression of skin lesions was observed at concentrations of 2% or less.

2. Ocular Herpesvirus Infections

Recurrent herpesvirus infections of the eye remain a serious problem and a leading cause of blindness. The rabbit eye provides an experimental model for corneal ulceration and deep stromal disease. SHIPKOWITZ et al. (1973) found that experimentally induced corneal lesions in rabbits were significantly reduced in severity by topical application of 0.5%–5.0% formulations of phosphonoacetate. Other laboratories have confirmed these studies and compared the drug with idoxuridine, currently used for clinical management of patients (MEYER et al. 1976; GERSTEIN et al. 1975; GORDON et al. 1977). The studies showed that 5% phosphonoacetate formulations were as effective as 0.5% idoxuridine in suppressing lesions and viral replication. Phosphonoacetate was also effective in the treatment of idoxuridine-resistant herpetic keratitis (MEYER et al. 1976). The same study showed that topically applied phosphonoacetate had no therapeutic effect on herpetic iritis; however, intravenous administration (150 mg/kg/day) or subconjuctival injection (100 mg/day) was effective in treating iritis.

Phosphonoacetate 5% formulations applied to the eye four times a day were well tolerated in all the reported studies, and no significant epithelial toxicities were observed. The rabbit eye appears to be more tolerant than hairless mouse skin to the high ionic strength of phosphonoacetic acid.

3. Herpes Genitalis

Chemotherapy with phosphonoacetate of genital HSV infections in female mice, female hamsters, and male and female capuchin monkeys *(Cebus apella* and *C. al-*

Table 7. Efficacy studies of phosphonoacetic acid in experimentally infected animals

Disease model	Animal	Virus[a]	Efficacy measurement	Drug route	References
Cutaneous lesions	Mouse	HSV-2	Survival	Topical/oral	Shipkowitz et al. (1973)
	Athymic mouse	HSV-1	Survival	Topical	Descamps et al. (1979)
	Hairless mouse	HSV-1	Lesion size	Topical	Klein and Friedman-Kien (1975)
					Harris and Boyd (1977)
	Guinea pig	HSV-1	Vesicle count	Topical	McCarty and Jarratt (1979)
					Alenius and Oberg (1978)
Keratitis/iritis	Rabbit	HSV-1	Corneal ulceration	Topical	Shipkowitz et al. (1973)
					Gerstein et al. (1975)
	Rabbit	HSV-1	Lesion severity	Topical/intravenous/subconjunctival	Meyer et al. (1976)
Genitalis	Mouse	HSV-1	Lesion severity/virus titer	Topical	Gordon et al. (1977)
	Mouse	HSV-2	Survival/virus titer	Intravaginal	Kern et al. (1977)
	Hamster	HSV-2	Survival/virus titer	Intravaginal/subcutaneous	Renis (1977)
Encephalitis	Capuchin monkey	HSV-2	Survival/virus titer	Topical	Palmer et al. (1977)
	Hamster	HSV-2	Survival	Intraperitoneal	Overby et al. (1977)
	Mouse	HSV-1	Survival/virus titer	Subcutaneous	Fitzwilliam and Griffith (1976)
	Rat	HSV-1	Survival/virus titer	Cerebrospinal	F. Y. Aoki et al., personal communication (1978)
Systemic	Mouse	SMON	Mortality/virus titer	Subcutaneous	Nishibe and Inoue (1978)
	Mouse	HSV-1	Mortality	Intraperitoneal	Lefkowitz et al. (1976)
	Mouse	CMV	Mortality/virus titer	Intraperitoneal	Overall et al. (1976)
	Mouse	HSV-1	Virus titer	Topical	Wohlenberg et al. (1976)
Latency Lymphoproliferation	Chicken	MDV	Mortality/paralysis	Oral	Lee et al. (1976)
Varicella	Patas monkey	Simian varicella virus	Symptoms/virus titer	Intramuscular	Felsenfeld et al. (1978)
Skin lesions	Rabbit	Vaccinia virus	Lesion severity	Topical	Friedman-Kien et al. (1976)
		Shope fibroma virus	Tumor severity	Topical	Friedman-Kien et al. (1976)

[a] HSV: Herpes simplex virus; SMON: subacute myelo-opticoneuropathy virus; CMV: cytomegalovirus MDV: Marek's disease virus

Table 8. Effects of antiviral compounds on the incidence of herpetic skin lesions and mortality of athymic hairless mice inoculated intracutaneously[a] with herpes simplex virus 1 (strain KOS) (Descamps et al. 1979)

Compound	Mice with epidermal lesions (necrosis of at least 5–10 mm in length)/mice alive at day indicated									Mean survival time (days)
	4	6	8	10	12	14	16	18	20	
Control	0/30	23/30	24/24	13/13	7/7	3/3	2/2	1/1	0	10
Trisodium phosphonoformate	0/10	2/10	1/8	1/8	5/6	4/5	3/4	3/3	1/1	14
Phosphonoacetic acid	0/10	0/10	0/10	1/10	4/10	3/9	2/8	1/7	1/6	>20
5-Iodo-2'-deoxyuridine	0/10	5/10	9/10	5/5	1/1	1/1	1/1	1/1	1/1	10
5'-Iodo-2'-deoxycytidine	0/10	3/10	5/10	6/7	4/4	2/2	2/2	1/1	1/1	11.5
5'-Amino-5-iodo-2',5'-dideoxy-uridine	0/10	8/10	9/9	3/3	2/2	1/1	0	0	0	9
5-Ethyl-2'-deoxyuridine	0/10	2/10	9/9	6/6	3/3	0	0	0	0	11
5-Propyl-2'-deoxyuridine	0/10	2/10	7/7	4/4	3/3	1/1	0	0	0	9
5-Propynyloxy-2'-deoxyuridine	0/10	0/10	8/10	4/4	3/3	2/2	2/2	2/2	0	9.5
E-5-(2-bromovinyl)-2'-deoxy-uridine	0/10	1/10	0/10	5/10	8/8	7/7	5/5	5/5	2/2	17
Thymidine arabinoside	0/10	1/10	6/9	6/7	2/3	3/3	2/2	0	0	11
Cytosine arabinoside	0/10	8/10	9/10	6/6	2/2	0	0	0	0	11
Adenine arabinoside	0/10	3/10	8/10	6/6	4/4	4/4	2/2	1/1	0	13
Acycloguanosine	0/10	0/10	2/10	2/9	5/9	5/7	4/6	2/4	2/3	17

[a] Athymic hairless mice, 25-day-old, weighing about 16–18 g were inoculated intracutaneously in the lumbar area with herpes simplex virus 1 strain KOS (approximately $10^{4.7}$ pfu/mouse) and treated topically twice daily for 6 days, starting immediately after virus inoculation, with a water-soluble ointment containing 1% active ingredient

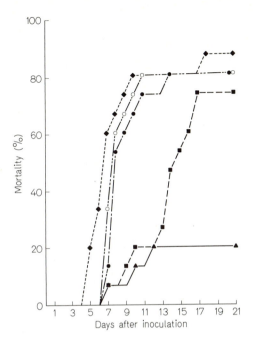

Fig. 7. Effect of intravaginal treatment with saline *(diamonds)*, ara-C *(open circles)*, IdUrd *(full circles)*, ara-A *(squares)*, and phosphonoacetic acid *(triangles)* on genital HSV-2 infection of female hamsters. Each hamster received 15 treatments beginning on day 0. RENIS (1977)

bifrons) have been reported. The mouse and hamster studies compared therapeutic activity of phosphonoacetate with other antiviral agents. KERN et al. (1977) reported that phosphonoacetate was effective when administered intravaginally in mice but Ara-A and adenine arabinoside monophosphate (Ara-AMP) were not. RENIS (1977) did a broader comparative study in HSV-infected female hamsters. He found that either phosphonoacetate or Ara-A was more effective than cytosine arabinoside (Ara-C) or 5-iodo-2′-deoxyuridine. Phosphonoacetate was more effective than Ara-A if treatment was initiated 1 h after infection. Activity was greatly reduced if initiation of treatment was delayed 24 h. Comparisons of the four antiviral agents in the study are shown in Fig. 7.

Phosphonoacetate was not an effective treatment for primary herpesvirus skin lesions on the genitalia of capuchin monkeys (PALMER et al. 1977). The drug was applied topically at the time of appearance of a lesion at the inoculation site. Concentrations of 2% and 5% proved extensively irritating. There were some reductions in lesion size and duration, but the differences from placebo-treated animals were not stastically significant.

4. Herpesvirus Infections of the Central Nervous System

Encephalitis is a life-threatening consequence of some herpesvirus infections. Systemic antiviral therapy is often ineffective because of the blood–brain barrier and

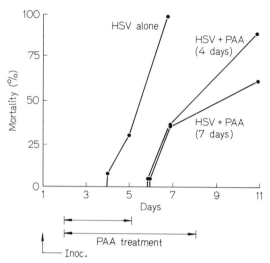

Fig. 8. Mortality rate among mice with encephalitis caused by herpes simplex virus (HSV) treated with phosphonoacetic acid (PAA; 750 mg/kg daily) for 4 or 7 days. (Fitzwilliam and Griffith JF 1976)

lack of specific and potent antiviral drugs. Therefore, it has been of some interest to evaluate the efficacy of phosphonoacetate in animals with herpetic central nervous system infections. Investigations have been carried out in hamsters, mice, and rats inoculated intracerebrally with virus. Overby et al. (1977) infected Syrian hamsters with 10^5 pfu of HSV-2 directly into the brain and began treatment 2 h later with daily intraperitoneal or subcutaneous injections of 200 mg phosphonoacetate. The survival rates were 10% in untreated controls, and 70% in the intraperitoneally treated animals. The drug was not effective by subcutaneous administration.

Similar studies were performed in rats by F. Y. Aoki, G. Trepanier, G. Lussier (unpublished work, 1978). In these studies, phosphonoacetate (2.0 mg/kg/day) was injected by cannula directly into the brain of infected animals, or at 500 mg/kg/day intraperitoneally. Both regimens were effective in increasing average survival times to 12.4 days from 7.0 days in untreated controls.

Fitzwilliam and Griffith (1976) used a mouse model of herpesvirus encephalitis to compare antiviral activity of tilorone hydrochloride (an interferon inducer) and phosphonoacetic acid. The untreated animals experienced a diffuse overwhelming infection and death occurred in 7 days. Tilorone hydrochloride did not alter the fatal course of encephalitis. In comparison, subcutaneous administration of phosphonoacetic acis (750 mg/kg/day) for 7 days resulted in a long-term survival rate of about 35% (Fig. 8).

Inoue (1975) has characterized a new type of human herpesvirus associated with subacute myelo-optico neuropathy (SMON) disease. SMON virus appears to be a variant of avian infectious laryngotracheitis virus that may have adapted to humans. Nishibe and Inoue (1978) showed that the virus was sensitive to phosphonoacetate, further suggesting that it is a herpesvirus. The virus replicates in the brain of suckling mice if injected intracerebrally at birth. When phosphonoacetate (2.5 mg/day) was given subcutaneously beginning on the tenth day after inoculation, the incubation period of the disease was effectively delayed.

The effectiveness of phosphonoacetate administered *systemically* against virus injected *directly into the brain* indicates that the drug reaches the site of viral replication across the blood–brain barrier. This also indicates that the drug exerts its antiviral activity directly in the brain and not by peripheral interactions.

5. Systemic Herpesvirus Infections

Two studies have evaluated the efficacy of phosphonoacetate in systemic herpesvirus infections. LEFKOWITZ et al. (1976) infected mice intraperitoneally with 2 median infective doses (ID_{50}) of HSV-1. The mice died 7–11 days afterwards with focal necrosis of the liver, polymorphonuclear cell infiltration, and lesions in the brain and lungs. Various antiviral drugs were given intraperitoneally, beginning 2 h after inoculation. The study demonstrated antiviral activity for Ara-A and interferon; but Ara-C, iododeoxyuridine, and phosphonoacetate had no antiviral effects. The authors suggest that their negative findings with phosphonoacetate could be due to "strain of virus or mice and routes of administration and dissemination of virus."

Murine, simian, and human cytomegalovirus (CMV) replication in tissue culture is inhibited by phosphonoacetic acid. OVERALL et al. (1976) compared Ara-A and phosphonoacetate for treatment of mice with lethal cytomegalovirus infections. Each drug was administered intraperitoneally at doses of 500 mg/kg/day or 250 mg/kg twice daily for 7 days, beginning 2, 24, or 48 h after infection. The treatment with Ara-A failed to alter the pathogenesis, or time and course of death. In contrast, phosphonoacetate treatment was effective if begun 2 or 24 h after infection. The mortality was reduced from 93% to 40% and the mean time of death increased from 6.1 to 8.2 days. The drug reduced viral replication in the brains and lungs of infected mice; however, the major life-sustaining effect was complete inhibition of replication of CMV in the liver.

6. Latent Herpesvirus Infections

Most of the studies of phosphonoacetate therapy of herpesvirus infections in animals have dealt with primary infections. Despite the uniformly positive finding with primary infections, it cannot be concluded that this drug would also alter infections arising from reactivation of latent viruses. WOHLENBERG et al. (1976) recovered latent HSV from sensory and autonomic ganglia of mice several months after recovery from primary infections. They found that topical treatment with phosphonoacetate at the time of infection markedly *reduced the incidence* of latent ganglionic infections with HSV. However, further treatment with phosphonoacetate at the original infection site *did not cure an already established* ganglionic latent infection. The results suggest further studies assessing whether continual cure of recurrent herpetic skin lesions might ultimately lead to decreased further recurrences.

7. Varicella Infections

FELSENFELD et al. (1978) investigated simian varicella virus (Delta herpesvirus) infections in Patas monkeys. Treatment with phosphonoacetate (200 mg/kg/day, intramuscularly) was begun 40 h after inoculation. In control groups, severe generalized wet dermatitis developed, and lesions healed in 40 days. No vesicles developed in the drug-treated group and the virus could not be isolated from lymphocytes. Antibodies to the virus were detected up to 3 weeks posttreatment, indicating that some virus replication may have occurred.

8. Lymphoproliferative Disease

In tissue culture, phosphonoacetate inhibits replication of herpesviruses associated with lymphocytic transformations. LEE et al. (1976) found that the drug completely inhibited replication of Marek's disease virus in duck embryo fibroblasts. In the same study, LEE and colleagues tested the effects of the drug on Marek's disease virus replication and Marek's disease lesions in chickens. One group of chickens was given phosphonoacetate intra-abdominally at 500 mg/kg/day for 5 days before inoculation, and thereafter every other day for 28 days. The treatment was not effective. The total disease incidence, the severity of the lesions, and contact transmission to cage mates were identical in treated and control groups.

9. Nonherpesvirus Infections

Two non-herpesvirus infections in rabbits have been investigated by FRIEDMAN-KIEN et al. (1976). Vaccinia virus and Shope fibroma virus are members of the poxvirus class and cause pustular lesions and benign tumors, respectively, when injected intradermally in rabbits. The number and severity of the lesions caused by both viruses were reduced by topical application of 2% phosphonoacetate solutions. Intraperitoneal injections of the drug were not effective for these infections.

10. Summary

In summary, observations in a variety of animal models have confirmed the anti-herpesvirus activity of phosphonoacetic acid observed in tissue culture. Direct application to lesion sites appears to be more effective for skin and ocular lesions than systemic administration. However, the drug reaches target organs after systemic administration, as shown by therapeutic effectiveness in central nervous system diseases induced by intracerebral inoculation of virus.

E. Pharmacologic and Clinical Studies

No formal publications are available on the toxicology, pharmacology, or clinical evaluations in humans for phosphonoacetic acid. In some of the animal model studies, investigators have recorded gross observations on toxicity and metabolism.

I. Metabolism

There is no evidence that phosphonoacetate is degraded or converted to other compounds in animals, or normal and virus-infected cells in culture. BOEZI (1979) reported that only the unmodified compound was recovered from a variety of cells treated with phosphonoacetate ^{3}H. In animal studies, using phosphonoacetate ^{14}C, BOPP et al. (1977) could not find any conversion to other compounds. Virtually all of the orally administered and injected drug is rapidly excreted intact in urine and feces.

II. Toxicology

No well-designed systematic toxicologic investigations of phosphonoacetate have been published. However, many of the animal studies on efficacy have led to incidental observations of gross toxic symptoms. SHIPKOWITZ et al. (1973) found that 300 mg/kg/day orally was well tolerated by mice, and KLEIN and FRIEDMAN-KIEN (1975) reported that the same dose was tolerated intraperitoneally. The median lethal dose (LD_{50}) dose for mice was 1,500 mg/kg/day (FITZWILLIAM and GRIFFITH 1976). For rats, F. Y. AOKI et al. (personal communication 1978) found that the acute single dose LD_{50} was 2,000–4,000 mg/kg. There were no gross evidences of systemic toxicity when MEYER et al. (1976) administered 150 mg/kg intravenously to rabbits. However, twice the dose (300 mg/kg) produced tetanic muscular spasms and death in some rabbits.

Epithelial tissues appear to be physically irritated by aqueous concentrations of phosphonoacetate above 2%. The erythema, probably due to the high ionic strength and acidity of the compound, disappears upon removal of the preparation. Phosphonoacetate appears to be well tolerated at 2%–5% when applied topically to rabbit eyes (GERSTEIN et al. 1975; MEYER et al. 1976). Fine punctate lesions of the corneal epithelium developed at the higher concentration, but they disappeared after cessation of treatment.

Phosphonoacetate was shown to be nonmutagenic in standard tests for revertants in *Salmonella typhimurium* TA-1535, 1537, or 1538 and with Fisher mouse lymphoma cells L51784, TK$^+$/− (BECKER et al. 1976). The studies also indicated nonmutagenicity in mice when 0.1 g was applied to hairless skin four times a day for periods up to 8 weeks. When ^{14}C-labeled drug was used, 71% of the dermally applied compound was adsorbed.

Radiolabeled phosphonoacetate is rapidly excreted by rodents and rabbits, but some becomes deposited in bone (KUNG et al. 1978). The deposit is in a chemically unmodified form, and the turnover appears to be slow (BOEZI 1979). Pharmacomenetic studies with phosphonoformate in mice showed that it was deposited also in bone and cartilage (HELGSTRAND et al. 1979). Upon histopathologic examination no abnormal features were found in bone of the treated animals.

III. Clinical Pharmacology

There are no reports of phosphonoacetate administration to humans. These studies must await complete and systematic evaluation of toxicology, pharmacology, and safety in animals.

F. Mechanism of Action

The antiviral specificity of phosphonoacetate for herpesviruses is highly suggestive that the site of action must be unique and essential for herpesvirus replication. Our initial observations led to the notion that the virus-induced DNA polymerase was a probable target. The chemical simplicity of phosphonoacetate and its similarity to pyrophosphate suggests that it may function as a competitive inhibitor of nucleic acid biosynthesis or nucleotide polymerization. In theory, the compound could react with biochemical substrates in the synthetic pathways, either directly or after conversion to an ester or amide. The relative lack of toxicity to normal cells at concentrations that completely inhibited virus replication conflicted with a mechanism involving major synthetic pathways necessary for cell viability. The compelling evidence led to a search for the mechanism within events programmed by the virus.

I. Inhibition of Herpesvirus-Induced DNA Polymerase

Our initial work in cell culture (Overby et al. 1974) showed that phosphonoacetate did not interfere with adsorption and penetration of the virus, but demonstrated that viral DNA synthesis was markedly repressed by the drug. Since late viral events depend on the appearance of progeny DNA, the mechanism of action was thus narrowed to early viral events related to the parental genome. At the molecular level, three possible targets appeared likely: inhibition of early viral transcription; inhibition of translation of viral messages; or interference with functions of products of the early transcripts. Mao et al. (1975) purified the DNA polymerase from HSV-infected W1-38 cells and showed that in a cell-free system viral polymerase activity was inhibited by 50% in the presence of 0.2 μg/ml phosphonoacetate. At these concentrations the normal cellular polymerases were not inhibited. Kinetic analyses of the cell-free nucleotide polymerization reactions by Mao and Robishaw (1975) clearly showed that the inhibition was noncompetitive with respect to each of the four nucleotide triphosphates and uncompetitive with respect to primer DNA. Enzyme–DNA primer complexes formed normally in the presence of inhibitory concentrations of phosphonoacetate. Mao and Robishaw's (1975) kinetic analyses led to the conclusion that phosphonoacetate specifically inhibited the addition of nucleotides to the growing polynucleotide chain in a viral enzyme polymerization reaction copying a template DNA strand.

Leinbach et al. (1976) proposed a specific mechanism for inhibition of the viral polymerase that accounts for the experimentally observed inhibition patterns. The proposal specifies that phosphonoacetate binds to the enzyme at the pyrophosphate binding site and thereby creates an alternate pathway. In a polymerization reaction, pyrophosphate is a product as the nucleotide triphosphate couples to a growing chain forming 3′–5′ phosphodiester bonds. Pyrophosphate is also a substrate in the pyrophosphate–deoxyribonucleoside triphosphate exchange reaction. A scheme for the alternate pathway inhibition mechanism is shown in Fig. 9. This mechanism predicts that phosphonoacetate should bind to the viral enzyme with measurable affinity and that a product, deoxynucleotide monophosphate phosphonoacetate (dNMP-PA), should be found in reaction mixtures containing phosphonoacetate. The putative dNMP-PA should also be a substrate for the viral en-

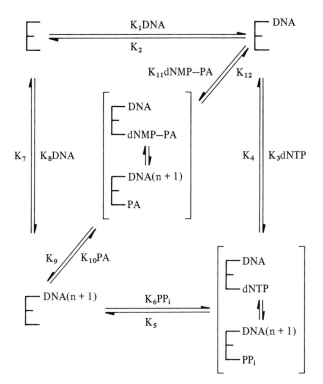

Fig. 9. Proposed mechanism of phosphonoacetate inhibition of herpesvirus-induced DNA polymerase. The basic reaction mechanism in the absence of phosphonoacetate (PA) is a modified ordered bimolecular–bimolecular mechanism. Initial velocity studies and the pyrophosphate (PPi) product inhibition studies presented here are consistent with this mechanism for the herpesvirus-induced DNA polymerase. The postulated compound, dNMP-PA, is a deoxyribonucleoside-5′monophosphate covalently linked to phosphonoacetate by a phosphodiester bond. (LEINBACH et al. 1976)

zyme. None of these predictions has been realized experimentally in support of the proposed mechanism (BOEZI 1979). In fact, the proposed substrate, dNMP-PA, was synthesized and it was not active as a substrate for herpesvirus DNA polymerase.

The exact molecular mechanism for phosphonoacetate inhibition of DNA polymerases has not been completely defined with experimental verification. As indicated, in the discussion of structure–activity relationships, the structural requirements for activity are rigorous in terms of ionic and secondary structure characteristics. The mechanisms must eventually account for this chemical specificity as well as for the biologic specificity of inhibiting polymerizations catalyzed by virus-coded DNA polymerases.

II. Genetic Resistance

The most convincing evidence for direct inhibition of herpesvirus-coded DNA polymerase by phosphonoacetate arises from work with resistant mutants. Viruses resistant to phosphonoacetate have been reported by Klein (1975), Klein and Friedman-Kien (1975), Hay and Subak-Sharpe (1976), Becker et al. (1977), Honess and Watson (1977), Overby et al. (1977), Jofre et al. (1977), Lee et al. (1978), Purifoy and Powell (1977), and Duff et al. (1978). The isolated DNA polymerases from cells infected with resistant viruses have a corresponding resistance to phosphonoacetate in cell-free reactions. A DNA-negative, temperature-sensitive mutant of HSV-1, *ts*D9, has been characterized by two groups and shown to be conditionally defective both in the structural gene for DNA polymerase and phosphonoacetate resistance (Jofre et al. 1977; Purifoy and Powell 1977). Revertants of the phenotypes were phosphonoacetate sensitive and temperature insensitive. The coincidence of genetic loci for phosphonoacetate resistance and temperature sensitivity for the *ts*D9 mutant confirm that at least one polypeptide component of the viral DNA polymerase is the target for phosphonoacetate action. Knipe et al. (1979) transferred the genetic locus for phosphonoacetate resistance from one HSV genome to another and mapped the locus at or near 0.45–0.49 map units on the HSV genome. These studies identify the genetic locus for sensitivity to phosphonoacetate.

Becker et al. (1977) found resistant mutants at the rate of 1 in 10^4 pfu after mutagenizing HSV with 5-bromodeoxyuridine. The isolation of mutants after mutagenization appears straightforward. However, the ease of isolation of spontaneous resistant strains from laboratory stocks of herpes simplex virus poses a question of their origin. A single passage of wild-type stocks in the presence of phosphonoacetate may yield resistant viruses. Structural considerations and mutagenicity testing eliminate phosphonoacetic acid as a mutagen. Duff et al. (1978) showed that some resistant strains can arise by selective growth of relatively resistant genomes present in the wild-type stocks before phosphonoacetate treatment. Once the resistant strains were isolated and cloned, they were genetically stable for 20 passages in tissue culture. Although the resistance marker remained stable for any one plaque-purified strain, the level of resistance varied from 48% to 95% among the individual plaques when tested against the same level of drug. This property of acquired resistance was not general for all herpesviruses, because identical procedures for equine rhinopneumonitis virus did not yield resistant strains. Duff et al. (1978) were unable to isolate resistant HSV-2 strains surviving in hamster brain tissue after 10 days treating the animal with high levels of phosphonoacetate.

Characterization of resistant mutants has proved that the DNA polymerase is the site of action of phosphonoacetate for herpesviruses. The drug provides a valuable genetic marker. Clinical significance of resistance cannot be assessed until further animal and clinical studies in humans are available.

G. Summary and Perspectives

The discovery of the antiviral properties of phosphonoacetic acid has provided a new dimension for seeking effective viral therapeutics. The drug interferes with viral nucleic acid synthesis by inhibiting an early gene product of the virus, and inhibits only the herpesviruses or similar viruses inducing a virus-specific DNA polymerase. The findings suggest that other viruses carrying genes for virus-specific polymerases should be susceptible to other specific inhibitors. The simple structure of phosphonoacetate is not attractive for chemical manipulation aimed at optimizing or broadening the antiviral spectrum or therapeutic index. Activity of this drug does prove that a complex chemical structure is not necessary for exquisite specificity.

A number of unanswered questions still remain. The precise molecular mechanism of action needs to be firmly established, including proof of enzyme binding and identification of postulated biochemical intermediates. Studies in animals have not revealed significant toxicity at therapeutic dose levels and systematic toxicologic and pharmacologic studies have not been reported. The extent and source of spontaneous resistant mutants requires further clarifications and explanations to assess potential clinical significance.

Phosphonoacetate has many aspects of an idealized antiviral agent. It attacks a unique viral mechanism which is well understood at the molecular and genetic level. Animals can tolerate relatively high systemic effective therapeutic doses without gross symptoms. It is effective against every species of one class of viruses. Its chemistry is simple, and the molecule is metabolically inert.

The future of the drug in clinical medicine cannot be assessed until well-controlled, double-blind clinical trials occur and the information from them is available for evaluation. Regulatory, economic, and technical considerations all influence such investigations. Even if the drug is not used in human disease, its discovery has already contributed to our basic knowledge of viruses and so may provide in due time a truly useful rationale for virus therapy.

References

Adams A, Lindahl T (1975) Epstein-Barr virus genomes with properties of circular DNA molecules in carrier cells. Proc Natl Acad Sci USA 72:1477–1481

Alenius S, Oberg B (1978) Comparison of the therapeutic effects of five antiviral agents on cutaneous herpesvirus infection in guinea pigs. Arch Virol 58:277–288

Alenius S, Dinter Z, Oberg B (1978) Therapeutic effect of trisodium phosphonoformate on cutaneous herpesvirus infection in guinea pigs. Antimicrob Agents Chemother 14:408–413

Allaudeen HS, Bertino JR (1978) Inhibition of activities of DNA polymerase α, β, γ, and reverse transcriptase of L1210 cells by phosphonoacetic acid. Biochem Biophys Acta 520:490–497

Allen GP, O'Callaghan DJ, Randall CC (1977) Purification and characterization of equine herpesvirus-induced DNA polymerase. Virology 76:395–408

Barahona H, Daniel MD, Bekesi JG, Fraser CEO, King NW, Hunt RD, Ingalls JK, Jones TC (1977) In vitro suppression of herpesvirus saimiri replication by phosphonoacetic acid. Proc Soc Exp Biol Med 154:431–434

Becker BA, Bopp BA, Brusick DJ, Lehrer SB (1976) Non-mutagenicity of phosphonoacetic acid (disodium salt) in in vitro tests and in rodents (abstr nr 533). Fed Proc 35:533

Becker Y, Asher Y, Cohen Y, Weinberg-Zahlering E, Shlomai J (1977) Phosphonoacetic acid-resistant mutants of herpes simplex virus: effect of phosphonoacetic acid on virus replication and in vitro deoxyribonucleic acid synthesis in isolated nuclei. Antimicrob Agents Chemother 11:919–922

Berger NA, Kauff RA, Sikorski GW (1978) ATP-independent DNA synthesis in vaccinia-infected L cells. Biochim Biophys Acta 520:531–538

Berger NA, Sikorski GW, Adams JW (1979) Phosphonoacetate inhibition of deoxyribonucleic acid synthesis in intact and permeable eukaryotic cells. Biochem Pharmacol 28:2497–2501

Boezi JA (1979) The antiherpesvirus action of phosphonoacetate. Pharmacol Ther 4:231–243

Boezi JA, Lee LF, Blakesley RW, Koenig M, Towle HC (1974) Marek's disease herpesvirus-induced DNA polymerase. J Virol 14:1209–1219

Bolden A, Aucker J, Weissbach A (1975) Synthesis of herpes simplex virus, vaccinia virus, and adenovirus DNA in isolated HeLa cell nuclei. I. Effect of viral-specific antisera and phosphonoacetic acid. J Virol 16:1584–1592

Bolden A, Noy GP, Weissbach A (1977) DNA polymerase of mitochondria is a γ-polymerase. J Biol Chem 252:3351–3356

Bopp BA, Estep CB, Anderson DJ (1977) Disposition of disodium phosphonoacetate-^{14}C in rat, rabbit, dog, and monkey. Fed Proc 36:939

Crofts PC (1958) Compounds containing carbon-phosphorus bonds. Q Rev Chem Soc 12:341–366

Descamps J, De Clercq E, Barr PJ, Jones AS, Walker RT, Torrence PF, Shugar D (1979) Relative potencies of different anti-herpes agents in the topical treatment of cutaneous herpes simplex virus infection of athymic nude mice. Antimicrob Agents Chemother 16:680–682

Duff RG, Robishaw EE, Mao JCH, Overby LR (1978) Characteristics of herpes simplex virus resistance to disodium phosphonoacetate. Intervirology 9:193–205

Edenberg HJ, Anderson S, De Pamphilis ML (1978) Inveolvement of DNA polymerase α in simian virus 40 DNA replication. J Biol Chem 253:3273–3280

Elliott RM, Bateson A, Kelly DC (1980) Phosphonoacetic acid inhibition of frog virus 3 replication. J Virol 33:539–542

Felsenfeld AD, Abee CR, Gerone PJ, Soike KF, Williams SR (1978) Phosphonoacetic acid in the treatment of simian varicella. Antimicrob Agents Chemother 14:331–335

Fitzwilliam JF, Griffith JF (1976) Experimental encephalitis caused by herpes simplex virus: comparison of treatment with tilorone hydrochloride and phosphonoacetic acid. J Infect Dis 133:A221–A225

Friedman-Kien AE, Fondak AA, Klein RJ (1976) Phosphonoacetic acid treatment of Shope fibroma and vaccinia virus skin infections in rabbits. J Invest Dermatol 66:99–102

Gerstein DD, Dawson CR, Oh JO (1975) Phosphonoacetic acid in the treatment of experimental herpes simplex keratitis. Antimicrob Agents Chemother 7:285–288

Gil-Fernández C, Paez E, Vilas P, Gancedo AG (1979) Effect of disodium phosphonoacetate and iododeoxyuridine on the multiplication of African swine fever virus in vitro. Chemotherapy 25:162–169

Gordon YKJ, Lahav M, Photiou S, Becker Y (1977) Effect of phosphonoacetic acid in the treatment of experimental herpes simplex keratitis. Br J Ophthalmol 61:506–509

Harris SRB, Boyd MR (1977) The activity of iododeoxyuridine, adenine arabinoside, cytosine arabinoside, ribavirin, and phosphonoacetic acid against herpes virus in the hairless mouse model. J Antimicrob Chemother [Suppl A] 3:91–98

Hay J, Subak-Sharpe JH (1976) Mutants of herpes simplex virus types 1 and 2 that are resistant to phosphonoacetic acid induce altered DNA polymerase activities in infected cells. J Gen Virol 31:145–148

Heimer EP, Nussbaum AL (1977) Phosphonoacetic acid derivatives of nucleosides. U.S. Patent No. 4,056,673

Helgstrand E, Eriksson B, Johansson NG, Lannero B, Larsson A, Misiorny A, Noren JO, Bjoberg B, Stenberg K, Stening G, Stridh S, Oberg B, Alenius S, Philipson L (1978) Trisodium phosphonoformate,a new antiviral compound. Science 201:819–821

Helgstrand E, Oberg B, Alenius S (1979) Experimental studies on the antiherpetic agent phosphonoformic acid. Adv Ophthalmol 38:276–280

Herrin TR, Fairgrieve JS, Bower RR, ShipkowitzNL, Mao JCH (1977) Synthesis and anti-herpes simplex activity of analogs of phosphonoacetic acid. J Med Chem 20:660–663

Hess G, Arnold W, Meyer zum Buschenfelde K-H (1980) Inhibition of hepatitis-B-virus DNA polymerase by phosphonoformate: Studies on its mode of action. J Mol Virol 5:309–316

Hirai K, Watanabe Y (1976) Induction of α-type DNA polymerases in human cytomegalovirus-infected W1-38 cells. Biochim Biophys Acta 447:328–339

Honess RW, Watson DH (1977) Herpes simplex virus resistance and sensitivity to phosphonoacetic acid. J Virol 21:584–600

Huang ES (1975) Human cytomegalovirus. IV. Specific inhibition of virusinduced DNA
polymerase activity and viral DNA replication by phosphonoacetic acid. J Virol
16:1560–1565

Huang ES, Huang CH, Huong SM, Selgrade M (1976) Preferential inhibition of herpes-
group viruses by phosphonoacetic acid: effect on virus DNA synthesis and virus-induced DNA polymerase activity. Yale J Biol Med 49:93–98

Inoue YK (1975) An avian-related new herpesvirus infection in man – subacute myelo-op-
tico-neuropathy (SMON). Prog Med Virol 21:35–42

Jofre JT, Schaffer PA, Parris DS (1977) Genetics of resistance to phosphonoacetic acid in
strain KOS of herpes simplex virus type 1. J Virol 23:833–836

Kaplan PM, Greenman RL, Gerin JL, Purcell RH, Robinson WS (1973) DNA polymerase
associated with human hepatitis B antigen. J Virol 12:995–1005

Kern ER, Richards JT, Overall JC, Glasgow LA (1977) Genital herpesvirus hominis infection in mice. II. Treatment with phosphonoacetic acid, adenine arabinoside, and adenine arabinoside 5′-monophosphate. J Infect Dis 135:557–567

Kern ER, Glasgow LA, Overall JC, Reno JM, Boezi JA (1978) Treatment of experimental
herpesvirus infections with phosphonoformate and some comparisons with phosphonoacetate. Antimicrob Agents Chemother 14:817–823

Kier HM, Gold E (1963) Deoxyribonucleic acid nucleotidyl transferase and deoxyribonuclease from cultured cells infected with herpes simplex virus. Biochim Biophys Acta
72:263–276

Kier HM, Subak-Sharpe JH, Shedden WIH, Watson DH, Wildy P (1966) Immunological
evidence for a specific DNA polymerase produced after infection by herpes simplex
virus. Virology 30:154–157

Klein G (1972) Herpesviruses and oncogenesis. Proc Natl Acad Sci USA 69:1056–1064

Klein RJ (1975) Isolation of herpes simplex virus clones and drug resistant mutants in
microcultures. Arch Virol 49:73–80

Klein RJ, Friedman-Kien AE (1975) Phosphonoacetic acid-resistant herpes simplex virus
infection in hairless mice. Antimicrob Agents Chemother 7:289–293

Klein RJ, De Stefano E, Brady E, Friedman-Kien AE (1979) Latent infections of sensory
ganglia as influenced by phosphonoformate treatment of herpes simplex virus-induced
skin infections in hairless mice. Antimicrob Agents Chemother 16:266–270

Knipe DM, Ruyechan WT, Roizman B (1979) Molecular genetics of herpes simplex virus.
III. Fine mapping of a genetic locus determining resistance to phosphonoacetate by two
methods of marker transfer. J Virol 29:698–704

Knopf KW, Yamada M, Weissbach A (1976) HeLa cell DNA polymerase γ: further purification and properties of the enzyme. Biochemistry 15:4540–4548

Koment RW, Haines H (1978) Decreased antiviral effect of phosphonoacetic acid on the
poikilothermic herpesvirus of channel catfish disease. Proc Soc Exp Biol Med 159:21–24

Kung HF, Ackerhalt R, Blau M (1978) Uptake of TC-99M monophosphate complexes in
bone and myocardial necrosis in animals. J Nucl Med 19:1027–1031

Lee LF, Nazerian K, Leinbach SS, Reno JM, Boezi JA (1976) Effect of phosphonoacetate
on Marek's disease virus replication. J Natl Cancer Inst 56:823–827

Lee LF, Nazerian K, Witter R, Leinbach SS, Boezi JA (1978) Phosphonoacetate-resistant
mutant of herpesvirus of turkeys. J Natl Cancer Inst 60:1141–1145

Lefkowitz E, Worthington M, Conliffe MA, Baron S (1976) Comparative effectiveness of
six antiviral agents in herpes simplex type 1 infection of mice. Proc Soc Exp Biol Med
152:337–342

Leinbach SS, Reno JM, Lee LF, Isbell AF, Boezi JA (1976) Mechanism of phosphonoacetate inhibition of herpesvirus-induced DNA polymerase. Biochemistry 15:426–430

Lindahl T, Adams A, Bjursell G, Bornkamm GW, Kaschka-Dierich C, Jehn U (1976)
Covalently closed circular duplex DNA of Epstein-Barr virus in a human lymphoid cell
line. J Mol Biol 102:511–530

Manor D, Margalith M (1979) Phosphonoacetic acid: Inhibition of transformation of human cord blood lymphocytes by Epstein-Barr virus. Cancer Biochem Biophys 3:157–
162

Mao JCH, Robishaw EE (1975) Mode of inhibition of herpes simplex virus DNA polymerase by phosphonoacetate. Biochemistry 14:5475–5479

Mao JCH, Robishaw EE, Overby LR (1975) Inhibition of DNA polymerase from herpes simplex virus-infected W1-38 cells by phosphonoacetic acid. J Virol 15:1281–1283

Mar EC, Huang ES (1979) Comparative study of herpes group virus-induced DNA polymerases. Intervirology 12:73–83

Mar EC, Huang YS, Huang ES (1978) Purification and characterization of varicella-zoster virus-induced DNA polymerase. J Virol 26:249–256

Margalith M, Manor D, Goldblum N (1980a) On the continuous culturing of B.95-8 cells in the presence of phosphonoacetic acid. J Virol Methods 1:349–354

Margalith M, Manor D, Usieli V, Goldblum N (1980b) Phosphonoformate inhibits synthesis of Epstein-Barr virus (EBV) capsid antigen and transformation of human cord blood lymphocytes by EBV. Virology 102:226–230

Margalith M, Manor D, Agranat I, Bentor Y, Gelfand T, Goldblum N (1980c) Esters of phosphonopropionic and phosphonoacetic acids: Effect on synthesis of Epstein-Barr virus (EBV) antigens and on transformation of cord blood lymphocytes by EBV. Cancer Biochem Biophys 4:137–143

May DC, Miller RL, Rapp F (1977) The effect of phosphonoacetic acid on the in vitro replication of varicella-zoster virus. Intervirology 8:83–91

McCarty JR, Jarratt MT (1979) Topical phosphonoacetic acid treatment of cutaneous herpes simplex infections in the guinea pig. J Am Acad Dermatol 1:244–248

Menezes J, Patel P, Dussault H, Bourkas AE (1978) Comparative studies on the induction of virus-associated nuclear antigen and early antigen by lymphocyte-transforming (B95-8) and nontransforming (P3HR-1) strains of Epstein-Barr virus. Intervirology 9:86–94

Meyer RF, Varnell ED, Kaufman HE (1976) Phosphonoacetic acid in the treatment of experimental ocular herpes simplex infections. Antimicrob Agents Chemother 9:308–311

Moreno MA, Carrascosa AL, Ortin J, Vinuela E (1978) Inhibition of African swine fever virus replication by phosphonoacetic acid. J Gen Virol 39:253–258

Nazerian K, Lee LF (1976) Selective inhibition by phosphonoacetic acid of MDV DNA replication in a lymphoblastoid cell line. Virology 74:188–193

Newton AA (1979) Inhibition of the replication of herpes viruses by phosphonoacetate and related compounds. Adv Ophthalmol 38:267–275

Nishibe Y, Inoue YK (1978) Effects of phosphonoacetic acid on subacute myeloopticoneuropathy virus in vitro and in vivo. J Med Virol 2:225–229

Nordenfelt E, Helgstrand E, Oberg B (1979) Trisodium phosphonoformate inhibits hepatitis B Dane particle DNA polymerase. Acta Pathol Microbiol Scand [B] 87:75–76

Nylen P (1924) Beitrag zur Kenntnis der organischen Phosphorverbindungen. Chem Berichte 57B:1023–1035

Nyormoi O, Thorley-Lawson DA, Elkington J, Strominger JL (1976) Differential effect of phosphonoacetic acid by the expression of Epstein-Barr viral antigens and virus production. Proc Natl Acad Sci USA 73:1745–1748

Ohashi M, Taguchi T, Ikegami S (1978) Aphidicolin: a specific inhibitor of DNA polymerase in the cytosol of rat liver. Biochem Biophys Res Commun 82:1084–1090

Ooka T, Lenoir G, Daillie J (1979) Characterization of an Epstein-Barr virus-induced DNA polymerase. J Virol 29:1–10

Overall JC, Kern ER, Glasgow LA (1976) Effective antiviral chemotherapy in cytomegalovirus infection of mice. J Infect Dis 133:A237–A244

Overby LR, Robishaw EE, Schleicher JB, Rueter A, Shipkowitz NL, Mao JCH (1974) Inhibition of herpes simplex virus replication by phosphonoacetic acid. Antimicrob Agents Chemother 6:360–365

Overby LR, Duff RG, Mao JCH (1977) Antiviral potential of phosphonoacetic acid. Ann NY Acad Sci 284:310–320

Palmer AE, London WT, Sever JL (1977) Disodium phosphonoacetate in cream base as a possible topical treatment for skin lesions of herpes simplex virus in cebus monkeys. Antimicrob Agents Chemother 12:510–512

Patel P, Menezes J (1979) Differential effect of phosphonoacetic acid on early antigen synthesis in two Epstein-Barr virus producer cell lines. Virology 92:236–239

Pearson GR, Beneke JS (1977) Inhibition of herpesvirus saimiri replication by phosphonoacetic acid, benzo(a)pyrene, and methylcholanthrene. Cancer Res 37:42–46

Powell KL, Purifoy DJM (1977) Nonstructural proteins of herpes simplex virus. I. Purification of the induced DNA polymerase. J Virol 24:618–626

Purifoy DJM, Powell KL (1977) Herpes simplex virus DNA polymerase as the site of phosphonoacetate sensitivity: temperature-sensitive mutants. J Virol 24:470–477

Purifoy DJM, Lewis RB, Powell KL (1977) Identification of the herpes simplex virus DNA polymerase gene. Nature 269:621–623

Renis HE (1977) Chemotherapy of genital herpes simplex virus type 2 infections of female hamsters. Antimicrob Agents Chemother 11:701–707

Reno JM, Lee LF, Boezi JA (1978) Inhibition of herpesvirus replication and herpesvirus-induced deoxyribonucleic acid polymerase by phosphonoformate. Antimicrob Agents Chemother 13:188–192

Rickinson AB, Epstein MA (1978) Sensitivity of the transforming and replicative functions of Epstein-Barr virus to inhibition by phosphonoacetate. J Gen Virol 40:409–420

Robberson DL, Kasamatsu H, Vinograd J (1972) Replication of mitochondrial DNA. Circular replicative intermediates in mouse L cells. Proc Natl Acad Sci USA 60:737–741

Sabourin CLK, Reno JM, Boezi JA (1978) Inhibition of eucaryotic DNA polymerases by phosphonoacetate and phosphonoformate. Arch Biochem Biophys 187:96–101

Seebeck T, Shaw JE, Pagano JS (1977) Synthesis of Epstein-Barr virus DNA in vitro: effects of phosphonoacetic acid, N-ethylmaleimide, and ATP. J Virol 21:435–438

Shannon W (1976) Selective inhibitors of RNA tumor virus replication in vitro and evaluation of candidate antiviral agents in vivo. Ann NY Acad Sci 284:472–502

Shipkowitz NL, Bower RR, Appell RN, Nordeen CW, Overby LR, Roderick WR, Schleicher JB, von Esch AM (1973) Suppression of herpes simplex virus infection by phosphonoacetic acid. Appl Microbiol 26:264–267

Spadari S, Weissbach A (1975) RNA-primed DNA synthesis: specific catalysis by HeLa cell DNA polymerase α. Proc Natl Acad Sci USA 72:503–507

Summers WC, Klein G (1976) Inhibition of Epstein-Barr virus DNA synthesis and late gene expression by phosphonoacetic acid. J Virol 18:151–155

Sundquist B, Oberg B (1979) Phosphonoformate inhibits reverse transcriptase. J Gen Virol 45:273–281

Thorley-Lawson D, Strominger JL (1976) Transformation of human lymphocytes by Epstein-Barr virus is inhibited by phosphonoacetic acid. Nature 263:332–334

Von Esch AM (1978) Amides of phosphonoacetic acid for treating herpes simplex virus type I and II infections. U.S. Patent No. 4,087,572

Wahren B, Oberg B (1979) Inhibition of cytomegalovirus late antigens by phosphonoformate. Intervirology 12:335–339

Wahren B, Oberg B (1980) Reversible inhibition of cytomegalovirus replication by phosphonoformate. Intervirology 14:7–15

Wang TSF, Fisher PA, Sedwick WD, Korn D (1975) Identification of a new DNA polymerase activity in human KB cells. J Biol Chem 250:5270–5272

Weissbach A (1979) The functional roles of mammalian DNA polymerase. Arch Biochem Biophys 198:386–396

Weissbach A, Schlabach A, Fridlender B, Bolden A (1971) DNA polymerases from human cells. Nature 231:167–170

Wohlenberg CR, Walz MA, Notkins AL (1976) Efficacy of phosphonoacetic acid on herpes simplex virus infection of sensory ganglia. Infect Immun 13:1519–1521

Yajima Y, Tanaka A, Nonoyama M (1976) Inhibition of productive replication of Epstein-Barr virus DNA by phosphonoacetic acid. Virology 71:352–354

Zur Hausen H (1975) Oncogenic herpes viruses. Biochim Biophys Acta 417:25–53

CHAPTER 12

Natural Products

P. E. CAME and B. A. STEINBERG

A. Introduction

Folk medicine is replete with references to herbal preparations and the therapeutic use of many naturally occurring substances. Some of these materials such as rauwolfia alkaloids, opium, belladonna, and digitalis continue to be used in modern medicine. With the exception of antibiotics, the use of natural substances in the area of infectious disease has not met with the success apparent in other areas of human disease. Until Pasteur, Koch, Semmelweiss, and others developed the germ theory of disease, there was no rational basis for an assault on the infectious process. The pioneering work of Koch brought an understanding of what bacteria can do as agents of disease and how their effect might be interrupted. This led to the field of chemotherapy with synthetic chemicals as possible therapeutic agents. With Fleming's serendipitous discovery of penicillin and its development by Chain and Florey came the antibiotic age with all its glowing promise. The search for other natural substances was not as intense as that for synthetic antibacterial agents or antibiotics. Nevertheless, there were individuals who attempted to uncover antiviral agents in the plant, animal, or marine world. It is our purpose in this chapter to relate what has been done and where it is leading. While the results up to now have not been overwhelmingly encouraging, a few substances with therapeutic possibilities have emerged and these offer optimism that others, perhaps superior, will result from additional research.

B. Amino Acids

Until the advent of techniques enabling the study of virus multiplication outside of the intact host, the effect of nutritional factors on virus replication and the disease process was empirical and difficult to interpret. One could withold various nutrients from the infected host and then could do little more than speculate on the mechanism of the response obtained. It was impossible to determine whether a reduction of viral replication resulted from the inability of the nutritionally compromised host to support virus multiplication or if the virus itself was affected directly. It had been reported that poliovirus was inhibited if the host animals were kept on a vitamin B_1-deficient or low calorie diet and this was confirmed by RASMUSSEN et al. (1944). JONES et al. (1946) reported that a tryptophan-deficient diet was more effective than a protein-deficient diet in producing a delay in the onset of poliomyelitis in mice. Subsequently, with the development of tissue culture techniques, many more of the amino acids and their analogs were tested for possible prophylactic or therapeutic value against virus diseases. The results of these studies have not led to therapeutic approaches of unequivocal practical value. The observations have, however, provided insight into the relationship of nutritional needs of the cell during infection. Some of the more recent investigations with lysine and amino acid analogs indicate that these substances may yet prove to be effective and convenient for the control of certain viral diseases.

I. Lysine

PEARSON and WINZLER (1949), using a Maitland culture system, grew Theiler GD VII mouse encephalitis virus in the presence of various amino acids (MOLDAVE et al. 1951; PEARSON et al. 1952). Lysine was a moderately active virus inhibitor in this system. The activity of lysine was confirmed at the relatively high concentration of 1 mg/ml in the minced mouse brain system used by PEARSON and WINZLER, and it was also shown that it could be reversed with methionine (RAFELSON et al. 1950). Serine and ornithine were also active at 1 mg/ml but not as active as lysine; 3 mg/ml alanine, arginine, aspartic acid, cystine, glycine, histidine, phenylalanine, threonine, or tryptophan were active. Later, PEARSON et al. (1955) showed that DL-ethionine and DL-methionine partially reversed the activity of lysine. RAFELSON et al. (1950) also demonstrated that infection with mouse encephalitis virus caused an increase in phosphate uptake by phospholipids and protein-bound phosphorus fractions of brain tissue. At 1 mg/ml, lysine did not substantially change the incorporation into the phospholipid fraction, but it drastically reduced the level of phosphate in the protein-bound fraction. Again, methionine was able partially to reverse the effect of lysine, but had no effect by itself on phosphorus uptake into either fraction.

Other workers found that lysine and arginine were inhibitory to mumps virus as well as the A/PR8 and B/Lee strains of influenza virus. L-Lysine was found to be twice as active as the DL-form (EATON et al. 1951). Although very high levels of lysine were used (2 mg/ml), there was no detectable virucidal effect on either the mumps or influenza viruses. Large virus inocula were able to overcome the inhibitory effects of the lysine and lysine did not interfere with the hemagglutinating properties of influenza virus.

KATZ et al. (1975) found that an acyl derivative of lysine, dicarbobenzoxy-L-lysine sodium, inhibited the growth of parainfluenza virus in vitro but did not exert an effect on SV40, vaccinia virus, poliovirus 1, Semliki Forest, eastern equine encephalomyelitis, or western equine encephalomyelitis viruses. The mode of action of the lysine derivative or carbobenzyl-L-aspartic acid, β-benzyl ester potassium, and N-3-phenylpropionyl-S-benzyl-L-cysteine potassium, which were also active, was not determined. In earlier studies, TANKERSLEY (1964) reported that lysine was not required for the growth of herpesvirus and, in fact, was inhibitory. Lysine-free Eagle's medium was more supportive of herpesvirus growth than complete medium (Table 1). Other studies had shown that the herpesvirus-infected cells contain less lysine than noninfected cells. Based on these observations and others, KAGAN (1974) gave patients L-lysine orally at the first indication of the onset of either oral or vulvar lesions of herpesvirus infection. This treatment reportedly led to a rapid resolution of the lesions. Doses of 390 mg/patient produced no overt toxicity.

Table 1. Effect of single amino acid deficiencies on herpesvirus yield from infected cells in serum-free medium (geometric mean of four experiments) (Tankersley 1964)

Amino acid deficiency	Virus yield (log pfu)
Histidine	1.80
Arginine	2.00
Tryptophan	2.60
Glutamine	2.80
Threonine	3.10
Valine	3.15
Methionine	3.40
Leucine	3.45
Phenylalanine	3.55
Tyrosine	3.70
Cysteine	4.00
Isoleucine	4.50
Eagle's medium[a]	4.60
Lysine	4.70

[a] Complete medium

GRIFFITH et al. (1978) undertook a multicentered study of lysine therapy in which herpesvirus-infected patients were given 800–1,000 mg daily during an overt infection and 300–500 mg daily as a maintenance dose. Dietary restriction was not imposed, but curtailment of arginine-rich foods (nuts, seeds, chocolate) while on the lysine regimen was recommended. The results were encouraging, showing rapid control of the infection as evidenced by disappearance of pain and the failure of new vesicles to appear. The infection quickly returned if the dosage of lysine was reduced below a critical limit (approximately 500 mg/day). The authors pointed out that the histone surrounding the DNA of the eukaryotic cells contains 28% lysine and only 3%–4% arginine, whereas the capsid coat around the virus DNA has more arginine than lysine. KAPLAN et al. (1970) had indicated that the different coding of cellular and viral DNA can explain the preferred utilization of arginine to lysine in herpes-infected cells. KINKADE (1971), in support of this viewpoint, indicated that lysine-rich histones are necessary for the structural integrity of nuclear DNA in the eukaryotic cells. KAPLAN et al. (1970) found that, prior to onset of cytopathogenicity, cells under the direction of viral DNA shifted from normal synthesis to the manufacture of protein with a preponderance of arginine compared with lysine. The changeover occurred, according to the authors, because the cell was manufacturing virus-specific proteins rather than cell-specific material. Although some doubts concerning its clinical efficacy have been expressed, studies using lysine therapy continue.

II. Phenylalanine and Phenylalanine Analogs

THOMPSON (1947) used Maitland cultures of chick embryo tissues to grow vaccinia virus and studied amino acid analogs and other substances as possible inhibitors of viral synthesis. The amino acid analogs he used were: aminomethane sulfonic acid (analog of glycine), α-aminoisobutane sulfonic acid (analogue of valine), α-aminophenylmethane sulfonic acid (analog of phenylalanine), and methoxinine (analog of methionine). All of the analogs were active as inhibitors of vaccinia virus growth at 1 mg/ml but not at 0.1 mg/ml.

THOMPSON and WILKIN (1948), also using the Maitland culture system, examined the effect of β-2-thienylalanine on vaccinia virus growth. The compound previously had been shown to interfere with the growth of *Escherichia coli* and *Saccharomyces cerevisiae*. Phenylalanine, at 50 µg/ml, had no effect on viral multiplication, but comparable doses of thienylalanine were inhibitory. In addition, the addition of phenylalanine to the medium containing thienylalanine neutralized the effect of the amino acid analog. Methionine used in the same manner, i.e., to reverse the activity of thienylalanine, was not effective. In contrast to the observation made by THOMPSON and WILKIN, PEARSON and WINZLER (1949) did not find phenylalanine antagonistic to the antiviral properties of β-2-thienylalanine. They did find that β-2-thienylalanine and β-2-furyl-DL-alanine were very active as virus inhibitors. L-Arginine, cystine, cysteine, glycine, histidine, leucine, proline, and alanine were not active.

In the studies by RAFELSON et al. (1950) cited earlier, in which uptake of labeled phosphorus was used as an indicator of virus replication in minced mouse brain, DL-2-thiophenylalanine was the most active of the substances tested and had no effect on the incorporation of phosphate in noninfected brain. The amino acid analog inhibited the stimulation of phosphorus incorporation by virus-infected tissue, and the inhibition of both incorporation and virus growth was not reversed by the addition of phenylalanine. The authors speculated that excess amino acid levels may interfere with the turnover of phosphorus essential for virus synthesis in brain tissue.

CUSHING and MORGAN (1952) found that β-2-thienylalanine at 0.5 mg/ml in minced chick embryo heart tissue culture was ineffective when tested against influenza or mumps virus. Phenylalanine was active against mouse encephalitis virus, as were a number of other amino acids (PEARSON et al. 1952), but at a high level (3 mg/ml). p-Fluorophenylalanine (FPA) and its stereoisomers were active at a lower but still high level (1 mg/ml). β-2-Thienylalanine, when tested in mice for protective activity, was not active. BROWN (1952) tested β-2-thienylalanine against the Lansing strain of poliovirus in tissue culture. The analog was active and was partially reversed by the addition of phenylalanine.

BROWN et al. (1961) reported that p-fluorophenylalanine inhibited the production of virus and infectious RNA from cells infected with foot-and-mouth disease virus (Fig. 1). In addition, phenylalanine reversed the activity of the analog. LEVINTOW et al. (1962) found that 5 µg/ml FPA prevented the maturation of poliovirus in HeLa cells but permitted the synthesis of infectious RNA. Reversal of the FPA effect by phenylalanine allowed for virus maturation with a shorter lag period which suggested that events early in the viral replication cycle proceeded even in the presence of FPA. WECKER et al. (1962) and SCHARFF and LEVINTOW (1963) noted a parallel inhibition of viral antigens and viral RNA by high levels of FPA with poliovirus and postulated a mutual dependency of viral antigens and viral RNA synthesis. At low FPA levels, even if the viral proteins contained FPA rather than phenylalanine, they were functional proteins, as evidenced by the pro-

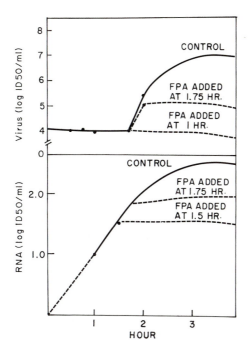

Fig. 1. Effect of adding 1,000 μ*M* p-fluorophenylalanine to infected cells at different times during the growth cycle of foot-and-mouth disease virus. (BROWN et al. 1961)

duction of viral RNA. At high levels, the FPA interfered with and probably halted the synthesis of protein and, consequently, the RNA synthesis as well. JACOBSON and BALTIMORE (1968) have shown that FPA is incorporated into poliovirus precursor protein and blocks the proteolytic cleavage leading to the generation of function proteins. These results suggest that inhibition of proteolytic cleavage is the mechanism by which FPA blocks poliovirus replication. The replicative cycle of poliovirus is described in Chap. 8.

KIT et al. (1963) found that FPA markedly inhibited thymidine kinase (TK) activity in vaccinia-infected mouse fibroblasts; however, normal mouse fibroblasts were similarly affected by FPA. These effects of FPA were reversed by phenylalanine. WECKER (1965) studied the effect of FPA, L-ethionine, and 7-azatryptophan on the growth of RNA viruses. The effect of FPA in these studies was similar to that already described, relative to the processes of viral maturation and infectious RNA production. The activity of FPA was further confirmed by LOH and PAYNE (1965) and DYM and BECKER (1969), among others, and the range of activity was extended to herpesvirus.

An amino acid-related compound, *N*-phenylacetoaminomethylene-DL-nitrophenylalanine, was tested for activity in a Friend (leukemia) virus-mouse system by FUJITA et al. (1979). It significantly inhibited virus-induced splenomegaly, reduced viable virus titers in plasma and spleen tissue, and prolonged survival time. The compound was also active in tissue cultures at its maximum tolerated dose. The analog may be an inhibitor of viral RNA synthesis or interfere with cell trans-

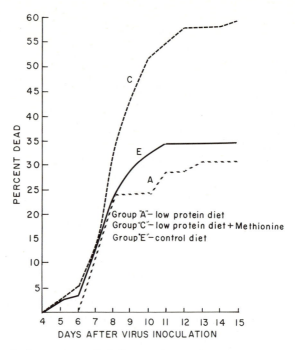

Fig. 2. Mortality of mice on controlled diets (with or without methionine) after infection with swine influenza virus. Curve A = low protein diet; C = low protein diet plus methionine; E = control diet. (Sprunt 1948)

formation enzyme systems. Treatment of infected mice may be delayed for as long as 24 h postinfection without loss of protection, which suggests an interference with the completion of viral replication.

III. Methionine and Methionine Analogs

Sprunt (1948) reported that methionine given intraperitoneally at high levels (Fig. 2) increased the susceptibility of mice on controlled diets to swine influenza. He concluded that methionine may make cells more susceptible to virus or interfere with antibody production. The inhibitory effect of methoxinine–methionine combinations on the growth of influenza A/PR8 virus in chorioallantoic (CA) membrane was investigated by Ackermann (1951). He posited that the amino acid analogs may have reduced the concentration of a normal substrate by competing with it for active sites in a critical enzyme system. Methoxinine, at 1.3 mg/ml, almost completely suppressed the growth of influenza virus, and at 0.3 mg/ml, there still was marked inhibition. The activity of methoxinine was completely blocked by DL-methionine. DL-Ethionine was also suppressive and was similarly reversed by the addition of methionine. The isomers of DL-methionine were tested for their antagonism to the antiviral effect of methoxinine. D-Methionine was without activity, whereas L-methionine was as active as the racemic mixture. Ackermann also determined that methoxinine was not virucidal and it was shown that methoxinine

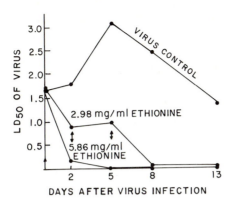

Fig. 3. Growth of Lansing poliovirus in human embryonic brain tissue culture. (BROWN and ACKERMANN 1951)

did not inhibit viral attachment since activity was well defined, even when methoxinine was added as late as 3 h postinfection. The CA membrane in the presence of methoxinine had the same respiratory rate as normal CA tissue, suggesting the lack of significant toxicity. In addition, when the methoxinine was washed from the tissues and 4.2 mg/ml methionine added, the tissue supported virus growth.

In a poliomyelitis virus–minced human brain tissue system, BROWN and ACKERMANN (1951) examined the effect of DL-ethionine on virus proliferation. Very large doses of approximately 6 and 3 mg/ml of the analog were markedly inhibitory to virus growth. If the last ethionine addition, which was made on days 2 and 5 after virus infection, was withheld, the tissues were able to support normal virus growth (Fig. 3). The addition of methionine to the flasks containing ethionine led to a partial reversal of the inhibitory effect. This observation may be better understood in light of the finding by JACOBSON and BALTIMORE (1968) which showed that incorporation of amino acid analogs may inhibit proteolytic cleavage and, concomitantly, poliovirus replication.

THOMPSON and LAVENDER (1953) medicated mice infected with Semliki Forest virus with DL-ethionine. The mice were infected either intraperitoneally or intracerebrally and medicated either in the diet or intraperitoneally. Ethionine was not active against intracerebral infection, but had a therapeutic effect against the intraperitoneally induced infection. Methionine fed in addition to ethionine did not uniformly reverse the therapeutic activity of the ethionine. GIFFORD et al. (1954) found, however, that DL-ethionine did not affect poliovirus growth in HeLa cells except at those levels which shut down cellular respiration. The ethionine-induced inhibition of respiration was only partly reversed by methionine. At approximately the same time, ACKERMANN and MAASSAB (1954) examined the effect of methoxinine on the growth of influenza A/PR8 virus strain in cultures of allantoic membranes in Warburg flasks. A compound related to tyrosine, α-amino-p-methoxyphenylmethane sulfonic acid (see Sect. B.IV), was also tested for its antiviral effect. This compound, but not methoxinine, had been reported to inhibit the incipient stages of viral development as well as impairing the release of mature virus. The results of their studies indicated that the sulfonic acid analog inhibited

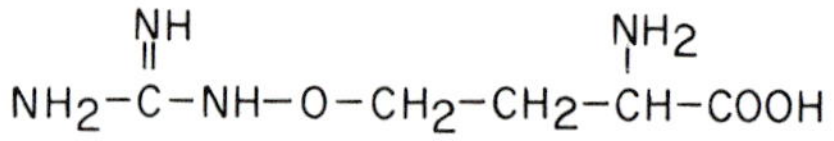

$$\text{NH}_2-\overset{\overset{\displaystyle NH}{\|}}{C}-NH-O-CH_2-CH_2-\overset{\overset{\displaystyle NH_2}{|}}{CH}-COOH$$

CANAVANINE

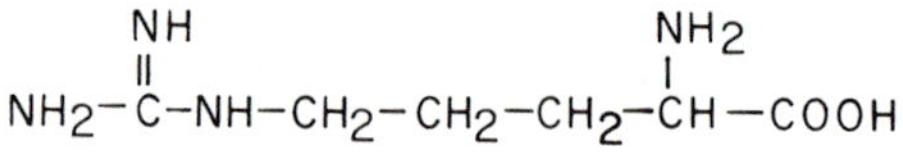

$$\text{NH}_2-\overset{\overset{\displaystyle NH}{\|}}{C}-NH-CH_2-CH_2-CH_2-\overset{\overset{\displaystyle NH_2}{|}}{CH}-COOH$$

ARGININE

Fig. 4. Structures of canavanine and arginine

absorption and penetration, whereas methoxinine had no effect on these stages. Methoxinine, however, had a profound effect on the latent period of virus maturation. Later phases in viral maturation were not affected by either sulfonic acid or methoxinine. Finally, α-amino-p-methoxyphenylmethane sulfonic acid was inhibitory at the virus release stage, whereas methoxinine was not.

In studies on the activity of lysine and its antagonism by ethionine and methionine, PEARSON et al. (1955) also showed that methoxinine was active against mouse encephalitis and its activity was antagonized by methionine. Other methionine antagonists were methionine sulfoxime, norleucine, and allylglycine, the activities of all of which were reversible by methionine. WECKER (1965) determined that ethionine dissociated the formation of infectious viral RNA from that of infectious virions. The infectious virion production was reduced by 90% with 125 µg/ml ethionine; however, infectious viral RNA activity was not affected even if the level of amino acid analog was raised to 600 µg/ml. 7-Azatryptophan behaved in a similar manner.

IV. Miscellaneous Amino Acids and Analogs

Ornithine and arginine were shown to be active against influenza virus by EATON et al. (1951) who concluded that the most active amino acids were those containing two amino groups. LWOFF (1965) also observed that L-arginine and L-ornithine inhibit the replication of poliovirus. The possible relationship of amino groups and the guanidino group to antiviral activity is discussed in Chap. 8. The effect of arginine was not reversed by RNA, adenylic acid, methionine, or creatinine. Furthermore, arginine, like lysine, did not interfere with the hemagglutinating or infective properties of the viruses.

Canavanine, an amino acid occurring in jack beans, was tested for its effect on the growth of influenza virus by PILCHER et al. (1955). Canavanine is a close structural analog of arginine (Fig. 4) and had shown activity against various fungi and bacteria. When it was injected into the allantoic cavity of chick embryos 1 h prior to infection with influenza B virus, there was marked inhibition of virus growth. A high dose (20 mg) was the optimum dosage while lower levels of the amino acid produced a dose-related response. In vitro, the compound inhibited the virus and its antiviral activity was reversed by arginine. The compound was not active against influenza A/PR8 virus or mumps virus. DUDA (1975) found that cana-

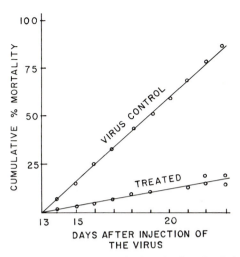

Fig. 5. Inhibition of rabies infection in rats by β-phenylserine. Pooled results of several experiments. Controls received no β-phenylserine. Treated animals were given the amino acid at a dose of 15 mg/day intraperitoneally for 10–14 days, starting either 4 days prior to, or 24 h after infection. (PONS and PRESTON 1961)

vanine induced the synthesis of a Sindbis virus capsid protein of somewhat larger molecular weight than that of controls. This abnormal capsid protein, however, did not affect the formation of nucleocapsids and virus particles, nor was the titer of the virus found to be different from that of normal Sindbis virus.

α-Aminosulfonic acids had been known as inhibitors of bacterial growth and also of coliphage. ACKERMANN (1952), using three α-amino sulfonic acids that resemble tyrosine and phenylalanine, tested their effects on the growth of influenza virus in tissue culture, embryonated eggs, and mice. α-Aminophenylmethane sulfonic acid and α-amino-p-methoxyphenylmethane sulfonic acid were tested for virucidal activity and were completely inactive at levels of 2.0 mg/ml. At 0.2 mg/ml, however, both compounds markedly supressed viral multiplication and were active at levels as low as 0.16 mg/ml. In embryonated eggs, the maximum tolerated dose of both inhibitors was 28 mg. A dose of 4 mg showed some viral inhibitory effect and 8 mg completely inhibited virus replication. In mice infected intracerebrally with influenza virus, the compounds were protective when administered by the same route but were inactive if given by other parenteral routes or in the diet.

The activity of the α-aminosulfonic acids was not reversible by their corresponding amino acids. Evidence has been presented that these compounds interfere with penetration and release of influenza virus at concentrations exerting little or no interference with normal cellular metabolism. Fragments of the α-aminosulfonic acids, such as NH_4^+, bisulfate ion, or aldehyde precursors were not active, thus indicating the essentiality of the intact structure. Their activity was not confined to a specific amino acid, but rather to functional groups present in a number of amino acids.

PONS and PRESTON (1961) found that β-phenylserine protected rats from lethal infection of rabies virus (Fig. 5). The rat produces most of its tyrosine from phenylalanine and β-phenylserine may inhibit phenylalanine hydroxylase. The authors

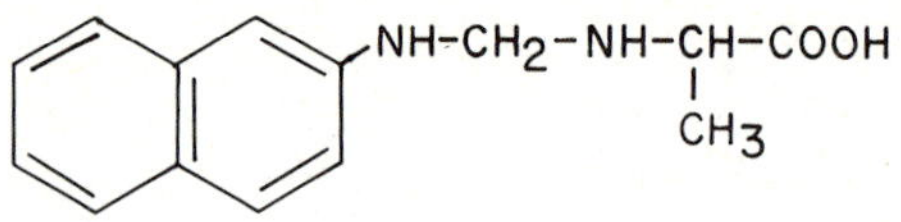

NH-CH$_2$-NH-CH-COOH
                    |
                    CH$_3$

N-β-Naphthylaminomethyl-L-α-alanine

SO$_2$-NH-CH$_2$-CH$_2$-COOH

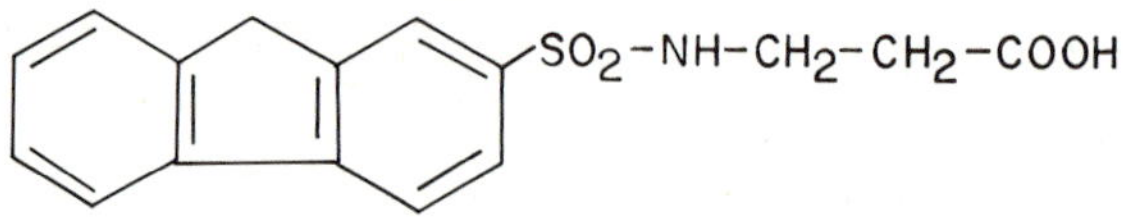

N-2-Fluorenesulfonyl-β-alanine

Fig. 6. Structures of *N*-β-naphthylaminomethyl-L-α-alanine and *N*-2-fluorenesulfonyl-β-alanine

speculated that the amino acid analog inhibited multiplication of virus by interfering with the incorporation of phenylalanine or tyrosine into new virus protein. The activity of these amino acids reversed the inhibitory activity of β-phenylserine. Compounds related to β-phenylserine but lacking either an amino, hydroxyl, or phenyl group were inactive.

D-Penicillamine, a valine analog, exhibits specific antipoliovirus activity in vitro (minimum effective dose: 33 µg/ml in KB cells) according to Gessa et al. (1966). The mode of action of the compound is unclear and it possesses little or no activity against herpesvirus, vaccinia virus, or vesicular stomatitis virus. The stereoisomer, L-penicillamine, is devoid of any activity and the antiviral activity of the D-isomer is not related to activities the two isomers show, i.e., copper chelating and pyridoxidine antagonism. This amino acid analog is presently being marketed for such diseases as cystinuria, Wilson's disease, and rheumatoid arthritis at the recommended doses (500–750 mg/day). The manufacturers have made no claims relative to antiviral activity.

Fujita (1973) tested two amino acid analogs which possessed therapeutic value against influenza virus in mice. *N*-β-Naphthylaminomethyl-L-α-alanine and N-2-fluorenesulfonyl-β-alanine (Fig. 6) were used to medicate mice infected with the A2/Adachi strain of influenza virus, starting 3 days postinfection. Both compounds reduced lung consolidation and mortality by a significant amount. Amantadine, tested under similar conditions, was not as effective.

C. Vitamin C

Following the publication of *Vitamin C and the Common Cold* in 1971 by Pauling, came a series of clinical trials designed to determine if vitamin C (asorbic acid) had a beneficial effect on the clinical manifestations of the common cold. Anderson et al. (1972) conducted a large-scale double-blind study using at least 1,000 volunteers. Subjects, recruited from various hospital staffs, schools, and industrial plants, were instructed to take 4 tablets/day (placebo or 250 mg vitamin C) in divided doses and to increase their intake to 16 tablets/day for the first 3 days of any illness. The study continued over a period of 60 days. In terms of average number of colds and days of sickness per subject, the vitamin group experienced less illness than the placebo group, but the differences were not statistically significant. There was, however, a difference in the number of subjects who remained free of illness throughout the study. Subjects receiving vitamin C experienced approximately 30% fewer total days of disability. In a study using more than 2,000 subjects, AN-DERSON et al. (1974) tested vitamin C for its prophylactic and/or therapeutic value on the common cold. There was some indication of reduced severity of disease, but it was not a large, statistically significant effect. A number of dose levels were used, but there was no evidence of a dose-related response. The authors concluded that ascorbic acid may have a beneficial effect if taken daily in doses of less than 1 g/day.

COULEHAN et al. (1974) investigated the effect of ascorbic acid against the common cold in a closed population at a Navajo boarding school. The study included determination of ascorbic acid blood levels, and a significant rise in circulating ascorbic acid values was seen when 1 or 2 g was taken daily. There were no significant differences in morbidity. In this study, however, there was a suggestion that the days of morbidity were lessened. When COULEHAN et al. (1976) expanded their earlier studies, vitamin C at doses of 1 g/day did not appear to be either therapeutically or prophylactically effective against upper respiratory disease. KARLOWSKI et al. (1975) found that ascorbic acid had a minor influence on duration and severity of colds in a double-blind study conducted at the National Institutes of Health in Bethesda, Maryland. They concluded that the differences seen might well be explained by a break in the protocol which was constructed to provide double-blind conditions. MILLER et al. (1977) performed a double-blind study using 44 school-age monozygotic twins. The vitamin did not significantly effect the cold symptoms.

Recently, MANZELLA and ROBERTS (1980) investigated the activity of ascorbic acid and hyperthermia on phytohemagglutinin transformation responsiveness of human peripheral leukocytes when exposed to influenza A virus, parainfluenza virus, adenovirus, respiratory syncytial virus, and rhinovirus. They found that the effects of ascorbic acid and hyperthermia were complementary and speculated that ascorbic acid might favorably influence the course of viral respiratory infections if antipyretic therapy is not used concomitantly. Their work suggests that vitamin C may exert immune enhancing activity.

D. Flavonoids

APPLE et al. (1975) found that flavonoids, which are phenylalanine metabolites, were active at doses of $< 10^{-7}$ mol/ml against Rous sarcoma virus and reduced the incidence of tumors in chicks by greater than 75%. The active flavonoids are those with an OH group in the 3 position and are potent inhibitors of viral reverse transcriptase. BELADI et al. (1977) tested a number of flavonoids against a variety of viruses. The structures are shown in Fig. 7. Two were virucidal for pseudorabies virus (morin and quercetin), whereas rutin was not. Quercetin was also virucidal for parainfluenza virus 3 and herpes simplex virus (HSV), but not for poliovirus 1 and adenovirus 3. Only moderate activity was noted in tissue culture. The authors disputed the earlier findings of APPLE et al. (1975) by indicating that activity was

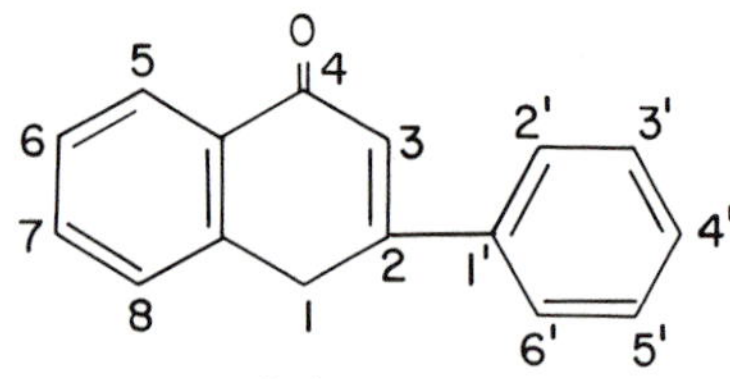

Quercetin –3,3',4',5,7 OH
Apigenin –4',5,7 OH
Fisetin   –3,3',4',7 OH
Luteolin –3',4',5,7 OH
Morin   –2',3,4',5,7 OH
Rutin   –Quercetin–3–glycoside

Fig. 7. Structure of quercetin and other flavonoids

not restricted to flavonoids with the hydroxyl in the 3 position. They point out that hydroxyl groups at C-3' and C-4' or C-2', and C-4' seem to be essential for antiviral activity, while the presence of glycosides at C-3 decreases the antiviral activity. MUSCI et al. (1978) found that the flavonoids exert their effect only on enveloped viruses and, although many flavonoids possess some degree of antiviral activity, the structure–activity relationship within the group is still somewhat obscure. VECKENSTEDT et al. (1978) tested quercetin and morin against Mengo virus infection in mice. Both were effective when given orally at doses of 40 mg/kg, but inactive via the subcutaneous route (Fig. 8). Medication was effective only if given prophylactically. Flavonoids with 3-glycoside moieties (quercetin and rutin) were ineffective.

E. Polysaccharides

Viral infections may be controlled by interference with virus attachment and penetration. Some polysaccharides are active by this means and are nonspecific in activity, i.e., their range of activity is not restricted to certain specific virus–cell systems.

I. Sulfated Polysaccharides

In 1947, HORSFALL and MCCARTY described the protective effect of dual infection with certain bacteria on the course of a virus infection in mice. Using such genera as *Streptococcus*, *Pneumococcus*, *Hemophilus*, and *Escherichia*, the authors were able to demonstrate a favorable modification of the infectious process due to pneumonia virus of mice (PVM). Extracts of these bacteria were also active and additional studies indicated that polysaccharides were the active moiety. As a result, polysaccharide preparations from *Streptococcus*, *Klebsiella*, *Shigella*, agar, and blood group A substance were administered intranasally to mice, and all inhibited the growth of PVM. Heparin (see Sect. E.II) was reported to lack antiviral activity.

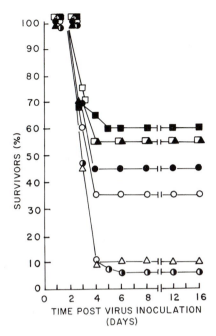

Fig. 8. Dose–response relationship of quercetin on the outcome of lethal Mengo virus encephalitis in mice. In both control and treatment groups, 20 animals were infected intraperitoneally with 10 LD_{50} virus and treated with placebo *(half-full circles)*, 10 *(open triangles)*, 20 *(open circles)*, 30 *(full circles)*, 40 *(open squares)*, 50 *(full squares)*, or 60 *(full triangles)* mg kg^{-1} day^{-1} quercetin. Drug was administered orally, beginning immediately before virus inoculation, twice daily every 12 h for 4 days. Mice were observed for 14 days or until death. (VECKENSTEDT et al. 1978)

GREEN and WOOLLEY (1947) examined the effect of apple pectin as well as flaxseed mucilage, blood group A substance, red blood cell extract, gum myrrh, and gum acacia on infection with influenza virus. Apple pectin inhibited not only hemagglutination by influenza A/PR8 virus, but also protected chick embryos from viral growth. They concluded that the polysaccharide affected the viral receptors on the red blood cells and also those on the cells lining the allantoic membrane. Alginic acid, a polymannuride, which is chemically and physically similar to apple pectin, was unable to affect either hemagglutination or infectivity. Many of these substances which inhibit agglutination are polysaccharides, rich in galacturonic acid. However, the polygalacturonide moiety is not essential since gum acacia and blood group A substance were also inhibitory but contain no galacturonic acid. Simple carbohydrates were inactive.

TAKEMORI and NOMURA (1960) discovered that the minute plaque forming mutants of poliovirus were inhibited by an extract of agar; the factor in the agar inhibited viral replication and was responsible for the small size of the plaques. TAKEMOTO and LIEBHABER (1961) and LIEBHABER and TAKEMOTO (1962) extended this observation to include encephalomyocarditis virus (EMC). They found that the multiplication of EMC in monolayer cultures grown in liquid medium proceded rapidly and completely destroyed the cell sheet, whereas under agar, two distinct plaque types appeared. The smaller plaque mutant (r$^+$) grew more slowly under agar than the large plaque mutant (r), but in liquid culture, the r$^+$ mutant multiplied much more rapidly than the r mutant. The inhibitory moiety was found to be a sulfated polysaccharide. SCHULZE and SCHLESINGER (1963) also characterized an inhibitory component of agar as a sulfated polysaccharide. It inhibited dengue fever virus in mice as well as plaque forming ability and hemagglutinating capacity. The sulfated polysaccharide combined directly with the virus and inhibited hemagglutination, but its exact mechanism of protection in the infectious process was not demonstrated. TAKEMOTO and FABISCH (1964) tested a synthetic sulfated polysaccharide, sodium dextran sulfate, as well as agar, and found that both restricted the growth of herpesvirus in liquid culture as well as under agar. TAKEMOTO and SPICER (1965) showed that some natural and synthetic polysaccharides were able to interact with the surfaces of cultured cells, and suggested that the antiviral action may be the result of virus–polyanion complexes plus an interaction with the host cell which had also taken up the inhibitor. HeLa cells, pretreated with polysaccharide, failed to support the growth of herpesvirus. The inhibition of herpesvirus and poliovirus may be a result of the interaction of the polyanion with viral receptor sites.

II. Heparin

Heparin has also been shown to interfere with the replication of HSV (TAKEMOTO and LIEBHABER 1962; and TAKEMOTO and FABISCH 1964). VAHERI and CANTELL (1963) reported that HSV was inhibited in vitro by heparin but mumps virus, Newcastle disease virus, measles virus, vaccinia virus, adenovirus 1 and 11, echovirus 9 and 13, and polioviruses were not affected. Infectious virus was recovered from a heparin solution by dilution, demonstrating that the virus–heparin complex was reversible and that heparin was not virucidal. Furthermore, only slight inhibition of virus multiplication was observed if the heparin was added 1 h after the virus, suggesting that heparin affected the early interaction of HSV and the cell. NAHMIAS and KIBRICK (1963, 1964) also demonstrated that heparin acts during the early stages of infection; virus replication took place if heparin was added after 1 h post-infection. HADHAZY et al. (1966) showed that neither heparin nor hyaluronic acid inhibited influenza or parainfluenza, but heparin prevented herpesvirus infection of cultured cells. In mechanism of action studies, HOCHBERG and BECKER (1968) found that heparin prevented adsorption of herpesvirus to cells and once virus had penetrated, it had no effect.

III. Intestinal Mucopolysaccharides

An extract of mouse intestine was found to inhibit the growth of encephalomyelitis in mice (MANDEL and RACKER 1953). MANDEL (1957) was able to demonstrate that the inhibitory material was a mucopolysaccharide that interacted with virions electrostatically. The complex was readily dissociated by decreasing the electrolyte concentration. PIAZZA (1964) found that the viral content of the intestines of mice infected with mouse hepatitis virus (MHV) varied with the distance from the liver. Mice with MHV median lethal dose (LD$_{50}$) infectivity titer of $10^{7.5}$ in liver and $10^{6.1}$ in bile had infectivity titers of 10^1 at the distal end of the small intestine and in unexpelled feces. Further studies (PIAZZA et al. 1965) indicated that the inhibitor is peculiar to mouse or rat intestinal tissue and is present in the first section of the mucosa of the small intestine. In subsequent studies, PIAZZA et al. (1967) found that the mucopolysaccharide was strongly active against rubella and mouse hepatitis viruses but showed only weak activity against influenza virus, measles virus, coxsackievirus A9, infectious bronchitis virus of chickens, and SV40. There was no activity against poliovirus, echovirus 11, or Newcastle disease virus.

The antiviral activity of these naturally occurring sulfated polymers has been difficult to demonstrate in vivo but has prompted interest in the evaluation of some chemically similar synthetic polymers. Polyvinyl sulfate, for one, has demonstrated in vitro and in vivo antiviral activity but its toxicity precluded trials in humans (CAME et al. 1969).

F. Substances from Microorganisms

A large number of antiviral substances derived from various microorganisms has been described over the past 30 years. The structures and mechanisms of action of some are known, others have been only partially identified and hypotheses concerning their mode of action have been proposed. There are still others about which only the most rudimentary knowledge is available. Many of the substances are metabolic inhibitors; some have been referred to as microbial toxins, others have been widely used as biologic tools, since their potent activity is not sufficiently selective to permit their use as prophylactic or therapeutic antiviral entities. Among these are: actinomycin, cytochalasin, daunomycin, and rifamycin. The study of these substances has provided considerable insight into the understanding of virus-specific replicative events. Adenine arabinoside (Ara-A) is perhaps the only substance originally obtained from a microorganism (a *Streptomyces* sp.) that has been approved by the U.S. Food and Drug Administration for limited use in humans. Detailed information concerning this drug can be found in Chap. 3. Most of the following substances were selected by virtue of their being well-studied agents that have contributed significantly to our knowledge base. It should be recognized that they represent only a small number of the compounds, derived from microorganisms, that show antiviral properties.

I. Fungal Products

1. Aphidicolin

This substance was described by BRUNDRET et al. (1972) as a tetracyclic diterpenoid substance and was obtained from *Cephalosporium aphilicola*. Aphidicolin has not been widely studied, but BUCKNALL et al. (1973) reported that it inhibited HSV in cell culture and infected rabbit eyes. OHASHI et al. (1978) examined the effects of the compound on several DNA polymerases, and showed that aphidicolin is inhibitory to the α DNA-dependent DNA polymerase of a mammalian cell but failed to show activity with mammalian nuclear DNA polymerase, mitochondrial DNA polymerase, the DNA polymerase from *E. coli*, or RNA-dependent DNA polymerase from avian myeloblastosis virus. The mechanism by which this substance inhibits the replication of HSV in vitro and in vivo is not yet completely understood.

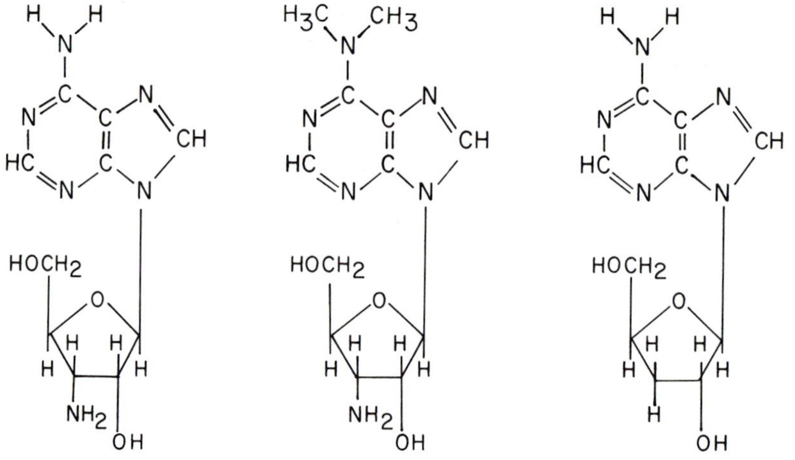

3'-Amino-3'-   Puromycin   Cordycepin
deoxyadenosine   Aminonucleoside

Fig. 9. Structure of three purine 3'-deoxyribonucleosides

2. Cordycepin

This antibiotic, isolated from a culture filtrate of *Cordyceps militaris*, bears a close relationship to 3'-amino-3'-deoxyadenosine and puromycin, as shown in Fig. 9. Both of the latter substances have also been isolated from culture filtrates of microorganisms and, in addition, have been chemically synthesized. All three agents and some of their analogs interfere with protein and nucleic acid biosynthesis. Initial interest in these substances was prompted by antitumor activity seen in rodents, but the potent nephrotoxicity of puromycin and related compounds soon became apparent, and cordycepin has been used only as a laboratory tool.

In studies with chicken embryo cells infected with Newcastle disease virus, WEISS and BRATT (1975) reported that cordycepin preferentially inhibited incorporation of uridine into 50 S virus-specific RNA at concentrations that did not inhibit 18–22 S mRNA. The resultant marked inhibition of infectious Newcastle disease virus production was interpreted as being due to a reduction in the accumulation of 50 S viral RNA and not to a general inhibition of poly(A) synthesis. EHRENFELD (1974) had shown that vesicular stomatitis virus is not inhibited by concentrations of the drug that inhibit certain species of cellular RNA synthesis. In studies employing picornaviruses, PANICALI and NAIR (1978) showed that cordycepin (as 3'-deoxyadenosine triphosphate) promptly competes specifically with ATP and prevents incorporation of AMP residues into poliovirus-specific and human rhinovirus-specific RNA. Their findings support the interpretation of RNA chain termination as the mechanism of inhibition of picornavirus-specific RNA. In addition, other reports describing the mechanism of action of the antibiotic have been published (MAHY et al. 1973; NAIR and PANICALI 1976).

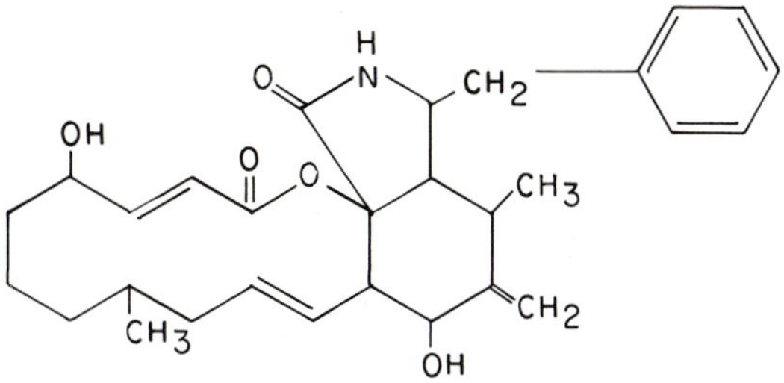

Fig. 10. Structure of cytochalasin B

This adenosine analog will probably continue to be employed to study the differences and similarities of the synthetic sequences of different viruses and may provide a better understanding of how one can separate viral-specific events from those which occur in eukaryotic cells.

3. Cytochalasin B

The cytochalasins are a class of mold metabolites exhibiting inhibitory effects on a wide variety of cellular functions. There are at least six members of this class, some of which (A, B, and F) have been isolated from *Helminthosporium dermatoideum*. Cytochalasin B (Fig. 10), which inhibits hexose transport in cells, has been used to study virus-specific glycoprotein synthesis. RICHTER and FALKE (1973) and DIX and COURTNEY (1976) have shown that cytochalasin B significantly inhibits the production of infectious herpes simplex virus 1 over a wide range of concentrations. They postulated that the inhibition of glycosylation and, thus, impaired viral glycoprotein synthesis was responsible for the reduced infectivity rather than a nonspecific toxic effect of the drug.

Cytochalasin B has been shown to inhibit the active transport of certain monosaccharides across the plasma membrane (BLOCH 1973). It is noteworthy that cytochalasin D, which is very similar to cytochalasin B, has been shown to enhance the infectivity of poliovirus and parainfluenza virus while decreasing the infectivity of adenovirus (DEITCH et al. 1973 a, b). Cytochalasin B has not been considered as a chemotherapeutic agent since it is not sufficiently selective in its antiviral properties. Its mechanism of depressing glycoprotein synthesis appears different from that of 2-deoxy-D-glucose. Additional studies with cytochalasin B may help define the sequence of events controlling the role of carbohydrates in the replication of certain viruses. Other activities of the antibiotic on cellular functions can be found in the reports of ESTERENSEN (1971), SPOONER et al. (1971), and ZIGMOND and HIRSCH (1972).

4. Gliotoxin, Aranotin, Sporidesmin, and Chetomin

Gliotoxin, produced by a number of molds, possesses antiviral activity against polioviruses, rhinoviruses, echoviruses, and other RNA viruses (RIGHTSEL et al.

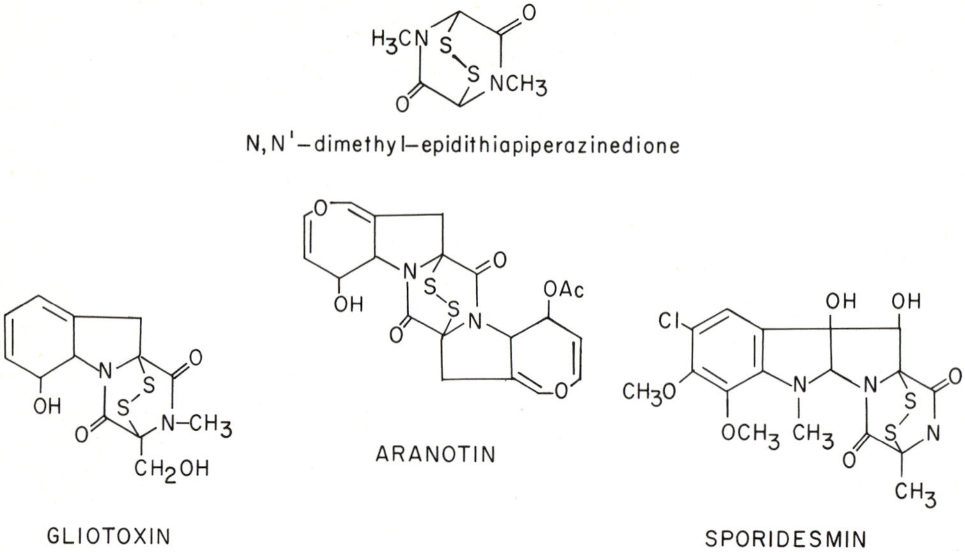

N,N'−dimethyl−epidithiapiperazinedione

ARANOTIN

GLIOTOXIN

SPORIDESMIN

Fig. 11. Structures of gliotoxin, aranotin, and sporidesmin together with that of *N,N'*-di-methylepidithiapiperazinedione

1964; Larin et al. 1965). Gliotoxin was reported to inhibit RNA-dependent synthesis of RNA in a specific irreversible fashion (Miller et al. 1968) and, more recently, to inhibit reverse transcriptase (Ottenheijm et al. 1978). The structure of gliotoxin is shown in Fig. 11, as are the structures of sporidesmin and aranotin as well as epidithiadioxopiperazine.

Aranotin was described by Neuss et al. (1968) and acetylaranotin by Trown et al. (1968). The Neuss group isolated aranotin from *Arachniotus aureus* Eidam and Trown and his colleagues obtained the acetylated derivative from *Aspergillus terreus*. As can be seen from the chemical structures, the aranotin moiety (and also some of its related metabolites) is found in gliotoxin (Bell et al. 1958), a metabolite from *Gliocladium fimbriatum* or *Trichoderma viride*.

The ability of acetylaranotin to inhibit the replication of viral RNA resided in the epidithiapiperazinedione moiety of the molecule. Trown and Bilello (1972) reported that gliotoxin, acetylaranotin, and the synthetic compound, dimethylepidithiapiperazinedione, most probably inhibit the activity of viral RNA polymerase directly rather than inhibition of its synthesis. Ottenheijm et al. (1978), as we have noted, reported the inhibition of reverse transcriptase or RNA-directed DNA polymerase activity.

Sporidesmin and its metabolites were isolated in 1963 by Ronaldson et al., although chetomin, a related compound, was probably isolated earlier from cultures of *Chaetomium cochliodes* by Waksman and Bugie (1944). It was later shown that gliotoxins, sporidesmins, and chetomin inhibit *Bacillus subtilis*. In view of the fact that all three of the agents contain a common moiety, epidithiadiketopiperazine, it would not be surprising if these agents also inhibited the RNA-containing viruses to the same extent. Gliotoxin and its analogs have been shown to interfere with the

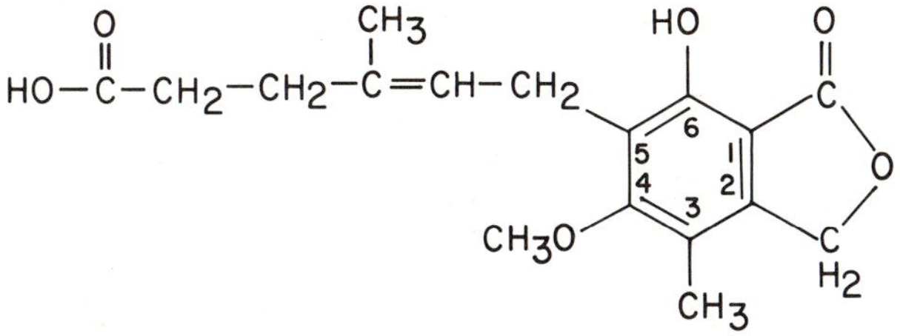

$$HO-\overset{\overset{\text{O}}{\|}}{C}-CH_2-CH_2-\overset{\overset{\text{CH}_3}{|}}{C}=CH-CH_2$$

Fig. 12. Structure of mycophenolic acid

RNA-directed DNA polymerase activity associated with Moloney (leukemia) virus.

Unfortunately, the antibiotics and metabolites sharing these structural similarities have been shown to be remarkably toxic and they do not possess practical value as therapeutic agents. No recent publications provide hope that modifications of the active center of these molecules may decrease toxicity and allow other biologic activities to remain.

5. Mycophenolic Acid

This substance (Fig. 12) has been obtained from a number of species of *Penicillium* and has been reported by PLANTEROSE (1969) to inhibit plaque formation by vaccinia, herpes simplex, Semliki Forest, encephalomyocarditis, and influenza A viruses, and coxsackievirus. Since cultures of chick embryo fibroblasts or hamster kidneys were inhibited at concentrations as low as $0.3–1.0$ μg/ml, it is probable that the virus inhibition was a result of cellular toxicity; the antiviral mode of action is not known. WILLIAMS et al. (1968) also found that mycophenolic acid exhibited in vitro activity, but antiviral activity could not be demonstrated in vivo. Mycophenolic acid also possesses antibacterial activity, but has never proven acceptable therapeutically.

6. Tenuazonic Acid

This compound was initially isolated from *Alternaria tenuis* and was subsequently obtained from culture filtrates of *Aspergillus* spp. The sodium salt, sodium tenuazonate, inhibited plaque production by measles, vaccinia, and herpes simplex viruses, echovirus 9, and polioviruses, but it was inactive against polyoma, rabies, and Friend viruses (MILLER et al. 1963). Toxicology studies were conducted with the compounds, but additional reports have not appeared.

II. Bacterial Products

1. Streptomyces
a) *Actinomycin D* (Dactinomycin)

Only brief mention of this widely studied agent will be made here since its ability to inhibit nucleic acid synthesis and the replication of certain viruses has been re-

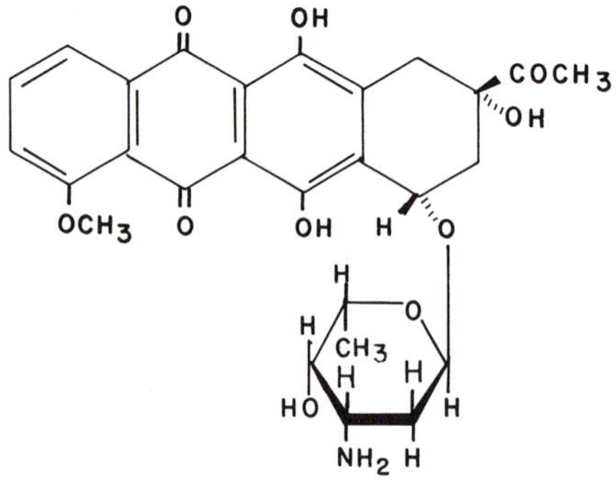

Fig. 13. Structure of daunorubicin

viewed elsewhere (GOLDBERG and FRIEDMAN 1971; TEMIN 1971). This antibiotic was isolated from broth cultures of *Streptomyces parvullus* and the actinomycins were originally recognized by their ability to inhibit the growth of bacteria. It became readily apparent that these agents would have no place in antibacterial therapy owing to their very substantial toxicity. Except for its use in cancer therapy, actinomycin D has been primarily employed to investigate the biosynthesis of macromolecules in virus-infected and noninfected eukaryotic and prokaryotic cells. The drug acts by binding to DNA, thereby inhibiting DNA-dependent RNA synthesis. Investigators have used actinomycin D to inhibit RNA synthesis of the host cell in order to study the synthesis of certain virus-specific RNA species which may proceed in the presence of the antibiotic (REICH et al. 1969). This antibiotic will undoubtedly continue to be used primarily for laboratory studies of viral replicative events.

b) *Adenine Arabinoside* (Ara-A, Vidarabine, 9-β-Arabinofuranosyladenine)

The antiviral activity of this clinically useful substance is detailed in Chap. 3 and is mentioned here simply to point out that investigators at Parke, Davis and Company and Southern Research Institute, independently, found Ara-A in concentrates of *Streptomyces antibioticus* culture medium. BERGMANN and FEENEY (1950, 1951) had described the isolation of 1-β-D-arabinofuranosyl derivatives of thymine and uracil from sponges.

c) *Daunomycin* (Daunorubicin, Rubidomycin)

This antibiotic has been isolated from cultures of *Streptomyces peucetius* and *Streptomyces coeruleorubidus* and is shown in Fig. 13. Daunomycin, an antibiotic of the anthracycline group, acts chiefly on DNA and DNA-dependent RNA synthesis (COHEN et al. 1969). It is closely related to, and shares characteristics with, adriamycin, which is currently used as an antitumor agent in humans. Certain bacterial viruses are inhibited by this antibiotic (PARISI and SOLLER 1964). CALENDI et al. (1966) reported that daunomycin inhibited a double-stranded DNA bacteriophage, but did not interfere with the multiplication of single-stranded DNA bacteriophages.

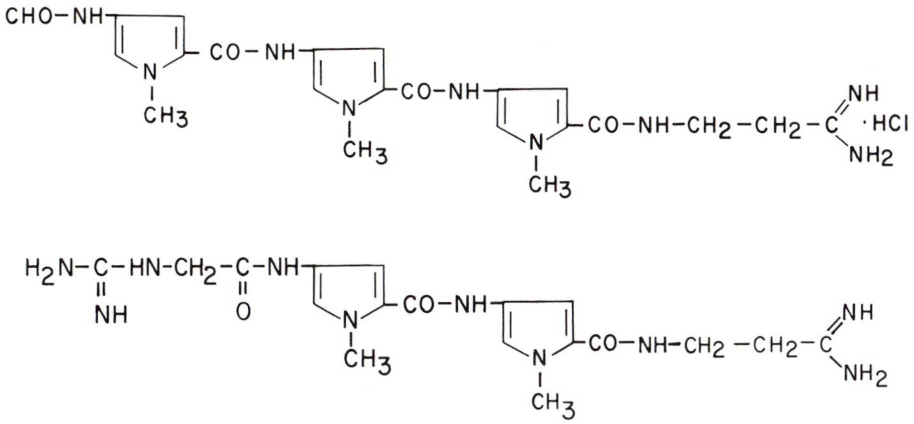

Fig. 14. Structures of distamycin A and netropsin

More recently, it was shown that HSV is inhibited in vitro by daunomycin (DI MARCO et al. 1968; COHEN et al. 1969). This inhibitor of nucleic acid biosynthesis also interferes with the replication of vaccinia virus in vitro (COHEN et al. 1969, 1971) and CASAZZA et al. (1971) have reported that daunomycin inhibits foci formation by Moloney virus in mouse embryo monolayers. The mechanism of action of daunomycin lies in its ability to form a strong complex with DNA. PIGRAM et al. (1972) have provided data supporting intercalation of the drug. It presumably acts by inhibiting the template functions of DNA to prevent replication and/or transcription of messenger RNA. Although daunomycin has been used to treat a variety of human cancers, the toxicity of daunomycin has precluded its use against most of the less life-threatening infections caused by viruses.

Recently, SHORTRIDGE and SQUIRES (1977) suggested that daunomycin might achieve clinical use by judicious local application in adenovirus-mediated ocular infections. Their suggestion arose from the observation that concentrations as low as 0.05 µg/ml, a noncytotoxic level, prevented replication of adenovirus in HeLa cells. If these findings can be confirmed, daunomycin, unlike many other antiviral antibiotics, might possibly serve as more than a laboratory tool for study of virus replication.

d) *Distamycin and Netropsin*

Distamycin is a product of *Streptomyces distallicus* fermentation and a related antibiotic, netropsin, is produced by *Streptomyces netropsis* (Fig. 14). Distamycin A forms complexes with DNA, and KOTLER and BECKER (1971) reported that it inhibited the reverse transcriptase of oncornaviruses. Antiviral activity has been reported in vitro and in vivo in the laboratory against vaccinia, herpes simplex, mouse hepatitis, Shope fibroma, and other viruses as well as in humans when applied topically for the treatment of chickenpox, herpes zoster, and eruptions resulting from smallpox vaccination (HAHN 1975). Well-controlled, double-blind clinical

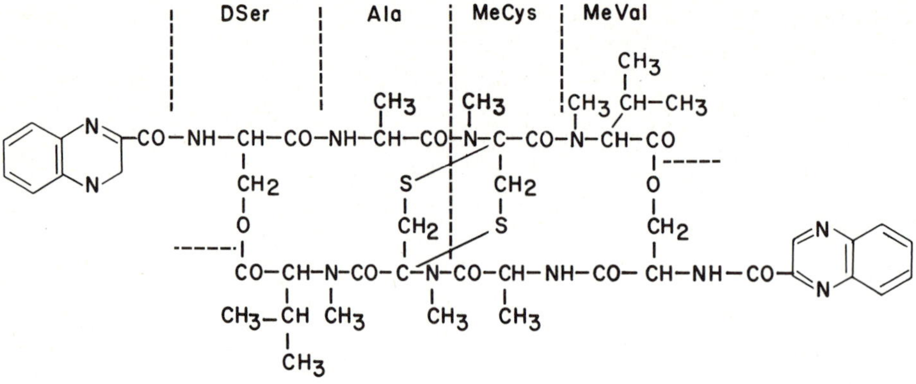

Fig. 15. Structure of quinomycin A

studies in humans have not yet been conducted. Netropsin was also shown to be active against vaccinia in laboratory studies by Schabel et al. (1953).

e) *Neuraminin*

Few reports describe this specific viral inhibitor which was isolated from a *Streptomyces* sp. by Lin et al. (1975 a, b). It does not inhibit neuraminidases of bacterial origin but does inhibit neuraminidases from several viruses. It has a differential activity against neuraminidases derived from influenza virus and Newcastle disease virus (Lin et al. 1977). The structure of neuraminin is not known; it has a high molecular weight and consists largely of glucose and mannose with a small amount (12%) of protein.

f) *Rifamycin*

This antibiotic was isolated from *Streptomyces mediterranei* and received considerable attention as an antiviral substance. A complete description can be found in Chap. 13.

g) *Quinomycin* (Levomycin, Actinoleukin, Echinomycin, X-948)

The quinomycins are a family of antibiotics that contain a quinoloxine moiety, and the structure of quinomycin A is shown in Fig. 15. Quinomycins are produced by a variety of *Streptomyces* including *S. aureus*, *S. echinatus*, *S. griseolus*, *S. flavochromogenes*, *S. lavendulae*, and an actinomycin-producing strain of *S. flaveolus*. Quinomycins A, B, and C all show potent in vitro activity against gram-positive bacteria and mycoplasms in addition to antitumor activity (Katagiri et al. 1975).

Tsunoda (1962) showed that quinomycin A, an actinomycin-like antibiotic, was prophylactically effective in mice infected with the MEF 1 and type 2 strains of poliovirus. If treatment was delayed until the day of infection or thereafter, no protection was noted. Ward et al. (1965) provided data suggesting that quinomycin A inhibited DNA-directed RNA synthesis and that an inhibitory complex was formed between the antibiotic and DNA and concluded that quinomycin A inhibited the synthesis of RNA in a fashion similar to actinomycin. This mode of action is consistent with the inhibitory action of quinomycin A against *E. coli* bacteriophages (SATO et al. 1969). Although qunomycin A has shown activity against numerous tumors in animals, it has not been evaluated in humans. It appears that it may be sufficiently similar in its action to actinomycin D to be used as a substance to study macromolecular biosynthesis in virus-infected cells.

h) *Tunicamycin*

This antibiotic was discovered among 4,000 *Actinomyces* isolates screened from soil samples. This glucosamine-containing antibiotic, which was derived from *Streptomyces lysosuperficus*, inhibits HSV in cell culture and Newcastle disease virus, both in cell monolayers and in embryonated eggs (TAKATSUKI and TAMURA 1971). LEAVITT et al. (1977) have reported that tunicamycin inhibits the glycosylation of viral proteins and the multiplication of Sindbis virus and vesicular stomatitis virus, two RNA viruses that are assembled by budding from cellular membranes. The antiviral activity of tunicamycin can be reversed by some aminosugars. Two other agents that inhibit glycoprotein biosynthesis, D-glucosamine and 2-deoxy-D-glucose, have been shown to interfere with the replication of another enveloped virus, influenza virus (KLENK et al. 1972).

Because 2-deoxy-D-glucose, D-glucosamine, and possibly tunicamycin affect cellular processes in addition to the specific glycosylation of virus glycoproteins, it might be anticipated that they may not be effective antiviral agents in clinical use. However, in an unconfirmed recent study, BLOUGH and GIUNTOLI (1979) reported that topical application of 2-deoxy-D-glucose is effective against genital herpesvirus infection.

j) *Incompletely Defined Substances*

In addition to the antibiotics and metabolic inhibitors of eukaryotic cells discussed previously, there are a number of less completely characterized substances described in a review by PIENTA and GROUPÉ (1964). They include an antibiotic called ehrlichin obtained from a strain of *Streptomyces lavendulae*, another material, viscosin, from *Pseudomonas viscosa*, and a crystalline nitrogenous substance from *Nocardia formica* that protected mice from influenza and several other viruses.

2. Other Bacteria

There are few, if any, reports of well-defined antiviral substances derived from bacteria other than the *Streptomyces* and other well-known antibiotic producers. A report that polysaccharides from *Klebsiella pneumoniae* suppressed the pneumonia caused by infection with pneumonia virus of mice (PVM) appeared as early as 1947, but the spectrum of activity of the substance was narrow and its mechanism of action was not completely determined (HORSFALL and McCARTHY 1947). See Sect. E.I for greater detail.

An undefined substance obtained from cultures of *Achromobacter* sp. that protected mice from the pneumonia resulting from infection with influenza A virus was described by GROUPÉ et al. (1952); however, subsequent reports on the nature of the material did not appear. The material was not inhibitory to numerous bacteria and was not virucidal. CUTTING et al. (1960) reported an extract from *Propionibacterium freudenreichii* that protected mice from infection with Columbia SK virus. The structure and the mechanism of action of this substance, called propionin, was not determined. An inhibitory factor with in vitro activity against Sindbis and chikungunya viruses in cultures of human amnion and chick embryo cells was isolated from a *Corynebacterium* sp. by CARVER and NAFICY (1962). They suggested that the factor was a protein and showed that it did not inhibit in vitro replication of several unrelated viruses. CARVER and ROSEN (1964) reported that material obtained from cultures of *E. coli* inhibited multiplication of vaccinia virus in vitro. In the next year, workers in the same laboratories described a bacterial constituent, obtained from an unidentified *Staphylococcus* sp. with properties compatible with those of a polysaccharide (GRESSER and GROGAN 1965). The substance inhibited Sindbis, western equine encephalitis, and West Nile viruses in human cell cultures, but not vaccinia virus, herpes simplex virus, echoviruses 2 and 11, poliovirus, or measles virus. Additional work on these particular substances has not appeared but, recently, HOTTA et al. (1977) reported an antiviral substance extracted from *Streptococcus faecalis* that inhibits the replication of viruses both in vitro and in vivo. The antiviral substance was fractionated and assayed against HSV in HeLa cell monolayers. Mice infected with HSV were protected by this substance and it also suppressed the development of virus-induced tumors in suckling hamsters infected with adenovirus 12. The uncharacterized substance did not induce interferon when injected into mice, nor did it increase resistance of L cells to challenge with vesicular stomatitis virus.

While these several investigations did not lead to the discovery of well-characterized materials of bacterial origin nor much substantive insight into their mechanism of action, one can glean sufficient information to hope that potential inhibitors of viral replication may be present in some bacteria or their culture broths. In view of the many well-documented biologic activities associated with endotoxin, it would be prudent to rule it out as the active substance from bacteria-derived antiviral substances.

G. Substances from Botanical Sources

Investigations spanning several decades have resulted in the isolation of substances from plants that exert antiviral activity in cell culture as well as in infected animals, but an agent with sufficient promise to enter clinical evaluation for viral infections has not yet been described. Results of broad spectrum programs suggest, however, that certain plants may exist which could provide a source of materials for development as antiviral drugs (GOULET et al. 1960; COCHRAN et al. 1966; FARNSWORTH 1966; FONG et al. 1972; VAN DEN BERGHE et al. 1978). The structures of many of the active substances are not known, nor is much known about how they act, but there are enough available data about a few of the materials to consider briefly.

I. Alkaloids

Extracts of Chinese herbs and medicinal plants from the Pacific area have shown antiviral activity in vitro and in vivo against encephalomyocarditis, Columbia SK, lymphocytic choriomeningitis, and vaccinia viruses in a series of studies (CUTTING et al. 1965; FURUSAWA and CUTTING 1966, 1970; FURUSAWA et al. 1967, 1968). These workers examined extracts from hundreds of plants and found two with activity against both Columbia SK and lymphocytic choriomeningitis viruses in mice. One such agent, from bulbs of *Narcissus tazetta*, was isolated and tentatively identified as the alkaloid, narcissidine. The second agent, from *Sambucus sieboldiana*, was not identified but was reported to have a molecular weight approximating 3,000–10,000 daltons. The mechanism of action of the substances was not determined, but both were capable of interfering with the replication of KB cells at concentrations exceeding those which resulted in the reduction of viral multiplication.

More recently, FURUSAWA et al. (1979) have reported the isolation of pretazettine, the major alkaloid from *Narcissus tazetta*, and described its antiviral activity in AKR leukemia virus-infected cells as well as its ability to decrease the systemic titer of AKR virus in mice. It was proposed (SUZUKI et al. 1974) that the alkaloid was a potent inhibitor of viral reverse transcriptase. Since there are several alkaloids in the narcissus bulbs, it is not possible to determine retrospectively which one or which combination may have been responsible for the activity seen in the earlier studies with Columbia SK virus and the other nononcogenic viruses studied.

Another alkaloid called taspine, isolated from an exudate from the tree *Croton lechleri* (family Euphorbiaceae), has also been reported to inhibit the RNA-directed DNA polymerase activity of avian myeloblastosis virus, Rauscher leukemia virus, and simian sarcoma virus, probably by interaction with the template primer, poly(rA)·oglio(dT), used to assay the polymerase enzymes (SETHI 1977). Studies in cell culture may reveal whether such inhibition of DNA polymerase activity is sufficiently selective to inhibit virus growth without interfering with host biosynthetic processes.

FARNSWORTH et al. (1968) reported that nine alkaloids from *Catharanthus* spp. exhibited activity against vaccinia and poliovirus in monolayers of green monkey kidney cells. The mechanism of action of the alkaloids, which had already been recognized as possessing antitumor activity, was not investigated. TAYLOR et al. (1954) reported the presence of antiviral activity in plant extracts, but the identity of the active moiety was not determined. The activity of the unidentified agent was recognized by its ability to inhibit vaccinia, influenza, and eastern equine encephalomyelitis viruses in infected eggs.

One of the most studied antiviral alkaloids is camptothecin. The structure of this compound, which was isolated from the tree, *Camptotheca acuminata*, is shown in Fig. 16. It is an effective inhibitor of adenovirus replication, but like most antiviral substances, camptothecin inhibits cellular as well as viral processes. It inhibits the synthesis of DNA and RNA in HeLa cells at concentrations that do not initially influence protein synthesis (HORWITZ et al. 1971). Camptothecin has also been reported to inhibit the replication of vaccinia virus (HORWITZ et al. 1972), herpes simplex virus (BECKER and OLSHEVSKY 1973), and has an indirect inhibitory ef-

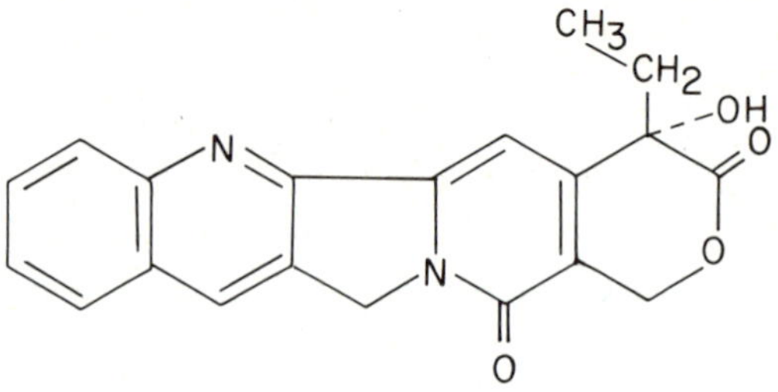

Fig. 16. Structure of camptothecin

fect on the replication of influenza virus (Minor and Dimmock 1975). This alkaloid has little, if any, effect on poliovirus replication at nontoxic concentrations.

In adenovirus-infected HeLa cells, camptothecin inhibits DNA synthesis and, intracellularly, causes breaks in preformed viral DNA (Horwitz and Brayton 1972). After camptothecin is removed, the nicked or partially degraded DNA is repaired and can serve as a template for further DNA synthesis. This compound exerts antitumor activity in animals, and has been evaluated as an antineoplastic agent in humans, but is not a candidate for antiviral therapy. The toxicity generally associated with many of the alkaloids precludes their use as agents for antiviral chemotherapy in humans, and it is possible that their ability to interfere with certain mitotic events contributes to the antiviral activities associated with them.

II. Tannins

Tannic acid, gallotannin, or tannins occur in the bark and fruit of many plants. The chemistry of these agents is variable and complex and some of the tannins consist of phenols of moderately complex structure. The antiviral activity of tannic acid was reported as early as 1934 by Olitsky and Cox who showed that tannic acid instilled intranasally in animals prevented infection with equine encephalomyelitis virus and poliovirus. It was not possible to determine the mechanism of action of the tannins with the methodology available at that time, although their astringent properties were considered to play a role. Subsequently, Green (1948, 1949) provided experimental evidence that showed that tannic acid inactivated influenza virus in vitro and inhibited the replication of influenza virus in ovo. The tannic acid he used was obtained commercially and presumably had been extracted from nutgalls and from black tea. High levels of tannic acid were required to afford protection and the material was toxic. Other studies with a member of the mint family, *Melissa officinalis*, the source of lemon or bee balm, revealed that extracts of *Melissa* spp. exhibited antiviral activity in cell culture and embryonated eggs against Newcastle disease, Semliki Forest, vaccinia, and herpes simplex viruses (Cohen et al. 1964). The activity was suggested to be due to a tannin or a tannin-like polyphenol. In subsequent studies, Herrmann and Kucera (1967) showed that extracts of various plants of the mint family (Labiatae) also had antiviral activity against Newcastle disease virus and suggested that they all might contain a common tannin. It was also shown, however, that certain tannin-free preparations exhibited antiviral activity. This other active substance was thought to be a nontannin polyphenol. It was learned later that the nontannin component was a unique polyphenol composed of units of caffeic acid, 3,4-dihydroxycinnamic acid (KUCERA and HERRMANN 1967). Caffeic acid was shown to inactivate virus on direct contact. However, they did not attribute the antiviral activity of the extracts to caffeic acid per se, but indicated that a biphenol could be responsible for the antiviral activity. POLLIKOFF et al. (1965) reported that caffeic acid, and its sodium salt, inhibited the replication of the A/PR8 strain of influenza virus in mice, as evidenced by increased survival and extension of survival time. Clinical trials against influenza virus infection in humans were conducted with caffeic acid, but no protection was seen.

KONOWALCHUK and SPEIRS (1976, 1978 a, b) have reported that commercial apple juice, grape juice, and wines, as well as some other beverages, were virucidal for HSV and various enteric viruses, including poliovirus. They also noted that certain grapes and apples are relatively rich in tannic acid and polyphenols. Their studies indicated that the virucidal substance in these fruits was most probably due to the phenolic concentration contributed by the tannic acid content.

III. Lignosulfonates

WARD and TANKERSLEY (1980) described a polymer obtained from wood, lignosulfonate, that possessed topical antiherpesvirus activity. This compound, which may exist in the form of a variety of cationic salts, is composed of repeating phenylpropane units. The material has been formulated in a variety of preparations and shown to be effective in vitro against herpes simplex virus 1 and 2, and also against herpesvirus in mice and guinea pigs infected intravaginally. Lignosulfonates have also been found to protect mice and guinea pigs from herpetic infections in other laboratories, both in vitro and in vivo. Sodium lignosulfonate (Georgia-Pacific Corporation), in a cream preparation gently massaged into the infected area of herpetic lesions in guinea pigs, was able to reduce the severity of the disease. Lignosulfonates in eye ointment have proved to be irritating and unsuitable for use against herpetic keratoconjunctivitis in rabbits. If the laboratory work by WARD and TANKERSLEY (1980) can be successfully extended to humans, the polymers may represent a means of effective therapy against herpesviruses.

IV. Other Substances

Numerous reports of "antiviral extracts" from plants and other natural sources not cited in the preceding sections can be found in the literature, but many were not sufficiently detailed to reveal the chemical nature of the substances or their mechanism of action. However, there are a few reports in which an antiviral substance of plant origin has been identified and these have provided some small measure of optimism that a continued search for antiviral agents from natural sources could be fruitful. Some examples appear in the following sections.

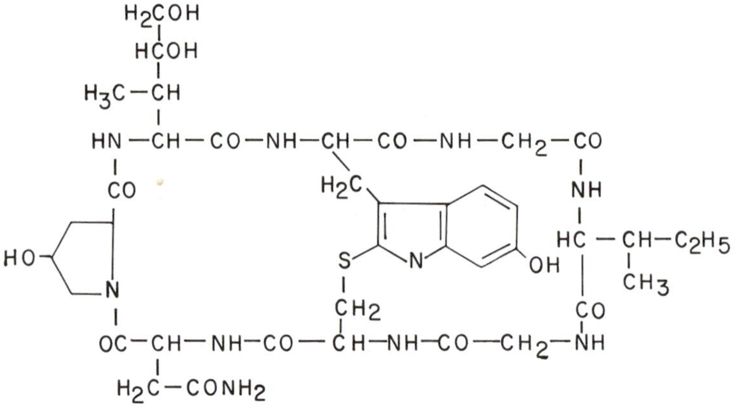

$$H_2COH$$
$$HCOH$$
$$H_3C-CH$$

HN —CH— CO—NH—CH— CO —NH —CH$_2$—CO

CO H$_2$C NH

HO— HC — CH—C$_2$H$_5$

N S N OH CH$_3$

CH$_2$ CO

OC—CH—NH—CO— CH—NH—CO—CH$_2$—NH

H$_2$C—CONH$_2$

Fig. 17. Structure of α-amanitin

1. α-Amanitin

This substance (Fig. 17) was isolated from *Amanita phalloides* and, although it is toxic, has been reported to inhibit the replication of Rous sarcoma virus (ZANETTI et al. 1971) and influenza virus (MAHY et al. 1972). TATA et al. (1972) reported that α-amanitin inhibited cellular DNA-dependent RNA polymerase, which suggests that its antiviral activity may be associated with its ability to interfere with RNA synthesis.

2. Calcium Elenolate

This compound is obtained from extracts of the olive plant, *Olea europaea*. The crystalline form has shown a high degree of virucidal activity against a broad spectrum of viruses, but has showed the greatest activity against enveloped viruses (RENIS 1969). On the basis of its virucidal activity, it was administered intranasally and was protective in hamsters experimentally infected with parainfluenza virus. The compound had to be given within minutes of intranasal virus instillation to show maximum efficacy (SORET 1969). Presumably, the presence of the compound in the nasal turbinates and other portions of the respiratory tree destroyed the virus on contact. It was relatively well tolerated by the nasal tissues at concentrations that inactivated virus although mucociliary action would probably reduce its concentration to ineffective levels in a relatively short period.

3. Glycyrrhizic Acid

In a screening program including roots of *Glycyrrhiza glabra* it was discovered that a component inhibited several DNA and RNA viruses. POMPEI et al. (1979) identified the active moeity as glycyrrhizic acid.

H. Substances from Marine Flora and Fauna

An area of biomedical investigation which has been only superficially explored is that concerning products or substances made from or by marine organisms. The examination of algae, shellfish, and other marine life has given rise to at least one material now used as an antiviral agent. BERGMANN and FEENEY (1950, 1951) isolated the nucleosides spongothymidine, spongouridine, and spongosine from a Caribbean sponge, *Cryptotethya crypta*, and the compounds served as models for the synthesis of D-arabinosyl cytosine and adenine arabinoside (Ara-A). See Chap. 3 for a fuller description of the antiviral profile of Ara-A.

The majority of antiviral material isolated from or produced by marine flora is generally polysaccharide in nature. GERBER et al. (1958) noted that when insoluble experimental compounds were suspended in 0.25% agar and injected into embryonated eggs infected with influenza B virus, there was erratic, minimal protective activity. The agar was suspect since different batches gave different results. The authors tested aqueous extracts of seaweeds *Gelidium cartilagenium*, a source of agar, and *Chondrus crispus*, the source of carrageenin, as possible producers of this antiviral activity. The extracts, which gave positive chemical test reactions typical of polysaccharides composed principally of D-galactose units, were active against influenza B and mumps viruses in embryonated eggs, but were inactive when tested in a system in which influenza A or Newcastle disease viruses were used. KATHAN (1965) also examined extracts of kelp and isolated a glycoprotein which inhibited neuraminidase and prevented attachment of influenza virus. The extract was protective to embryonated eggs as late as 6 h postinfection and inhibited not only the viral hemagglutinins but also the infectivity titer. Purification of the extract did not increase the activity and, consequently, the exact nature of the inhibition was not determined.

Marine algae from two related species of Chordophyta, *Cryptosyphonia woodii* and *Farlowia mollis*, were collected off the California coast by DEIG et al. (1974). Extracts of algal homogenates were prepared and tested against HSV-1 and HSV-2. Antiherpetic activity was present in these extracts and there was no direct inactivation of virus, nor was interferon induced. No significant activity was seen with eleven other RNA and DNA viruses. Later work by this group (EHRESMANN et al. 1977) extended the original findings to include eight members of the Rhodophyta family which also possess antiherpes activity. An additional species, *Constantinea simplex*, yielded substances which interfered with the infectivity of coxsackievirus B5. Closer examination of these antiviral substances demonstrated that the active agent was a polysaccharide.

RICHARDS et al. (1978) tested extracts of *Constaninea simplex* and *Farlowia mollis* for antiviral activity in tissue culture and in mice. In vitro, the extracts were capable of inhibiting HSV-1 and HSV-2, vaccinia virus, and vesicular stomatitis virus, but not encephalomyocarditis virus, Semliki Forest virus, or murine cytomegalovirus. The extracts were prophylactically active in vivo if given to mice infected intracerebrally, intraperitoneally, or intranasally with herpesvirus 2. Neither preparation was active therapeutically nor were they active if mice were infected intravaginally with HSV-2. As with the other algal extracts, the active material appeared to be a polysaccharide.

Li (1960) discovered that the abalone *(Haliotis refescens)* contained an antibacterial substance and a material active against poliovirus. Mice fed commercial canned abalone juice were protected, to a limited extent, from the lethal effects of an intraspinal or intracerebral infection with poliovirus. The antiviral material was thermostable and nondialyzable. Li et al. (1962) extended the original observation to include a fractionation of the abalone juice and extension of the antiviral activity to influenza A virus. The active materials, later named paolin II and fraction C, appeared to be protein in nature although not digested by pepsin, and were capable of protecting mice from lethal infections with poliovirus and influenza B virus (Der Marderosian 1969). Similar antiviral materials have been isolated from the oyster, squid, conch, clam, and sea snail. In addition, an extract from shellfish has demonstrated in vivo antitumor effect (Schmeer 1964; Schmeer and Huala 1965). Apparently, the same substance showing activity against the sarcoma 180 tumors was also protective against lethal virus-induced mouse leukemia (Judge 1966).

Marine life is often difficult to obtain and propagate in the laboratory, and these technical factors could limit its appeal as a simple and convenient investigational area. Marine organisms have not yet proven to be particularly fruitful, but it is noteworthy that at least one clinically useful antiviral agent, adenine arabinoside, had its origin in a sea sponge.

I. Other Substances

I. Vitamin A

Auperin et al. (1980) reported the virucidal activity of vitamin A analog against herpes simplex virus 2. Less that 0.6 mg/ml of the analogs destroyed 50% of virus activity within 30 min. The analogs with various polar head groups and *cis*-unsaturated fatty acid chains of 14–20 carbon atoms, were not cytopathic and were generally more active against lipid-containing viruses, although it was reported that 2.25 mg/ml inactivated SV40 virus. Activity was inhibited by 1% serum albumin and 50 µg/ml lecithin. Calcium ions (which may cause a slight destablization of the virus structure, thus potentiating the virucidal activity) appeared to increase the activity of vitamin A against herpesvirus.

II. Milk

Human milk has been known for many years to contain antiviral substances unrelated to antibody content. Sabin and Fieldsteel (1962) found that human milk neutralized the activity of such viruses as Japanese B encephalitis, St. Louis encephalitis, West Nile, dengue, yellow fever, western equine encephalomyelitis virus, and herpesvirus. The activity was not antibody related, since it was: (a) resistant to heating at 100 °C for 30 min; (b) present in the cream fraction; and (c) not found in the protein fractions normally associated with poliomyelitis antibody in human or bovine milk. Subsequently, Sarkar et al. (1973) showed that human milk inhibited the growth of murine mammary tumor virus in cell culture. Fieldsteel (1974) confirmed earlier studies and extended his observations to show that human milk contains a potent, lipid-like substance that inhibits splenomegaly induced by both Friend and Rauscher leukemia viruses. The lipid component of milk and colostrum has also been shown to reduce the plaque forming activity of all dengue virus types (FALKER et al. 1975). The antiviral substance remained present in the milk obtained as long as 10 months postpartum. The inhibitor did not inhibit virus if added to cells after the infection was initiated and may exert its effect directly on the virus.

MATTHEWS et al. (1976) also detected an antiviral component in human and cows' milk which is, apparently, not related to antibody or any other known virus inhibitor. Using vesicular stomatitis virus in a plaque assay system, they found that as little as 5% of either human or cows' milk reduced the plaque count by 50%. The greatest effect was seen when the milk was mixed with the virus at the time that the cultures were challenged. Influenza and rhinoviruses were also inhibited although there were wide strain differences within each group. The active principal was unaffected by buffered saline dialysis or acid hydrolysis for 30 min and it was removed by ether extraction. Although the activity was not affected by heating at 56 °C for 30 min, boiling was destructive. Dried milk formulas were uniformly inactive and the milk components, lactoferrin and lysozyme, were not antiviral. The butterfat content of milk was not critical since skimmed milk was also active. The authors suggested that milk may reversibly alter the properties of the cell surface, thus interfering with virus entry.

WELSH et al. (1979) used Semliki Forest virus to detect antiviral activity in human milk. Fractionation of the milk revealed the presence of a heat-stable, lipid-associated substance in a majority of the samples tested. Bovine and synthetic milks lacked activity. The monoglyceride and free fatty acid fractions contained the activity. Subsequently, WELSH and MAY (1979) reported that nonenveloped viruses were unaffected by the antiviral lipids. Preliminary electron microscopic studies suggested that the mode of action of the lipid is via disruption of the virus envelope. The presence of the lipid-associated antiviral factor in addition to interferon and antibodies in human milk prompted WELSH and his associates to call for renewed interest in breast feeding of infants.

III. Mosquito Tissues

Tissue cultures of *Aedes albopictus* cells persistently infected with Sindbis virus produced a low molecular weight material which reduced the yield of virus in mosquito cells (RIEDEL and BROWN 1979). The inhibitor was inactivated by treatment with proteases, but it was not affected by rabbit antiserum to Sindbis virus. The as yet uncharacterized antiviral substance does not appear to affect attachment of virus to mosquito or BHK-21 cells and acts, probably, at some later stage.

IV. Cobra Venom

SANDERS et al. (1953) examined the effect of detoxified cobra venom from Indian and Cape cobras on the pathogenesis of poliomyelitis virus in monkeys and mice. Treatment with the neurotoxoids interfered with poliovirus infection in rhesus monkeys, but not in mice. The highly neurotropic toxoids produced chromatolysis in motorneurons when given in massive doses and induced an inhibition of succinic dehydrogenase and a decrease in cytochrome oxidase activity. Both of these effects were closely associated with a state of refractivity to poliovirus. Sanders et al. (1958)prepared other toxoids, notably from the South American rattlesnake and combined them with cobra venom toxoid. The combinations protected monkeys from poliovirus infection.

The interest in cobra venom was maintained by Clark et al. (1962) who used the Sanders neurotoxoid to treat herpes keratitis. Using the cobra–rattlesnake venom toxoid combination, the authors medicated their private-practice patients. In these uncontrolled studies, they found that the toxoid produced corneal clearing and restoration of corneal sensitivity. Purification of cobra venom by Sephadex chromatography was carried out by Miller et al. (1977) and sixteen components were separated. Some of the fractions were neurotoxic, and only these were active in inhibiting poliovirus plaque formation in BHK-21 cells. It seems unlikely that the neurotoxins will provide a safe or efficacious approach to the control of viral diseases.

V. Neuraminidase Inhibitors

Neuraminidase is a component of paramyxoviruses, and of influenza, mumps, and Newcastle disease viruses. The function of the enzyme is not completely understood, although it has been proposed that neuraminidase facilitates the release of virus from the glycoprotein inhibitors of the respiratory tract (Palese et al. 1977).

As early as 1950, Tamm and Horsfall described urinary mucoprotein as a specific substrate for neuraminidase which reduced the infectivity of influenza viruses. Drzeniek (1966) found that substances such as DNA, RNA, pig submaxillary mucin, and heparin inhibit neuraminidase activity in vitro. Lin et al. (1975a, b) were able to isolate a high molecular weight glycoprotein from a *Streptomyces* sp. which inhibited influenza virus neuraminidase at extremely low concentrations, but they did not identify its structure. Panosialin is a neuraminidase inhibitor isolated by Aoyagi et al. (1975). Its activity is nonspecific and, chemically, it behaves like a polyanion, the activity of which can be reversed by the addition of polycations or protein (Siastatin A and B are) inhibitors isolated from *Streptomyces* spp. and characterized by Umezawa et al. (1974) and Aoyagi et al. (1975). An ovine aminoglycoprotein isolated by Campbell et al. (1967) inhibited NDV in a plaque reduction assay. Palese and Schulman (1977) showed that lectins, such as concanavalin A, bind nonspecifically to cellular and viral glycoproteins and inhibit viral replication.

Many investigators have sought virus-specific neuraminidase inhibitors as substances which might prove useful in combating influenza virus infections, but we are unaware that any have been evaluated clinically. Unless neuraminidase inhibitors with unique specificity are found, their potential usefulness is open to question since they may act on the host neuraminidases, interfere with normal sialylation processes, and produce undesirable side effects.

Acknowledgment. We gratefully acknowledge the excellent assistance of Peter Furlani and Carol Rapsard in locating important references. Dr. James Cornett generously provided criticism and suggestions and his help led to numerous improvements of the chapter.

References

Ackermann WW (1951) The role of l-methionine in virus propagation. J Exp Med 93:337–343

Ackermann WW (1952) α-aminosulfonic acids and viral propagation. Proc Soc Exp Biol Med 80:362–367

Ackermann WW, Maassab HF (1954) Growth characteristics of influenza virus: biochemical differentiation of stages of development. J Exp Med 100:329–339

Anderson TW, Reid DBW, Beaton GH (1972) Vitamin C and the common cold: a double-blind trial. Can Med Assoc J 107:503–508

Anderson TW, Suranyi G, Beaton GH (1974) The effect on winter illness of large doses of vitamin C. Can Med Assoc J 111:31–36

Aoyagi T, Komiyama T, Nerome K, Takeuchi T, Umezawa H (1975) Characterization of myxovirus sialidase. Experientia 31:896–898

Apple MA, Fischer P, Wong W, Paganelli J, Harasymiv I, Osofsky L (1975) Inhibition of oncorna virus reverse transcriptase by plant flavonoids. Proc Am Assoc Cancer Res 16:198

Auperin DD, Reinhardt A, Sands JA, Snipes W, Taylor WD (1980) Characterization of viruicidal activities of retinoids. In: Nelson JD, Grassi C (eds) Proc. 11th Int. Congr. Chemother. and 19th Intersci. Conf. on Antimicrob. Agents and Chemother. American Society of Microbiology, Washington, D.C., p 1368

Becker Y, Olshevsky U (1973) Inhibition of herpes simplex virus replication by camptothecin. Is J Med Sci 9:1578–81

Béládi I, Pusztai R, Mucsi I, Bakay M, Gabor M (1977) Activity of some flavonoids against viruses. Ann NY Acad Sci 284:358–364

Bell MR, Johnson JR, Wildi BS, Woodward RB (1958) The structure of gliotozin. J Am Chem Soc 80:1001

Bergmann W, Feeney RJ (1950) The isolation of a new thymine pentoside from sponges. J Am Chem Soc 72:2809–2810

Bergmann W, Feeney RJ (1951) Contributions to the study of marine products. XXXII. The nucleosides of sponges. J Org Chem 16:981–987

Bloch R (1973) Inhibition of glucose transport in human erythrocytes by cytochalasin B. Biochemistry 12:4799–4801

Blough HA, Giuntoli RL (1979) Successful treatment of human genital herpes infections with 2-deoxy-d-glucose. J AMA 241:2798–2801

Brown F, Planterose DN, Stewart DL (1961) Effect of p-fluorophenylalanine on the multiplication of foot-and-mouth disease. Nature 191:414–415

Brown GC (1952) The influence of chemicals on the propagation of poliomyelitis virus in tissue culture. J Immunol 69:441–450

Brown GC, Ackermann WW (1951) Effect of DL-ethionine on poliomyelitis growth in tissue culture. Proc Soc Exp Biol Med 77:367–369

Brundret KM, Dalziel W, Hesp B, Jarvis JAJ, Neidle S (1972) X-Ray crystallographic determination of the structure of the antibiotic aphidicolin: a tetracycline diterpenoid containing new ring system. J Chem Soc D Chem Commun 1027–1028

Bucknall RA, Moores H, Simms R, Hesp B (1973) Antiviral effects of aphidicolin, a new antibiotic produced by Cephalosporium aphidicola. Antimicrob Agents Chemother 4:294–298

Calendi E, Dettori R, Neri MG (1966) Filamentous sex-specific bacteriophages of E. coli K-12. IV. Studies on physico-chemical characteristics of bacteriophage Ec9. G Microbiol 14:227–241

Came PE, Lieberman M, Pascale A, Shimonaski G (1969) Antiviral activity of an interferon inducing synthetic polymer. Proc Soc Exp Biol Med 131:443–446

Campbell BJ, Schneider A, Howe D, Durand D (1967) Structural aspects of ovine α₁-glycoprotein, an inhibitor of Newcastle disease virus. Biochim Biophys Acta 148:137–145

Carver DH, Naficy K (1962) Inhibition of arborviruses (Group A) by a protein-like constituent of a corynebacterium. Proc Soc Exp Biol Med 111:356–360

Carver DH, Rosen FS (1964)Viral inhibitors of biological origin. II. A viral inhibitory factor obtained from E. coli 0111 and inhibition of viral replication by nucleic acid derivatives. Proc Soc Exp Biol Med 116:575–579

Casazza AM, Di Marco A, Di Cuonzo G (1971) Interference of daunomycin and adriamycin on the growth and repression of murine sarcoma virus (Maloney)-tumors in mice. Cancer Res 31:1971–1976

Clark WB, Baldone JA, Thomas CI (1962) The use of Sander's Neurotoxid I (modified snake venom) in the treatment of recurrent herpes simplex of the cornea. South Med J 55:947–951

Cochran KW, Nishikawa Teke ES (1966) Botanical sources of influenza inhibitors. Antimicrob Agents Chemother 515–520

Cohen A, Harley EH, Rees NR (1969) Antiviral effect of daunomycin. Nature 222:36–38

Cohen A, Crook LE, Nees NR (1971) Effect of daunomycin on vaccinia nucleic acid synthesis. Int. Virol. 2. 2nd Int. Congr. Virol. Budapest 1971. Basel, Karger, p 282

Cohen RA, Kucera LS, Herrmann EC Jr (1964) Antiviral activity of Melissa officinalis (Lemon Balm) extract. Proc Soc Exp Biol Med 117:431–434

Coulehan J, Reisinger KS, Rogers KD, Bradley DW (1974) Vitamin C prophylaxis in a boarding school. N Engl J Med 290:6–10

Coulehan JL, Eberhard S, Kapner L, Taylor F, Rogers K, Garry P (1976) Vitamin C and acute illness in Navajo school children. N Engl J Med 295:973–977

Cushing RT, Morgan HR (1952) Effects of some metabolic analogues on growth of mumps and influenza viruses in tissue culture. Proc Soc Exp Biol Med 79:497–500

Cutting W, Furst A, Read D, Grant D, Cords H, Megna J, Butterworth E (1960) Antiviral extracts from propionibacteria. Antibiot Chemother 10:623–625

Cutting WE, Furusawa E, Furusawa S, Woo YK (1965) Antiviral activity of herbs on Columbia SK in mice, and LCM, vaccinia and adeno, type 12 viruses in vitro. Proc Soc Exp Biol Med 120:330–333

Deig EF, Ehresmann DW, Hatch MT, Riedlinger DJ (1974) Inhibition of herpesvirus replication by marine algae extracts. Antimicrob Agents Chemother 6:524–525

Deitch AD, Godman GC, Tanenbaum SW (1973a) Cytochalasin D enhances the infectivity of poliovirus. Proc Soc Exp Biol Med 144:60–64

Deitch AD, Sawicki SG, Godman GC, Tanenbaum SW (1973b) Enhancement of viral infectivity by cytochalasin. Virology 56:417–428

Der Marderosian A (1969) Marine pharmaceuticals. J Pharm Sci 58:1–33

Di Marco A, Terni M, Silentrini R, Scarpinato B, Biagioli E, Antonelli A (1968) Effect of daunomycin on herpes virus hominis in human cells. G Microbiol 16:25–38

Dix RD, Courtney RJ (1976) Effects of cytochalasin B on herpes simplex virus, type 1 replication. Virology 70:127–135

Drzeniek R (1966) Inhibition of neuraminidase by polyanions. Nature 211:1205–1206

Duda E (1975) The effect of canavanine on the capsid protein of sindbis virus. Med Biol 53:365–367

Dym H, Becker Y (1969) Effect of p-fluorophenylalanine on the replication of herpes simplex virus. Isr J Med Sci 5:1083–1086

Eaton MD, Magasanik B, Perry ME, Karibian D (1951) Inhibition of influenza and mumps viruses in tissue culture by basic amino acids. Proc Soc Exp Biol Med 77:505–508

Ehrenfeld E (1974) Polyadenylation of vesicular stomatitis virus mRNA. J Virol 13:1055–1060

Ehresmann DW, Deig EF, Hatch MT, Di Salvo LH, Vedros NA (1977) Antiviral substances from California marine algae. J Phycol 13:37–40

Esterensen RD (1971) Cytochalasin BI: Effect on cytokinesis of Novikoff hepatoma cells. Proc Soc Exp Biol Med 136:1256–1260

Falker WA Jr, Diwan AR, Halstead SB (1975) A lipid inhibitor of dengue virus in human colostrum and milk. Arch Virol 47:3–10

Farnsworth NR (1966) Biological and phytochemical screening of plants. J Pharm Sci 55:225–276

Farnsworth NR, Svoboda GH, Blomster RN (1968) Antiviral activity of selected catharanthus alkaloids. J Pharm Sci 57:2174–2175

Fieldsteel AH (1974) Nonspecific anti-viral substances in human milk active against arbovirus and murine leukemia virus. Cancer Res 34:712–715

Fong HHS, Farnsworth NR, Henry LK, Svoboda GH, Yates MJ (1972) Biological and phytochemical evaluation of plants. Lloydia 35:35–48

Fujita H (1973) Dual effect on the mechanism of action of anti-influenza virus amino acid analogues. Antimicrob Agents Chemother 3:57–62

Fujita H, Sakurai T, Toyoshima S (1979) Antiviral effect of N-phenylacetoamino-methylene-DL-p-nitrophenylalanine (A-101) on murine leukemia viruses. J Natl Cancer Inst 62:565–568

Furusawa E, Cutting W (1966) Antiviral activity of higher plants in LCM infection in vitro and in vivo. Proc Soc Exp Biol Med 122:280–282

Furusawa E, Cutting W (1970) The higher plants with antiviral and antilethal activity on virus infections in mice. Ann NY Acad Sci 173:668–679

Furusawa E, Ramanathan S, Furusawa S, Woo Y, Cutting W (1967) Antiviral activity of higher plants and propionin in LCM infection. Proc Soc Exp Biol Med 125:234–239

Furusawa E, Furusawa S, Kroposki M, Cutting W (1968) Activity of S. sieboldiana on Col SK and LCM virus infection in mice. Proc Soc Exp Biol Med 128:1196–1199

Furusawa E, Lockwood RH, Furusawa S, Lum MKM, Lee JYB (1979) Therapeutic activity of Pretazettine, a narcissus alkaloid, on spontaneous AKR leukemia. Chemotherapy 25:308–315

Gerber P, Dutcher JD, Adams EV, Sherman JH (1958) Protective effect of seaweed extracts for chick embryos infected with influenza B or mumps virus. Proc Soc Exp Biol Med 99:590–593

Gessa GL, Loddo B, Brotzu M, Schiro ML, Tagliamonte A, Spanedda A, Bo G, Ferrari W (1960) Selective inhibition of poliovirus growth by D-penicillamine in vitro. Virology 30:618–622

Gifford GE, Robertson HE, Syverton JT (1954) Application of manometric method to testing chemical agents in vitro for interference with poliomyelitis virus synthesis. Proc Exp Biol Med 86:515–522

Goldberg IH, Friedman PA (1971) Antibiotics and nucleic acids. Annu Rev Biochem 40:775–810

Goulet NR, Cochran KW, Brown GC (1960) Differential and specific inhibition of ECHO viruses by plant extracts. Proc Soc Exp Biol Med 103:96–100

Green RH (1948) Inhibition of multiplication of influenza virus by tannic acid. Proc Soc Exp Biol Med 67:483–484

Green RH (1949) Inhibition of multiplication of influenza virus by extracts of tea. Proc Soc Exp Biol Med 71:84–85

Green RH, Woolley DW (1947) Inhibition by certain polysaccharides of hemagglutination and multiplication of influenza virus. J Exp Med 86:55–64

Gresser I, Grogan EA (1965) Inhibition of arboviruses by a constituent of staphyloccus. Proc Soc Exp Biol Med 119:1176–1181

Griffith RS, Norins AI, Kagan C (1978) A multicentered study of lysine therapy in herpes simplex infection. Dermatologica 156:257–267

Groupé V, Pugh LH, Levine AS (1952) Suppression of viral pneumonia in mice by a microbial product (APM). Proc Soc Exp Biol Med 80:710–714

Hadhazy G, Horvath E, Gergely L (1966) Simultaneous inhibitory action on virus multiplication of interferon and some natural mucopolysaccharides (heparin, hyaluronic acid). Acta Microbiol Hung 13:193–196

Hahn FE (1975) Distamycin A and netropsin. In: Corcoran JW, Hahn FE (eds) Antibiotics III. Mechanism of action of antimicrobial and antitumor agents. Springer, Berlin Heidelberg New York, p 79

Herrmann EC, Kucera LS (1967) Antiviral substances in plants of the mint family (Labiatae). III. Peppermint (Mentha piperita) and other mint plants. Proc Soc Exp Biol Med 124:874–878

Hochberg E, Becker Y (1968) Adsorption, penetration, and uncoating of herpes simplex virus. J Gen Virol 2:231–241

Horsfall FI Jr, McCarty M (1947) The modifying effects of certain substances of bacterial origin on the course of infection with pneumonia virus of mice (PVM). J Exp Med 85:623–646

Horwitz MS, Brayton C (1972) Camptothecin: mechanism of inhibition of adenovirus formation. Virology 48:690–698

Horwitz SB, Chang CK, Grollman AP (1971) Studies on camptothecin: 1. Effects on nucleic acid and protein synthesis. Mol Pharmacol 7:632–644

Horwitz SB, Chang CK, Grollman AP (1972) Antiviral action of camptothecin. Antimicrob Agents Chemother 2:395–401

Hotta S, Kojima M, Fujisaki M, Uchida S, Kuroda H, Hamada C (1977) An antiviral substance extracted from Streptococcus faecalis. Nature 268:733–734

Jacobson MF, Baltimore D (1968) Polypeptide cleavage in the formation of poliovirus proteins. Proc Natl Acad Sci USA 61:77–84

Jones JH, Foster C, Henle W, Alexander D (1946) Dietary deficiencies and poliomyelitis. Effects of low protein and low tryptophan diets on the response of mice to the Lansing strain of poliomyelitis virus. Arch Biochem 11:481–487

Judge JR (1966) Inhibition of effects of leukemogenic viruses in mice by extracts of Mercenaria mercenaria. Proc Soc Exp Biol Med 123:299–302

Kagan C (1974) Lysine therapy for herpes simplex. Lancet I:137

Kaplan AS, Shimono H, Ben-Porat T (1970) Synthesis of proteins in cells infected with herpesvirus. Virology 40:90–101

Karlowski TR, Chalmers TC, Frenkel LD, Kapikian AZ, Lewis TL, Lynch JM (1975) Ascorbic acid for the common cold: a prophylactic and therapeutic trial. JAMA 231:1038–1042

Katagiri K, Yoshida T, Sato K (1975) Quinoxaline antibiotics. In: Corcoran JW, Hahn FE (eds) Antibiotics III. Mechanism of action of antimicrobial and antitumor agents. Springer, Berlin Heidelberg New York, p 234

Kathan RH (1965) Kelp extracts as antiviral substances. Ann NY Acad Sci 130:390–397

Katz E, Margalith E, Winer B (1975) Inhibition of the growth of hemadsorption 2 virus by three acyl derivatives of amino acids. Antimicrob Agents Chemother 7:717–718

Kinkade JM Jr (1971) Differences in the quantitative distribution of lysine-rich histone in neoplastic and normal tissue. Proc Soc Exp Biol Med 137:1131–1134

Kit S, Piekarski LJ, Dubbs DR (1963) Induction of thymidine kinase by vaccinia-infected mouse fibroblasts. J Mol Biol 6:22–33

Klenk HD, Scholtissek C, Rott R (1972) Inhibition of glycoprotein biosynthesis of influenza virus by D-glucosamine and 2-deoxy-D-glucose. Virology 49:723–734

Konowalchuk J, Speirs JI (1976) Virus inactivation by grapes and wines. Appl Environ Microbiol 32:757–763

Konowalchuk J, Speirs JI (1978a) Antiviral effect of apple beverages. Appl Environ Microbiol 36:798–801

Konowalchuk J, Speirs JI (1978b) Antiviral effect of commercial juices and beverages. Appl Environ Microbiol 35:1219–1220

Kotler M, Becker Y (1971) Rifampicin and distamycin A as inhibitors of Rous sarcoma virus reverse transcriptase. Nature 234:212–214

Kucera LS, Herrmann EC Jr (1967) Antiviral substances in plants of the mint family (labiatae). I. Tannin of Melissa officinalis. II. Non-tannin polyphenol of Melissa officinalis. Proc Soc Exp Biol Med 124:865–878

Larin NM, Copping MP, Herbst-Laier RH, Roberts B, Wenham RBM (1965) Antiviral activity of gliotoxin. Chemotherapy 10:12–23

Leavitt R, Schlesinger S, Kornfield S (1977) Tunicamycin inhibits glycosylation and multiplication of sindbis and vesicular stomatitis viruses. J Virol 21:375–385

Levintow L, Thoren MM, Darnell JE, Hooper JL (1962) Effect of p-fluorophenylalanine and puromycin on the replication of poliovirus. Virology 16:220–229

Li CP (1960) Antimicrobial effects of abalone juice. Proc Soc Exp Biol Med 103:522–524

Li CP, Prescott B, Jahnes WG (1962) Antiviral activity of a fraction of abalone juice. Proc Soc Exp Biol Med 109:532–538

Liebhaber H, Takemoto KK (1962) The basis for morphologic differences in plaques produced by variants of EMC virus. Bacteriol Proc 62:139

Lin W, Oishi K, Aida K (1975 a) A new screening method of viral neuraminidase inhibitors. Agric Biol Chem 39:759–765

Lin W, Oishi K, Aida K (1975 b) Isolation purification and physical and chemical properties of neuraminidase inhibitor No 289. Agric Biol Chem 39:923–930

Lin W, Oishi K, Aida K (1977) Specific inhibition of viral neuraminidases by an inhibitor, neuraminin, produced by streptomyces sp. Virology 78:108–114

Loh PC, Payne FE (1965) Effect of p-fluorophenylalanine on the synthesis of vaccinia virus. Virology 25:560–574

Lwoff A (1965) The specific effectors of viral development. Biochem J 96:289–302

Mahy BWJ, Hastie ND, Armstrong S (1972) Inhibition of influenza virus replication by α-amanitin: mode of action. Proc Natl Acad Sci 69:1421–1424

Mahy BWJ, Cox NJ, Armstrong SJ, Barry RD (1973) Multiplication of influenza virus in the presence of cordycepin, an inhibitor of cellular RNA synthesis. Nature 243:172–174

Mandel B (1957) Inhibition of Theiler's encephalomyelitis virus (GDVII strain) of mice by an intestinal mucopolysacharide. Virology 3:444–463

Mandel Racker B (1953) Inhibition of Theiler's encephalomyelitis virus (GD VII strain) of mice by an intestinal mucopolysaccharide. I. Biological properties and mechanism of action. J Exp Med 98:399–415, 417–426

Manzella JP, Roberts NJ Jr (1980) Effects of ascorbic acid and hyperthermia on human leukocytes exposed to respiratory viruses. In: Nelson J, Grassi D (eds) Current chemoterapy and infectious disease. American Society for Microbiology, Washington, D.C., p 1350

Matthews ThJ, Lawrence MK, Nair CDG, Tyrell DAJ (1976) Antiviral activity in milk of possible clinical importance. Lancet II:1387–1389

Miller FA, Rightsel WA, Sloan BJ, Ehrlich J, French JC, Bartz QR, Dixon GJ (1963) Activity of tenuazonic acid. Nature 200:1338–1339

Miller KD, Miller GG, Sanders M, Fellowes ON (1977) Inhibition of virus-induced plaque formation by a toxic derivative of purified cobra neurotoxins. Biochim Biophys Acta 496:192–196

Miller JZ, Nance WE, Norton JA, Wolen RL, Griffith RS (1977) Therapeutic effect of vitamin C: a co-twin control study. JAMA 237:248–251

Miller PA, Milstrey KP, Trown PW (1968) Specific inhibition of viral ribonucleic acid replication by gliotoxin. Science 159:431–432

Minor PD, Dimmock NJ (1975) Inhibition of synthesis of influenza virus proteins: evidence for two host-cell-dependent events during multiplication. Virology 67:114–123

Moldave K, Winzler RJ, Pearson HE (1951) Effect of lysine on metabolism of minced one-day-old mouse brain and propagation of Theiler's GD VII virus. Fed Proc 10:225

Musci I, Béládi I, Presztai R, Bahery M, Gabor M (1978) Antiviral effect of flavonoids. In: Proc Hung Bioflavonoid Symposium, 5 th Chem. Abs. 89:401–449

Nahmias AJ, Kibrick S (1963) Inhibitory effect of heparin on certain viruses. Bacteriol Proc 63:145

Nahmias AJ, Kibrick S (1964) Inhibitory effect of heparin on herpes simplex virus. J Bacteriol 87:1060–1066

Nair CN, Panicali DL (1976) Polyadenylate sequences of human rhinovirus and poliovirus RNA and cordycepin sensitivity of virus replication. J Virol 20:170–176

Neuss N, Boeck LD, Brannon DR, Cline JC, Delong DC, Gorman M et al. (1968) Aranotin and related metabolites from *Arachniotus aureus* (Eidam) Schroeter. IV. Fermentation, isolation, stucture, elucidation, biosynthesis, and antiviral properties. Antimicrob Agents Chemother 213

Ohashi M, Taguchi T, Ikeganic S (1978) Aphidicolin: a specific inhibitor of DNA polymerases in the cytosol of rat liver. Biochem Biophys Res Commun 82:1048–1090

Olitsky PK, Cox HR (1934) Temporary prevention by chemical means of intranasal infection of mice with equine encephalomyelitis virus. Science 80:566–567

Ottenheijm HCJ, Herscheid JDM, Tijhuis MW, Nivard RJF, DeClercq E, Prick PAJ (1978) Gliotoxin analogues as inhibitors of reverse transcriptase. 2. Resolution and x-ray crystal structure determination. J Med Chem 21:799–804, 796–799

Palese P, Schulman JL (1977) Inhibitors of viral neuraminidase as potential antiviral drugs. In: Oxford JS (ed) Chemoprophylaxis and viral infections of the respiratory tract. CRC Press, Cleveland, Ohio, p 189

Palese P, Bucher D, Kilbourne ED (1973) Applications of a synthetic neuraminidase substrate. Appl Microbiol 25:195–201

Panicali DL, Nair CN (1978) Effect of cordycepin triposphate on in vitro RNA synthesis by picornavirus polymerase complexes. J Virol 25(1):124–128

Parisi B, Soller A (1964) Studies on the antiphage activity of daunomycin. GG Microbiol 12:183–194

Pauling L (1971) Vitamin C and the common cold. JAMA 216:332

Pearson HE, Winzler RJ (1949) Amino acids, analogues, and the propagation of Theiler's GD VII virus in mouse brain tissue culture. Fed Proc 8:409

Pearson HE, Lagerborg DL, Winzler RJ (1952) Effects of certain amino acids and related compounds on propagation of mouse encephalomyelitis virus. Proc Soc Exp Biol Med 79:409–411

Pearson HE, Lagerborg DL, Winzler RJ, Visser DW (1955) Methionine compounds and growth of mouse encephalomyelitis virus in tissue culture. J Bacteriol 69:225

Piazza M (1964) Inactivation of MHV-3 virus by intestinal content and intestine of normal mice. Nature 203:1196–1197

Piazza M, Amaido A, Pane G (1965) Distribution of the intestinal factor of normal mice which inactivates murine hepatitis virus. Nature 208:1009–1010

Piazza M, Pane G, Picciotto L, Lombardi D (1967) Effect on the infectivity of various viruses by the intestinal factor of normal mice which inactivates murine hepatitis virus. Nature 213:293–294

Pienta RJ, Groupé V (1964) Experiences with experimental chemotherapy of viral diseases. In: Schnitzer RJ, Hawkins F (eds) Experimental chemotherapy, vol III. pp 525–586

Pigram WJ, Fuller W, Hamilton LD (1972) Stereochemistry of intercalation: interaction of daunomycin with DNA. Nature 235:17–19

Pilcher KS, Soike KF, Smith VH, Trosper F, Folston B (1955) Inhibition of multiplication of Lee influenza virus by canavanine. Proc Soc Exp Biol Med 88:79–86

Planterose DN (1969) Antiviral and cytotoxic effects of mycophenolic acid. J Gen Virol 4:629–630

Pollikoff R, Liberman M, Cochran KW, Pascale AM (1965) Effect of caffeic acid on mouse and ferret lung infected with influenza A virus. Antimicrob Agents Chemother 561–566

Pompei K, Ornella F, Marccidis MA, Pani A, Loddo B (1979) Glycyrrhizic acid inhibits virus growth and inactivates virus particles. Nature 281:689–690

Pons MW, Preston WS (1961) The in vivo inhibition by β-phenylserine of rabies, myxoma and vaccinia viruses. Virology 15:164–172

Rafelson ME Jr, Pearson HE, Winzler RJ (1950) The effects of certain amino acids and metabolic antagonists on propagation of Theiler's GD VII virus and P^{32} uptake by minced one-day-old mouse brain. Arch Biochem 29:69–74

Rasmussen AF Jr, Waisman HA, Elvehjem CA, Clark PF (1944) Influence of the level of thiamine uptake on the susceptibility of mice to poliomyelitis virus. J Infect Dis 74:41–47

Reich E, Franklin RM, Skatkin AJ, Tatum EL (1969) Effect of actinomycin D on cellular nucleic acid synthesis and virus production. Science 134:556–557

Renis HE (1969) In vitro antiviral activity of calcium elenolate. Antimicrob Agents Chemother 167–172

Richards JT, Kern ER, Glasgow LA, Overall JC Jr, Deign EF, Hatch MT (1978) Antiviral activity of extracts from marine algae. Antimicrob Agents Chemother 14:24–30

Richter IE, Falke D (1973) Scanning electron microscopic observations of the inhibition of herpes-induced grant cell formation by Cpd 48/80 and cytochalasin B. Fourth Congress of the European Society of Pathology, Budapest

Riedel B, Brown DT (1979) Novel antiviral activity found in the media of sindbis virus-persistently infected mosquito *(aedes albopictus)* cell cultures. J Virol 29:51–60

Rightsel WA, Schneider HG, Sloan BJ, Graf PR, Miller FA, Bartz QR, Ehrlich J, Dixon GJ (1964) Antiviral activity of gliotoxin and gliotoxin acetate. Nature 204:1333–1334

Ronaldson JW, Taylor A, White EP, Abraham RJ (1963) Sporadesmins. I. Isolation and characterization of sporadesmins and sporadesmin B. J Chem Soc 3172–3180

Sabin AB, Fieldsteel AH (1962) Antipoliomyelitic activity of human and bovine colostrum and milk. Pediatr 29:105–115

Sanders M, Soret MG, Akin BA (1953) Neurotoxoid interference with two human strains of poliomyelitis in Rhesus monkeys. Ann NY Acad Sci 58(1):1–12

Sanders M, Soret MG, Akin BA, Roizin L (1958) Neurotoxoid interference in *Macacus rhesus* infected intramuscularly with poliovirus. Science 127:594–596

Sakar NH, Charney J, Dion AS, Moore DH (1973) Effect of human milk on the mouse mammary tumor virus. Cancer Res 33:626–629

Sato K, Niinomi Y, Kaagiri K, Matsukage A, Minagawa T (1969) Prevention of phage multiplication by quinonmycin A. Biochim Biophys Acta 174:230–238

Schabel FM Jr, Laster WR, Brockman RW, Skipper HE (1953) Observations on antiviral activity of netropsin. Proc Soc Exp Biol Med 83:1–3

Scharff MD, Levintow L (1963) Quantitative study of the formation of poliovirus antigens in infected HeLa cells. Virology 19:491–500

Schmeer MR (1964) Growth inhibiting agents from mercenaria extracts: chemical and biological properties. Science 144:413–414

Schmeer MR, Huala C (1965) Mercenene: in vivo effects of mollusk extracts on sarcoma 180. Ann NY Acad Sci 118:605–610

Schulze IT, Schlesinger RW (1963) Inhibition of infectious and hemagglutinating properties of type 2 dengue virus by aqueous agar extracts. Virology 19:49–57

Sethi ML (1977) Inhibition of RNA-directed DNA polymerase activity of RNA tumor viruses by taspine. Can J Pharmacol Sci 12:7–9

Shortridge KF, Squires S (1977) Effect of daunorubicin on the growth of adenovirus. J Antimicrob Chemother 3:133–139

Soret MG (1969) Antiviral activity of calcium elenolate on parainfluenza infection of hamsters. Antimicrob Agents Chemother 160–166

Spooner BS, Yamada KM, Wessells NR (1971) Microfilaments and cell locomotion. J Cell Biol 49:596–613

Sprunt DH (1948) Incrased susceptibility of mice to swine influenza as a result of methionine injections. Proc Soc Exp Biol Med 67:319–321

Suzuki N, Tani S, Furusawa S, Furusawa E (1974) Therapeutic activity of narcissus alkaloids on Rauscher leukemia. Antiviral effect in vitro and rational drug combination in vivo. Proc Soc Exp Biol Med 145:771–777

Takatsuki A, Tamura G (1971) Tunicamycin, a new antibiotic. III. Reversal of the antiviral activity of tunicamycin by aminosugars and their derivatives. J Antibiot (Tokyo) 24:232–238

Takemori N, Nomura S (1960) Mutation of poliovirus with respect to size of plaque. II. Reverse mutation of minute plaque mutant. Virology 12:171–184

Takemoto KK, Fabisch P (1964) Inhibition of herpes virus by natural and synthetic acid polysaccharides. Proc Soc Exp Biol Med 116:140–144

Takemoto KK, Liebhaber H (1961) Virus-polysaccharide interactions. 1. An ager polysaccharide determining plaque morphology of EMC-virus. Virology 14:456–462

Takemoto KK, Liebhaber H (1962) The inhibition effect of sulfated polysaccharides on viral multiplication. Fed Proc Fed Am Soc Exp Biol 21(2):461

Takemoto KK, Spicer SS (1965) Effects of natural and synthetic sulfated polysaccharides on viruses and cells. Ann NY Acad Sci 130:365–373

Tamm I, Horsfall FL Jr (1950) Characterization and separation of an inhibitor of viral hemagglutination present in urine. Proc Soc Exp Med 74:108–114

Tankersley RW Jr (1964) Amino acid requirements of herpes simplex virus in human cells. J Bacteriol 87:609–613

Tata JR, Hamilton MJ, Shields D (1972) Effect of α-amanitin in vivo on RNA polymerase and nuclear RNA synthesis. Nature 238:161–164

Taylor A, McKenna GF, Burlage HM, Stokes DM (1954) Plant extracts tested against egg cultivated viruses. Tex Rep Biol Med 12:551–557

Temin AM (1971) Mechanism of cell transformation by RNA tumor viruses. Annu Rev Microbiol 25:609–648

Thompson RL (1947) The effect of metabolites, metabolite antagonists, and enzymeinhibitors on the growth of vaccinia virus in Maitland type of tissue cultures. J Immunol 55:345–352

Thompson RL, Lavender AR (1953) Effect of ethionine and other materials on Semliki Forest virus infection in the mouse. Proc Soc Exp Biol Med 84:483–486

Thompson RL, Wilkin ML (1948) Inhibition of growth of the vaccinia virus by β-2-thienylalanine and its reversal by phenylalanine. Proc Soc Exp Biol Med 68:434–436

Trown PW, Bilello JA (1972) Mechanism of action of gliotoxin: elimination of activity by sulfhydryl compounds. Antimicrob Agents Chemother 2:261–266

Trown PW, Lindh HF, Milstrey K, Gallo VM, Mayberry BR, Lindsay HL, Miller PA (1968) LL-S88α An antiviral substance produced by *Aspergillus terreus*. Antimicrob Agents Chemother 225–228

Tsunoda A (1962) Chemoprophylaxis of poliomyelitis in mice with quinomycin. J Antibiot (Tokyo) [Ser] 15:60–66

Umezawa H, Aoyagi T, Komiyama T, Morishima H, Hamada M, Takeuchi T (1974) Purification and characterization of a sialidase inhibitor, siastatin, produced by streptomyces. Jpn J Antibiot 27:963–969

Vaheri A, Cantell K (1963) The effect of heparin on herpes simplex virus. Virology 21:661–662

Van Den Berghe DA, Ieven M, Mertens F, Vlietinck AJ (1978) Screening of higher plants for biological activities. II. Antiviral activity. Lloydia 41:463–471

Veckenstedt A, Beladi A, Musci I (1978) Effect of treatment with certain flavonoids in mengo virus-induced encephalitis in mice. Arch Virol 57:255–260

Waksman SA, Bugie E (1944) Chaetomin, a new antibiotic substance produced by Chaetomium cochliodes. Formation and properties. J Bacteriol 48:527–530

Ward DC, Reich E, Goldberg IH (1965) Base specificity in the interaction of polynucleotides with antibiotic drugs. Science 149:1259–1263

Ward JW, Tankersley RW Jr (1980) Method of combating herpes simplex viruses with lignosulfonates. U.S. Patent No. 4,185,097, Jan. 22

Wecker E (1965) Direct inhibition of protein synthesis and its effect on the growth of RNA viruses. Ann NY Acad Sci 130:259–266

Wecker E, Hummeler K, Goetz O (1962) Relationship between viral RNA and viral protein synthesis. Virology 17:110–117

Weiss SR, Bratt MA (1975) Effect of cordycepin (3-deoxyadenosine) and virus-specific RNA species synthesized in Newcastle disease virus-infected cells. J Virol 16:1575–1583

Welsh JK, May JT (1979) Anti-infective properties of breast milk. J Pediatr 94:1–9

Welsh JK, Skurrie IJ, May JT (1978) Use of Semliki Forest virus to identify lipid mediated antiviral activity and anti-alphavirus immunoglobulin A in human milk. Infect Immun 19:395–401

Williams RH, Lively DH, DeLong DC, Cline JC, Sweeney MJ, Poore GA, Larsen SH (1968) Mycophenolic acid: antiviral and antitumor properties. J Antibiot 21:463–464

Zanetti M, Foa L, Costanzo F, La Placa M (1971) Specific inhibition of Rous sarcoma virus by α-amanitin. Arch Ges Virusforsch 34:255–260

Zigmond SH, Hirsh JG (1972) Effects of cytocholasin B on polymorphonuclear leukocyte locomotion, phagocytosis, and glycolysis. Exp Cell Res 73:383–393

CHAPTER 13

Rifamycins

C. GURGO, S. BRIDGES, and M. GREEN

A. Introduction

The term rifamycins indicates a large group of related compounds sharing as a common structural feature, a naphthohydroquinone chromophore spanned by a an aliphatic ansa chain. Originally, a mixture of five compounds, designated rifamycins A–E, was isolated from the fermentation broth of *Nocardia mediterranei* (SENSI et al. 1959 a, b). It was subsequently found that one of the compounds, rifamycin B, was produced almost exclusively when sodium diethylbarbiturate was present in the fermentation medium (MARGALITH and PAGANI 1961). Chemical modification of this compound, particularly in the 3 position, yielded additional compounds with more extensive antimicrobial activity. The best known of these is the derivative 3-(4-methylpiperazinoiminomethyl) rifamycin SV, or more simply, rifampicin.

On the basis of extensive work with *Escherichia coli*, it is assumed that the mechanism by which rifampicin inhibits bacterial multiplication is by blocking RNA synthesis through a specific interaction between the drug and the bacterial DNA-dependent RNA polymerase. The enzyme is inhibited in vitro at very low levels of drug (0.01–0.1 µg/ml). When used at higher levels (100 µg/ml), rifampicin has been shown to have antiviral activity against several mammalian viruses, the most extensively studied being the poxviruses. The mechanism by which poxviruses are inhibited is not completely understood. Multiple effects have been identified; these include a block of virus assembly, inhibition of precursor polypeptide cleavage, and inhibition of an RNA polymerase activity. However, the virion-associated RNA polymerase of poxviruses does not appear to be the target of the drug.

Several semisynthetic rifamycin derivatives inhibit the RNA-dependent DNA polymerase (reverse transcriptase) of retroviruses, and virus replication and cell transformation by these viruses as well. Although many studies suggest that the antiviral activity of these compounds against retroviruses is related to their ability to inhibit the enzyme, not all the observed effects can be reduced to a unique interaction between the drugs and the viral polymerase. Effective inhibitors of the reverse transcriptase are also inhibitors of other polymerizing enzymes.

Previously published reviews dealing with various aspects of the structure and activity of rifamycins include: general aspects (WEHRLI and STAEHELIN 1971; RIVA and SILVESTRI 1972); biosynthesis and chemistry of rifamycins and related compounds (SENSI 1975; BRUFANI 1977; WEHRLI 1977); structure–activity relationships (LANCINI and ZANICHELLI 1977); antipolymerase activity (GURGO 1977, 1980). In this article, we will focus on the antiviral properties of rifamycins and related ansamycins.

B. Activity of Rifamycins on Bacteria

Rifampicin is active against gram-positive bacteria, gram-negative bacteria, and mycobacteria (see BINDA et al. 1971, for a comprehensive review on the subject). Effective concentrations of the drug for the various groups are, respectively: <0.1 µg/ml, 0.1–1 µg/ml, and 1–5 µg/ml. Enterobacteria such as *E. coli* are less sensitive, and concentrations of 10 µg/ml are required for growth inhibition. Rifampicin inhibits bacterial growth, acting at the level of RNA synthesis (LANCINI and SARTORI 1968). Inhibition of protein synthesis follows as a consequence of polyribosome decay (SCHLESSINGER et al. 1969; GURGO et al. 1971 a). Inhibition of RNA synthesis is achieved through a tight but reversible binding of the drug to the bacterial DNA-dependent RNA polymerase; one molecule of drug for each enzyme molecule is sufficient to achieve inhibition.

I. Structural Requirements for Activity

Very likely, hydrogen bonds, lipophilic and π–π interactions are involved in the binding of rifampicin to the bacterial RNA polymerase. Studies of the tertiary structure of the drug molecule indicate that the four hydroxyl groups, at positions C-1 and C-8 of the naphthohydroquinone ring and C-21 and C-23 of the ansa chain (Fig. 1), are on the same side of the molecule (BRUFANI et al. 1974). They are likely involved in binding, through hydrogen bond interactions, to suitable groups of a complementary region of the RNA polymerase. These hydroxyl groups are essential for antipolymerase and biologic activity. Kinetic studies of the interaction of rifampicin with RNA polymerase in various solvents suggest that the bonds forming the drug–enzyme complex are largely lipophilic in nature (WEHRLI et al. 1976). It is possible that π–π bonds between the naphthohydroquinone nucleus of the drug and aromatic nuclei of appropriate amino acids might serve to stabilize the drug–enzyme interaction.

The ansa chain confers rigidity on the drug molecule, thus guaranteeing the geometric configuration of the four hydroxyl groups already mentioned. Hydrogenation of the double bonds of the chain increases structural flexibility and reduces the antipolymerase activity. Opening of the chain or attachment to a different position of the naphthohydroquinone ring system completely abolishes the antipolymerase activity (reviewed in SENSI 1975; BRUFANI 1977; LANCINI and ZANICHELLI 1977; WEHRLI 1977).

II. Mechanism of Inhibition of RNA Polymerase

In the bacterial system, several sequential steps in RNA transcription have been identified. They include: (1) formation of a binary complex between RNA polymerase and DNA (preinitiation); (2) binding of the first two nucleotides to the initiation and elongation sites and formation of the first phosphodiester bond (initiation); (3) sequential addition of nucleoside monophosphates to the hydroxyl group of the growing chain (elongation); and (4) release of a complete RNA chain (termination), followed by dissociation of the enzyme–template complex (CHAMBERLIN 1976).

The mechanism of inhibition of the bacterial polymerase has been the subject of several review articles (RIVA and SILVESTRI 1972; WEHRLI et al. 1976; GURGO

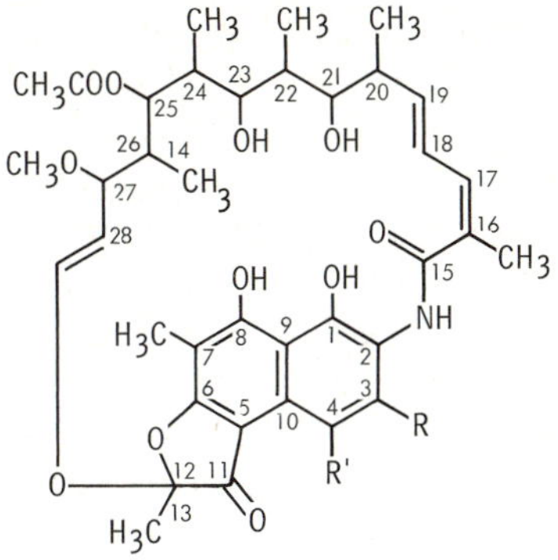

COMPOUND	R	R'
RIFAMYCIN B	-H	$-OCH_2COOH$
RIFAMPICIN	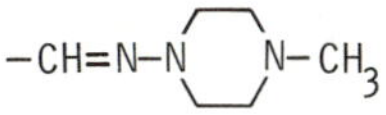	-OH
RIFAMYCIN SV	-H	-OH
AF/AP	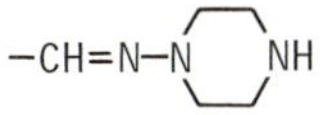	-OH
AF/ABDMP	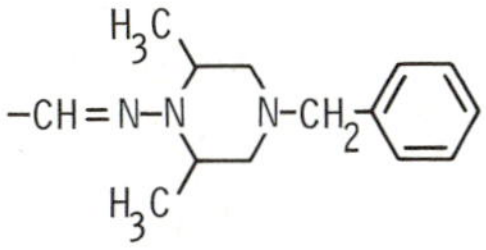	-OH
AF/DNFI	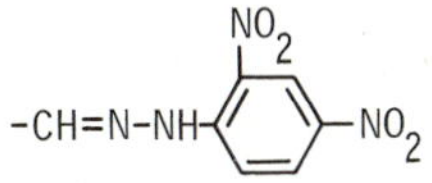	-OH
AF-05	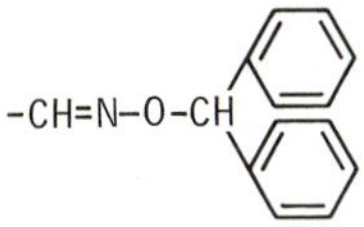	-OH
AF-013	$-CH=N-O-(CH_2)_7CH_3$	-OH
C-27	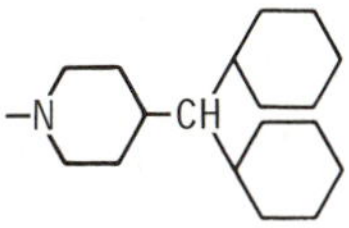	-OH
R-8_2	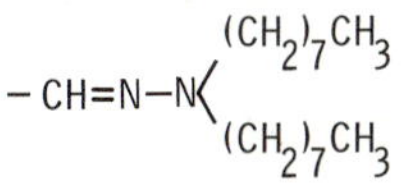	-OH

Fig. 1. Structures of rifamycins. The structures of several compounds most widely studied are illustrated. For structures of other derivatives mentioned in this article, see LANCINI and ZANICHELLI (1977). The numbering system is that of V. PRELOG. (OPPOLZER et al. 1964)

1980). Briefly, rifampicin binds to the free enzyme without inhibiting the subsequent formation of enzyme–DNA complex. The drug also binds to the polymerase when it is associated with template; the rate constant for this binding is two orders of magnitude lower than the rate constant of the binding reaction with the free enzyme. It has been proposed that the apparent template protection is the result of competition between the inactivation and the much faster polymerization. Once the enzyme is engaged in the process of chain elongation, rifampicin has no further inhibitory effect. It has been generally accepted that rifampicin inhibits initiation, and several models involving interactions at different steps have been proposed. For example, it has been suggested that rifampicin: (1) competes with a purine triphosphate for binding to the initiation site; (2) inhibits the formation of an enzymatically active enzyme–DNA complex; or (3) inhibits the formation of the first phosphodiester bond. In studying the steady state synthesis of pppApU at a promoter region of λ DNA, Johnston and McClure (1976), however, found that rifampicin does not inhibit the synthesis of the dinucleotide tetraphosphate and that the drug inhibits, instead, elongation, by completely blocking the formation of the second phosphodiester bond.

III. Effects on Psittacosis–Lymphogranuloma–Trachoma Agents

It has also been reported that rifampicin inhibits the replication of trachoma agent and the related psittacosis–lymphogranuloma agents, i.e. the PLT group of organisms (Becker and Zakay-Rones 1969; Becker et al. 1969). While these organisms have now been characterized as bacteria rather than viruses (reviewed by Becker 1978), they share with the latter the inability to replicate outside a host cell. Rifampicin is active during an initial stage of trachoma development, characterized by intense RNA synthetic activity, presumably by interacting with the DNA-dependent RNA polymerase present in the "elementary bodies" (infectious particles) (Becker et al. 1970). In cells treated with emetine to eliminate host protein synthesis, it was found that rifampicin (1 µg/ml) almost completely abolished trachoma-directed protein synthetic activity (Becker and Asher 1972). In cell cultures in vitro, rifampicin and a related hydrazone derivative inhibited the development of trachoma agent by 100% at 0.01 µg/ml; in embryonated eggs, rifampicin was active against the same agent at 5–10 µg. Rifampicin was an effective treatment for an established trachoma infection in the baboon when used at 200 µg/day, applied locally, for several weeks (Becker et al. 1969), and there is also evidence that the compound may be useful in treating trachoma infections in humans (Darougar et al. 1977). Rifamycin SV, several additional 3-substituted rifamycin SV derivatives, rifamycin B, and 8-O-acetylrifamycin S were also tested for activity in vitro and in vivo (in embryonated eggs); 10–100-fold higher doses were required for an effect equivalent to that seen with rifampicin (Becker et al. 1970; Becker 1971).

C. Activity of Rifamycins on Bacterial Viruses

I. Effect on DNA Bacteriophages

DNA bacteriophages which use the bacterial DNA-dependent RNA polymerase for transcription, albeit modified or altered by phage functions, are sensitive to rifampicin throughout their multiplication cycle. These include the *E. coli* bacterio-phages T4 (HASELKORN et al. 1969) and λ (TAKEDA et al. 1969), and *Bacillus subtilis* bacteriophages SPO1 (GEIDUSCHEK and SKLAR 1969) and β22 (HEMPHILL et al. 1969). RNA synthesis is severely inhibited by the addition of rifampicin at any time during the cycle, while the yield is progressively less affected with time after infection. *E. coli* and *B. subtilis* mutants which have rifampicin-resistant RNA polymerase support in a normal way the growth of such bacteriophages in the presence of the drug.

Other bacteriophages, such as T3 and T7, are sensitive to rifampicin only during the early stage of replication (CHAMBERLIN et al. 1970; MAITRA 1971). In this case, early bacteriophage gene transcription is carried out by the host cell polymerase, while late gene transcription is carried out by a phage-coded polymerase which is resistant to rifampicin.

The replication of single-stranded DNA bacteriophages can be inhibited at two points by rifampicin. With M13, the in vitro conversion of the single-stranded DNA form to double-stranded replicative form (RF) is sensitive to rifampicin (BRUTLAG et al. 1971), because the drug blocks the enzymatic activity which mediates primer synthesis required for this step (WICKNER et al. 1972); RF replication is not sensitive to rifampicin. With φX174, rifampicin does not affect the formation of RF from single-stranded bacteriophage DNA (SILVERSTEIN and BILLEN 1971); primer synthesis is carried out by a rifampicin-resistant RNA polymerase (SCHEKMAN et al. 1972; BOUCHÉ et al. 1975). Further replication of the parental RF into progeny RF is, however, sensitive to rifampicin when the drug is added before infection (SILVERSTEIN and BILLEN 1971), apparently because primer synthesis is also required at this step and is mediated by a sensitive enzyme (HIGASHI and KOMANO 1977).

Rifampicin inhibits the synthesis of MVL51, a group of nonlytic mycoplasma viruses containing single-stranded circular DNA. The host *Acholeplasma laidlawii* is rifampicin resistant (DAS and MANILOFF 1976). In this system, DNA replication involves several intermediates: (1) RFI, a covalently closed circular double-stranded DNA; and (2) RFII, a nicked form of RFI, which are precursors of (3) SSI, a circular, single-stranded progeny viral DNA. Rifampicin has no effect on the formation of RFI, RFII, or SSI molecules; it blocks the movement of SSI into mature virus, that is, it functions at the level of assembly. When rifampicin is removed, viral assembly occurs and mature particles are released. It was shown that synthesis of some virus-specific RNA was inhibited in the presence of rifampicin, suggesting that virus-specific transcription is required for assembly. To explain the occurrence of rifampicin sensitivity in a resistant host, it was hypothesized that the virus might modify the host polymerase, rendering it sensitive.

II. Effect on RNA Bacteriophages

The development of the RNA bacteriophages such as f2, Qβ, and MS2 in *E. coli* is unaffected if rifampicin is added at 4 min or later after infection (FROMAGEOT and ZINDER 1968; JOCKUSCH et al. 1970). Addition of rifampicin before or shortly after infection (at 50–100 µg/ml) interferes with the intracellular growth of the bacteriophages (FROMAGEOT and ZINDER 1968; PASSENT and KAESBERG 1971; ENGEL-

Berg 1972; Meir and Hofschneider 1972; Rothwell and Yamazaki 1972) and release of mature particles (Engelberg and Soudry 1971a). In host cells having a resistant DNA-dependent RNA polymerase, neither the development nor release is affected (Marino et al. 1968; Passent and Kaesberg 1971; Engelberg and Soudry 1971b).

There are at least two mechanisms by which the drug inhibits intracellular development of the mature particle. In the case of $Q\beta$, rifampicin appears to function by strongly reducing the rate of bacteriophage assembly; bacteriophage-directed RNA and protein synthesis are not affected (Passent and Kaesberg 1971). On the basis of these findings, it was suggested that a host-coded protein is involved in $Q\beta$ assembly. On the other hand, with f2, MS2, and R17, which are serologically related among themselves but distinct from $Q\beta$, growth appears to be inhibited at the level of bacteriophage RNA synthesis (Engelberg et al. 1975). Each bacteriophage, however, is inhibited in a slightly different way. With f2, the drug interferes with the synthesis of the negative-strand RNA, while it has no effect on the synthesis of progeny positive-strand RNA; with MS2, the drug affects the synthesis of progeny positive-strand RNA and weakly affects the synthesis of the negative-strand RNA; with R17, both steps of RNA replication are partially inhibited. The action of rifampicin thus appears to be related to one or more bacterial proteins which are essential for the first step of f2 RNA replication, the second step of MS2 replication, and are partially needed for both steps of R17 replication.

Another effect that has been reported recently concerns the action of the drug on infectivity. When f2 bacteriophage is incubated in vitro with high concentrations of the drug (500 µg/ml), for 3–4 h, infectivity is reduced to 10% of untreated samples (Naimski and Chroboczek 1977). One molecule of drug binds to each particle, while three molecules bind to the naked RNA component; no binding to isolated bacteriophage proteins was noted. It was shown that the native secondary structure of the RNA was essential for binding. Rifampicin-complexed RNA was unable to infect *E. coli* spheroplasts.

D. Activity of Rifamycins on Mammalian Viruses

I. Growth Inhibition of Mammalian Viruses by Rifampicin

It was reported by Heller et al. (1969) that, at doses between 50 and 100 µg/ml, rifampicin inhibited the growth of vaccinia virus in mouse embryo cells; independently, Subak-Sharpe et al. (1969) reported that the drug blocked the production of mature vaccinia virus in BHK cells. When screened against many strains of the major groups of mammalian viruses, rifampicin was shown to inhibit plaque formation by adenovirus in addition to all strains of vaccinia, cowpox, and smallpox that were tested (Subak-Sharpe et al. 1969). However, there was no growth inhibition noted, at the highest dose used (150 µg/ml), in the case of the large DNA viruses, herpes simplex and pseudorabies viruses, the small DNA tumor viruses SV40 and polyoma, nor for a variety of RNA viruses, including reovirus, equine rhinopneumositis virus, poliovirus 1, coxsackievirus B6, influenza AO virus, encephalomyocarditis virus (Subak-Sharpe et al. 1969), and vesicular stomatitis virus (Heller et al. 1969; Subak-Sharpe et al. 1969).

II. Mechanism of Vaccinia Virus Growth Inhibition by Rifampicin

A considerable part of this chapter will be devoted to the discussion of the effects of rifamycins on the growth of vaccinia virus (previously reviewed by FOLLETT and PENNINGTON 1973), since much attention has been focused on this subject in the literature. Rifampicin has been shown to be active against all poxviruses studied, with the exception of Cotia virus (UEDA et al. 1978). Unless otherwise noted, the drug was present, at 100 μg/ml, from the time of infection. It should be kept in mind that vaccinia virus replicates in the cytoplasm of infected cells and, unlike most mammalian viruses, is responsible for the synthesis of its own lipoprotein envelope, the fatty acid component of which is different from that of the host cell membrane (DALES and MOSBACH 1968). This difference offers a potential site of selective attack, particularly for lipophilic compounds such as rifamycins.

1. Effect on DNA Synthesis of Vaccinia-Infected Cells

In several studies on the effect of rifampicin on virus-directed macromolecular synthesis, it was found that rifampicin depressed thymidine ^{3}H incorporation in cytoplasmic fractions of treated, vaccinia-infected cells, the extent of which was variable from slight depression (Moss et al. 1969 b) to values of 30%–50% (SUBAK-SHARPE et al. 1969; BEN-ISHAI et al. 1969; NAGAYAMA et al. 1970), depending on the cell line and possibly the vaccinia virus strain used. Several observations, described as follows, make it unlikely, however, that this effect is relevant to virus growth inhibition.

a. The sequential appearance, size, and location of viral "factories" were found to be identical in rifampicin-treated, virus-infected cells to those found in untreated, infected cells. DNA in these cytoplasmic inclusions was identified by electron microscopic autoradiography of thymidine ^{3}H-labeled cells (NAGAYAMA et al. 1970), and more recently by the extremely sensitive technique of fluorescence microscopy in which the "factories" were stained with a fluorescent DNA-binding compound (ESTEBAN 1977).

b. A full yield of infectious virus was obtained using DNA made during 4.5 h rifampicin treatment when 5-fluorodeoxyuridine (FUDR) was added prior to the removal of rifampicin, to prevent further DNA synthesis (Moss et al. 1969 b).

c. The synthesis of various vaccinia virus DNA intermediates proceeds normally in the presence of rifampicin. Briefly, vaccinia virus DNA replication involves the discontinuous synthesis of small fragments (10–12 S), the formation of intermediate sized molecules (30–50 S) by ligation, the maturation into full length (70–72 S) unit-sized, single-stranded DNA, and finally the introduction of cross-links between complementary strands (GESHELIN and BERNS 1974) and the formation of mature, double-stranded molecules (92–94 S and 102–104 S; ESTEBAN and HOLOWZAK 1977). When the distributions of these forms synthesized in the presence and absence of rifampicin were compared (ESTEBAN 1977), no differences were noted, ruling out the possibility that a step in DNA replication was a target of the inhibitor. Of particular importance was the finding that cross-linking occurred in the presence of rifampicin, since the blocking of this terminal event of DNA synthesis might well have explained a subsequent failure in virus assembly.

2. Effect on mRNA Synthesis

In the initial studies on the mechanism by which rifampicin mediates vaccinia growth inhibition, SUBAK-SHARPE et al. (1969) and POGO (1971) noted a reduction in uridine ^{3}H incorporation in the cytoplasm of vaccinia-infected, rifampicin-treated cells, while no such effect was observed in the presence of the drug when rifampicin-resistant mutants were used (SUBAK-SHARPE et al. 1969). This finding was of particular interest since it was already known that rifampicin inhibits bacterial growth by interfering with the RNA polymerase and that the vaccinia virus contains a DNA-dependent RNA polymerase within the mature virion (MUNYON et al. 1967; KATES and McAUSLAN 1967). It was immediately suggested that the inhibition of vaccinia virus growth observed in the presence of rifampicin could be the result of the interaction of the drug with the viral enzyme (SUBAK-SHARPE et al. 1969; HELLER et al. 1969).

POGO (1971) demonstrated that, in the continuous presence of rifampicin, uridine ^{3}H incorporation was inhibited 40% 4 h after infection and as much as 57% at later times. Several viral enzymatic activities, previously characterized as late functions, did not increase in particulate fractions with time after infection; these included two DNases, nucleotide phophorylase, and RNA polymerase (McAUSLAN 1969; NAGAYAMA et al. 1970; KATZ et al. 1970). Two early activities, poly d(AT) primable RNA polymerase and thymidine kinase were unaffected. Furthermore, when the RNA polymerase activity in particulate cytoplasmic fractions was examined, it was found to be sensitive to rifampicin, most profoundly so 6–8 h after infection (POGO 1971).

On the contrary, MOSS et al. (1969 a) reported two findings that seemed to exclude the possibility that the site of action of the drug was at the transcriptional level: (1) the rate of synthesis and the sedimentation properties of viral mRNA from the cytoplasm of cells pulse labeled at different times after infection did not change in the presence of the drug; and (2) core particle RNA polymerase activity was not inhibited by the drug. These results were obtained with drug concentrations (100 µg/ml) that almost completely inhibited the production of virus, detectable as infectious units or labeled particles. Similarly, other investigators found no quantitative difference in the uridine ^{3}H incorporation measured at the peak of viral mRNA synthesis (McAUSLAN 1969; BEN-ISHAI et al. 1969), i.e., 3–4 h after infection, in the presence of rifampicin, nor in its ability to bind to ribosomes and form virus-specific polysomes (BEN-ISHAI et al. 1969).

Further studies utilized inhibitors of protein and DNA synthesis to investigate the proposed transcriptional block. When vaccinia-infected cells are treated with actidione, a protein synthesis inhibitor, viral DNA is not released from the core and is not replicated, and "early" mRNA is continuously transcribed. Under these conditions, no difference was seen in the uridine ^{3}H incorporation in the presence and absence of rifampicin (McAUSLAN 1969). However, in similar experiments in which DNA synthesis was blocked by FUDR, uridine ^{3}H incorporation was depressed by about 40% when rifampicin was present. Under conditions where DNA synthesis is blocked, viral DNA is uncoated and released into the cytoplasm, though not replicated. To explain the observed effect of rifampicin, it was speculated that after uncoating: (1) interaction of rifampicin with the viral RNA polymerase becomes possible and can result in a partial inhibition of RNA synthesis;

or perhaps (2) a different viral polymerase is induced which is involved in the transcription of specific classes of viral RNA and which is rifampicin sensitive.

While there is some degree of controversy over the effect of rifampicin on various aspects of transcription, there is agreement on the point that, when tested in vitro, the drug does not inhibit the RNA polymerase found in purified virions or cores (MCAUSLAN 1969; MOSS et al. 1969 a; BEN-ISHAI et al. 1969; COSTANZO et al. 1970; POGO 1971; SZILÁGYI and PENNINGTON 1971). Whether another RNA polymerase, sensitive to rifampicin, exists or not is unclear. Recently, a viral RNA polymerase has been extensively purified from the cytoplasm of vaccinia-infected cells (NEVINS and JOKLIK 1977). It is a complex enzyme composed of seven subunits, three of which comigrate with virion structural proteins on SDS–polyacrylamide gels. It appears to be an "early" enzyme, on the basis of the migration of the three easily identifiable subunits, since they are found in gels at a position characteristic of polypeptides synthesized early after infection. The enzyme transcribes poly d(AT) in addition to native and denatured DNA templates and is resistant to concentrations of rifampicin as high as 200 μg/ml.

3. Effect on Protein Synthesis

There is widespread agreement that rifampicin has no effect on early virus-directed protein synthesis; the effect on late synthesis is a function of the poxvirus tested. In the case of vaccinia, it was found that rifampicin markedly depressed the rate of late protein synthesis by accelerating the generalized decline which occurs 7–8 h after infection (MOSS et al. 1969 a, b; BEN-ISHAI et al. 1969; TAN and MCAUSLAN 1970). As judged by immunodiffusion and acrylamide gel elecrophoresis, it appeared, however, that all viral proteins were synthesized in the presence of rifampicin (MOSS et al. 1969 a). When cowpox was substituted for vaccinia virus, only a slight inhibition in the rate of protein synthesis was observed at times late after infection (TAN and MCAUSLAN 1970). Thus there was no evidence for the idea that rifampicin functions by preventing late protein synthesis; it could not be ruled out, however, that rifampicin inhibits the synthesis of an essential viral protein (or proteins) normally present in amounts not easily detectable by the methods utilized. With regard to this point, in a recent study, over 100 vaccinia virus polypeptides were visualized by two-dimensional gel electrophoresis (ESSANI and DALES 1979) and it seems likely that others will be identified as the technology improves.

4. Effect on Virus Assembly

a) Blockade of Assembly in the Presence of Rifampicin

At the electron microscopic level (as reviewed by DALES and MOSBACH 1968), assembly of vaccinia virus begins with the de novo formation of virus envelopes at about 3–3.5 h after infection. Initially, they exist as short segments of trilaminar "unit" membrane, coated externally with a dense layer of spicules. The segments first appear as arcs and gradually become three-dimensional spheres which enclose DNA and proteins. The differentiation of the nucleoprotein core within a membrane barrier follows, and the virion takes on its characteristic mature form.

In the presence of rifampicin, however, Moss et al. (1969 b) demonstrated that radioactively labeled vaccinia virus DNA remained in a DNase-sensitive form at the top of the gradient rather than sedimenting with the marker virus, despite the fact that the entire viral genome and a broad spectrum of viral proteins had been synthesized. By electron microscopy, it was revealed that, in the presence of rifampicin, there was an accumulation of irregularly shaped areas of electron-dense material surrounded by trilaminar membrane which lacked the characteristic outer spicule layer of the poxvirus envelope. In a series of papers which followed (GRIMLEY et al. 1970; PENNINGTON et al. 1970; NAGAYAMA et al. 1970), the block of morphogenesis was explored in great detail with general agreement on the abnormal structures observed. As described by GRIMLEY et al. (1970), viroplasmic regions indistinguishable from those seen in untreated virus-infected cells appear 2 h after infection. They differentiate into discrete domains of condensed material, partially delineated by uncoated membranes, increasing in number until protein synthesis rapidly declines, i.e., 6–8 h after infection. After 24 h in the presence of rifampicin, many membranes are detached from the domains and are found in micellar or laminar forms in the cytoplasm. Only rarely are normal developmental forms found. Other structures seen in the cytoplasm of rifampicin-treated cells include areas of fibrous material in the viroplasmic matrix and dense filamentous material condensed into paracrystalline aggregates (DNA). If rifampicin is added at 4–6 h after infection, instead of at the time of infection, maturation proceeds in the presence of the drug, and membrane-limited domains coexist with normal mature and immature forms.

b) Reversal of Rifampicin-Induced Assembly Block

The effect of rifampicin on morphogenesis is rapidly reversed. Within 5 min after the removal of rifampicin, membrane coating (addition of spicules) is nearly complete and membrane segments assume their typical curved contour. Large numbers of immature particles are present within 10 min, and the formation and differentiation of the cores has begun. By 2 h, mature virions are observed. Re-addition of rifampicin before complete conversion of the blocked forms to immature forms has occurred, i.e., before 10 min, results in a smaller number of progeny than if it is re-added after complete conversion (Moss et al. 1971). New envelope formation is again blocked, but early stage forms continue to mature ultrastructurally and infectious virus is progressively formed in the presence of the drug.

c) Effect of RNA and Protein Synthesis Inhibitors on Virus Maturation After Rifampicin Removal

To ascertain whether the removal of the block in virus morphogenesis caused by rifampicin was contingent on new protein synthesis, inhibitors of the synthesis of RNA (actinomycin D) or protein (streptovitacin A or cycloheximide) were added prior to or at the time of the removal of rifampicin, and the appearance of infectious virus or particles was monitored some time later. Presumably, this information could discriminate between the two proposed mechanisms: (1) that rifampicin acts specifically at the stage of virus assembly, by binding to a structural, maturational, or enzymatic function that is needed for assembly, and does not interfere with later steps in biogenesis; or (2) that rifampicin acts at the level of transcription or translation and blocks maturation by preventing the appearance of proteins required for maturation.

Depending on the time of addition after infection, inhibitors of RNA and protein synthesis can be used to separate several stages of viral biogenesis (DALES and MOSBACH 1968). For example, formation of viral membranes can be blocked if an inhibitor of RNA synthesis or protein synthesis is added before transcription of the relevant mRNA or translation of the corresponding membrane protein has occurred, that is, before 2 h for actinomycin D or 3 h for streptovitacin A in the vaccinia virus–L cell system. If these inhibitors are added at 2.5 or 3.5 h, respectively, biogenesis of membranes and immature forms occurs, but the formation of mature progeny is blocked. After all vaccinia-specific material has been synthesized, inhibition of protein synthesis does not interfere with assembly of infectious progeny.

A variety of experiments were done by Moss and collaborators, who were proponents of the first mechanism, to assess the need for protein synthesis for the maturation of virus particles after the removal of rifampicin. They showed that, in HeLa cells infected with vaccinia virus, the conversion of precursor membranes to viral envelopes was obtained when inhibitors of protein synthesis were added before the removal of the drug, at levels sufficient to suppress amino acid incorporation by 98% within 10 min. The degree of maturation achieved in the progeny was shown to depend on the time of drug removal (Moss et al. 1971). If rifampicin was removed 4 h after infection, conversion of membranes to viral envelopes occurred, but maturation to later stage virus was prevented when cycloheximide or streptovitacin A was added 10 min or 1 h before rifampicin was removed. If rifampicin was removed late in the virus growth cycle, between 6 and 8 h, some mature virus was obtained; presumably, a sufficient number of proteins required for maturation had accumulated prior to the addition of inhibitor. The formation of infectious progeny virus initiated upon removal of rifampicin continued for 1 h at the same rate in the presence or absence of cycloheximide (Moss et al. 1969b). At 4 h after the removal of rifampicin, the number of mature virus particles was 10%–20% of that observed in the absence of protein synthesis inhibitors, as judged by electron microscopy (Moss et al. 1971). TAN and MCAUSLAN (1970) also reported a limited amount of assembly of cowpox virions when rifampicin was removed 12 h after infection in the presence of cycloheximide, although the particles appeared slightly denser than normal virions.

Neither infectious virus (NAGAYAMA et al. 1970) nor mature particles (PENNINGTON et al. 1970) were observed by two other groups of investigators when inhibitors of protein synthesis were added at the time of rifampicin removal; in the latter case, however, envelope assembly occurred and immature virus particles formed. NAGAYAMA et al. (1970) used the vaccinia virus–L cell system, an incubation period of 6 h in the presence of rifampicin, followed by 6 h without rifampicin, but in the presence of streptovitacin A; PENNINGTON et al. (1970) used a vaccinia virus–BHK cell system, and incubation of 17 h with rifampicin, followed by 6 h in the absence of rifampicin, but in the presence of puromycin or cycloheximide.

Both Moss et al. (1971) and NAGAYAMA et al. (1970) found that actinomycin D did not prevent the conversion of precursor membranes into viral envelopes after the removal of rifampicin, although mature particles did not form. The former group suggested that, by binding to DNA, actinomycin might block maturation by interfering with packing, while the latter group interpreted the finding as supportive of the second mechanism by which inhibitors of transcription or translation block further maturation.

5. Inhibition of Precursor Polypeptide Cleavage

In pulse-chase experiments on cells infected with vaccinia virus, it was demonstrated that rifampicin prevents the disappearance of the two precursor polypeptides, P4a and P4b, and the appearance of two polypeptides (4a and 4b) of lower molecular weight, which are the two major structural components of the viral core (KATZ and MOSS 1970a; PENNINGTON 1973; MOSS and ROSENBLUM 1973). Rifampicin was used to accumulate P4a and P4b (MOSS and ROSENBLUM 1973), and tryptic peptide analysis established a precursor–product relationship between P4a, P4b, and 4a, 4b, respectively, thus indicating that the drug inhibits maturation of the two core proteins by blocking the cleavage of their precursors.

It was suggested by Moss and collaborators that this effect was secondary to the block in envelope assembly observed in the presence of rifampicin, since it had been shown earlier that cleavage most likely occurs during the formation of the viral core (KATZ and MOSS 1970a), a stage in morphogenesis which follows envelope assembly. As discussed previously, when rifampicin is added at the time of infection and removed sometime thereafter, envelope assembly occurs rapidly; however, KATZ and MOSS (1970b) report that 4a does not appear in significant amounts for 30–60 min.

6. Antivaccinia Activity of Various Rifamycin Derivatives

Attention was focused on the side chain component of rifampicin as being responsible for the antiviral activity, since no specific inhibition was found with a variety of analogs (see Fig. 1 and Table 1 for structures and nomenclature), including: rifamycin SV (the parent compound of rifampicin, with no side chain at the 3 position of the ring structure), M/27, and rifazine, tested on vaccinia-infected BHK cells (SUBAK-SHARPE et al. 1969); several hydrazone derivatives closely related to rifampicin, M/27, and rifamycin SV, tested on Shope fibroma virus (a poxvirus; ZAKAY-RONES and BECKER 1970); and 27 compounds, among which were amides and hydrazides of rifamycin B (substituted at the 4 position of the ring structure), pyrrole rifamycins, oxime and hydrazone derivatives of 3-formylrifamycin SV, tested on vaccinia virus, herpesvirus, and other viruses grown in chick cells (THIRY and LANCINI 1970). The latter investigators reported antivaccinia activity associated with the isolated side chain of rifampicin, 1-amino-4-methyl-piperazine (THIRY and LANCINI 1970; LANCINI et al. 1971); at 200–300 µg/ml, this compound blocked growth in chick cells. With another system, vaccinia-infected BHK cells, the side chain was unable to maintain the rifampicin-induced maturation block, at 1 mg/ml, nor did it affect plaque formation at nontoxic doses (FOLLETT and PENNINGTON 1971). THIRY and LANCINI (1972) later found that the mechanism of the effect they had observed with the side chain was different from that of rifampicin; it was most likely related to an effect on the cell rather than the virus.

Since many of the compounds were found to be cytotoxic, reducing yields of rifampicin-resistant as well as wild-type vaccinia virus, their relative activities were judged by their ability to cause maturation block after short-term incubation (GRIMLEY and MOSS 1971), or to maintain a rifampicin-induced maturation block (PENNINGTON and FOLLETT 1971). Among a group of 3-substituted rifamycin SV derivatives tested by these investigators, AF/AP, AF/AMI, and AF were active in both assay systems at concentrations between 50 and 200 µg/ml; the effects were shown to be readily reversible. The unsubstituted rifamycin SV did not cause maturation arrest at any dose tested, and only partially maintained the rifampicin-induced maturation block at a dose of 1 mg/ml. The latter finding was also true for AF/ABDMP, a compound closely related to rifampicin. In general, it was not possible to find a correlation between the magnitude of the antiviral activity and the chemical structure of the side chain. By varying the chemical group at the 4 position of the piperazine ring of rifampicin, MOSS et al. (1972) found that minimal shortening or lengthening of the chain led to loss of activity. A derivative slightly more active than rifampicin was obtained when the CH_3 of rifampicin was substituted by an NH_2 group.

Further studies examined the ability of several rifamycin derivatives and related antibiotics to inhibit the RNA polymerase activity of purified vaccinia virus, since GURGO et al. (1971 b) had shown that the RNA-dependent DNA polymerase of RNA tumor viruses could be inhibited by several such compounds. Although it was possible to find inhibitors of the vaccinia virus RNA polymerase, the antiviral activity did not appear to be the consequence of the inhibition of this enzyme, since the polymerases from rifampicin-resistant mutants and from the wild-type virus were equally inhibited by these compounds at doses higher than those required to block the growth of the wild-type virus (SZILÁGYI and PENNINGTON 1971).

7. Effect of Rifampicin on Experimental Vaccinia Infections

The effect of rifampicin on the vaccination reaction was studied in humans; local application of a 10% ointment or 15% cream was effective in blocking the development of a reaction in about 50% of the subjects tested (MOSHKOWITZ et al. 1971). Those treated orally (12 mg/kg body weight) showed a positive reaction although there was a 2-day delay with respect to control subjects before 100% reactors were scored.

III. Effect of Rifampicin on DNA Viruses Other Than Vaccinia

The activity of rifampicin has been tested on representatives of two other groups of double-stranded DNA viruses, herpesviruses and adenoviruses. Unlike poxviruses, these replicate and assemble in the nucleus of the host cell. Herpesviruses acquire a lipoprotein envelope as they mature by budding through the host nuclear membrane; adenoviruses are not enveloped.

1. Herpesviruses

While the growth of herpes simplex virus is not affected by rifampicin (SUBAK-SHARPE et al. 1969; HALSTED et al. 1972; FURUKAWA et al. 1975), two other herpesviruses, cytomegalovirus and varicella zoster virus, are sensitive in the dose range of 50–150 µg/ml (HALSTED et al. 1972; FURUKAWA et al. 1975). With regard to cytomegalovirus, rifampicin does not inhibit viral events occurring during the eclipse period; thus if the drug is removed prior to 48 h after infection (before the time of onset of DNA synthesis) there is no difference in the time of appearance or final titer of virus between treated and untreated cultures (FURUKAWA et al. 1975). In the presence of the drug, virus-related inclusion bodies do not form, and the characteristic increase in viral RNA synthesis, at about 16 h after infection, and viral DNA synthesis, at 48 h, do not occur. Early cytopathic effects (6–12 h post-infection) are manifest normally in rifampicin-treated cultures as are cytomegalovirus-associated antigens. After the removal of rifampicin, RNA synthesis can be detected within 2 h, while DNA synthesis is not detected until 14 h. Although it is not clear by what molecular mechanism rifampicin functions in inhibiting virus multiplication, FURUKAWA et al. (1975) suggest that the drug may interfere with the synthesis of specific classes of mRNA.

2. Adenoviruses

Except for a preliminary report by SUBAK-SHARPE et al. (1969) that rifampicin inhibited adenovirus 1 growth in HeLa cells (at 50–100 µg/ml), all other reports have been essentially negative. Adenoviruses 3, 4, and 7 were tested by McCORMICK et al. (1972), and adenoviruses 1, 3, 4, 12, and 19 were tested by WIGAND et al. (1974). In vivo, rifampicin was shown to decrease the incidence of tumors induced by adenovirus 12 in male, but not female, newborn hamsters (TOOLAN and LEDINKO 1972). Doses of 0.1 and 0.2 µg were administered to each hamster, in single or multiple weekly subcutaneous injections; toxic effects were noted which resulted in the death of some animals.

IV. Effect of Rifampicin on RNA Viruses Other Than Retroviruses

As mentioned earlier, in the screening by SUBAK-SHARPE et al. (1969) rifampicin had no effect on a variety of RNA viruses. Since that study, however, conditions have been found under which an inhibitory effect can be demonstrated for two picornaviruses, poliovirus and foot-and-mouth disease virus; in addition, a rifampicin-sensitive mutant of vesicular stomatitis virus, a rhabdovirus, has been isolated and described. Viruses belonging to these two groups have single-stranded RNA genomes and replicate and assemble in the cytoplasm. Rhabdoviruses are enveloped; picornaviruses are not.

1. Picornaviruses

While poliovirus is not inhibited by rifampicin when grown in monolayer culture (SUBAK-SHARPE et al. 1969), GRADO and OHLBAUM (1973) made the interesting observation that poliovirus and another picornavirus, foot-and-mouth disease virus, are inhibited 90%–95% when grown in suspension culture in the presence of 20 µg/ml rifampicin. Rifampicin did not cause particle inactivation since it was equally effective when added before or after virus adsorption, nor was the inhibition due to toxic effects on the host cell. The difference observed between monolayer and suspension cultures was attributed to membrane alterations generated during the enzymatic preparation of the latter cultures. As with the poxvirus system, the effect of rifampicin was reversible; removal of the drug resulted in the rapid production of virus. This observation suggested to the authors that the drug might function by blocking precursor polypeptide cleavage, an effect previously described for vaccinia virus. Since the picornavirus genome is translated as one large polyprotein which is subsequently cleaved to form structural proteins, and enzymes involved in genome replication as well, such a mechanism would be an efficient way to block virus multiplication. To our knowledge, this finding has not been followed up.

2. Vesicular Stomatitis Virus

A spontaneous rifampicin-sensitive mutant was isolated by MOREAU (1974) from wild-type vesicular stomatitis virus (VSV), which is, as previously mentioned, rifampicin resistant. The mechanism of the inhibitory effect was examined in a cell-free system, and it was found that the viral transcriptase activity was completely inhibited by rifampicin, at an early stage of the transcription process. However, in cells, inhibition of the total VSV-directed RNA synthesis was only decreased by 50%. In the latter case, the synthesis of 13–18 S mRNA was found to be preferentially inhibited in the presence of the drug (100–200 µg/ml), while no change was evident in the amount of 42 S replicative RNA or 28 S mRNA (MOREAU and SANZEY 1977). Viral proteins accumulated in the cytoplasm when rifampicin was present during the first half of the replication cycle (1–4 h postinfection); no such effect was observed when the drug was present at the end of the cycle (4–7 h postinfection). Analysis of the viral proteins synthesized when the drug was present during the first part of the cycle revealed alterations in the relative amounts of two proteins; the quantity of one protein was elevated while that of the other was diminished. The latter protein, which in the case of the wild-type virus is normally inserted into the cell membrane immediately after synthesis, was found predominantly in the free form in cells infected with the mutant in the presence or absence of rifampicin. The authors concluded that the primary defect in the sensitive mutant was in the transcriptase. This mutation, in the presence of rifampicin, resulted in transcriptional and translational abnormalities. The fact that a virus membrane protein did not associate normally with the cell membrane suggested that enveloping of the virus might also be defective in this mutant.

V. Inhibition of Retrovirus Functions by Rifamycins

The retroviruses are a group of RNA viruses, widely distributed among vertebrates, which possess an enzyme capable of transcribing RNA into DNA. This enzyme, the reverse transcriptase or RNA-dependent DNA polymerase, was first discovered by TEMIN and MIZUTANI (1970) in Rous sarcoma virus and by BALTIMORE (1970) in Rauscher leukemia virus, and subsequently in many other retroviruses (GREEN et al. 1970; SPIEGELMAN et al. 1970). Briefly, the enzyme is involved in the replication of the retroviruses, a multistep process in which both viral and cellular functions participate (reviewed by BISHOP 1978). The single-stranded RNA genome is transcribed into DNA, passing through an RNA–DNA hybrid (ROKUTANDA et al. 1970; SPIEGELMAN et al. 1970) to a double-stranded DNA form which integrates into the cellular genome. This proviral DNA is subsequently transcribed by a cellular polymerase into RNA, which in part serves as mRNA for the synthesis of viral proteins, in part as genome for virus progeny. Following assembly, progeny bud through the host cell plasma membrane, acquiring their characteristic envelope.

Many retroviruses are oncogenic. They induce neoplastic transformation of fibroblasts in vitro, a property which is specified by the viral *src* gene, and transformation of a variety of cell types in vivo, depending on the particular virus. Other retroviruses acquire oncogenic potential by genetic recombination with cellular genes and/or other viruses of the host; the mechanism by which this oncogenicity is mediated is not clearly understood.

Because the replication cycle of these viruses is complex, there are many potential sites at which their multiplication can be blocked by antiviral agents. The fact that reverse transcription is an obligatory function for virus replication and cell transformation renders the search for specific inhibitors of this enzyme particularly worthwhile. The finding of such inhibitors would be invaluable for studying the possible role of this type of enzyme in normal cellular processes, as proposed by TEMIN (1971), as well as in human oncogenesis. Ansamycin compounds appear suitable for this purpose because of the mechanism by which they express antibacterial activity, that is, by specifically interacting with the bacterial polymerase, and because of their activity, albeit modest, against vaccinia and some representatives of the herpesvirus family.

Interest in the ansamycins as antiviral agents was stimulated by the finding that chemical modification of rifampicin, which is inactive against the reverse transcriptase of RNA tumor viruses, yielded compounds which were effective inhibitors of the enzyme (GURGO et al. 1971 b; GREEN et al. 1971) as well as the RNA-dependent DNA polymerase activity present in human leukemia cells (GALLO et al. 1970, 1971). Subsequently, large-scale screening programs were carried out to identify additional, more powerful inhibitors (GURGO et al. 1972; YANG et al. 1972), new derivatives were synthesized and tested for efficacy (TISCHLER et al. 1973, 1974; FROLOVA et al. 1977), and the mechanism of inhibition of the reverse transcriptase was investigated (GURGO et al. 1974, 1975; WU and GALLO 1974; GURGO and GRANDGENETT 1977; FROLOVA et al. 1977). As will be discussed in Sect. 4, several compounds were systematically tested in cell culture and found to inhibit virus replication and cell transformation and to have selective cytotoxicity for transformed cells; in animal model systems, they were found to delay the onset or prevent the occurrence of experimental neoplasms induced by RNA tumor viruses and chemical carcinogens and to have growth inhibitory activity for some established tumor lines in vitro and in vivo.

1. Search for Selective Inhibitors of the Reverse Transcriptase

In the initial studies, it was found that rifampicin was inactive against the reverse transcriptase of retroviruses; removal of the methyl group from the amino-piperazine side chain or substitution of the methyl with a benzyl group provided

Table 1. Nomenclature of selected rifamycin derivatives

Laboratory code	Chemical name
AF/AMP (Rifampicin)	3-(4-Methylpiperazinoiminomethyl)-rifamycin SV
AF/AP (N-demethylrifampicin)	3-(Piperazinoiminomethyl)-rifamycin SV
AF/ABDMP (DMB)	3-(4-Benzyl-2,6-dimethylpiperazinoimino-methyl)-rifamycin SV
AF/DNFI	3-(2,4-Dinitrophenylhydrazonomethyl)-rifamycin SV
AF/CPEDI	3-(Cyclopentadecylhydrazonomethyl)-rifamycin SV
AF/DPI	3-(Dipropylhydrazonomethyl)-rifamycin SV
AF	3-Formylrifamycin SV
AF–013	3-Formylrifamycin SV: 0-n-octyloxime
AF–05	3-Formylrifamycin SV: 0-(diphenylmethyl)-oxime
PR/19	3′-Acetyl-1′-benzyl-2′-methylpyrrolo-[3,2-c]-4-desoxyrifamycin SV
C–27	3-(4-Dicyclohexylmethylpiperidyl)-rifamycin SV
R–8$_2$	3-(Dioctylhydrazonomethyl)-rifamycin SV
M/27	Rifamide

a weak (AF/AP) and an effective (AF/ABDMP) inhibitor of the viral enzyme, respectively (GURGO et al. 1971 b; see Fig. 1 and Table 1 for structures and nomenclature). On the basis of this finding, several hundred rifamycins were systematically screened in order to identify more powerful inhibitors. Of the compounds tested, the most effective belonged to the oxime and hydrazone derivatives of rifamycin SV (GURGO et al. 1972; YANG et al. 1972) and to the 3-cyclic amine derivatives (GREEN et al. 1972). When potent inhibitors of the viral reverse transcriptase were tested against purified mammalian DNA polymerases (YANG et al. 1972; GALLO et al. 1972; GREEN et al. 1972, 1974a, b), little selectivity was observed.

Subsequently, SETHI and OKANO (1976) further investigated the selectivity of the inhibitory effects by examining the relative inhibition of several additional enzymes by a group of 20 compounds. These enzymes included: simian sarcoma virus (SSV) DNA polymerase; cytoplasmic DNA polymerases α and β, nuclear RNA polymerases I and II, and cytoplasmic poly(A) polymerase, all from mouse embryos; and fructose-1,6 diphosphatase. Drugs and enzymes were preincubated in the presence of bovine serum albumin (BSA). AF-05, AF-013, and a formylhydrazone derivative were the most effective inhibitors of all the polymerases. AF/DNFI was the most selective, since at the highest concentration used, 100 µg/ml, it failed to inhibit cellular DNA polymerases, was a moderate inhibitor of the other polymerases, and at 40 µg/ml inhibited the viral enzyme by 50%. None of the compounds used inhibited fructose-1,6 diphosphatase.

FROLOVA et al. (1977) also reported the finding of selective inhibitors among a group of ten newly synthesized hydrazone derivatives of rifamycin SV. The inhibitory activity of the drugs against purified avian myeloblastosis virus (AMV) DNA polymerase was compared with that against E. coli DNA polymerase and calf thymus DNA polymerase β. Among the compounds tested, the 3-(ethylhydrazonomethyl) rifamycin SV, CH_3-CH_2-NH-N$=$CH-R, was inactive, but a slight modification converted this compound into a strong inhibitor of the viral polymerase. The latter derivative, 3-(monoallylhydrazonomethyl) rifamycin SV or $CH_2=$

CH-CH$_2$-NH-N$=$CH-R, was a selective inhibitor inasmuch as it was a very weak inhibitor of the bacterial and cellular DNA polymerases. Other compounds, such as 3-(2,3,6-trinitrophenylhydrazonomethyl) rifamycin SV, were strong inhibitors of all the polymerases tested, with an EC$_{50}$ (concentration giving 50% inhibition) of 13–15 µg/ml.

Forty-four 3- and 4-substituted compounds were tested at various concentrations against purified reverse transcriptase, terminal transferase, and DNA polymerases α, β, and γ (Dicioccio and Srivastava 1978). The rifamycins utilized in these studies included 3-iminomethyl, 3-formylhydrazone, 3-formyloxime, 3,4-pyrrole derivatives, and various other compounds substituted in the 3 or 4 positions. It was confirmed that the most effective inhibitors of the reverse transcriptase were derivatives with long carbon chains in the 3 position. The introduction of an aromatic moiety in the side chain did not always confer increased activity as was the case with rifampicin and the related compound AF/ABDMP. Strong inhibitors of the reverse transcriptase were also strong inhibitors of purified cell DNA polymerases when comparable protein concentrations were used. However, it was demonstrated that rifamycins bind more tightly to the reverse transcriptase than to mammalian DNA polymerases, and that they are, therefore, selective inhibitors of the viral enzyme. This was shown by using BSA as a competitor of the binding reaction between drug and enzyme. When BSA was added at 250 µg/ml to assay mixtures containing representative derivatives, at inhibitory concentrations, the reverse transcriptase and terminal transferase were inhibited as efficiently as in the absence of BSA. On the contrary, DNA polymerases α, β, and γ were not inhibited under these conditions. Thus, in a population of proteins containing the reverse transcriptase, terminal transferase, and cellular DNA polymerases, the first two would be selectively inhibited.

2. Correlation Between Lipophilicity and Antipolymerase Activity

The effective reverse transcriptase inhibitors identified in the screening studies shared as a common structural feature a bulky, lipophilic substituent in the 3 position. In order to investigate the relationship between lipophilicity and efficacy on the reverse transcriptase systematically, Tischler et al. (1974) designed two groups of derivatives: (1) a series of rifazacyclo derivatives containing in the di-substituted hydrazone group cyclic aliphatic chains of varying sizes; and (2) an analogous series of rifazone derivatives containing two aliphatic chains of equal, but increasing lengths. When the lipophilicity of these compounds was examined, a direct correlation was found between the number of carbon atoms in the side chain and the lipophilicity, as measured by a reversed phase thin layer chromatographic technique. Furthermore, the effectiveness of these compounds against the reverse transcriptase increased as a function of increasing lipophilicity. The ability to inhibit the viral enzyme selectively, in comparison with the bacterial DNA polymerase, also increased with increasing lipophilicity (Thompson et al. 1974).

Wu et al. (1980) recently carried out a similar study with a group of 22 selected compounds representing a wide range of lipophilicities and molecular sizes. The effect of the compounds, which included hydrazone and oxime derivatives, was tested on purified SSV reverse transcriptase and α and β mammalian DNA polymerases. The results of the study showed that the activity of the compounds was linearly related to the partition coefficient, an index of lipophilicity. In agreement with TISCHLER's observation, increasing size and lipophilicity favored increased inhibitory activity against the reverse transcriptase. The viral enzyme was generally more sensitive than the mammalian polymerases, but none of the compounds tested was strongly selective. The most selective was 3-(diethylaminomethyl) rifamycin SV which inhibited the cellular polymerases with EC_{50} values 25 times that for the reverse transcriptase. This derivative was among the least hydrophobic of the derivatives tested.

It seems appropriate to mention here that some controversy existed in the past concerning the ability of lipophilic inhibitors of the reverse transcriptase to inhibit enzymes nonspecifically when the drugs are used at high concentrations (RIVA et al. 1972; GERARD et al. 1973). Careful studies by GERARD and co-workers demonstrated that a battery of nonpolymerizing enzymes were not inhibited by selected rifamycins at very high molecular ratios of drug to enzyme, while several polymerizing enzymes were inhibited at much lower ratios. Effects observed at very high drug concentrations of lipophilic derivatives should be cautiously considered, since it is known that these compounds tend to form aggregates under such conditions.

3. Mechanism of Inhibition of the Reverse Transcriptase

Several rifamycin SV derivatives, chosen from among the most effective inhibitors of the reverse transcriptase, were utilized to study the mechanism by which the enzyme is inhibited. These included: AF/ABDMP, AF/DNFI, AF-013, and C-27. The type of drug–enzyme interaction, as well as the step of transcription sensitive to the action of the drugs, was investigated.

Analysis of the effect of the various derivatives on the initial velocity of polymerization demonstrated that these compounds bind to the enzyme with a cooperative type of interaction (GURGO et al. 1974). Hill analysis of kinetic data suggested the binding of several molecules to a hydrophobic region distant from the active center. The inhibitors do not compete with deoxytriphosphate substrates or template–primer for binding on the enzyme (GURGO et al. 1974; WU and GALLO 1974; FROLOVA et al. 1977). The degree of interaction and the number of bound drug molecules, estimated to be from three to seven by Hill analysis, varies with the structure of the compound. Direct measurement with radioactively labeled AF/ ABDMP demonstrated that a minimum of two molecules bind tightly to each molecule of enzyme (WU and GALLO 1974). The binding of the drug to the enzyme is reversible (GURGO et al. 1974; WU and GALLO 1974).

The rate constant of inactivation of the reverse transcriptase by AF/DNFI was one order of magnitude lower than the rate constant of inactivation of *E. coli* RNA polymerase by rifampicin. Preincubation of the enzyme with template–primer confers protection to the enzyme when drug and substrates are added simultaneously; if drug is added before substrate, the subsequent inhibition depends on the time of incubation of the enzyme–template complex with the drug and on the drug concentration. The rate constant of inactivation of the enzyme–template complex was one order of magnitude lower than that of the free enzyme. In analogy with the bacterial system, the apparent template protection effect is the result of a rapid formation of enzyme–template complex and to a reduced rate of inactivation of the enzyme–template complex by the drug with respect to that of the free enzyme. The enzyme is in its most resistant form when bound to the template and growing product.

The derivatives AF-013, AF/DNFI, and C-27, which have major differences in the structure of the side chain component, were compared for their ability to inhibit the enzyme when added during the reaction of polymerization (Gurgo and Grandgenett 1977). These compounds, which have comparable activity when added prior to the template, can be distinguished on the basis of their behavior when added during the reaction of DNA synthesis. C-27 had no effect on the size of the DNA chains already initiated, at a dose 50 times that necessary to give 50% inhibition (EC_{50}) if added before template and primer; no new chains are initiated. At much lower doses, i.e., 2–4 times the EC_{50}, AF-013 and AF/DNFI inhibited elongation, as judged by the reduction of the size of the DNA synthesized in the presence of the drug. Thus it appears that C-27 is a selective inhibitor of an initial step of polymerization. With a different approach, Milavetz et al. (1976) likewise observed that different rifamycin derivatives and analogs inhibit the reverse transcriptase at different stages of transcription. According to their studies: (1) rifamycin SV and related compounds such as streptovaricin C inhibit the reverse transcriptase by preventing the dissociation of the enzyme from the template; (2) AF/ABDMP prevents the formation of the enzyme–template–primer complex; and (3) AF-013 increases the dissociation of reverse transcriptase from template and template–primer. These findings support the idea that the antipolymerase activity of rifamycins can be modulated by structural modification to provide derivatives with increased specificity.

4. Effects of Rifamycins on Virus Replication and Cell Transformation

Several rifamycins have been reported to inhibit virus replication and/or cell transformation. As for the former, the antiviral effects identified were expressed: (1) soon after infection, in such a manner as to suggest an interaction of the drug with the reverse transcriptase; (2) concomitant with the appearance of the transformed phenotype, suggesting inhibition of cellular functions involved in virus replication, perhaps at the transcriptional level; or (3) as a result of cumulative effects which lead to the production of noninfectious particles. As for the effect of rifamycins on transformation, in some instances this has been attributed to interference with an initial event, such as inhibition of reverse transcriptase activity; in other cases as the consequence of cytotoxicity arising with morphological and metabolic changes of the transformed cells. As will be discussed in this section, a variety of inhibitory effects have been noted in cell culture; to a certain extent, this may be a reflection of the major structural differences of the rifamycins utilized in these studies.

a) Correlation Between Inhibition of Reverse Transcriptase and Inhibition of Viral Functions

A positive correlation was observed between the ability of several 3-substituted rifamycins to inhibit the reverse transcriptase activity of RNA tumor viruses and their ability to inhibit: (1) in vitro replication of Rauscher leukemia virus (RLV) and focus formation induced by Moloney sarcoma virus (TING et al. 1972); and (2) in vivo RLV-induced leukomogenesis, as judged by splenomegaly (WU et al. 1973). Virus preparations were preincubated with the drugs at 100 μg/ml for 30 min at 37 °C. Before the treated samples were used to infect cells in vitro or to inject mice for in vivo studies, they were diluted in order to avoid cytotoxic effects in the former case and to reduce the amount of free drug injected in the latter case. Among the most active compounds tested were AF/ABDP, AF/DNFI, and AF-013; less active were rifamycin SV, AF/AP, and PR/3. Rifampicin, which is not an inhibitor of the reverse transcriptase, was a moderate inhibitor of splenomegaly. It was suggested that this could have been due to a metabolic conversion of the drug to AF/AP (CRICCHIO et al. 1975). On the basis of these experiments, it was inferred that the drugs acted through a blockade of reverse transcriptase activity, thus inhibiting a viral function essential for cell transformation in vitro and malignant transformation of lymphocytes in vivo. It could not be excluded, however, that other factors essential to virus replication and cell transformation might also be sensitive to the drugs (GALLO 1971). GIELKINS et al. (1972) likewise reported an effect of rifampicin on RLV-induced leukemogenesis, when the drug was administered orally at high doses, whereas SINKOVICS (1971) found AF/AP, but not rifampicin, to be active in the same system when a dose of 3 mg/day was injected intraperitoneally.

An analogous positive correlation was found by GREEN et al. (1972) between the ability of several 3-cyclic amine derivatives of rifamycin SV to inhibit the reverse transcriptase in vitro and block focus formation in BALB/3T3 cells infected with Moloney sarcoma virus. The compounds were present in the medium from 1 h after infection until the medium change 3–4 days later; the assay for focus formation was done 6 days after infection. The drugs were active on transformation at concentrations of 1–5 μg/ml with only slight effects on cell proliferation noted. The compounds which were active against both the viral transcriptase and transformation were also inhibitory for a DNA polymerase from the mammalian KB cell line, although 5–10 times higher concentrations were required for an effect comparable to that seen with the viral enzyme. Because of this finding, it was not clear whether the effect on cell transformation was due to inhibition of the viral enzyme, cell polymerase, or possibly both. A subsequent report showed that several of the most active compounds also inhibited splenomegaly induced by Friend virus when they were injected in multiple doses from the time of virus inoculation (RANA et al. 1975).

AF/ABDMP, a strong inhibitor of the reverse transcriptase, has been found to be effective on both virus replication and cell transformation. CALVIN et al. (1971) first reported the effect of this drug on Moloney sarcoma virus infection of BALB/3T3 cells. When AF/ABDMP was added at 10 μg/ml after virus adsorption, foci of transformation were completely suppressed, infectious virus reduced by a factor of 50, and cell proliferation by a factor of 3, at 7 days after infection. The latter effect was not considered sufficiently severe to account for the strong effect on transformation.

Using the same system and varying the time of drug addition, HACKETT et al. (1972) found that 24 h exposure of the infected cells to 3 μg/ml, a dose noninhibitory for cell growth, was sufficient to prevent transformation, provided that it was added between 36 and 72 h after infection. Once transformation was established, the drug was no longer effective. Complete inhibition of virus growth was achieved when cells were infected at low multiplicity; at high multiplicity, the inhibitory effect was overcome. In another report, 6 µg/ml AF/ABDMP inhibited, by 70%–80%, focus formation induced by Moloney leukemia virus on UBC-1 cells, a BALB/3T3-derived line transformable by Moloney leukemia virus. A moderate reduction (20%–30%) of XC plaques induced by Moloney leukemia virus was also observed (HACKETT and SYLVESTER 1972a, b).

In order to rule out the possibility that the effect of AF/ABDMP on transformation and virus replication was the result of cytotoxic effects, SMITH and HACKETT(1974) selected a variant of BALB/3T3 which grows in the presence of the drug. The plating efficiency of the resistant cell line was unaffected by the presence of AF/ABDMP (10 µg/ml) and amphotericin B (1 µg/ml) while the growth of the parental BALB/3T3 line was completely inhibited. In the presence of the drugs, transformation induced by Moloney sarcoma virus was completely blocked; transformation of the same cells by the DNA virus SV40 was not affected. The authors suggested that the antiviral effect was the result of an interaction of the drug with the viral reverse transcriptase.

An interesting in vivo effect of AF/ABDMP was reported by JOSS et al. (1973) who observed a significant delay in the onset and subsequent growth of chemically induced mammary tumors in rats treated with the drug. Intraperitoneal injections of 4–10 mg were given at 7-day intervals for 20 days after the administration of the chemical carcinogen, benzanthracene. R-8_2 was less effective than AF/ABDMP, and RC-16, dirifampin, and rifampicin were ineffective (HUGHES and CALVIN 1976).

It is possible that the effect was due to antiviral activity of the drug, since there is evidence to support the idea that chemical carcinogenesis involves the activation of latent viruses (IGEL et al. 1969). Considering, however, the selective cytotoxicity of several rifamycins for cells morphologically transformed in tissue culture by retroviruses and for malignant versus normal activated lymphocytes (SMITH et al. 1972), antitumor activity observed in laboratory animals could be the consequence of cytotoxicity. For example, effects of rifamycin SV on the growth of a transplantable tumor, the Walker 256 carcinosarcoma, could be correlated with the in vitro cytotoxicity of the drug on three tumor lines (ADAMSON 1971). The ability of these drugs to mediate cytotoxicity might in part be due to their antipolymerase activity, as extensively demonstrated with the inhibition of various mammalian polymerizing enzymes (reviewed in GURGO 1980) and in tissue culture with the inhibition of RNA and DNA synthesis when the drugs are used at sufficiently high concentrations.

b) Inhibition of Virus Replication

In this section are reported studies in which the observed antiviral activity of rifamycin derivatives is unlikely to be mediated by interaction of the drugs with the viral reverse transcriptase, and appears, instead, to be due to interference with later steps in virus multiplication, with cellular functions involved in virus replication, or to multiple effects.

Two oxime derivatives, AF-05 and AF-013, were shown to inhibit the replication of Rous sarcoma virus selectively (Schmidt-Ruppin strain) in transformed chick cells (BARLATI and VIGIER 1972 a, b). The derivatives were added at 20 µg/ml at the time of infection, but their effect on free virus production was not evident until 2–3 days later, concomitant with the appearance of the transformed pheno-type. The drugs had no effect on the ability of virus to cause transformation, al-though the foci formed were smaller in size. In order to demonstrate that the sen-sitivity of virus production depended on the transformed phenotype, a tempera-ture-sensitive mutant was used which replicates at 37° and 41 °C, but maintains the transformed state only at the permissive temperature (37 °C). After transformation had occurred at 37 °C, the cells were divided into two parts and incubated 24 h at 37° or 41 °C; in the latter case, the transformed phenotype disappeared. The incu-bation was continued an additional 24 h in the presence of AF-013, and the free virus titer was then determined. Virus production was inhibited in the mutant-transformed cells maintained at 37 °C and in cells transformed by wild-type virus maintained at either temperature; no inhibition was observed in the mutant-trans-formed cells "detransformed" by incubation at 41 °C. The inhibition was not due to the production of virus with decreased infectivity, since a reduction in physical particles accompanied the reduction in free virus titers. The drugs did not appear to be cytotoxic to normal or transformed cells at the dose used to inhibit virus rep-lication, and DNA synthesis was not significantly altered. The authors suggested that synthesis of viral RNA, or later steps in virus multiplication, such as viral pro-tein synthesis or assembly, could be the target of the drug.

R-8_2, a potent inhibitor of the reverse transcriptase, has been shown to have antiviral activity as well. Growth of established Rous sarcoma virus-transformed cells in the presence of 15 µg/ml R-8_2 reduced the infectivity of the progeny by 99% after 1 day, whereas particle production was reduced much more slowly. The re-duction in the number of particles was attributed to a cytotoxic effect on trans-formed cells, since it was not seen when the cells were infected with a transforma-tion defective strain of Rous sarcoma virus (SZABO et al. 1976). In an earlier report (BISSELL et al. 1974), R-8_2 had been shown to be selectively cytotoxic for trans-formed cells.

Analysis of the particles formed in the presence of R-8_2 revealed a decrease in their average buoyant density, from 1.16 to 1.14 g/ml (SZABO and BISSELL 1978); the particles were deficient in 60–70 S RNA and contained, instead, low molecular weight RNA. Control experiments, in which mature Rous sarcoma virus was incu-bated with the drug, excluded the possibility that simple binding of the highly li-pophilic drug could result in the disruption of the normal structure and consequent loss of infectivity. The lack of 60–70 S RNA appeared to be the ultimate cause of the loss of infectivity. It was suggested that R-8_2, an inhibitor of polymerases, might interfere with viral RNA transcription. The abnormal density of the parti-cles could be due to interference of the drug with assembly or the failure of a full complement of proteins to be synthesized. R-8_2 also inhibited focus formation when added at 3–10 µg/ml shortly after infection (BISSELL et al. 1974). It appeared that this was the result of cumulative effects, including inhibition of reverse tran-scriptase activity, cytotoxicity for transformed cells, and production of noninfec-tious particles.

SHANNON et al. (1974) studied the effect of rifamycin SV and several strong in-hibitors of the reverse transcriptase on Gross virus replication in NIH Swiss mouse embryo cells, using the UV-XC plaque reduction assay. Rifamycin SV, although a weak inhibitor of the viral enzyme, was the most effective compound in achieving good antiviral effects at noncytotoxic doses. A linear dose-dependent effect was observed between 0.1 and 10 µg/ml, with 50% inhibition of plaque formation at 1 µg/ml. Cell viability was strongly impaired after 4 days exposure to the other derivatives – AF-05, AF/DPI, and AF/CPEDI – at 10 µg/ml. No significant antiviral effect was obtained in this system at noncytotoxic concentrations of these drugs.

c) Effects on Cell Transformation

Diggelman and Weissman (1969) reported that rifampicin strongly inhibited transformation of chick fibroblasts by Rous sarcoma virus, as measured by focus formation. The drug was used at 60 µg/ml, a concentration that was not cytotoxic to normal chick cells and only slightly inhibitory to production of Rous sarcoma virus. Experiments in which the drug was present during different time periods after infection demonstrated that there was a critical period, from 36 to 60 h, during which the drug was active. If the drug was added late after infection, presumably after transformation had occurred, there was no effect on focus formation.

According to Vaheri and Hanafusa (1971), rifampicin suppresses focus formation induced by Rous sarcoma virus via an effect on the growth of transformed cells rather than an effect on the transforming event. When rifampicin or its derivative AF/AP was added at 60–80 µg/ml prior to infection, the drugs had little if any effect on transformation, as judged by morphological and metabolic markers, or on virus replication. If added to cultures of established transformed cells, the drugs were inhibitory to focus formation at 20–40 µg/ml; both the number of foci and the number of cells per focus were reduced by 50% or more, depending on the drug and its concentration. Since, in the system used, each focus develops from the multiplication of one transformed cell and not by recruitment of neighboring cells by infection, the effect on focus formation reflects only effects on growth of the transformed cell and not on virus production by that cell. After 3 days incubation with 60 µg/ml of rifampicin, the viability of transformed cells was severely reduced, whereas the growth and viability of uninfected chick fibroblasts were unaffected by similar treatment. AF/AP was slightly less toxic. The selective cytotoxic effect on transformed cells was not due to increased uptake of the drug, since normal and transformed cells accumulated comparable amounts of labeled rifampicin.

Another study on this subject by Robinson and Robinson (1971) found that rifampicin was also toxic to normal chick fibroblasts. It is probable that the discrepancies in the results reported by these groups of investigators are due to differences in the experimental conditions used, and that the effect of rifampicin on focus formation is the result of an inhibitory effect on proliferation of transformed cells.

Several naturally occurring rifamycins were shown to inhibit the transformation of human fetal spleen cells by feline sarcoma virus (FSV; O'Connor et al. 1974). Rifamycins SV and S depressed focus formation by 100% and 50%, respectively, when added at 4 µg/ml shortly after infection; rifamycins O and B were less effective, in that order (Figs. 1 and 2). None of these rifamycins significantly inhibited poly(A)·oligo d(T)-directed reverse transcriptase activity of simian sarcoma virus, nor did they affect cellular DNA and RNA polymerases at drug levels of 100 µg/ml. Among the 3-substituted rifamycin SV derivatives tested, rifampicin and a group of compounds with strong activity against the reverse transcriptase and cellular polymerases (AF-013, AF/ABDMP, and AF/DNFI) behaved as moderate inhibitors of focus formation. The plot of inhibition of focus formation versus drug concentration was relatively flat compared with that obtained for rifamycins SV, S, and O over the range tested (1–8 µg/ml). In mouse 3T3 cells infected with Moloney sarcoma virus, the results obtained with the two groups of drugs were more comparable. The drugs were used below the threshold of cytotoxicity, as judged by effects on cell growth and on the incorporation of labeled precursors into RNA, DNA, and protein; effects on one or more of these parameters were manifested at 10 µg/ml with some of the derivatives.

Rifamycin S significantly decreased the virus yield of 3T3 cells infected with Moloney sarcoma virus when added shortly after infection at 4–6 µg/ml, but had no effect on virus yield when added to cultures of previously transformed, actively virus-shedding cells. It was suggested that the rifamycins inhibited morphological transformation by interfering with an early viral function at a stage between penetration and replication.

E. Pharmacology of Rifampicin

It is beyond the scope of this chapter to review the enormous literature on the pharmacologic aspects of the rifamycins; a comprehensive summary of animal and human studies done at the time of the introduction of rifampicin into antibacterial therapy has been published by BINDA et al. (1971). Some relevant considerations will, however, be presented.

Briefly, after oral doses of rifampicin which are standard for long-term treatment of tuberculosis (600 mg/day), serum levels of the drug increase over a period of several hours, then peak, and rapidly decline throughout the remainder of the 24-h period. Depending on the particular schedule of administration, peaks of up to 25 µg/ml can be obtained, but these are exceptional and are not maintained for extended periods of time. Some attempts have been made to increase the mean serum levels of the drug by administering probenecid, a substance used to exend the half-life of other antibiotics, in combination with rifampicin. A report was made by KENWRIGHT and LEVI (1973) that the use of probenecid resulted in a 100% increase in serum levels of rifampicin in humans. In this study, the maximum levels obtained were about 8 µg/ml, even with the use of probenecid, when 300 mg rifampicin was administered orally. A subsequent study did not confirm the effect (FALLON et al. 1975). As mentioned earlier in this review, the concentrations of rifampicin required for effects in vitro against vaccinia virus are in the range of 100 µg/ml. Considering the information available in the literature concerning the maximal levels obtainable, there seems to be no place for the therapeutic application of rifampicin for viral infections in humans, at the present.

F. Antiviral Activity of Other Ansamycins

The streptovaricins, tolypomycins, and geldanamycin are antibiotics which are chemically closely related to rifamycins; they all contain an aromatic nucleus

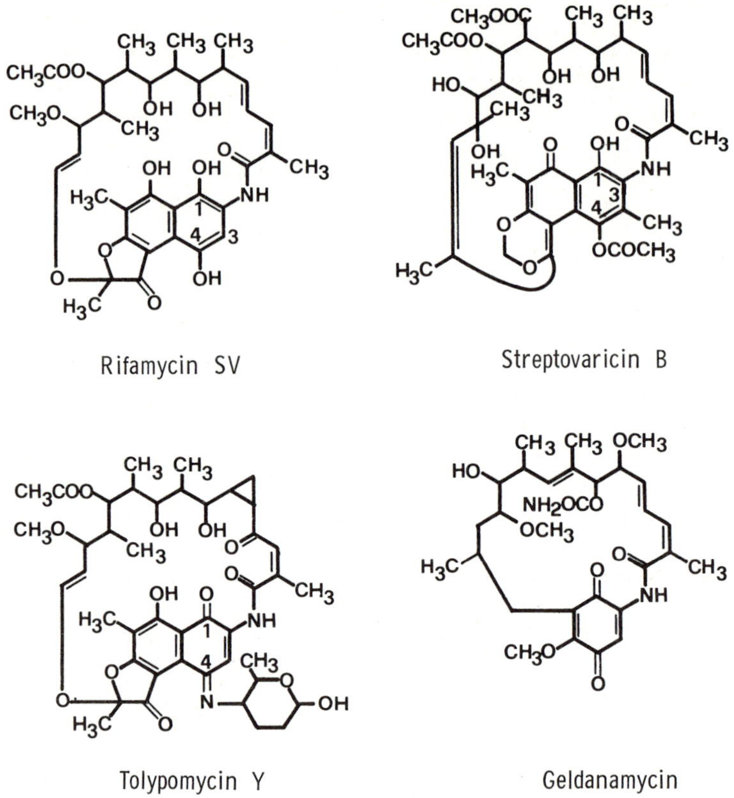

Fig. 2. Structures of ansamycins. The structures of rifamycin SV and related ansamycin antibiotics are illustrated. For the structures of other naturally occurring ansamycins, see Wehrli (1977) and Brufani (1977)

spanned by an aliphatic ansa bridge (Fig. 2). The former two compounds inhibit the bacterial RNA polymerase (Mizuno et al. 1968 a, b), although to a lesser extent than rifampicin. Both drugs competitively inhibit the binding of rifampicin to the bacterial enzyme, thus demonstrating that all three bind to the same site (Wehrli and Staehelin 1971). Rifampicin, streptovaricins, and tolypomycin Y are highly active against gram-positive bacteria; rifampicin and streptovaricins also against *Mycobacterium tuberculosis*. The streptovaricins have not been widely used as antibiotics because of their smaller therapeutic efficiency and higher toxicity compared with rifampicin; tolypomycin Y is chemically unstable and thus has not been introduced into therapeutic use (Brufani 1977). Geldanamycin has primarily antiparasitic activity.

I. Streptovaricins

The streptovaricins are a group of antibiotics produced by *Streptomyces spectabilis*. Like rifamycins, they possess a naphthalene chromophore spanned by an ansa bridge. The eight components (A–G, J) which can be isolated from the strep-tovaricin complex differ from one another in the extent of oxidation and acetyla-tion (see RINEHART 1972; BRUFANI 1977; WEHRLI 1977 for reviews).

1. Effects on Vaccinia Virus

SUBAK-SHARPE et al. (1969) reported that streptovaricin, at 100 µg/ml, had no ef-fect on vaccinia growth in BHK cells. In a subsequent study, however, QUINTRELL and MCAUSLAN (1970) found that the streptovaricin complex was effective in blocking the growth of cowpox virus in HeLa cells and chick embryo fibroblasts at levels between 2 and 10 µg/ml. The numbers of vaccinia and rabbitpox plaques were relatively unaffected by the same doses of the drug, but the size was reduced by 50%, indicating a possible inhibition. Streptovaricins A and C, the major com-ponents of the complex, were without effect on any of the three viruses tested in either cell system. Thus, it was suggested that the active component was a minor species of the complex.

In contrast to rifampicin, streptovaricin was an inhibitor of an early function in this system. When added at the time of infection, it markedly reduced the rate of viral DNA synthesis; if added 1 h after infection, i.e., after the initiation of DNA synthesis, it was less effective. Although high concentrations of the drug did not inhibit RNA synthesis carried on by viral cores in vitro, that carried on by un-coated viral cores in vivo was greatly reduced by 5–10 µg/ml streptovaricin, indi-cating an effect on early mRNA synthesis. The finding that streptovaricin inhibits an early viral function very likely explains the apparent conflict between the reports of SUBAK-SHARPE et al. (1969) and QUINTRELL and MCAUSLAN (1970); the former investigators added the drug after a 1-h virus adsorption period, presumably after early events were under way. In the assay system of PENNINGTON and FOLLETT (1971), streptovaricin showed only a weak ability to maintain the rifampicin-in-duced maturation block of vaccinia in BHK cells; concentrations of 1 mg/ml were required.

2. Effect on Retrovirus Functions

CARTER et al. (1971) demonstrated a relatively selective effect on cell transforma-tion by streptovaricin inhibitors of the reverse transcriptase. Streptovaricin com-plex and purified streptovaricin D partially inhibited transformation of BALB/3T3 cells by Moloney sarcoma virus at noncytotoxic drug levels, 2 and 20 µg/ml, respectively. Streptovaricin A, which is not an inhibitor of the reverse transcrip-tase, did not affect focus formation, even at doses close to cytotoxicity (80 µg/ml). Inhibition of an initial viral function was suggested, since the drugs were ineffective when added 24 h after infection.

Oral administration of streptovaricin complex, at 1.5 mg kg^{-1} day^{-1}, reduced Rauscher leukemia virus-induced splenomegaly in mice by a factor of two (BORDEN et al. 1971). This dose resulted in a relatively constant serum level of 1–3 µg/ml; it was not toxic, as judged by final body weight, nor did it reduce spleen weight in uninfected mice. It had no effect on the formation of splenic foci by normal he-matopoietic cells nor did it affect splenomegaly induced by L1210, a transplantable murine lymphoma. Thus the results argued against a direct cytotoxic effect of streptovaricin and suggested, instead, that the drug functioned by blocking a virus-induced event, probably involving the reverse transcriptase of Rauscher leukemia virus.

II. Tolypomycins

The tolypomycins are antibiotics produced by *Streptomyces tolypophorus*. One of the components, tolopomycin Y, has been isolated and found to be related to rifamycin S (KISHI et al. 1972). The aromatic part of the molecule, prepared by hydrolysis, is identical to a component obtained by chemical degradation of the iminoethyl ester of rifamycin S, thus demonstrating that tolypomycins and rifamycins have the same naphthoquinone moiety. Tolypomycin R, at 300 µg/ml, was capable of maintaining the maturation block produced by rifampicin in vaccinia-infected BHK cells (PENNINGTON and FOLLETT 1971).

III. Geldanamycin and Related Compounds

Geldanamycin is produced by *Streptomyces hygroscopicus*. It differs from the other described ansamycins, both in the aromatic moiety, which is a benzoquinone ring, and in the aliphatic ansa chain; it follows, however, the same biosynthetic pathway as rifamycins and streptovaricins. Two additional groups of ansamycins have been described which are structurally related to geldanamycin: (1) the maytansinoids, of plant origin (KUPCHAN et al. 1972); and (2) the ansamitocins, which are produced by a strain of *Nocardia* (HIGASHIDE et al. 1977). These antibiotics have a chlorine-subsituted benzene ring as the aromatic nucleus and an ansa bridge (KUP-CHAN et al. 1972; ASAI et al. 1979). Maytansine and geldanamycin have been reported to inhibit transformation of mouse cells infected with Moloney sarcoma virus (O'CONNOR et al. 1975). Maytansine and the ansamitocins have been shown to have activity against a variety of experimental murine tumors and appear to function as antimitotic agents (REMILLARD et al. 1975; ADAMSON et al. 1976; KUP-CHAN et al. 1978; OOTSU et al. 1980).

G. Concluding Remarks

The finding of specific antiviral compounds with a broad range of antiviral activity is a tantalizing prospect, but thus far an unrealized objective. Because mammalian viruses differ with respect to their mechanisms of replication, genetic complexity, associated enzymes, and presence and composition of envelopes and other possible targets, it is unlikely that a compound with broad spectrum antiviral activity will be discovered, or designed from preexisting compounds. Moreover, the fact that viruses utilize some host cell functions in their multiplication cycle renders more difficult the finding of specific antiviral compounds, much in the same way that it is difficult to find drugs specifically cytotoxic for malignant cells.

Rifamycins have been viewed with interest as a potential source of antiviral agents. They are well known for their antibacterial activity which is achieved through inhibition of the DNA-dependent RNA polymerase. Rifampicin also inhibits the growth of many DNA and RNA bacteriophages which utilize the bacterial polymerase for transcription. As has been documented in this review, rifampicin has activity against poxviruses. This activity appears to be specific to this group of viruses since, with few exceptions, the drug is inactive against other DNA viruses and RNA viruses. Although the effect of rifampicin on vaccinia virus multiplication has been the object of many studies, the mechanism by which the block in maturation is mediated is not, as yet, clearly understood. The high drug levels required preclude any clinical application of this compound for poxvirus infections. Attempts to use derivatives active in vitro against the viral polymerase did not provide better antivaccinia agents.

Rifampicin does not interfere specifically with retrovirus replication, and the observed effect on focus formation appears to be related to a preferential cytotoxicity for transformed cells. The possibility of blocking virus replication and cell transformation by inhibiting the activity of the RNA-dependent DNA polymerase contained within the virion was suggested by the finding that the reverse transcriptase of retroviruses and a similar activity present in human leukemic blasts were inhibited by analogs of rifampicin. Subsequent findings that purified DNA polymerases and, in general, polymerizing enzymes were also inhibited did not reduce the initial interest in this class of compounds, since it was known that viruses induce or carry polymerases different from the cellular polymerases.

The work of TING et al. (1972) and WU et al. (1973) suggested that, if drug and virus are allowed to interact closely, a positive correlation between the ability to inhibit virus replication and cell transformation in vitro and in vivo and the ability to inhibit the reverse transcriptase is obtained. However, when various derivatives are added to cell cultures infected with retroviruses, such correlation is not always observed, very likely because of cellular restraints imposed upon derivatives with different structural components. Moreover, it appears that when cytotoxic effects are carefully avoided, rifamycins express antiviral activity by interacting with various steps in virus replication or with cell functions implicated in virus replication, as seems to be the case with the parental antibiotics rifamycin S and SV, which are very weak inhibitors of the viral reverse transcriptase, or with potent inhibitors such as AF-013 and R-8_2. As for the effect on cell transformation, the effectiveness of strong inhibitors of the reverse transcriptase, like AF/ABDMP, varies according to the system used, and in some cases it has been reported that modest or weak inhibitors of the viral enzyme are more effective than strong inhibitors in blocking focus formation. Because of major structural differences in the drugs, and the different responses of various biologic systems, it is not possible to reduce the modes of action of rifamycins to a unique, basic mechanism.

It should be stressed that, thus far, numerous studies have not identified any specific inhibitors of the reverse transcriptase or of any cellular polymerase, with the exception of a few examples of relative selectivity. In particular, the study by WU et al. (1980) demonstrated that increasing the lipophilicity of the compounds does not provide more specific inhibitors. It seems reasonable to assume that, if rifamycin derivatives are to be designed with increased anti-reverse trancriptase activity, the mechanism by which different selected rifamycins inhibit the viral enzyme should be further investigated, since it appears that various derivatives and the parental rifamycin SV inhibit via different mechanisms. It is possible that modifications in the ansa ring and in the chromophore moiety would allow a better fit between the drug and reverse transcriptase. While such modifications may be difficult to obtain chemically, it is not excluded that such compounds could be provided by microorganisms under appropriate growth conditions. Naturally occurring ansamycins which have interesting biologic activity have been described in the literature; examples of such compounds are streptovaricins and tolypomycins (which share the same biosynthetic pathway as rifamycins) and geldanamycin and maytansine. Variants of these compounds continue to be isolated; thus, the search for antiviral and antipolymerase compounds from among the ansamycins has not yet been exhausted.

Acknowledgments. We thank Prof. G. Lancini for useful discussions. We thank Ms. Carolyn E. Mulhall for help in the preparation of the manuscript. This work was supported by the Progetto Finalizzato Virus and by the Controllo della Crescita Neoplastica of the National Council of Research (C.N.R.) of Italy.

References

Adamson R (1971) Antitumor activity of two antiviral drugs – rifampicin and tilorone. Lancet I:398

Adamson RH, Sieber SM, Whang-Peng J, Wood HB (1976) Experimental studies with the antitumor agent maytansine. Proc Am Assoc Cancer Res 17:42

Asai M, Mizuta E, Izawa M, Haibara K, Kishi T (1979) Isolation, chemical characterization and structure of ansamitocin, a new antitumor ansamycin antibiotic. Tetrahedron 35:1079–1085

Baltimore D (1970) RNA-dependent DNA polymerase in virions of RNA tumor viruses. Nature 226:1209–1211

Barlati S, Vigier P (1972a) Effect of two rifamycin derivatives on the Rous sarcoma virus transformation system. J Gen Virol 17:221–225

Barlati S, Vigier P (1972b) Selective inhibition of Rous sarcoma virus production in transformed chick fibroblasts by two rifamycin derivatives. FEBS Letters 24:343–346

Becker Y (1971) Antitrachoma activity of rifamycin B and 8-0-acetylrifamycin S. Nature 231:115–116

Becker Y (1978) The *Chlamydia:* molecular biology of procaryotic obligate parasites of eucaryocytes. Microbiol Rev 42:274–306

Becker Y, Asher Y (1972) Synthesis of trachoma agent proteins in emetine-treated cells. J Bact 109:966–970

Becker Y, Zakay-Rones Z (1969) Rifampicin–A new antitrachoma agent. Nature 222:851–853

Becker Y, Asher Y, Himmel N, Zakay-Rones Z, Maythar B (1969) Rifampicin inhibition of trachoma agent in vivo. Nature 224:33–34

Becker Y, Asher Y, Himmel N, Zakay-Rones Z (1970) Antitrachoma activity of rifampicin and rifamycin SV derivatives. Nature 225:454–455

Ben-Ishai A, Heller E, Goldblum N, Becker Y (1969) Rifampicin and poxvirus replication. Nature 224:29–32

Binda G, Domenichini E, Gottardi A, Orlandi B, Ortelli E, Pacini B, Fowst G (1971) Rifampicin, a general review. Arzneimittel-Forschung 12a:1907–1976

Bishop JM (1978) Retroviruses. Ann Rev Biochem 47:35–88

Bissell M, Hatie C, Tischler A, Calvin M (1974) Preferential inhibition of the growth of virus-transformed cells in culture by rifazone-8_2, a new rifamycin derivative. Proc Natl Acad Sci USA 71:2520–2524

Borden EC, Brockman WW, Carter WA (1971) Selective inhibition by streptovaricin of splenomegaly induced by Rauscher leukemia virus. Nature New Biol 232:214–216

Bouché J, Zechel K, Kornberg A (1975) *dna*G gene product, a rifampicin resistant RNA polymerase, initiates the conversion of a single-stranded coliphage DNA to its duplex replicative form. J Biol Chem 250:5995–6001

Brufani M (1977) The Ansamycins. In: Sammes PG (ed) Topics in antibiotic chemistry, vol 1. Aminoglycosides and ansamycins. Ellis Horwood, Chichester, pp 93–217

Brufani M, Cerrini S, Fedeli W, Vaciago A (1974) Rifamycins: an insight into biological activity based on structural investigations. J Mol Biol 87:409–435

Brutlag D, Schekman R, Kornberg A (1971) A possible role for RNA polymerase in the initiation of M13 DNA synthesis. Proc Natl Acad Sci USA 68:2826–2829

Calvin M, Joss UR, Hackett AJ, Owens RB (1971) Effect of rifampicin and two of its derivatives on cells infected with Moloney sarcoma virus. Proc Natl Acad Sci USA 68:1441–1443

Carter WA, Brockman WW, Borden EC (1971) Streptovaricins inhibit focus formation by MSV(MLV) complex. Nature New Biol 232:212–214

Chamberlin M (1976) RNA polymerase–An overview. In: Losick R, Chamberlin M (eds) RNA polymerase. Cold Spring Harbor Laboratory, New York, pp 17–67

Chamberlin M, McGrath J, Waskell L (1970) New RNA polymerase from *Escherichia coli* infected with bacteriophage T7. Nature 228:227–231

Costanzo F, Fiume L, La Placa M, Mannini-Palenzona A, Novello G, Stirpe F (1970) Ribonucleic acid polymerase induced by vaccinia virus: lack of inhibition by rifampicin and α-amanitin. J Virol 5:226–269

Cricchio R, Cietto G, Rossi E, Arioli V (1975) Farmaco Ed Sci 30:704

Dales S, Mosbach ED (1968) Vaccinia as a model for membrane biogenesis. Virol 35:564–583

Darougar S, Viswalingam M, Treharne JD, Kinnison JR, Jones BR (1977) Treatment of TRIC infection of the eye with rifampicin or chloramphenicol. Brit J Opthalm 61:255–259

Das J, Maniloff J (1976) Replication of mycoplasma virus MVL51. IV. Inhibition of viral synthesis by rifampin. J Virol 18:969–976

DiCioccio RA, Srivastava SBI (1978) Structure-activity relationships and specificity of inhibition of DNA polymerases from normal and leukemia cells of man and from simian sarcoma virus by rifamycin derivatives. J Natl Cancer Instit 61:1187–1194

Diggelman H, Weissman C (1969) Rifampicin inhibits focus formation in chick fibroblasts infected with Rous sarcoma virus. Nature 224:1277–1279

Engelberg H (1972) Inhibition of RNA bacteriophage replication by rifampicin. J Mol Biol 68:541–546

Engelberg H, Soudry E (1971 a) Inhibition of ribonucleic acid bacteriophage release from its host by rifampin. J Virol 7:847–848

Engelberg H, Soudry E (1971 b) Ribonucleic acid bacteriophage release: requirement for host-controlled protein synthesis. J Virol 8:257–264

Engelberg H, Brudo I, Israeli-Reches M (1975) Discriminative effect of rifampin on RNA replication of various RNA bacteriophages. J Virol 16:340–347

Essani K, Dales S (1979) Biogenesis of vaccinia: evidence for more than 100 polypeptides in the virion. Virol 95:385–394

Esteban M (1977) Rifampicin and vaccinia DNA. J Virol 21:796–801

Esteban M, Holowczak JA (1977) Replication of vaccinia DNA in mouse L cells. Virol 78:57–75

Fallon RJ, Lees AW, Allan GW, Smith J, Tyrrell WF (1975) Probenecid and rifampicin serum levels. Lancet II:792–794

Follett EAC, Pennington TH (1971) Antiviral effect of constituent parts of the rifampicin molecule. Nature 230:117–118

Follett EAC, Pennington TH (1973) The mode of action of rifamycins and related compounds on poxvirus. Advances in Virus Res 18:105–142

Frolova LY, Meldrays YA, Kochkina LL, Giller SA, Eremeyev AV, Grayevskaya NA, Kisselev LL (1977) DNA polymerase inhibitors. Rifamycin derivatives. Nucleic Acids Res 4:523–538

Fromageot H, Zinder N (1968) Growth of bacteriophage f2 in *E. coli* treated with rifampicin. Proc Natl Acad Sci USA 61:184–191

Furukawa T, Tanaka S, Plotkin SA (1975) Inhibition of human cytomegalovirus by rifampin. J Gen Virol 28:355–362

Gallo RC (1971) Reverse transcriptase, the DNA polymerase of oncogenic RNA viruses. Nature 234:194–198

Gallo RC, Yang SS, Ting RC (1970) RNA-dependent DNA polymerase of human acute leukaemic cells. Nature 228:927–929

Gallo RC, Yang SS, Smith RG, Herrera F, Ting RC, Bobrow SN, Davis C, Fujioka S (1971) RNA- and DNA-dependent DNA polymerases of human normal and leukemic cells. In: Silvestri L (ed) The biology of oncogenic viruses. North-Holland, Amsterdam, pp 210–220

Gallo RC, Smith RC, Whang-Peng J, Ting RC, Yang SS, Abrell JW (1972) RNA tumor viruses, DNA polymerases, and oncogenesis: some selective effects of rifampicin derivatives. Medicine 51:159–168

Geiduschek EP, Sklar J (1969) Continual requirement for a host RNA polymerase component in bacteriophage development. Nature 221:833–836

Gerard GF, Gurgo C, Grandgenett DP, Green M (1973) Rifamycin derivatives: specific inhibitors of nucleic acid polymerases. Biochem Biophys Res Commun 53:194–201

Geshelin P, Berns KI (1974) Characterization and localization of the naturally occurring cross-links in vaccinia virus DNA. J Mol Biol 88:785–796

Gielkins A, Burghouts J, Bloemendal H (1972) Inhibitory effect of rifampicin on Rauscher-virus-induced murine leukemia. Int J Cancer 9:595–598

Grado C, Ohlbaum A (1973) The effect of rifampicin, actinomycin D, and mitomycin C on poliovirus and foot-and-mouth disease virus replication. J Gen Virol 21:297–303

Green M, Rokutanda M, Fujinaga K, Ray RK, Rokutanda H, Gurgo C (1970) Mechanism of carcinogenesis by RNA tumor viruses. I. An RNA-dependent DNA polymerase in murine sarcoma cells. Proc Natl Acad Sci USA 67:385–393

Green M, Rokutanda M, Fujinaga K, Rokutanda H, Gurgo C, Ray RK, Parsons JT (1971) Synthesis of DNA by RNA tumor viruses and viral RNA by virus transformed cells. In: Silvestri L (ed) The biology of oncogenic viruses. North-Holland, Amsterdam, pp 193–205

Green M, Bragdon J, Rankin A (1972) 3-cyclic amine derivatives of rifamycin: strong inhibitors of the DNA polymerase activity of RNA tumor viruses. Proc Natl Acad Sci USA 69:1294–1298

Green M, Gerard GF, Grandgenett DP, Gurgo C, Rankin AM, Green MR, Cassel DM (1974a) Biochemical suppression of tumor virus activity. Cancer 34:1427–1438

Green M, Gurgo C, Gerard G, Grandgenett DP, Shimada K (1974b) Inhibition of DNA polymerases of RNA tumor viruses and cells by rifamycin SV derivatives. In: Molecular studies in viral neoplasia. William and Wilkins Co, Baltimore, pp 258–288

Grimley PM, Rosenblum EN, Mims SJ, Moss B (1970) Interruption by rifampicin of an early stage in vaccinia virus morphogenesis: accumulation of membranes which are precursors of virus envelopes. J Virol 6:519–533

Grimley PM, Moss B (1971) Similar effect of rifampicin derivatives on vaccinia virus morphogenesis. J Virol 8:225–231

Gurgo C (1977) Rifamycins as inhibitors of DNA and RNA polymerases. Pharm Ther Part A 2:139–169

Gurgo C (1980) Rifamycins as inhibitors of DNA and RNA polymerases. In: Sarin P, Gallo RC (eds) The international encyclopedia of pharmacology and therapeutics, section 103. Pergamon Press, Oxford, pp 159–189

Gurgo C, Grandgenett DP (1977) Different modes of inhibition of purified ribonucleic acid polymerase of avian myeloblastosis virus by rifamycin SV derivatives. Biochemistry 16:786–792

Gurgo C, Craig E, Schlessinger D, Afolayan A (1971a) Polyribosome metabolism in Escherichia coli starved for an amino acid. J Mol Biol 62:525–535

Gurgo C, Ray RK, Thiry L, Green M (1971b) Inhibition of the RNA and DNA dependent polymerase activities of RNA tumor viruses. Nature 229:111–114

Gurgo C, Ray RK, Green M (1972) Rifamycin derivatives strongly inhibiting RNA-DNA polymerase (reverse transcriptase) of murine sarcoma viruses. J Natl Cancer Instit 49:61–79

Gurgo C, Grandgenett DP, Gerard GF, Green M (1974) Interaction of purified ribonucleic acid directed deoxyribonucleic acid polymerase of avian myeloblastosis virus and murine sarcoma-leukemia virus with a rifamycin SV derivative. Biochemistry 13:708–713

Gurgo C, Grandgenett DP, Gerard GF, Green M (1975) Mechanism of inhibition of RNA tumor virus reverse transcriptase by rifamycin SV derivatives. In: Kolber A (ed) Tumor virus-host cell interaction. Plenum, New York, pp 273–291

Hackett AJ, Sylvester SS (1972a) Cell line derived from BALB/3T3 that is transformed by murine leukemia virus: a focus assay for leukemia virus. Nature New Biol 239:164–166

Hackett AJ, Sylvester SS (1972b) Inhibition of MLV-induced transformation in BALB/3T3 derived cells. Nature New Biol 239:166–167

Hackett AJ, Owens RB, Calvin M, Joss U (1972) Inhibition of MSV viral function by rifampicin derivatives. Medicine 51:175–180

Halsted C, Minnefor A, Lietman P (1972) Inhibition of cytomegalovirus by rifampin. J Infectious Dis 125:552–555

Haselkorn R, Vogel M, Brown R (1969) Conservation of the rifamycin sensitivity of transcription during T4 development. Nature 221:836–838

Heller E, Argaman M, Levy H, Goldblum N (1969) Selective inhibition of vaccinia virus by the antibiotic rifampicin. Nature 222:273–274

Hemphill H, Whiteley H, Brown L, Doi R (1969) The effect of rifampin on the production of β22 phage by Bacillus subtilis. Biochem Biophys Res Commun 37:559–566

Higashi A, Komano T (1977) Inhibition of bacteriophage ϕX174 replicative-form DNA replication by rifampicin. Agric Biol Chem 41:383–388

Higashide E, Asai M, Ootsu K, Tanida S, Kozai Y, Hasegawa T, Kishi T, Sugino Y, Yoneda M (1977) Ansamitocin, a group of novel maytansinoid antibiotics with antitumor properties from Nocardia. Nature 270:721–722

Hughes AM, Calvin M (1976) Effect of some rifamycin derivatives on chemically induced mammary tumors in rats. Cancer Letters 2:5–10

Igel HJ, Huebner RJ, Turner HC, Kotin P, Falk HL (1969) Mouse leukemia virus activation by chemical carcinogens. Science 166:1624–1626

Jockusch H, Ball LA, Kaesbert P (1970) Synthesis of polypeptides directed by the RNA of phage Qβ. Virol 42:401–414

Johnston DE, McClure WR (1976) Abortive initiation of in vitro RNA synthesis on bacteriophage λ DNA. In: Losick R, Chamberlin M (eds) RNA polymerase. Cold Spring Harbor Laboratory, New York, pp 413–428

Joss UR, Hughes AM, Calvin M (1973) Effect of dimethylbenzyldesmethylrifampicin (DMB) on chemically induced mammary tumors in rats. Nature New Biol 242:88–90

Kates JR, McAuslan BR (1967) Poxvirus DNA-dependent RNA polymerase. Proc Natl Acad Sci USA 58:134–141

Katz E, Moss B (1970a) Formation of a vaccinia virus structural polypeptide from a higher molecular weight precursor: inhibition by rifampicin. Proc Natl Acad Sci USA 66:677–684

Katz E, Moss B (1970b) Vaccinia virus structural polypeptide derived from a high-molecular-weight precursor: formation and integration into virus particles. J Virol 6:717–726

Katz E, Grimley P, Moss B (1970) Reversal of antiviral effects of rifampicin. Nature 227:1050–1051

Kenwright S, Levi AJ (1973) Impairment of hepatic uptake of rifamycin antibiotics by probenecid and its therapeutic implications. Lancet II:1401–1405

Kishi T, Yamana H, Muroi M, Harada S, Asai M, Hasegawa T, Mizuno K (1972) Tolypomycin, a new antibiotic. III. Isolation and characterization of tolypomycin Y. J Antibiotics 25:11

Kupchan SM, Komoda Y, Court WA, Thomas GT, Smith RM, Karim A, Gilmore CJ, Haltiwanger RC, Bryan RF (1972) Maytansine, a novel antileukemic ansa macrolide from Maytenus ovatus. J Am Chem Soc 94:1354–1356

Kupchan SM, Sneden AT, Branfman AR, Howie GA, Rebhun LI, McIvor WE, Wang RW, Schnaitman TC (1978) Structural requirements for antileukemic activity among the naturally occurring and semisynthetic maytansinoids. J Med Chem 21:31–37

Lancini GC, Sartori G (1968) Rifamycins. LXI. In vivo inhibition of RNA synthesis by rifamycins. Experientia 24:1105–1106

Lancini GC, Zanichelli W (1977) Structure-activity relationships in rifamycins. In: Perlman D (ed) Structure-activity relationships among the semisynthetic antibiotics. Academic Press, New York, pp 531–600

Lancini GC, Cricchio R, Thiry L (1971) Antiviral activity of rifamycins and N-amino-piperazines. J Antibiotics 24:64–66

Maitra U (1971) Induction of a new RNA polymerase in *Escherichia coli* infected with bacteriophage T3. Biochem Biophys Res Commun 43:443–450

Margalith P, Pagani H (1961) Rifomycins. XIV. Production of rifomycin B. Appli Microbiol 9:325–334

Marino P, Baldi I, Tocchini-Valentini G (1968) Effect of rifamycin on DNA dependent RNA polymerase and on RNA phage growth. Cold Spring Harbor Symp Quant Biol 33:125–127

McAuslan BR (1969) Rifampicin inhibition of vaccinia replication. Biochem Biophys Res Commun 37:289–295

McCormick DP, Wenzel RP, Smith EP, Beam WE (1972) Failure of rifampicin to inhibit adenovirus replication. Antimicrob Ag Chemother 2:326–328

Meir D, Hofschneider P (1972) Effect of rifampicin on the growth of bacteriophage M12. FEBS Letters 25:179–183

Milavetz B, Horoszewicz J, Rinehart K, Carter W (1976) An immobilized template assay of reverse transcriptase inhibition by ansamycins. Proc Am Assoc Cancer Res 17:179

Mizuno S, Yamazaki H, Nitta K, Umezawa H (1968a) Inhibition of DNA-dependent RNA polymerase reaction of *E. coli* by streptovaricin. Biochim Biophys Acta 157:322–332

Mizuno S, Yamazaki H, Nitta K, Umezawa H (1968b) Inhibition of initiation of DNA-dependent RNA synthesis. Biochem Biophys Res Commun 30:379–385

Moreau M (1974) Inhibition of a vesicular stomatitis virus mutant by rifampin. J Virol 14:517–521

Moreau M, Sanzey B (1977) Rifampin-susceptible mutant of vesicular stomatitis virus: protein and RNA synthesis. J Virol 21:41–53

Moshkowitz A, Goldblum N, Heller E (1971) Studies on the antiviral effect of rifampicin in volunteers. Nature 229:422–424

Moss B, Rosenblum ED (1973) Protein cleavage and poxvirus morphogenesis: tryptic peptide analysis of core precursors accumulated by blocking assembly with rifampicin. J Mol Biol 81:267–269

Moss B, Katz E, Rosenblum EN (1969a) Vaccinia virus directed RNA and protein synthesis in the presence of rifampicin. Biochem Biophys Res Commun 36:858–865

Moss B, Rosenblum ED, Katz E, Grimley PM (1969b) Rifampicin: a specific inhibitor of vaccinia virus assembly. Nature 224:1280–1284

Moss B, Rosenblum EN, Grimley PM (1971) Assembly of vaccinia virus particles from polypeptides made in the presence of rifampicin. Virol 45:123–134

Moss B, Rosenblum E, Grimley P, Mims S (1972) Rifamycins: modulation of specific anti-poxviral activity by small substitutions on the piperazinyliminomethyl side chain. Antimicrob Ag Chemother 2:181–185

Munyon W, Paoletti E, Grace JT (1967) RNA polymerase in purified infectious vaccinia. Proc Natl Acad Sci USA 58:2280–2287

Nagayama A, Pogo BGT, Dales S (1970) Biogenesis of vaccinia: separation of early stages from maturation by means of rifampicin. Virol 40:1039–1051

Naimski P, Chroboczek J (1977) Effect of rifampicin on the infectivity of RNA bacteriophage f2. Eur J Biochem 76:419–423

Nevins JR, Joklik WK (1977) Isolation of and properties of the vaccinia virus DNA-dependent RNA polymerase. J Biol Chem 252:6930–6938

O'Connor T, Schiop-Stansly P, Sethi VS, Hadidi A, Okano P (1974) Antiviral antibiotics: inhibition of focus-formation in human or mouse cell cultures by sarcoma-inducing oncornaviruses with rifamycins. Intervirol 3:63–83

O'Connor TE, Aldrich C, Hadidi A, Lomax N, Okano P, Sethi S, Wood HB (1975) Maytansine and geldanamycin inhibition of transformation of mouse cell cultures infected with murine sarcoma virus. Proc Am Assoc Cancer Res 16:29

Ootsu K, Kozai Y, Takeuchi M, Ikeyama S, Igarashi K, Tsukamoto K, Sugino Y, Tashiro T, Tsukagoshi S, Sakurai Y (1980) Effects of new antimitotic antibiotics, ansamitocins, on the growth of murine tumors in vivo and on the assembly of microtubules in vitro. Cancer Res 40:1707–1717

Oppolzer W, Prelog V, Sensi P (1964) Konstitution des Rifamycins B und verwandter Rifamycine. Experientia 20:336–339

Passent J, Kaesberg P (1971) Effect of rifampin on the development of ribonucleic acid bacteriophage Qβ. J Virol 8:286–292

Pennington TH, Follett EAC (1971) Inhibition of poxvirus maturation by rifamycin derivatives and related compounds. J Virol 7:821–829

Pennington TH, Follett EAC, Szilagyi JF (1970) Events in vaccinia virus-infected cells following the reversal of the antiviral action of rifampicin. J Gen Virol 9:225–237

Pennington TH (1973) Vaccinia virus morphogenesis: a comparison of virus-induced antigens and polypeptides. J Gen Virol 19:65–79

Pogo BGT (1971) Biogenesis of vaccinia: effect of rifampicin on transcription. Virol 44:576–581

Quintrell NA, McAuslan BR (1970) Inhibition of poxvirus replication by streptovaricin. J Virol 6:485–491

Rana M, Pinkerton H, Rankin A (1975) Effect of rifamycin and tilorone derivatives on Friend virus leukemia in mice. Proc Soc Exp Biol Med 150:32–35

Remillard S, Rebhun L, Howie GA, Kupchan SM (1975) Antimitotic activity of the potent inhibitor maytansine. Science 189:1002–1005

Rinehart KL (1972) Antibiotics with ansa rings. Accounts of Chemical Research 5:57–64

Riva S, Silvestri L (1972) Rifamycins: a general view. Ann Rev Microbiol 26:199–224

Riva S, Fietta A, Silvestri LG (1972) Mechanism of action of a rifamycin derivative (AF-013) which is active on the nucleic acid polymerases insensitive to rifampicin. Biochem Biophys Res Commun 49:1263–1271

Robinson H, Robinson W (1971) Inhibition of growth of uninfected and Rous sarcoma virus-infected chick embryo fibroblasts by rifampicin. J Natl Ca Instit 46:785–788

Rokutanda M, Rokutanda H, Green M, Fujinaga K, Ray RK, Gurgo C (1970) Formation of viral RNA-DNA hybrid molecules by the DNA polymerase of sarcoma-leukemia viruses. Nature 227:1026–1028

Rothwell J, Yamazaki H (1972) Limited production of R17 ribonucleic acid phage in the presence of rifampicin. Biochemistry 11:3333–3338

Schekman R, Wickner W, Westergaard O, Brutlag D, Geider K, Bertsch L, Kornberg A (1972) Initiation of DNA synthesis: synthesis of φX174 replicative form requires RNA synthesis resistant to rifampicin. Proc Natl Acad Sci USA 69:2691–2695

Schlessinger D, Gurgo C, Luzzato L, Apirion D (1969) Polyribosome metabolism in growing and nongrowing E. coli. Cold Spring Harbor Symp Quant Biol 34:231–242

Sensi P (1975) Recent progress in the chemistry and biochemistry of rifamycins. Pure and Applied Chem 41:15–29

Sensi P, Margalith P, Timbal M (1959a) Rifomycin, a new antibiotic-preliminary report. Farmaco, Ed Sci 14:146–147

Sensi P, Greco A, Ballotta R (1959b) Rifomycins. I. Isolation and properties of rifomycin B and rifomycin complex. Antibiotics Ann, pp 262–270

Sethi VS, Okano P (1976) Interaction of rifamycins with mammalian nucleic acid polymerizing enzymes. Biochim Biophys Acta 454:230–247

Shannon W, Westbrook L, Schabel F (1974) Inhibition of Gross murine leukemia virus replication by rifamycin SV and certain of its derivatives in vitro. Intervirol 3:84–96

Silverstein S, Billen D (1971) Transcription: role in the initiation and replication of DNA synthesis in Escherichia coli and φX174. Biochim Biophys Acta 247:383–390

Sinkovics J (1971) Antitumor activity of L-asparaginase and rifampicin. Lancet II:48–49

Smith HS, Hackett AJ (1974) The specificity of dimethylbenzylrifampicin as an inhibitor of viral induced transformation. Proc Natl Acad Sci USA 71:2770–2772

Smith R, Whang-Peng J, Gallo RC, Levine P, Ting RC (1972) Selective toxicity of rifamycin derivatives for leukaemic human leucocytes. Nature New Biol 236:166–171

Spiegelman S, Burney A, Das MR, Keydar J, Schlom J, Travnicek M, Watson K (1970) Characterization of the products of RNA-directed DNA polymerases in oncogenic RNA viruses. Nature 227:563–567

Subak-Sharpe JH, Timbury MC, Williams JF (1969) Rifampicin inhibits the growth of some mammalian viruses. Nature 222:341–345

Szabo C, Bissell MJ (1978) Antiviral action of a rifamycin derivative: formation of Rous sarcoma virus particles deficient in 60 to 70S RNA. J Virol 25:944–947

Szabo C, Bissell MJ, Calvin M (1976) Inhibition of infectious Rous sarcoma virus production by a rifamycin derivative. J Virol 18:445–453

Szilágyi JF, Pennington TH (1971) Effect of rifamycins and related antibiotics on the deoxyribonucleic acid-dependent ribonucleic acid polymerase of vaccinia virus particles. J Virol 8:133–141

Takeda Y, Oyama Y, Nakajima K, Yura T (1969) Role of host RNA polymerase for lambda phage development. Biochem Biophys Res Commun 36:533–538

Tan KB, McAuslan BR (1970) Effect of rifampicin on poxvirus protein synthesis. J Virol 6:326–332

Temin H (1971) The protovirus hypothesis: speculations on the significance of RNA-directed DNA synthesis for normal development and for carcinogenesis. J Natl Cancer Instit 46:III–VII

Temin H, Mizutani S (1970) RNA-dependent DNA polymerase in virions of Rous sarcoma virus. Nature 226:1211–1213

Thiry L, Lancini G (1970) Inhibition of vaccinia virus growth by 1-methyl-4-amino-piperazine. Nature 227:1048–1050

Thiry L, Lancini G (1972) Mode of action of rifamycin and aminopiperazine derivatives on animal viruses and cells. FEBS Symp 22:177–192

Thompson FM, Tischler AN, Adams J, Calvin M (1974) Inhibition of three nucleotide polymerases by rifamycin derivatives. Proc Natl Acad Sci USA 71:107–109

Ting RC, Yang SS, Gallo RC (1972) Reverse transcriptase, RNA tumor virus transformation and derivatives of rifamycin SV. Nature New Biol 236:163–166

Tischler AN, Joss UR, Thompson FM, Calvin M (1973) Synthesis of some rifamycin derivatives as inhibitors of RNA-instructed DNA polymerase function. J Med Chem 16:1071–1075

Tischler AN, Thompson FM, Libertini LJ, Calvin M (1974) Rifamycin derivatives as inhibitors of a ribonucleic acid instructed deoxyribonucleic acid polymerase function. Effect of lipophilicity. J Med Chem 17:948–952

Toolan H, Ledinko N (1972) Effect of rifampicin on the development of tumors induced by adenovirus in male hamsters. Nature New Biol 237:200–202

Ueda Y, Dumbell KR, Tsuruhara T, Tagaya I (1978) Studies on Cotia virus–an unclassified poxvirus. J Gen Virol 40:263–276

Vaheri A, Hanafusa H (1971) Effect of rifampicin and a derivative on cells transformed by Rous sarcoma virus. Cancer Res 31:2032–2036

Wehrli W (1977) Ansamycins: chemistry, biosynthesis, and biological activity. Topics in Current Chemistry 72:22–49

Wehrli W, Staehelin M (1971) Actions of the rifamycins. Bact Rev 35:290–309

Wehrli W, Handschin J, Wunderli W (1976) Interaction between rifampicin and DNA dependent RNA polymerase of *E. coli*. In: Losick R, Chamberlin M (eds) RNA polymerase. Cold Spring Harbor Laboratory, New York, pp 397–412

Wickner W, Brutlag D, Schekman R, Kornberg A (1972) RNA synthesis initiates in vitro conversion of M13 DNA to its replicative form. Proc Natl Acad Sci 69:965–969

Wigand R, Vujic A, Schöner M (1974) Inhibition of adenovirus multiplication by rifamycin derivatives. Acta Virol 18:113–120

Wu AM, Gallo RC (1974) Interaction between murine type-C virus RNA-directed DNA polymerases and rifamycin derivatives. Biochim Biophys Acta 340:419–436

Wu AM, Ting RCY, Gallo RC (1973) RNA-directed DNA polymerase and virus-induced leukemia in mice. Proc Natl Acad Sci USA 70:1298–1302

Wu RS, Wolpert-DeFilippes MK, Quinn FR (1980) Quantitative structure-activity correlations of rifamycins as inhibitors of viral RNA-directed DNA polymerase and mammalian α and β DNA polymerases. J Med Chem 23:256–261

Yang SS, Herrera F, Smith R, Reitz M, Lancini G, Ting R, Gallo RC (1972) Rifamycin antibiotics: inhibitors of Rauscher murine leukemia virus reverse transcriptase and of purified DNA polymerases from human normal and leukemic lymphoblasts. J Natl Cancer Instit 49:7–25

Zakay-Rones Z, Becker Y (1970) Anti-poxvirus activity of rifampicin associated with hydrazone side chain. Nature 226:1162–1163

Subject Index

Handbook of Experimental Pharmacology

Continuation of "Handbuch der experimentellen Pharmakologie"

Editorial Board
G.V.R.Born, A.Farah,
H.Herken, A.D.Welch

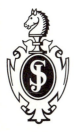

Springer-Verlag
Berlin
Heidelberg
New York

Handbook of Experimental Pharmacology

Continuation of "Handbuch der experimentellen Pharmakologie"

Editorial Board
G. V. R. Born, A. Farah,
H. Herken, A. D. Welch

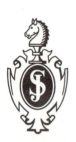

Springer-Verlag
Berlin
Heidelberg
New York